Practice Standards

of ASHP

1997–1998

American

Society of

Health-System

Pharmacists

Editor, Joseph H. Deffenbaugh, M.P.H.

Published by the American Society of Health-System Pharmacists, 7272 Wisconsin Avenue, Bethesda, MD 20814.

ASHP® is a service mark of the American Society of Health-System Pharmacists™, Inc.; registered in the U.S. Patent and Trademark Office.

ISBN: 1-879907-75-5

Printed in the United States of America.

Contents

Acknowledgments vi

Introduction vii

ASHP's Project Catalyst ix

ASHP Statements

ASHP Mission Statement 2

Pharmacy and Therapeutics Committee, ASHP Statement on the 3

Formulary System, ASHP Statement on the 5

Economic Status Program, ASHP Statement on Its 7

Continuing Education, ASHP Statement on 9

Unit Dose Drug Distribution, ASHP Statement on 10

Infection Control, ASHP Statement on the Pharmacist's Role in 11

Third-Party Compensation for Clinical Services by Pharmacists, ASHP Statement on 13

Pharmacokinetic Services, ASHP Statement on the Pharmacist's Role in Clinical 14

Research in Organized Health-Care Settings, ASHP Statement on Pharmaceutical 15

Patient Education Programs, ASHP Statement on the Pharmacist's Role in 16

Drug Delivery Systems and Administration Devices, ASHP Statement on the
Pharmacist's Role with Respect to 17

Distribution and Control of Drug Products, ASHP Statement on the Pharmacist's Responsibility for 19

Unlabeled Uses, ASHP Statement on the Use of Medications for 20

Pharmaceutical Care, ASHP Statement on 22

Principles for Including Medications and Pharmaceutical Care in Health Care Systems,
ASHP Statement on 25

Patient-Focused Care, ASHP Statement on the Role of the Pharmacist in 26

ASHP Guidelines

Selecting Pharmaceutical Manufacturers and Suppliers, ASHP Guidelines for 30

* Pharmacist-Conducted Patient Education and Counseling, ASHP Guidelines on 32

Minimum Standard for Pharmacies in Hospitals, ASHP Guidelines: 35

Research in Organized Health-Care Settings, ASHP Guidelines for Pharmaceutical 41

Documenting Pharmaceutical Care in Patient Medical Records, ASHP Guidelines for
Obtaining Authorization for 43

Investigational Drugs in Organized Health-Care Settings, ASHP Guidelines for the Use of 45

Compensation for Clinical Services by Pharmacists, ASHP Guidelines for Implementing and Obtaining 49

Medication-Use Evaluation, ASHP Guidelines on 51

Ambulatory Patients, ASHP Guidelines on Pharmaceutical Services for 54

Adverse Drug Reaction Monitoring and Reporting, ASHP Guidelines on 58

Relationships with Industry, ASHP Guidelines on Pharmacists' 61

Formulary System Management, ASHP Guidelines on 62

Medication Errors in Hospitals, ASHP Guidelines on Preventing 66

Home Care, ASHP Guidelines on the Pharmacist's Role in 76

* Indicates documents that have been added or revised since the 1996–97 edition.

ASHP Guidelines—continued

Vendors' Representatives in Organized Health Care Systems, ASHP Guidelines for
Pharmacists on the Activities of 81

Pediatric Pharmaceutical Services in Organized Health Care Systems, ASHP Guidelines for Providing 83

Correctional Facilities, ASHP Guidelines on Pharmaceutical Services in 86

Standardized Method for Pharmaceutical Care, ASHP Guidelines on a 90

Provision of Medication Information by Pharmacists, ASHP Guidelines on the 93

* Clinical Care Plans, ASHP Guidelines on the Pharmacist's Role in the Development of 96

ASHP Technical Assistance Bulletins

Drug Distribution and Control, ASHP Technical Assistance Bulletin on Hospital 102

Single Unit and Unit Dose Packages of Drugs, ASHP Technical Assistance Bulletin on 111

Controlled Substances in Organized Health-Care Settings, ASHP Technical Assistance
Bulletin on Use of 113

Repackaging Oral Solids and Liquids in Single Unit and Unit Dose Packages,
ASHP Technical Assistance Bulletin on 124

Drug Formularies, ASHP Technical Assistance Bulletin on 126

Outcome Competencies and Training Guidelines for Institutional Pharmacy Technician Training
Programs, ASHP Technical Assistance Bulletin on 129

Evaluation of Drugs for Formularies, ASHP Technical Assistance Bulletin on the 134

Cytotoxic and Hazardous Drugs, ASHP Technical Assistance Bulletin on Handling 136

Cost-Containment Strategies for Pharmacies in Organized Health-Care Settings,
ASHP Technical Assistance Bulletin on Assessing 153

Surgery and Anesthesiology Pharmaceutical Services, ASHP Technical Assistance Bulletin on 159

Immunization, ASHP Technical Assistance Bulletin on the Pharmacist's Role in 165

Ophthalmic Products, ASHP Technical Assistance Bulletin on Pharmacy-Prepared 169

Quality Assurance for Pharmacy-Prepared Sterile Products, ASHP Technical Assistance Bulletin on 171

Compounding Nonsterile Products in Pharmacies, ASHP Technical Assistance Bulletin on 182

Recruitment, Selection, and Retention of Pharmacy Personnel, ASHP Technical Assistance
Bulletin on the 189

ASHP Therapeutic Position Statements

International Normalized Ratio System to Monitor Oral Anticoagulant Therapy,
ASHP Therapeutic Position Statement on the Use of the 194

Sodium Chloride Injection to Maintain Patency of Peripheral Indwelling Intermittent Infusion
Devices, ASHP Therapeutic Position Statement on the Institutional Use of 0.9% 197

* Strategies for Identifying and Preventing Pneumococcal Resistance
ASHP Therapeutic Position Statement on 199

* Strategies for Preventing and Treating Multidrug-Resistant Tuberculosis
ASHP Therapeutic Position Statement on 202

Strict Glycemic Control in Selected Patients with Insulin-Dependent Diabetes Mellitus,
ASHP Therapeutic Position Statement on 205

ASHP Therapeutic Guidelines

* Angiotensin-Converting-Enzyme Inhibitors in Patients with Left Ventricular Dysfunction,
ASHP Therapeutic Guidelines on 208

Antimicrobial Prophylaxis in Surgery, ASHP Therapeutic Guidelines on 221

Nonsurgical Antimicrobial Prophylaxis, ASHP Therapeutic Guidelines on 251

* Indicates documents that have been added or revised since the 1996–97 edition.

ASHP Residency Accreditation Regulations and Standards

Residencies and Fellowships, Definitions of Pharmacy 274

Clinical Fellowship Training Programs, Guidelines for 276

Accreditation of Pharmacy Residencies, ASHP Regulations on 277

** Residency in Pharmacy Practice (with Emphasis on Pharmaceutical Care),
ASHP Accreditation Standard for 280

Specialized Pharmacy Residency Training (with Guide to Interpretation),
ASHP Accreditation Standard for 288

Drug Information Practice, ASHP Supplemental Standard and Learning Objectives
for Residency Training in 295

Geriatric Pharmacy Practice, ASHP Supplemental Standard and Learning Objectives
for Residency Training in 301

Nuclear Pharmacy (with Guide to Interpretation), ASHP Accreditation Standard
for Residency Training in 304

Nutritional Support Pharmacy Practice, ASHP Supplemental Standard and
Learning Objectives for Residency Training in 313

Oncology Pharmacy Practice, ASHP Supplemental Standard and Learning Objectives
for Residency Training in 317

Pediatric Pharmacy Practice, ASHP Supplemental Standard and Learning Objectives
for Residency Training in 321

Adult Internal Medicine Pharmacy Practice, ASHP Supplemental Standard and Learning
Objectives for Residency Training in 326

Psychopharmacy Practice, ASHP Supplemental Standard and Learning Objectives
for Residency Training in 329

Hospital Pharmacy Administration, ASHP Supplemental Standard and Learning Objectives
for Residency Training in 337

Clinical Pharmacokinetics Practice, ASHP Supplemental Standard and Learning Objectives
for Residency Training in 341

Critical Care Pharmacy Practice, ASHP Supplemental Standard and Learning Objectives
for Residency Training in 345

Primary Care Pharmacy Practice, ASHP Supplemental Standard and Learning Objectives
for Residency Training in 349

Pharmacotherapy Practice, ASHP Supplemental Standard and Learning Objectives
for Residency Training in 353

Infectious Diseases Pharmacy Practice, ASHP Supplemental Standard and Learning Objectives
for Residency Training in 361

ASHP Technician Training Program Accreditation Regulations and Standards

Hospital Pharmacy Technician Training Programs, ASHP Regulations on Accreditation of 370

Pharmacy Technician Training Programs, ASHP Accreditation Standard for 373

ASHP-Endorsed Documents

Code of Ethics for Pharmacists 378

White Paper on Pharmacy Technicians 379

Index

Index 383

ASHP Policies

ASHP Policies 389

* Indicates documents that have been added or revised since the 1996–97 edition.
** Supplemental goals and learning objectives have been developed for residencies in pharmacy practice that are
centered in each of the following practice sites: hospital care, home care, long-term care, and managed care. Copies
of the supplemental documents may be obtained by contacting the ASHP Accreditation Services Division.

Acknowledgments

ASHP gratefully acknowledges the following individuals who donated their expertise in developing recently approved practice standards:

Marianne Billeter, Pharm.D., BCPS
Michael B. Bottorff, Pharm.D.
Steven C. Ebert, Pharm.D.
Gregory C. Gousse, M.S., FASHP
Daniel E. Hilleman, Pharm.D.
Karen E. Koch, Pharm.D., BCPS
Larry M. Lopez, Pharm.D.
Mary Lynn McPherson, Pharm.D., BCPS
Mark A. Munger, Pharm.D.
Paul E. Nolan, Jr., Pharm.D., FASHP
J. Herbert Patterson, Pharm.D., FASHP
Laura L. Stevenson, Pharm.D., M.S.
James E. Tisdale, Pharm.D.

Introduction

The American Society of Health-System Pharmacists (ASHP) is the 30,000-member national professional association that represents pharmacists who practice in hospitals, health maintenance organizations, long-term care facilities, home care agencies, and other components of health care systems. ASHP has extensive publishing and educational programs designed to help members improve their delivery of pharmaceutical care, and the society is a national accrediting organization for pharmacy residency and pharmacy technician training programs.

ASHP, since its founding, has developed official professional guidance documents about pharmacy practice, first for hospitals, and then for the continuum of practice settings in health systems. Since 1983, these documents have been compiled in the book, *Practice Standards of ASHP*. This compendium of practice standards initially contained ASHP Statements, Guidelines, Technical Assistance Bulletins, and Residency Accreditation Regulations and Standards. ASHP Therapeutic Guidelines and Therapeutic Position Statements were added in 1991. There is a gradation in detail among practice standards, with Statements expressing basic philosophy, Guidelines offering programmatic advice, and Technical Assistance Bulletins offering more reference information and detailed programmatic advice. Of the two types of therapeutic documents, Therapeutic Guidelines are thorough discussions of drug use and Therapeutic Position Statements are concise responses to specific therapeutic issues. Selected ASHP-endorsed documents were added to the 1996–1997 edition.

Practice standards originate with an ASHP council or commission. ASHP Statements, because of their broad, philosophical nature, are approved by the ASHP Board of Directors (BOD) and the ASHP House of Delegates (HOD). The other types of practice standards are approved only by the BOD. All practice standards constitute ASHP policy.

The *Practice Standards of ASHP 1997–1998* edition includes a companion document, ASHP Policies, which is a reverse chronological catalog of policy positions adopted by the HOD. These short pronouncements, intended to address professional practice, generally originate with an ASHP council or by resolution. Often a principle established in an HOD policy position is elaborated on in an official practice standard. This addition of policy positions adopted by the HOD creates, for the first time, a consolidated reference of all ASHP's official professional policies.

These official professional policies represent a consensus of professional judgment, expert opinion, and documented evidence. They provide guidance and direction to ASHP members and pharmacy practitioners and to other audiences that affect pharmacy practice. Their use may help to comply with federal and state laws and regulations, to meet accreditation requirements, and to improve practice. They are written to establish reasonable goals, to be progressive and challenging, yet attainable in applicable practice settings. They generally do not represent minimum levels of practice, unless titled as such, and should not be viewed as ASHP requirements, except those for residency accreditation.

The use of ASHP's practice standards by members and other practitioners is strictly voluntary. The content of individual documents should be assessed and adapted based on independent judgment to meet the needs of local practice settings.

The need for authoritative guidance in pharmacy practice has grown with changes in health care and with the shifting influences from regulatory, accrediting, risk-management, financing, and other bodies. Immediate development of new (or revisions to existing) practice standards in response to environmental changes is typically not attempted. Other ASHP activities and services, such as educational sessions at national meetings and *American Journal of Health-System Pharmacy* (*AJHP*) articles, provide more timely information that may be helpful, until sufficient experience is gained to serve as the basis for a practice standard.

Definitions

The types of practice standards included in this publication are defined as follows:

ASHP Statement: A declaration and explanation of basic philosophy or principle.

ASHP Guidelines: General advice on the implementation of pharmacy practice programs.

ASHP Technical Assistance Bulletin: Specific, detailed advice on pharmacy programs or functions as developed by an ASHP staff division in consultation with experts.

ASHP Therapeutic Guidelines: Thorough, systematically developed advice for health-care professionals on appropriate use of medications for specific clinical circumstances.

ASHP Therapeutic Position Statement: Concise statements that respond to specific therapeutic issues of concern to health care consumers and pharmacists.

ASHP Residency Accreditation Regulations and Standards: Requirements for ASHP-accredited postgraduate residency and technician training programs.

Development

The responsible ASHP council or commission chooses to develop a practice standard after considering whether the topic: a) has achieved some stability and an actual norm of practice has evolved; b) is relevant to the practice of a significant portion of ASHP's members; c) is within the purview of pharmacy practice in health systems; d) is without other sufficient guidance; and e) does not pose significant legal risks to ASHP. The processes used to draft and review new or revised practice standards vary depending on the body responsible for their development and on the type of practice standard. These are described below. Once approved, the practice standard becomes an official ASHP policy and is published in *AJHP* and incorporated into the next edition of *Practice Standards of ASHP*.

ASHP Statements, Guidelines, and Technical Assistance Bulletins. Any of the ASHP policy recommending bodies (councils and commissions) may initiate and oversee the development of ASHP Statements, Guidelines, and Technical Assistance Bulletins; however, those that are practice-related usually fall within the purview of the Council on

Professional Affairs. The development of these documents generally includes the following steps:

1. A group of experts on a given topic is assigned to develop a preliminary draft. Drafters are selected based on demonstrated knowledge of the topic and their practice settings. Most often, the drafters are ASHP members.
2. The draft is sent by ASHP to reviewers who have interest and expertise in the given topic. Reviewers consist of members and selected individuals knowledgeable in the content area, representatives of various ASHP bodies, and other professional organizations. A draft of particular interest to ASHP's membership may be published in *AJHP* or discussed at an open hearing or in a network forum during an ASHP Annual, Midyear Clinical, or Home Care Meeting to solicit comments. In the future, drafts will be posted on ASHP's Web site to solicit comments.
3. Based on the comments, a revised draft is submitted to the appropriate ASHP policy-recommending body for action. If the draft meets the criteria for content and quality, that body recommends that the ASHP Board of Directors approve the document. ASHP Statements must be approved by both the ASHP Board of Directors and the ASHP House of Delegates. ASHP Guidelines and Technical Assistance Bulletins must be approved by the ASHP Board of Directors.

ASHP Therapeutic Guidelines and Position Statements. The Commission on Therapeutics has responsibility for the development of ASHP Therapeutic Guidelines and ASHP Therapeutic Position Statements.

Therapeutic Guidelines. The development of these documents generally includes the following steps:

1. When the Commission on Therapeutics (COT) identifies a topic for Therapeutic Guidelines development, ASHP formally solicits proposals for a contractual arrangement with an individual, group, or organization to draft the guidelines document and coordinate its review. The contractor works with a multidisciplinary panel of 6–10 experts appointed by ASHP who have diverse backgrounds relevant to the topic.
2. A systematic analysis of the literature is performed, and scientific evidence is evaluated based on predetermined criteria. Recommendations in the document are based on scientific evidence or expert consensus. When expert judgment must be used, the document indicates the scientific reasoning that influenced the decision. Scientific evidence takes precedence over expert judgement. Each recommendation is accompanied by projections of the relevant health and cost outcomes that could result.
3. The expert panel and COT review each draft of the guidelines document and provide comments. This process is repeated until the expert panel and COT are satisfied with the content of the document.
4. ASHP solicits multidisciplinary input on the draft. Reviewers consist of members and selected individuals knowledgeable in the content area, representatives of various ASHP bodies, and other professional organizations.
5. Once the above processes are completed, COT recommends that the ASHP Board of Directors approve it.

ASHP Therapeutic Position Statements (TPS). The development of these documents generally includes the following steps:

1. One or more experts on a given topic is (are) assigned to draft the TPS. Drafters are selected based on demonstrated knowledge of the topic and their practice setting. Most often, the drafters are ASHP members.
2. The proposed draft document is reviewed by COT, which may suggest modifications. This process is repeated until COT is satisfied with the content of the document.
3. ASHP solicits multidisciplinary input on the draft. Reviewers consist of members and selected individuals knowledgeable in the content area, representatives of various ASHP bodies, and other professional organizations.
4. Once the above processes are completed, COT finalizes the draft and recommends that the ASHP Board of Directors approve it.

ASHP Residency Accreditation Regulations and Standards. The Commission on Credentialing has responsibility for the development of ASHP Residency Accreditation Regulations and Standards.

Timeliness

The goal is to have an approvable draft within one year of the initial decision to develop a new or revised practice standard. Development usually takes from one to three years, depending on availability of drafters, strength of evidence, and accumulated practice experience, and on the extent of reviews and revisions. ASHP practice standards are dynamic. They are reviewed and revised as needed, generally every five years.

Access to Practice Standards

Besides publishing in *AJHP* and the *Practice Standards of ASHP*, most practice standards are available on ASHP's Fax On-Demand Service by calling (301) 664-8888. They soon will be available through ASHP's Web site at http://www.ashp.org.

Opportunities to be a Part of Practice Standards Development

ASHP members determine the needs for practice standards. They write and review the drafts. And, as members of policy-recommending bodies, the Board of Directors, and House of Delegates, they approve the documents.

ASHP members are encouraged to take an active role in the development of practice standards by suggesting ideas for new documents or modifications to current ones, volunteering to be drafters or reviewers, and completing survey and evaluation forms. Members may comment on or express their interests in participating in the development of practice standards by contacting the Editor, Joseph H. Deffenbaugh, M.P.H., R.Ph., Professional Practice Associate, Professional Practice and Scientific Affairs Division at ASHP, telephone (301) 657-3000, Ext. 1250, or e-mail jdeffenb@ashp.org.

ASHP's Project Catalyst

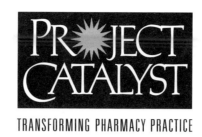

Project Catalyst is ASHP's landmark initiative designed to help pharmacists implement pharmaceutical care in their practices. It is a major element in achieving ASHP's Vision Statement. One of ASHP's commitments toward fostering pharmaceutical care is to create progressive practice standards that stimulate improvements in the quality of medication use. In some way, all of ASHP's practice standards contribute to pharmaceutical care. The following practice standards, however, are specific tools developed to support the provision of pharmaceutical care:

ASHP Statements

- ✔ Patient-Focused Care, The Role of the Pharmacist in
- ✔ Patient Education Programs, The Pharmacist's Role in
- ✔ Pharmaceutical Care
- ✔ Clinical Pharmacokinetic Services, The Pharmacist's Role in
- ✔ Principles for Including Medications and Pharmaceutical Care in Health Care Systems

ASHP Guidelines

- ✔ Developing Critical Care Plans, The Pharmacist's Role in
- ✔ Documenting Pharmaceutical Care in Patient Medical Records, Obtaining Authorization for
- ✔ Home Care, The Pharmacist's Role in
- ✔ Medication Information, Provision by Pharmacists
- ✔ Medication-Use Evaluation
- ✔ Patient Counseling, Pharmacist-Conducted
- ✔ Pharmaceutical Care, Standardized Method for
- ✔ Pharmacist-Conducted Patient Education and Counseling

ASHP
Statements

ASHP Mission Statement

Statement

The mission of ASHP is to represent its members and to provide leadership that will enable pharmacists in organized health-care settings to (1) extend pharmaceutical care focused on achieving positive patient outcomes through drug therapy; (2) provide services that foster the efficacy, safety, and cost-effectiveness of drug use; (3) contribute to programs and services that emphasize the health needs of the public and the prevention of disease; and (4) promote pharmacy as an essential component of the health-care team.

Goals

In support of the mission statement, ASHP has established the following goals:

1. To advance rational, patient-oriented drug therapy.
2. To promote pharmacists as integral members of the health-care team in order to allow full utilization of their clinical and drug use control functions that would be beneficial in each health-care setting.
3. To serve as a primary advocate for advancing professional practice, increasing the cost-effectiveness of pharmaceutical services, and improving the quality of patient care.
4. To advocate the pharmacist's value to patients in ensuring that appropriate clinical services and drug use control processes are applied to their benefit.
5. To promote good health by fostering the optimal and responsible use of drugs, including prevention of improper or uncontrolled use of drugs.
6. To assure sufficient, competent manpower in the profession by offering education and training programs.
7. To contribute to continuing educational programs for pharmacy practitioners.
8. To provide leadership in the identification, analysis, and evaluation of health-care trends and in the development of public policy and to address legislative and regulatory initiatives of concern to pharmacy.
9. To facilitate research in health and pharmaceutical sciences and services.
10. To facilitate information exchange between the members, health-care professions, and consumers.
11. To maintain lines of communication between the organization and its membership so that needs are accurately represented and to provide a full complement of services and products to the membership.

Approved by the ASHP House of Delegates, June 3, 1992.

The bibliographic citation for this document is as follows: American Society of Hospital Pharmacists. ASHP mission statement. *Am J Hosp Pharm.* 1992; 49:2003.

ASHP Statement on the Pharmacy and Therapeutics Committee

The multiplicity of drugs available and the complexities surrounding their safe and effective use make it necessary for organized health-care settings to have a sound program for maximizing rational drug use. The pharmacy and therapeutics (P&T) committee, or its equivalent, is the organizational keystone to this program.

The P&T committee evaluates the clinical use of drugs, develops policies for managing drug use and drug administration, and manages the formulary system. This committee is composed of physicians, pharmacists, and other health professionals selected with the guidance of the medical staff. It is a policy-recommending body to the medical staff and the administration of the organization on matters related to the therapeutic use of drugs.

Purposes

The primary purposes of the P&T committee are

1. *Policy Development.* The committee formulates policies regarding evaluation, selection, and therapeutic use of drugs and related devices.[a]
2. *Education.* The committee recommends or assists in the formulation of programs designed to meet the needs of the professional staff (physicians, nurses, pharmacists, and other health-care practitioners) for complete current knowledge on matters related to drugs and drug use.

Organization and Operation

While the composition and operation of the P&T committee might vary among specific practice sites, the following generally will apply:

1. The P&T committee should be composed of at least the following voting members: physicians, pharmacists, nurses, administrators, quality-assurance coordinators, and others as appropriate. The size of the committee may vary depending on the scope of services provided by the organization. Committee members should be appointed by a governing unit or authorized official of the organized medical staff.
2. A chairperson from among the physician representatives should be appointed. A pharmacist should be designated as secretary.
3. They should meet regularly, at least six times per year, and more often when necessary.
4. The committee should invite to its meetings persons within or outside the organization who can contribute specialized or unique knowledge, skills, and judgments.
5. An agenda and supplementary materials (including minutes of the previous meeting) should be prepared by the secretary and submitted to committee members in sufficient time before each meeting for them to review the material properly.
6. The minutes of committee meetings should be prepared by the secretary and maintained in the permanent records of the organization.
7. Recommendations of the committee should be presented to the medical staff or its appropriate committee for adoption or recommendation.
8. Liaison with other organizational committees concerned with drug use should be maintained.
9. Actions of the committee should be routinely communicated to the various health-care personnel involved in the care of the patient.
10. The committee should be organized and operated in a manner that ensures the objectivity and credibility of its recommendations. The committee should establish a conflict of interest policy with respect to committee recommendations and actions.
11. In formulating drug use policies for the organization, the committee should be attentive to the content and changes in pertinent guidelines and policies of professional organizations and standards-setting bodies such as the American Society of Hospital Pharmacists, the American Hospital Association, medical and nursing associations, the Joint Commission on Accreditation of Healthcare Organizations, governmental agencies, and others as appropriate.

Functions and Scope

The basic organization of each health-care setting and its medical staff may influence the specific functions and scope of the P&T committee. The following list of committee functions is offered as a guide:

1. To serve in an evaluative, educational, and advisory capacity to the medical staff and organizational administration in all matters pertaining to the use of drugs (including investigational drugs).
2. To develop a formulary of drugs accepted for use in the organization and provide for its constant revision. The selection of items to be included in the formulary should be based on objective evaluation of their relative therapeutic merits, safety, and cost. The committee should minimize duplication of the same basic drug type, drug entity, or drug product.[b]
3. To establish programs and procedures that help ensure safe and effective drug therapy.
4. To establish programs and procedures that help ensure cost-effective drug therapy.
5. To establish or plan suitable educational programs for the organization's professional staff on matters related to drug use.
6. To participate in quality-assurance activities related to distribution, administration, and use of medications.
7. To monitor and evaluate adverse drug (including, but not limited to, biologics and vaccines) reactions in the health-care setting and to make appropriate recommendations to prevent their occurrence.
8. To initiate or direct (or both) drug use evaluation programs and studies, review the results of such activities, and make appropriate recommendations to optimize drug use.

9. To advise the pharmacy department in the implementation of effective drug distribution and control procedures.

10. To disseminate information on its actions and approved recommendations to all organizational health-care staff.

---

[a]For additional information, see the "ASHP Statement on the Formulary System" (*Am J Hosp Pharm*. 1983; 40:1384–5) and the "ASHP Technical Assistance Bulletin on the Evaluation of Drugs for Formularies" (*Am J Hosp Pharm*. 1988; 45:386–7).

[b]For additional information, see the "ASHP Technical Assistance Bulletin on Drug Formularies" (*Am J Hosp Pharm*. 1991; 48:791–3).

Approved by the ASHP Board of Directors, November 20, 1991, and by the ASHP House of Delegates, June 1, 1992. Revised by the ASHP Council on Professional Affairs. Supersedes previous versions approved by the House of Delegates, May 15, 1978, and June 6, 1984.

The bibliographic citation for this document is as follows: American Society of Hospital Pharmacists. ASHP statement on the pharmacy and therapeutics committee. *Am J Hosp Pharm*. 1992; 49:2008–9.

ASHP Statement on the Formulary System

Preamble

The care of patients in hospitals and other health-care facilities is often dependent on the effective use of drugs. The multiplicity of drugs available makes it mandatory that a sound program of drug usage be developed within the institution to ensure that patients receive the best possible care.

In the interest of better patient care, the institution should have a program of objective evaluation, selection, and use of medicinal agents in the facility. This program is the basis of appropriate, economical drug therapy. The formulary concept[a] is a method for providing such a program and has been utilized as such for many years.

To be effective, the formulary system must have the approval of the organized medical staff, the concurrence of individual staff members, and the functioning of a properly organized pharmacy and therapeutics (P&T) committee[b] of the medical staff. The basic policies and procedures governing the formulary system should be incorporated in the medical staff bylaws or in the medical staff rules and regulations.

The P&T committee represents the official organizational line of communication and liaison between the medical and pharmacy staffs. The committee is responsible to the medical staff as a whole, and its recommendations are subject to approval by the organized medical staff as well as to the normal administrative approval process.

This committee assists in the formulation of broad professional policies relating to drugs in institutions, including their evaluation or appraisal, selection, procurement, storage, distribution, and safe use.

Definition of Formulary and Formulary System

The *formulary* is a continually revised compilation of pharmaceuticals (plus important ancillary information) that reflects the current clinical judgment of the medical staff.[c]

The *formulary system* is a method whereby the medical staff of an institution, working through the P&T committee, evaluates, appraises, and selects from among the numerous available drug entities and drug products those that are considered most useful in patient care. Only those so selected are routinely available from the pharmacy. The formulary system is thus an important tool for assuring the quality of drug use and controlling its cost. The formulary system provides for the procuring, prescribing, dispensing, and administering of drugs under either their nonproprietary or proprietary names in instances where drugs have both names.

Guiding Principles

The following principles will serve as a guide to physicians, pharmacists, nurses, and administrators in hospitals and other facilities utilizing the formulary system:

1. The medical staff shall appoint a multidisciplinary P&T committee and outline its purposes, organization, function, and scope.

2. The formulary system shall be sponsored by the medical staff based on the recommendations of the P&T committee. The medical staff should adapt the principles of the system to the needs of the particular institution.

3. The medical staff shall adopt written policies and procedures governing the formulary system as developed by the P&T committee. Action of the medical staff is subject to the normal administrative approval process. These policies and procedures shall afford guidance in the evaluation or appraisal, selection, procurement, storage, distribution, safe use, and other matters relating to drugs and shall be published in the institution's formulary or other media available to all members of the medical staff.

4. Drugs should be included in the formulary by their nonproprietary names, even though proprietary names may be in common use in the institution. Prescribers should be strongly encouraged to prescribe drugs by their nonproprietary names.

5. Limiting the number of drug entities and drug products routinely available from the pharmacy can produce substantial patient-care and (particularly) financial benefits. These benefits are greatly increased through the use of *generic equivalents* (drug products considered to be identical with respect to their active components; e.g., two brands of tetracycline hydrochloride capsules) and *therapeutic equivalents* (drug products differing in composition or in their basic drug entity that are considered to have very similar pharmacologic and therapeutic activities; e.g., two different antacid products or two different alkylamine antihistamines). The P&T committee must set forth policies and procedures governing the dispensing of generics and therapeutic equivalents. These policies and procedures should include the following points:

   - That the pharmacist is responsible for selecting, from available generic equivalents, those drugs to be dispensed pursuant to a physician's order for a particular drug product.
   - That the prescriber has the option, at the time of prescribing, to specify the brand or supplier of drug to be dispensed for that particular medication order/prescription. The prescriber's decision should be based on pharmacologic or therapeutic considerations (or both) relative to that patient.
   - That the P&T committee is responsible for determining those drug products and entities (if any) that shall be considered therapeutic equivalents. The conditions and procedures for dispensing a therapeutic alternative in place of the prescribed drug shall be clearly delineated.

6. The institution shall make certain that its medical and nursing staffs are informed about the existence of the formulary system, the procedures governing its operation, and any changes in those procedures. Copies of the formulary must be readily available and accessible at all times.

7. Provision shall be made for appraisal and use of drugs not included in the formulary by the medical staff.

8. The pharmacist shall be responsible for specifications as to the quality, quantity, and source of supply of all drugs, chemicals, biologicals, and pharmaceutical preparations used in the diagnosis and treatment of patients. When applicable, such products should meet the standards of the *United States Pharmacopeia*.

Recommendation

A formulary system, based on these guiding principles, is important in drug therapy in institutions. In the interest of better and more economical patient care, its adoption by medical staffs is strongly recommended.

The policy of the American Medical Association on drug formularies and therapeutic interchange is consistent with this practice standard of ASHP (see *Am J Hosp Pharm.* 1994; 51:1808–10).

[a]The formulary system is adaptable for use in any type of health-care facility and is not limited to hospitals.

[b]For additional information, see the "ASHP Statement on the Pharmacy and Therapeutics Committee" (*Am J Hosp Pharm.* 1978; 35:813–4).

[c]For additional information, see the "ASHP Guidelines for Hospital Formularies" (*Am J Hosp Pharm.* 1978; 35:326–8).

Approved by the ASHP Board of Directors, November 18, 1982, and by the ASHP House of Delegates, June 7, 1983. Developed by the ASHP Council on Clinical Affairs. Supersedes the "ASHP Statement of Guiding Principles on the Operation of the Hospital Formulary System" approved by the Board of Directors, January 10, 1964.

The bibliographic citation for this document is as follows: American Society of Hospital Pharmacists. ASHP statement on the formulary system. *Am J Hosp Pharm.* 1983; 40:1384–5.

ASHP Statement on Its Economic Status Program

Policy on Economic Status

The professional and economic goals of the professional person are closely interrelated. Only in attainment of these goals can he assume the leadership role expected of him in the community, by his colleagues, and by other health professions. When satisfactory economic status is achieved, the professional can realize his maximum potential and apply his full energies to the needs of society.

The American Society of Hospital Pharmacists has, since its inception, concentrated on the professional responsibilities of hospital pharmacists through promotion of high standards of professional ethics, education, and attainments. Nevertheless, the economic interests of members of the Society were acknowledged several years ago when the *Mirror to Hospital Pharmacy* and the Society's Commission on Goals counseled ASHP to involve itself in activities dealing with the economic status of hospital pharmacists. Indeed, one of the goals of the Society's statement, "Goals for Hospital Pharmacy," adopted in 1964 is to: "Promote payment of realistic salaries to hospital pharmacists in both staff and managerial positions in order to attract and retain the services of career personnel." More recently, the Society conducted a salary survey to obtain factual data on the economic status of pharmacists in institutional practice.

The Society's concern for the economic welfare of its members complements the professional and scientific objectives presently set forth in the Constitution of the American Society of Hospital Pharmacists. Involvement by the Society in the economic well-being of its members is in the public interest since assurance of economic satisfaction tends to attract highly qualified pharmacists to institutional practice.

Salaries, working hours, and fringe benefits of hospital pharmacists should be commensurate with professional education, responsibility, and status and with the increased participation by hospital pharmacists in the actual planning and administration of pharmacy service and in the determination of policies which directly affect them. Both employers and employed pharmacists have an obligation to resolve employment issues fairly and in good faith.

The responsibilities of the individual are primary. However, as institutions and the delivery of health care grow in size and complexity, collective effort may be necessary to solve group economic problems. With this view, the Society must meet the needs of its members by embarking on a broad program of economic status which may include such activities as the compilation of statistical data, the preparation of model contracts, and, when necessary, mediation, conciliation, and arbitration. When economic problems of employment cannot be resolved by the individual practitioner or the pharmacy staff of a hospital, the Society's affiliated chapters, with the legal and financial assistance of ASHP, may find it necessary to engage in collective bargaining.

The Board of Directors of the American Society of Hospital Pharmacists, at its meeting of January 10–11, 1970, voted:

> To engage in collective bargaining by assisting affiliated chapters, upon request, in accordance with policies and guidelines as established by the House of Delegates of the American Society of Hospital Pharmacists; further,
> To adopt the statement, "Economic Status Program of the American Society of Hospital Pharmacists."

In accordance with this action, the following are guidelines for individual members, affiliated chapters, and ASHP.

Guidelines for Collective Bargaining

Individual Members

1. Hospital pharmacists must recognize their obligation to the patient, the institution, the profession, the allied health professions, and society.
2. Hospital pharmacists shall not deprive patients of pharmaceutical services by withholding their services in any form, including strikes, in support of economic demands.

Affiliated Chapters

1. Affiliated chapters may engage in collective bargaining, preferably through the statewide affiliated chapter. Any such activity shall be conducted solely in the name of, and by, the affiliated chapter.
2. Affiliated chapters may engage in collective bargaining when
   a. professional prerogatives of the pharmacists are endangered by the lack of effective representation; or
   b. wages or conditions of employment are below acceptable levels; or
   c. the environment in which the profession is practiced is not conducive to good patient care; and
   d. good faith attempts have failed to remedy the above situation(s).
3. Affiliated chapters will make available the services of negotiating contracts to active ASHP members. All hospital pharmacists who practice at the contracting institution may be represented. Hospital pharmacists being represented who are not members of the affiliated chapter and the American Society of Hospital Pharmacists must become members, if permitted by all applicable laws.
4. Affiliated chapters will accept or reject contracts as determined by a majority of the members in the bargaining unit.
5. Affiliated chapters will assess each hospital pharmacist a service fee for each contract negotiated, as determined by and paid to ASHP, to the extent permitted by applicable laws.
6. Affiliated chapters must follow procedures outlined by ASHP.

American Society of Hospital Pharmacists

1. The Society will coordinate collective bargaining ac-

tivities of affiliated chapters by providing

a.   statistical information and research assistance;

b.   legal assistance; and

c.   financial assistance when necessary.

Approved by the ASHP Board of Directors, January 11, 1970, and

by the ASHP House of Delegates, March 29, 1971.

The bibliographic citation for this document is as follows: American Society of Hospital Pharmacists. ASHP statement on its economic status program. *Am J Hosp Pharm.* 1971; 28:517–8.

ASHP Statement on Continuing Education

Next to integrity, competence is the first and most fundamental moral responsibility of all the health professions....Each of our professions must insist that competence will be reinforced through the years of practice. After the degree is conferred, continuing education is society's only real guarantee of the optimal quality of health care.

—Edmund D. Pellegrino

In an era of rapidly accelerating change in health-care delivery, the roles of pharmacy practitioners are being constantly redefined. As roles change, competency requirements change; and as pharmacy practitioners assume the increased responsibilities demanded in these new roles, they must make a corresponding commitment to improve their professional competence. Continuing education is a means by which practitioners can gain the knowledge and skills necessary to develop, maintain, and improve their professional competence.

In keeping with the mission of ASHP, the purpose of continuing education for health professionals is the improvement of patient care and health maintenance and the enrichment of health careers. Every practitioner should assume personal responsibility for maintaining and improving professional competence through lifelong, self-directed education. Every pharmacist should set personal educational objectives based on individual needs and career goals. One way to achieve these objectives is through continuing education experiences judiciously selected from among area, regional, and national resources. It should be the role of ASHP to facilitate the efforts of the pharmacist in self-directed education.

Objectives

The objectives for the continuing education services of the American Society of Hospital Pharmacists shall be

1. To help pharmacists develop a more complete understanding of the importance and methods of lifelong, self-directed education and to encourage and assist them toward this goal.
2. To help practitioners evaluate their professional performance, identify areas where improvement is needed, and set realistic and attainable educational goals.
3. To provide to practitioners information on available area, regional, and national educational resources which will help them achieve their personal educational objectives.
4. To assist pharmacists in selecting educational resources that most effectively fulfill their individual needs.
5. To provide to pharmacists continuing education resources in a variety of formats and media best suited for the subject matter and needs of the greater number of learners.

Authority

Matters relating to continuing education services will be considered by the Council on Educational Affairs and will be submitted to the Board of Directors for review.

Guidelines

The following guidelines are used in the development and conduct of continuing education programs and activities of the American Society of Hospital Pharmacists:

1. Continuing education programs will be planned and conducted in accordance with the Criteria for Quality of the Continuing Education Provider Approval Program of the American Council on Pharmaceutical Education.
2. ASHP will collaborate, when appropriate, with other professional organizations, agencies, and educational institutions in the planning and conduct of continuing education activities.
3. When appropriate, due consideration will be given to the curricular approach in the planning and implementation of continuing education activities.
4. ASHP may limit or restrict the enrollment for any continuing education program, depending on the nature and requirements of the particular program.
5. ASHP's overall continuing education activity is intended to be self-supporting; however, the benefit versus cost value to members of a specific educational program must also be considered.

Approved by the ASHP Board of Directors, November 15, 1989. Developed by the Council on Educational Affairs. Supersedes a previous version approved by the ASHP House of Delegates on May 15, 1978.

The bibliographic citation for this document is as follows: American Society of Hospital Pharmacists. ASHP statement on continuing education. *Am J Hosp Pharm.* 1990; 47:1855.

ASHP Statement on Unit Dose Drug Distribution

The unit dose system of medication distribution is a pharmacy-coordinated method of dispensing and controlling medications in organized health-care settings.

The unit dose system may differ in form, depending on the specific needs of the organization. However, the following distinctive elements are basic to all unit dose systems: medications are contained in single unit packages; they are dispensed in as ready-to-administer form as possible; and for most medications, not more than a 24-hour supply[a] of doses is delivered to or available at the patient-care area at any time.[1,2]

Numerous studies concerning unit dose drug distribution systems have been published over the past several decades. These studies indicate categorically that unit dose systems, with respect to other drug distribution methods, are (1) safer for the patient, (2) more efficient and economical for the organization, and (3) a more effective method of utilizing professional resources.

More specifically, the inherent advantages of unit dose systems over alternative distribution procedures are

1. A reduction in the incidence of medication errors.
2. A decrease in the total cost of medication-related activities.
3. A more efficient usage of pharmacy and nursing personnel, allowing for more direct patient-care involvement by pharmacists and nurses.
4. Improved overall drug control and drug use monitoring.
5. More accurate patient billings for drugs.
6. The elimination or minimization of drug credits.
7. Greater control by the pharmacist over pharmacy workload patterns and staff scheduling.
8. A reduction in the size of drug inventories located in patient-care areas.
9. Greater adaptability to computerized and automated procedures.

In view of these demonstrated benefits, the American Society of Hospital Pharmacists considers the unit dose system to be an essential part of drug distribution and control in organized health-care settings in which drug therapy is an integral component of health-care delivery.

References

1. Summerfield MR. Unit dose primer. Bethesda, MD: American Society of Hospital Pharmacists; 1983.
2. American Society of Hospital Pharmacists. ASHP technical assistance bulletin on hospital drug distribution and control. *Am J Hosp Pharm.* 1980; 37:1097–1103.

---

[a]In long-term care facilities, a larger supply of medication (e.g., 48 or 72 hours) may be acceptable.

Approved by the ASHP Board of Directors, November 16, 1988, and by the ASHP House of Delegates, June 5, 1989. Supersedes previous versions approved by the House of Delegates on June 8, 1981, and by the Board of Directors on April 19, 1975, and November 13–14, 1980.

The bibliographic citation for this document is as follows: American Society of Hospital Pharmacists. ASHP statement on unit dose drug distribution. *Am J Hosp Pharm.* 1989; 46:2346.

ASHP Statement on the
Pharmacist's Role in Infection Control

Purposes

The purposes of this statement are (1) to assert the Society's position that pharmacists should be included in the infection control activities of hospitals and other organized health-care settings, and (2) to enumerate the functions pharmacists should seek to carry out in conjunction with their infection control responsibilities.

Background

The importance of infection control programs in hospitals and other organized health-care settings is widely recognized. The standards of the Joint Commission on Accreditation of Hospitals[1] require that hospitals maintain active infection control programs and that responsibility for such programs be vested in multidisciplinary infection control (or equivalent) committees.

Among the basic responsibilities of the infection control committee are the following:

1. Development of written standards for hospital sanitation and asepsis.
2. Development and promulgation of procedures and techniques for meeting these standards and monitoring compliance with them.
3. Development and implementation of a system for eliciting, reporting, and evaluating data concerning infections in the hospital's patient and personnel populations.
4. Development and implementation, in cooperation with the pharmacy and therapeutics (P&T) committee, of a system for the routine surveillance and review of antimicrobial use within the hospital.

Since approval of the first ASHP statement on this subject in 1977,[2] the Society has advocated active participation by pharmacists in hospitals' infection control programs.[a]

ASHP's Position

ASHP believes that pharmacists, as health-care providers, have a clear responsibility to participate in infection control programs and that this responsibility arises from their education and training and particularly from their understanding and influence over antibiotic use in the hospital. Further, the Society believes that the pharmacist's effectiveness in infection control and antibiotic use review can best be realized through formal appropriate committees of the hospital and medical staff.

Functions

The responsibilities of pharmacists for infection control extend into the following areas: control of nosocomial infection, promotion of rational use of antimicrobial agents, and education.

Control of Nosocomial Infections. Pharmacists' responsibilities in this area can be met through the following functions:

1. Participating in the affairs of the infection control (or equivalent) committee.
2. Advising the hospital on the selection and use of appropriate antiseptics, disinfectants, and sterilants.
3. Establishing internal pharmacy policies, procedures, and quality control programs to prevent contamination of drug products prepared in or dispensed from the pharmacy department. Of paramount importance in this area are the preparation and handling of sterile products. Other considerations include (but are not limited to) provisions for cleaning various articles of pharmaceutical equipment (such as laminar airflow hoods, unit dose trays, and bulk compounding equipment) and establishment of appropriate personnel policies (e.g., limiting the activities of staff members who exhibit obvious symptoms of a cold, flu, or other infectious condition).
4. Encouraging the use of single dose packages of sterile drugs instead of multiple dose containers.
5. Recommending policies for the frequency of changing intravenous sets and other intravenous administration equipment and dressings.
6. Recommending proper storage of sterile products and multiple dose containers (if used).

Promotion of Rational Use of Antimicrobial Agents. An important clinical responsibility of the pharmacist is to promote the rational use of antibiotics and other antimicrobial agents. In the context of infection control, this responsibility extends to the establishment of measures for minimizing the development of resistant strains of microorganisms as well as for optimizing the chance of successful therapeutic outcomes in individual patients.

Functions related to this responsibility include

1. Working within the P&T committee structure to control the number and types of antibiotics and other antimicrobial agents admitted to the formulary. Both therapeutic and microbiological factors and cost-containment considerations should influence such decisions.
2. Collaborating with the medical staff in establishing policies related to prophylactic antibiotic use, restricted use of specific antibiotics, and other drug use policies related to antibiotics and other antimicrobial agents.
3. Establishing and operating (in conjunction with the medical staff) an ongoing concurrent-prospective antibiotic use review program for assessing and improving the quality of antimicrobial therapy.
4. Generating and analyzing quantitative data on antimicrobial drug use.
5. Working with the microbiology laboratory to improve microbial sensitivity screening tests and the reporting of their results.
6. Working with the appropriate individuals and committees in the institution who are responsible for se-

lecting and controlling intravenous sets, infusion devices, and other equipment and paraphernalia related to intravenous antibiotic administration.

Educational Activities. Pharmacists' responsibilities in this area extend to other health professionals as well as to patients and to the public. Specific functions include

1. Conducting inservice educational programs, clinical conferences, and other types of presentations for health professionals on appropriate topics, including (but not limited to) the following:
   a. Antimicrobial therapy.
   b. Decontaminating agents (disinfectants, antiseptics, and sterilants).
   c. Aseptic technique and procedures.
   d. Sterilization methods.
2. Educating and counseling inpatients, ambulatory care patients, and home care patients in the following areas:
   a. Importance of compliance with prescribed directions for antibiotics (and all other drugs).
   b. Other information necessary for safe and appropriate drug use (e.g., whether or not to take with meals).
   c. Instructions on storage conditions, including drugs administered through home care programs.
   d. Other infection control procedures to be followed in a home care patient's household.
3. Establishing and conducting ongoing quality-assurance activities and inservice presentations to pharmacy staff on appropriate topics, including but not limited to
   a. Aseptic techniques and procedures.
   b. Sterilization methods.
   c. Environmental quality control (e.g., laminar airflow hood checks).

4. Participating in public health education and awareness campaigns concerning control of the spread of infectious disease.

References

1. Accreditation manual for hospitals 1985. Chicago: Joint Commission on Accreditation of Hospitals; 1985.
2. American Society of Hospital Pharmacists. ASHP statement on the hospital pharmacist's role in infection control. *Am J Hosp Pharm.* 1978; 35:814–5.

---

[a]As of 1985, there had been no JCAH recommendation that a pharmacist be included on the infection control committee. The American Hospital Association, however, has endorsed the recommendation that infection control committees include a pharmacist.

Approved by the ASHP Board of Directors, November 20–21, 1985, and by the ASHP House of Delegates, June 4, 1986. Developed by the ASHP Council on Professional Affairs. Supersedes the previous statement, "ASHP Statement on the Hospital Pharmacist's Role in Infection Control," approved by the ASHP Board of Directors, November 14–15, 1977, and by the ASHP House of Delegates, May 15, 1978.

The bibliographic citation for this document is as follows: American Society of Hospital Pharmacists. ASHP statement on the pharmacist's role in infection control. *Am J Hosp Pharm.* 1986; 43:2006–8.

ASHP Statement on Third-Party Compensation for Clinical Services by Pharmacists

Historically, institutional pharmacists have been concerned primarily with dispensing drugs and secondarily with providing drug-related information. With the major increase in the number, potency, and toxicity of drugs in recent years, pharmacists are increasingly providing clinical services. This means that the primary focus of institutional pharmacy practice is shifting from a system of drug distribution to one of drug use control, which includes both drug distribution and provision of information. Therefore, a substantial portion of many pharmacies' total expenses and workload relates to patient service activities. These activities, which are not directly related to drug dispensing, are described in the "ASHP Statement on Clinical Functions in Institutional Pharmacy Practice."[1]

Clinical pharmacy services and rational drug therapy are essential components of total patient care and contributing factors to the reduction of patient-care costs. Federal and state legislation and regulations and numerous private standards[a] recognize the benefits of clinical pharmacy services and strongly encourage, if not require, the provision of these services to patients in organized health-care settings. To maintain clinical pharmacy services in organized health-care settings, the following principles should be noted by health-care administrators, third-party payers, and pharmacy managers:

1. Currently, many types of third-party payment systems are in use, including such diverse payment mechanisms as Medicare prospective pricing (e.g., diagnosis-related groups), capitated payments for health maintenance organizations, and cost-based reimbursement for commercial third-party insurance. Each third-party payer may use different payment or reimbursement mechanisms,[b] and each hospital's reimbursement may vary by its location, its primary third-party payer, and its case mix. Therefore, pharmacy managers must be cognizant of the types of compensation received by their individual hospitals and must structure their pharmaceutical services in a manner that permits identification and monitoring of costs versus benefits under each payment mechanism.

2. Regardless of the payment mechanism, clinical services are generally considered reimbursable or payable items when they are integral to the case management plan for each patient and when the costs and benefits of the service are carefully documented. Payment for clinical services may also be determined by the third-party payer's review and approval of the service. In the case of commercial insurers, those who are insured can direct that payment for clinical services be included in their policies.

3. Pharmacists should take the initiative in proposing clinical programs and documenting the health-care benefits of such programs. They should develop such services and cooperate with provider fiscal officers to document accurately the related costs. Services should also be consistent with regulatory agency, industry, and institutional standards of cost identification and allocation. Likewise, pharmacists should document the cost impact of such services on the entire drug use continuum, which includes the selection of a drug regimen, delivery of the drug product, its administration to the patient, and the monitoring of its effects. Pharmacy administrators must play a central role in identifying the clinical services that should be provided by their institution and ensuring that each service is consistent with professional standards.

4. Methods used to determine costs of clinical pharmacy services should be consistent with the methods used to determine costs of other patient-care services. The costs and charges associated with clinical pharmacy services should reflect the provider's reasonable fiscal needs for providing such services.

5. Mechanisms for charging patients for pharmaceutical services may take one of several forms. A patient charge mechanism for pharmaceutical services should be developed by the provider's fiscal officer and pharmacists, taking into account professional trends, management philosophy, and the implications of that patient charging mechanism for reimbursement or payment.

6. Reimbursement or payment for clinical services will usually be to the provider (i.e., the institution), not directly to the pharmacist. Generally, charges for pharmaceutical services will be rendered as part of the provider's bill to the patient. Pharmacy or pharmacist compensation for services generally should be resolved with the provider and may take any form that is acceptable to both parties.

Reference

1. American Society of Hospital Pharmacists. ASHP statement on clinical functions in institutional pharmacy practice. *Am J Hosp Pharm.* 1978; 35:813.

---

[a]An example is the "ASHP Statement on Clinical Pharmacy and Its Relationship to the Hospital" (*Am J Hosp Pharm.* 1971; 28:357).
[b]Generally, payment refers to prospective compensation, and reimbursement refers to retrospective compensation.

Approved by the ASHP House of Delegates, June 3, 1985, and by the Board of Directors, April 25, 1985. Developed by the ASHP Council on Administrative Affairs. Supersedes the "ASHP Statement on Reimbursement and Payment for Clinical Pharmacy Services," which was approved June 8, 1981.

The bibliographic citation for this document is as follows: American Society of Hospital Pharmacists. ASHP statement on third-party compensation for clinical services by pharmacists. *Am J Hosp Pharm.* 1985; 42:1580–1.

ASHP Statement on the Pharmacist's Role in Clinical Pharmacokinetic Services

Clinical pharmacokinetics is the process of applying pharmacokinetic principles to determine the dose and dosage frequency of specific drugs for specific patients. Application of these principles requires an understanding of the absorption, distribution, metabolism, and excretion characteristics of specific drugs in specific diseases. The influence of other factors including age, disease, diet, and the concomitant use of other drugs must also be understood. The development of patients' individualized dosage regimens should be based on integrated findings from the monitoring of both concentration–effect responses and pharmacological responses to drugs.

Pharmacists' clinical functions include drug therapy monitoring and the provision of clinical pharmacokinetic assessments.[1] Specific education, training, or experience is necessary to perform pharmacokinetic services. Pharmacists' responsibilities for participation in clinical pharmacokinetic services increase as the pharmacokinetic characteristics of drugs become clearly defined and as safe therapeutic concentration ranges for specific drugs are established. The need for clinical pharmacokinetic services is more pronounced when the range between minimal effectiveness and toxicity is narrow.

Pharmacists involved in clinical pharmacokinetic services should participate in the

1. Design of patient-specific drug dosage regimens based on the pharmacokinetic and pharmacological characteristics of the drugs used, the objectives of drug therapy, concurrent diseases and drug therapy, and other pertinent patient factors (e.g., age, laboratory data) that may affect the safety and effectiveness of drug therapy.
2. Monitoring and adjustment of dosage regimens based both on pharmacological responses and on biological fluid (e.g., plasma, serum, blood, cerebrospinal fluid) and tissue drug concentrations in conjunction with clinical signs and symptoms or other biochemical parameters.
3. Evaluation of unusual patient responses to drug therapy for possible pharmacokinetic and pharmacological explanations.
4. Communication of information on patient-specific drug therapy to physicians, nurses, and other clinical practitioners.
5. Education of pharmacists, physicians, nurses, and other clinical practitioners on pharmacokinetic principles.
6. Recommendation of procedures and assays for the analysis of drug concentrations in order to facilitate the evaluation of dosage regimens.
7. Formation of collaborative relationships with other individuals and departments involved in drug therapy monitoring to encourage the development and appropriate use of clinical pharmacokinetic services.
8. Development of quality-assurance programs to document improved therapeutic benefits, decreased toxicity, and economic benefits resulting from clinical pharmacokinetic services.
9. Design and conduct of research to expand clinical pharmacokinetic knowledge and its relationship to pharmacological responses, explore dose–response relationships for specific drugs, and contribute to the evaluation and expansion of clinical pharmacokinetic services.
10. Development and application of computer programs to enhance the accuracy and sophistication of pharmacokinetic modeling.

Reference

1. American Society of Hospital Pharmacists. ASHP statement on the pharmacist's clinical role in organized health-care settings. *Am J Hosp Pharm*. 1988; 45:890–1.

Approved by the ASHP House of Delegates, June 5, 1989, and the ASHP Board of Directors, November 16, 1988. Developed by the ASHP Council on Professional Affairs. Supersedes a previous version approved by the ASHP House of Delegates on June 7, 1982.

The bibliographic citation for this document is as follows: American Society of Hospital Pharmacists. ASHP statement on the pharmacist's role in clinical pharmacokinetic services. *Am J Hosp Pharm*. 1989; 46:2344.

ASHP Statement on Pharmaceutical Research in Organized Health-Care Settings

Pharmacy practice is grounded in the physicochemical, biological, and socioeconomic sciences. Hence, the continued and future success and self-esteem of the profession are dependent on the expanded knowledge base that can be produced through dynamic and rigorous scientific research and development. This research, to be meaningful and productive in terms of pharmacy's needs and goals in organized health-care settings, must include the participation of pharmacists practicing in those settings.

Pharmacists in organized health-care settings function in cooperation with other health-care professionals. They contribute a unique expertise to the drug-related aspects of patient care and take personal professional responsibility for the outcomes from the pharmaceutical care they provide to patients. Improvements in drug therapy depend on new knowledge generated by scientific research. Thus, pharmacists in organized health-care settings have a professional obligation to participate actively in and increase pharmacy-related and drug-related research efforts.[1,2]

Reflecting the collaborative nature of contemporary health care, this research should be multidisciplinary to be most beneficial. Thus, ASHP encourages pharmacists with a researchable idea or problem to seek the advice and active participation of people and organizations with scientific expertise such as

- College faculty (especially college of pharmacy faculty).
- Other staff and departments within the setting.
- Staff and departments in other health-care organizations.
- Industrial research personnel and laboratories.

It also is appropriate for pharmacists to function as principal investigators in research projects.

ASHP encourages pharmacists to increase their involvement in the following kinds of scientific research and development:

- Pharmaceutical research, including the development and testing of new drug dosage forms and drug preparation and administration methods and systems.

- Clinical research, such as the therapeutic characterization, evaluation, comparison, and outcomes of drug therapy and drug treatment regimens.
- Health services research and development, including behavioral and socioeconomic research such as research on cost–benefit issues in pharmaceutical care.
- Operations research, such as time and motion studies and evaluation of new and existing pharmacy programs and services.

This research will be a critical contribution of pharmacy to health care and must be fostered by all facets of the profession.

References

1. American Society of Hospital Pharmacists. ASHP guidelines for pharmaceutical research in organized health-care settings. *Am J Hosp Pharm.* 1989; 46:129–30.
2. American Society of Hospital Pharmacists. ASHP guidelines for the use of investigational drugs in organized health-care settings. *Am J Hosp Pharm.* 1991; 48:315–9.

Approved by the ASHP Board of Directors, November 14, 1990, and the ASHP House of Delegates, June 3, 1991. Revised by the ASHP Council on Professional Affairs. Supersedes a previous statement, "ASHP Statement on Institutional Pharmacy Research," approved by the ASHP House of Delegates on June 3, 1985, and the ASHP Board of Directors on November 14–15, 1984.

The bibliographic citation for this document is as follows: American Society of Hospital Pharmacists. ASHP statement on pharmaceutical research in organized health-care settings. *Am J Hosp Pharm.* 1991; 48:1781.

ASHP Statement on the Pharmacist's Role in Patient Education Programs

The American Society of Hospital Pharmacists strongly supports efforts to provide appropriate drug education to patients and the public. Further, ASHP believes that maximum benefits of patient education programs are realized when a cooperative multidisciplinary approach is used and that sharing of pertinent patient information by all participants is fundamental to the success of patient education services. While the objectives of patient education programs are uniform among health-care settings, the methods for executing programs may vary according to the requirements of each setting.

ASHP endorses the following activities of pharmacists in patient education programs:

1. Serving as members of appropriate committees involved in patient education (e.g., discharge planning committee and patient education committee).
2. Participating in the development of drug-related patient education material. Only materials that have been reviewed and approved by pharmacists in the setting should be used.
3. Advising other health-care practitioners on matters of patient drug education.
4. Helping to ensure that patient drug education is skillfully and sensitively communicated to patients from various socioeconomic backgrounds.
5. Participating in educational programs for pharmacists and other health-care practitioners involved in patient drug education.
6. Organizing and presenting the drug-related aspects of community health education programs.
7. Providing patient education and counseling regarding drug therapy and drug-related disease prevention.[1,2]

References

1. American Society of Hospital Pharmacists. ASHP statement on the pharmacist's clinical role in organized health-care settings. *Am J Hosp Pharm.* 1989; 46:805–6.
2. American Society of Hospital Pharmacists. ASHP guidelines on pharmacist-conducted patient counseling. *Am J Hosp Pharm.* 1984; 41:331.

Approved by the ASHP Board of Directors, November 14, 1990, and the ASHP House of Delegates, June 3, 1991. Revised by the ASHP Council on Professional Affairs. Supersedes a previous statement, "ASHP Statement on the Pharmacist's Role in Institutional Patient Education Programs," approved by the ASHP House of Delegates on June 3, 1985, and the ASHP Board of Directors on November 14–15, 1984.

The bibliographic citation for this document is as follows: American Society of Hospital Pharmacists. ASHP statement on the pharmacist's role in patient education programs. *Am J Hosp Pharm.* 1991; 48:1780.

ASHP Statement on the Pharmacist's Role with Respect to Drug Delivery Systems and Administration Devices

Technological advances in drug delivery systems and administration devices frequently enable improved control of drug administration. Such advances may offer numerous potential benefits to patients, including improved therapeutic outcomes in disease management, improved patient compliance with drug regimens, and greater efficiency and economy in disease therapy. These advances constitute an important aspect of pharmaceutical knowledge and are routinely incorporated into pharmacy practice as they occur.

A drug delivery system is defined as one in which a drug (one component of the system) is integrated with another chemical, a drug administration device, or a drug administration process to control the rate of drug release, the tissue site of drug release, or both. A drug administration device is an apparatus that is used for introducing a drug to the body or controlling its rate of introduction. Drug delivery systems include (but are not limited to) osmotic pumps, thermal isolation, transdermal patches, liposomal encapsulation, iontophoresis, phonophoresis, magnetic migration, and implantation. Drug administration devices include (but are not limited to) mechanical (e.g., balloon-driven), gravity-driven, and electromechanical pumps. Some of the latter are portable, implantable, computer controlled, or patient controlled. Some enable the simultaneous infusion of multiple drugs. Drug administration control devices include plasma concentration monitoring and administration rate monitoring devices, which incorporate computers.

Pharmacists bear a substantial responsibility for ensuring optimal clinical outcomes from drug therapy and are suited by education, training, clinical expertise, and practice activities to assume responsibility for the professional supervision of drug delivery systems and administration devices. As a natural extension of efforts to optimize drug use, pharmacists should participate in organizational and clinical decisions with regard to these systems and devices. Some decisions and activities in which pharmacists should participate follow. Others may be appropriate as well.

1. Research and development of innovative drug delivery systems and administration devices.
2. Evaluation and research to determine the direct and comparative efficacy, safety, and cost-effectiveness of specific drug delivery systems and administration devices.
3. In conjunction with pharmacy and therapeutics committees (or other appropriate medical staff committees), decisions to choose or exclude particular drug delivery systems and administration devices for use in specific organizational settings.
4. Development of organization-specific policies and procedures regarding the acquisition, storage, distribution, use, maintenance, and ongoing product quality control of drug delivery systems and administration devices.
5. Choice of a particular drug delivery system or administration device for use in a specific patient's drug therapy.
6. Direct communication with patients to instruct them in the use of such systems and devices and to gather information necessary to monitor the outcome of their therapy.
7. Monitoring of the ongoing clinical effectiveness and suitability of specific drug delivery systems or administration devices with respect to specific patients and the communication of clinically relevant observations and recommendations to prescribers and other health professionals involved in the patients' care.

Failures or malfunctions of drug administration devices may lead to patient harm. Reports of such problems should be made in accordance with the provisions of the Safe Medical Devices Act of 1990 (PL 101-629).

Recommendations for Additional Reading

Acevedo ML. Electronic flow control. *NITA*. 1983; 6:105–6.

Akers MJ. Current problems and innovations in intravenous drug delivery. Considerations in using the i.v. route for drug delivery. *Am J Hosp Pharm*. 1987; 44:2528–30.

Alexander MR. Current problems and innovations in intravenous drug delivery. Developing and implementing a contract for electronic infusion devices. *Am J Hosp Pharm*. 1987; 44:2553–6.

Anderson RW, Cohen JE, Cohen MR, et al. Hospital pharmacy symposium on new concepts in parenteral drug delivery. *Hosp Pharm*. 1986; 21:1033–55.

Baharloo M. Iontophoresis and phonophoresis: a role for the pharmacist. *Hosp Pharm*. 1987; 22:730–1.

Block LH, Shukla AJ. Drug delivery in the 1990s. *US Pharm*. 1986; 11(Oct):51–6, 58.

Boothe CD, Talley JR. Mechanical and electronic intravenous infusion devices. Part 1. *Infusion*. 1986; 10:6–8.

Chandrasekaran SK, Benson H, Urquhart J. Methods to achieve controlled drug delivery, the biomedical engineering approach. In: Robinson JR, ed. Sustained and controlled release drug delivery systems. New York: Marcel Dekker; 1978:557–93.

Colangelo A. Current problems and innovations in intravenous drug delivery. Drug preparation techniques for i.v. drug delivery systems. *Am J Hosp Pharm*. 1987; 44:2550–3.

Davis SR. Latest developments in drug delivery systems—abstracts. *Hosp Pharm*. 1987; 22:890–908.

Goodman MS, Wickham R. Venous access devices: oncology nurse overview. *Hosp Pharm*. 1985; 20:495–511.

Holm A, Campbell N. Role of institutional review boards in facilitating research, marketing of drugs and devices, and protecting human subjects. *Drug Dev Ind Pharm*. 1985; 11:1–12.

Juliano RL. Drug delivery systems. New York: Oxford University Press; 1980.

Kelly WN, Christensen LA. Selective patient criteria for the use of electronic infusion devices. *Am J IV Ther Clin Nutr*. 1983; 10(Mar):18, 19, 21, 25, 26, 29.

Kirschenbaum B, Klein S. Pharmacy-coordinated infusion

device evaluation. *Am J Hosp Pharm.* 1984; 41:1181–3.

Leff RD. Current problems and innovations in intravenous drug delivery. Features of i.v. devices and equipment that affect i.v. drug delivery. *Am J Hosp Pharm.* 1987; 44:2530–3.

Longer MA, Robinson JR. Sustained-release drug delivery systems. In: Gennaro AR, ed. Remington's pharmaceutical sciences. Easton, PA: Mack Publishing Company; 1985:1644–61.

McFarlane AE. Role for pharmacists in the provision of medical devices. *Aust J Hosp Pharm.* 1986; 16:78.

Mutschler E. Now and future of drug delivery systems. *Pharm Tech.* 1983(Suppl); 7:13–5.

Nahata MC. Current problems and innovations in intravenous drug delivery. Effect of i.v. drug delivery systems on pharmacokinetic monitoring. *Am J Hosp Pharm.* 1987; 44:2538–42.

Piecoro JJ Jr. Current problems and innovations in intravenous drug delivery. Development of an institutional i.v. drug delivery policy. *Am J Hosp Pharm.* 1987; 44:2557–9.

Polack AE, Roberts MS. Drug delivery systems. *Med J Aust.* 1986; 144:311–4.

Rapp RP. Current problems and innovations in intravenous drug delivery. Considering product features and costs in selecting a system for intermittent i.v. drug delivery. *Am J Hosp Pharm.* 1987; 44:2533–8.

Reilly KM. Current problems and innovations in intravenous drug delivery. Problems in administration techniques and dose measurement that influence accuracy of i.v. drug delivery. *Am J Hosp Pharm.* 1987; 44:2545–50.

Reiss RE. Volumetric IV pumps. *Pharm Tech.* 1983(Suppl); 7:46–9.

Self TH, Brooks JB, Lieberman P, et al. The value of demonstration and role of the pharmacist in teaching the correct use of pressurized bronchodilators. *Can Med Assoc J.* 1983; 128:129–31.

Selton MV. Implantable pumps. *CRC Crit Rev Biomed Eng.* 1987; 14:201–40.

Smith KL. Developments in drug delivery systems. *Hosp Pharm.* 1987; 22:905–6.

Talley JR. Mechanical and electronic intravenous infusion devices. Part 2. *Infusion.* 1986; 10:31–4.

Talley JR. Mechanical and electronic intravenous infusion devices. Part 3. *Infusion.* 1986; 10:58–62.

Talsma H, Crommelin DJA. Liposomes as drug delivery systems, part I: preparation. *Pharm Tech.* 1992(Oct); 16:98, 100, 102, 104, 106.

Urquhart J. Implantable pumps in drug delivery. *Pharm Tech.* 1983(Suppl); 7:53–4.

Zenk KE. Current problems and innovations in intravenous drug delivery. Intravenous drug delivery in infants with limited i.v. access and fluid restriction. *Am J Hosp Pharm.* 1987; 44:2542–5.

Approved by the ASHP Board of Directors, November 18, 1992, and the ASHP House of Delegates, June 9, 1993. Revised by the ASHP Council on Professional Affairs. Supersedes a previous version approved by the ASHP House of Delegates on June 5, 1989, and the ASHP Board of Directors on November 16, 1988.

The bibliographic citation for this document is as follows: American Society of Hospital Pharmacists. ASHP statement on the pharmacist's role with respect to drug delivery systems and administration devices. *Am J Hosp Pharm.* 1993; 50:1724–5.

ASHP Statement on the Pharmacist's Responsibility for Distribution and Control of Drug Products

A fundamental purpose of pharmaceutical services in any setting is to ensure the safe and appropriate use of drug products and drug-related devices. Fulfillment of this responsibility is enhanced through the pharmacist's involvement in all aspects of the use of drugs.[1]

This involvement should include decisions and actions with respect to the evaluation, procurement, storage, distribution, and administration of all drug products. The pharmacist is responsible for development, in consultation with appropriate other professionals, departments, and interdisciplinary committees in the setting, of all drug-use control policies. The pharmacist should be directly responsible for the control and distribution of all stocks of drugs.

The Federal Food, Drug, and Cosmetic Act defines the term *drug* as "(A) articles recognized in the official United States Pharmacopeia, official Homeopathic Pharmacopeia of the United States, or official National Formulary, or any supplement to any of them; and (B) articles intended for use in the diagnosis, cure, mitigation, treatment, or prevention of disease in man or other animals; and (C) articles (other than food) intended to affect the structure or any function of the body of man or other animals; and (D) articles intended for use as a component of any article specified in clauses (A), (B), or (C) of this paragraph; but does not include devices or their components, parts, or accessories."[2]

For purposes of this document, drugs include those used by inpatients and outpatients, large- and small-volume injections, radiopharmaceuticals, diagnostic agents including radiopaque contrast media, anesthetic gases, blood-fraction drugs, dialysis fluids, respiratory therapy drugs, biotechnologically produced drugs, investigational drugs, drug samples, drugs brought to the setting by patients or family, and other chemicals and biological substances administered to patients to evoke or enhance pharmacologic responses.

The pharmacist's responsibility for drug-use control extends throughout the setting served. This purview extends to all pharmacy satellite locations (inpatient and outpatient, including those serving the general public), emergency rooms, surgical and labor and delivery suites (and related areas such as recovery rooms), anesthesiology, nuclear medicine, radiology, dialysis areas, ambulatory care clinics and treatment (including surgery) areas, respiratory therapy areas, central sterile supply centers, blood banks, intensive care areas, cardiac catheterization suites, research areas, and all other areas in which drugs are handled and used. The pharmacist should be responsible for drug-use policies and routine inspection of all drug stocks, even if direct custody and distribution are not possible.

The pharmacist also has an advocacy responsibility with respect to decisions and policies about the use of drug-related devices as they affect drug therapy. As appropriate, the pharmacist may also be assigned direct responsibility for control and distribution of drug-related devices.[3] Drug-related devices include electromechanical pumps, devices for administration of injectable drugs, devices for monitoring plasma drug concentration, and devices for monitoring drug administration rate.

References

1. American Society of Hospital Pharmacists. ASHP guidelines: minimum standard for pharmacies in institutions. *Am J Hosp Pharm.* 1985; 42:372–5.
2. 21 U.S.C. §321 (g) (1).
3. American Society of Hospital Pharmacists. ASHP statement on the pharmacist's role with respect to drug delivery systems and administration devices. *Am J Hosp Pharm.* 1989; 46:802–4.

Approved by the ASHP Board of Directors, November 16, 1994. Supersedes a previous version dated June 3, 1992. Approved by the ASHP Board of Directors, November 16, 1994, and by the ASHP House of Delegates, June 5, 1995. Revised by the ASHP Council on Professional Affairs.

The bibliographic citation for this document is as follows: ASHP statement on the pharmacist's responsibility for distribution and control of drug products. In: *Practice Standards of ASHP 1996–97.* Deffenbaugh JH, ed. Bethesda, MD: American Society of Health-System Pharmacists; 1996.

ASHP Statement on the Use of Medications for Unlabeled Uses

The freedom and responsibility to make drug therapy decisions that are consistent with patient-care needs is a fundamental precept supported by ASHP. This activity is a professional duty of pharmacists not limited by language in Food and Drug Administration (FDA)-approved product labeling.

The prescribing, dispensing, and administration of FDA-approved drugs for uses, treatment regimens, or patient populations that are not reflected in FDA-approved product labeling often represent a therapeutic approach that has been extensively studied and reported in medical literature. Such uses are *not* indicative of inappropriate usage. Health-care professionals should appreciate the critical need for freedom in making drug therapy decisions and understand the implications of unlabeled uses. ASHP supports third-party reimbursement for FDA-approved drug products appropriately prescribed for unlabeled uses.

Definition of Unlabeled Use

The FDA approves drug products for marketing in the United States. Such a product approved for marketing is often termed an "FDA-approved drug." FDA also approves each drug product's labeling (container label, package insert, and certain advertising); the term "FDA-approved labeling" applies here. Drug uses that are not included in the indications or dosage regimens listed in the FDA-approved labeling are defined as "unlabeled uses." For purposes of this document, unlabeled use includes the use of a drug product in (1) doses, (2) patient populations, (3) indications, or (4) routes of administration that are not reflected in FDA-approved product labeling.

It is important to recognize that FDA cannot approve or disapprove physician prescribing practices of legally marketed drugs. FDA does regulate what manufacturers may recommend about uses in their products' labeling and what manufacturers can include in advertising and promotion.

The sometimes-used term "unapproved use" is a misnomer, implying that FDA regulates prescribing and dispensing activities. This term should be avoided.[1] Other terminology that is sometimes used to describe unlabeled use includes "off-label use," "out-of-label use," and "usage outside of labeling."

According to FDA, unlabeled use encompasses a range of situations that extend from inadequate to carefully conceived investigations, from hazardous to salutary uses, and from infrequent to widespread medical practice. Accepted medical practice often involves drug use that is not reflected in FDA-approved drug-product labeling.[2]

Health-Care Issues Related to Unlabeled Use

Access to Drug Therapies. The prescribing and dispensing of drugs for unlabeled uses are increasing.[3,4] In many clinical situations, unlabeled use represents the most appropriate therapy for patients. Failure to recognize this or, more importantly, regarding such use as "unapproved" or "experimental" may restrict access to necessary drug therapies.

Lack of Practice Standards. Well-defined medical practice standards that differentiate between experimental therapies and established practice will probably always be somewhat lacking, owing to the advancement of medical science and the dynamic nature of medical practice. Standards of practice for certain drug therapies, particularly biotechnologically produced drugs, cancer chemotherapy, and AIDS treatments, are continually evolving. The dynamic nature of these drug therapies makes it difficult for professional societies to review scientific data expediently and to develop standards that remain absolutely current.

Failure of Package Insert and FDA-Approved Labeling to Reflect Current Practice. For FDA-approved product labeling to be modified, scientific data must be submitted by a product's manufacturer to FDA to support any additional indication(s) and dosage regimen(s). Once they are submitted, FDA must review the data and make a decision to permit alteration of the package insert.

Knowing that unlabeled uses are permitted, and knowing that the accumulation and submission of scientific data to FDA to modify labeling is a time-consuming and often expensive process, some pharmaceutical manufacturers elect not to pursue labeling changes. Therefore, a product's labeling sometimes fails to represent the most current therapeutic information for a drug, and situations naturally occur when it is appropriate to prescribe drugs for unlabeled uses.

Pharmacist's Role

ASHP believes that pharmacists in organized health-care settings bear a significant responsibility for ensuring optimal outcomes from all drug therapy. With respect to unlabeled uses, the role of the pharmacist should be to

1. Fulfill the roles of patient advocate and drug information specialist.
2. Develop policies and procedures for evaluating drug orders (prescriptions) and dispensing drugs for unlabeled uses in their own work settings. Such policies and procedures might address the documentation of scientific support, adherence to accepted medical practice standards, or a description of medical necessity.
3. Develop proactive approaches to promote informed decisionmaking by third-party payers for health-care services.

Role of Drug Information Compendia

The Medicare Catastrophic Coverage Act of 1988 (now repealed) included the statements that "in carrying out the legislation, the Secretary [of Health and Human Services] shall establish standards for drug coverage. In establishing such standards, which are based on accepted medical practice, the Secretary shall incorporate standards from such current authoritative compendia as the Secretary may select."[5] Specific compendia recommended were the *AHFS*

Drug Information, AMA Drug Evaluations, and *USP Dispensing Information, Volume I.* Despite the repeal of the Act, some third-party payers have adopted guidelines that endorse these three compendia as authoritative information sources with respect to unlabeled uses for drug products.

Positions on Unlabeled Use

FDA Position. A statement entitled "Use of Approved Drugs for Unlabeled Indications" was published in the *FDA Drug Bulletin* in April 1982 to address the issues of appropriateness and legality of prescribing approved drugs for uses not included in FDA's approved labeling. This statement included the following:

> *The Food, Drug and Cosmetic Act does not limit the manner in which a physician may use an approved drug. Once a product has been approved for marketing, a physician may prescribe it for uses or in treatment regimens or patient populations that are not included in approved labeling. Such "unapproved" or, more precisely, "unlabeled" uses may be appropriate and rational in certain circumstances, and may, in fact, reflect approaches to drug therapy that have been extensively reported in medical literature.[1]*

Other Organizations. Other organizations that have published positions on the issue of unlabeled uses of drug products are the Health Care Financing Administration (HCFA),[6] the Blue Cross and Blue Shield Association of America (BC/BS),[7] and the Health Insurance Association of America (HIAA).[8]

The American Medical Association, American Society of Clinical Oncology, Association of American Cancer Institutes, Association of Community Cancer Centers, Candlelighters Childhood Cancer Foundation, Memorial Sloan Kettering Cancer Center, National Cancer Institute, and the National Institute of Allergy and Infectious Diseases jointly developed a consensus statement and recommendations regarding use and reimbursement of unlabeled uses of drug products.[9]

These statements are consistent with the ASHP position.

Reimbursement Issues

As a cost-containment measure, most third-party payers exclude coverage for experimental therapies. Drug therapy coverage decisions are complicated, because often it is difficult to differentiate among an accepted standard of practice, an evolving standard of practice, and investigational therapies. Data demonstrating medical necessity and improved patient outcome are often difficult to retrieve. Consequently, insurance carriers and managed care provid-

ers have sometimes elected to cover only those indications included in FDA-approved drug-product labeling and have frequently denied coverage for unlabeled uses of drug products.

ASHP believes that such coverage denials restrict patients from receiving medically necessary therapies that represent the best available treatment options. A growing number of insurance carriers are following the BC/BS and HIAA guidelines that encourage the use of the three authoritative drug compendia, peer-reviewed literature, and consultation with experts in research and clinical practice to make specific coverage decisions. ASHP supports informed decisionmaking that promotes third-party reimbursement for FDA-approved drug products appropriately prescribed for unlabeled uses.

References

1. Use of approved drugs for unlabeled indications. *FDA Drug Bull.* 1982, 12.4–5.
2. Nightingale SL. Use of drugs for unlabeled indications. *FDA Q Rep.* 1986(Sep); 269.
3. Mortenson LE. Audit indicates many uses of combination therapy are unlabeled. *J Cancer Program Manage.* 1988; 3:21–5.
4. Off-label drugs: initial results of a national survey. Washington, DC: U.S. General Accounting Office. 1991:1–27.
5. PL 100-360, 1988.
6. Health Care Financing Administration. Medicare carriers' manual. Section 2050.5. Washington, DC: U.S. Department of Health and Human Services; 1987 Aug.
7. Statement on coverage recommendation for FDA-approved drugs. Chicago: Blue Cross and Blue Shield Association; 1989 Oct 25.
8. Statement of the Health Insurance Association of America (HIAA) on coverage for unapproved drugs and drug-related costs. Presented to the National Committee to Review Current Procedures for Approval of New Drugs for Cancer and AIDS. 1989 Oct 25.
9. Cancer economics. *Cancer Lett.* 1989; Suppl(Jun):2–3.

Approved by the ASHP Board of Directors, November 20, 1991, and by the ASHP House of Delegates, June 1, 1992. Developed by the Council on Professional Affairs.

The bibliographic citation for this document is as follows: American Society of Hospital Pharmacists. ASHP statement on the use of medications for unlabeled uses. *Am J Hosp Pharm.* 1992; 49:2006–8.

ASHP Statement on Pharmaceutical Care

The purpose of this statement is to assist pharmacists in understanding pharmaceutical care. Such understanding must precede efforts to implement pharmaceutical care, which ASHP believes merit the highest priority in all practice settings.

Possibly the earliest published use of the term pharmaceutical care was by Brodie in the context of thoughts about drug use control and medication-related services.[1,2] It is a term that has been widely used and a concept about which much has been written and discussed in the pharmacy profession, especially since the publication of a paper by Hepler and Strand in 1990.[3-5] ASHP has formally endorsed the concept.[6] With varying terminology and nuances, the concept has also been acknowledged by other national pharmacy organizations.[7,8] Implementation of pharmaceutical care was the focus of a major ASHP conference in March 1993.

Many pharmacists have expressed enthusiasm for the concept of pharmaceutical care, but there has been substantial inconsistency in its description. Some have characterized it as merely a new name for clinical pharmacy; others have described it as anything that pharmacists do that may lead to beneficial results for patients.

ASHP believes that pharmaceutical care is an important new concept that represents growth in the profession beyond clinical pharmacy as often practiced and beyond other activities of pharmacists, including medication preparation and dispensing. All of these professional activities are important, however, and ASHP continues to be a strong proponent of the necessity for pharmacists' involvement in them. In practice, these activities should be integrated with and culminate in pharmaceutical care provided by individual pharmacists to individual patients.

In 1992, ASHP's members urged the development of an officially recognized ASHP definition of pharmaceutical care.[9] This statement provides a definition and elucidates some of the elements and implications of that definition. The definition that follows is an adaptation of a definition developed by Hepler and Strand.[3]

Definition

The mission of the pharmacist is to provide pharmaceutical care. Pharmaceutical care is the direct, responsible provision of medication-related care for the purpose of achieving definite outcomes that improve a patient's quality of life.

Principal Elements

The principal elements of pharmaceutical care are that it is *medication related*; it is *care* that is *directly provided* to the patient; it is provided to produce *definite outcomes*; these outcomes are intended to improve the patient's *quality of life*; and the provider accepts personal *responsibility* for the outcomes.

Medication Related. Pharmaceutical care involves not only medication therapy (the actual provision of medication) but also decisions about medication use for individual patients. As appropriate, this includes decisions *not* to use medication therapy as well as judgments about medication selection, dosages, routes and methods of administration, medi-

cation therapy monitoring, and the provision of medication-related information and counseling to individual patients.

Care. Central to the concept of care is caring, a personal concern for the well-being of another person. Overall patient care consists of integrated domains of care including (among others) medical care, nursing care, and pharmaceutical care. Health professionals in each of these disciplines possess unique expertise and must cooperate in the patient's overall care. At times, they share in the execution of the various types of care (including pharmaceutical care). To pharmaceutical care, however, the pharmacist contributes unique knowledge and skills to ensure optimal outcomes from the use of medications.

At the heart of any type of patient care, there exists a one-to-one relationship between a caregiver and a patient. In pharmaceutical care, the irreducible "unit" of care is one pharmacist in a direct professional relationship with one patient. In this relationship, the pharmacist provides care directly to the patient and for the benefit of the patient.

The health and well-being of the patient are paramount. The pharmacist makes a direct, personal, caring commitment to the individual patient and acts in the patient's best interest. The pharmacist cooperates directly with other professionals and the patient in designing, implementing, and monitoring a therapeutic plan intended to produce definite therapeutic outcomes that improve the patient's quality of life.

Outcomes. It is the goal of pharmaceutical care to improve an individual patient's quality of life through achievement of definite (predefined), medication-related therapeutic outcomes. The outcomes sought are

1. Cure of a patient's disease.
2. Elimination or reduction of a patient's symptomatology.
3. Arresting or slowing of a disease process.
4. Prevention of a disease or symptomatology.

This, in turn, involves three major functions: (1) identifying potential and actual medication-related problems, (2) resolving actual medication-related problems, and (3) preventing potential medication-related problems. A medication-related problem is an event or circumstance involving medication therapy that actually or potentially interferes with an optimum outcome for a specific patient. There are at least the following categories of medication-related problems:[3]

- *Untreated indications.* The patient has a medical problem that requires medication therapy (an indication for medication use) but is not receiving a medication for that indication.
- *Improper drug selection.* The patient has a medication indication but is taking the wrong medication.
- *Subtherapeutic dosage.* The patient has a medical problem that is being treated with too little of the correct medication.
- *Failure to receive medication.* The patient has a medical problem that is the result of not receiving a medication (e.g., for pharmaceutical, psychological, sociological, or economic reasons).
- *Overdosage.* The patient has a medical problem that is

being treated with too much of the correct medication (toxicity).

- *Adverse drug reactions.* The patient has a medical problem that is the result of an adverse drug reaction or adverse effect.
- *Drug interactions.* The patient has a medical problem that is the result of a drug–drug, drug–food, or drug–laboratory test interaction.
- *Medication use without indication.* The patient is taking a medication for no medically valid indication.

Patients may possess characteristics that interfere with the achievement of desired therapeutic outcomes. Patients may be noncompliant with prescribed medication use regimens, or there may be unpredictable variations in patients' biological responses. Thus, in an imperfect world, intended outcomes from medication-related therapy are not always achievable.

Patients bear a responsibility to help achieve the desired outcomes by engaging in behaviors that will contribute to—and not interfere with—the achievement of desired outcomes. Pharmacists and other health professionals have an obligation to educate patients about behaviors that will contribute to achieving desired outcomes.

Quality of Life. Some tools exist now for assessing a patient's quality of life. These tools are still evolving, and pharmacists should maintain familiarity with the literature on this subject.[10,11] A complete assessment of a patient's quality of life should include both objective and subjective (e.g., the patient's own) assessments. Patients should be involved, in an informed way, in establishing quality-of-life goals for their therapies.

Responsibility. The fundamental relationship in any type of patient care is a mutually beneficial exchange in which the patient grants authority to the provider and the provider gives competence and commitment to the patient (accepts responsibility).[3] Responsibility involves both moral trustworthiness and accountability.

In pharmaceutical care, the direct relationship between an individual pharmacist and an individual patient is that of a professional covenant in which the patient's safety and well-being are entrusted to the pharmacist, who commits to honoring that trust through competent professional actions that are in the patient's best interest. As an accountable member of the health-care team, the pharmacist must document the care provided.[4,7,12,13] The pharmacist is personally accountable for patient outcomes (the quality of care) that ensue from the pharmacist's actions and decisions.[1]

Implications

The idea that pharmacists should commit themselves to the achievement of definite outcomes for individual patients is an especially important element in the concept of pharmaceutical care. The expectation that pharmacists personally accept responsibility for individual patients' outcomes that result from the pharmacists' actions represents a significant advance in pharmacy's continuing professionalization. The provision of pharmaceutical care represents a maturation of pharmacy as a clinical profession and is a natural evolution of more mature clinical pharmacy activities of pharmacists.[14]

ASHP believes that pharmaceutical care is fundamental to the profession's purpose of helping people make the best

use of medications.[15] It is a unifying concept that transcends all types of patients and all categories of pharmacists and pharmacy organizations. Pharmaceutical care is applicable and achievable by pharmacists in all practice settings. The provision of pharmaceutical care is not limited to pharmacists in inpatient, outpatient, or community settings, nor to pharmacists with certain degrees, specialty certifications, residencies, or other credentials. It is not limited to those in academic or teaching settings. Pharmaceutical care is not a matter of formal credentials or place of work. Rather, it is a matter of a direct personal, professional, responsible relationship with a patient to ensure that the patient's use of medication is optimal and leads to improvements in the patient's quality of life.

Pharmacists should commit themselves to continuous care on behalf of individual patients. They bear responsibility for ensuring that the patient's care is ongoing despite work-shift changes, weekends, and holidays. An important implication is that a pharmacist providing pharmaceutical care may need to work as a member of a team of pharmacists who provide backup care when the primary responsible pharmacist is not available. Another is that the responsible pharmacist should work to ensure that continuity of care is maintained when a patient moves from one component of a health-care system to another (e.g., when a patient is hospitalized or discharged from a hospital to return to an ambulatory, community status). In the provision of pharmaceutical care, professional communication about the patient's needs between responsible pharmacists in each area of practice is, therefore, essential. ASHP believes that the development of recognized methods of practicing pharmaceutical care that will enhance such communication is an important priority for the profession.

Pharmaceutical care can be conceived as both a purpose for pharmacy practice and a purpose of medication use processes. That is, a fundamental professional reason that pharmacists engage in pharmacy practice should be to deliver pharmaceutical care. Furthermore, the medication use systems that pharmacists (and others) operate should be designed to support and enable the delivery of pharmaceutical care by individual pharmacists. ASHP believes that, in organized health-care settings, pharmaceutical care can be most successfully provided when it is part of the pharmacy department's central mission and when management activity is focused on facilitating the provision of pharmaceutical care by individual pharmacists. This approach, in which empowered frontline staff provide direct care to individual patients and are supported by managers, other pharmacists, and support systems, is new for many pharmacists and managers.

An important corollary to this approach is that pharmacists providing pharmaceutical care in organized health-care settings cannot provide such care alone. They must work in an interdependent fashion with colleagues in pharmacy and other disciplines, support systems and staff, and managers.[7] It is incumbent on pharmacists to design work systems and practices that appropriately focus the efforts of all activities and support systems on meeting the needs of patients. Some patients will require different levels of care, and it may be useful to structure work systems in light of those differences.[16,17] ASHP believes that the provision of pharmaceutical care and the development of effective work systems to document and support it are major priorities for the profession.

In the provision of pharmaceutical care, pharmacists use their unique perspective and knowledge of medication therapy to evaluate patients' actual and potential medication-related problems. To do this, they require direct access to clinical information about individual patients. They make judgments regarding medication use and then advocate optimal medication use for individual patients in cooperation with other professionals and in consideration of their unique professional knowledge and evaluations. Pharmaceutical care includes the active participation of the patient (and designated caregivers such as family members) in matters pertinent to medication use.

The acknowledgment of pharmacists' responsibility for therapeutic outcomes resulting from their actions does not contend that pharmacists have exclusive authority for matters related to medication use. Other health-care professionals, including physicians and nurses, have valuable and well-established, well-recognized roles in the medication use process. The pharmaceutical care concept does not diminish the roles or responsibilities of other health professionals, nor does it imply any usurping of authority by pharmacists. Pharmacists' actions in pharmaceutical care should be conducted and viewed as collaborative. The knowledge, skills, and traditions of pharmacists, however, make them legitimate leaders of efforts by health-care teams to improve patients' medication use.

Pharmaceutical care requires a direct relationship between a pharmacist and an individual patient. Some pharmacists and other pharmacy personnel engage in clinical and product-related pharmacy activities that do not involve a direct relationship with the patient. Properly designed, these activities can be supportive of pharmaceutical care, but ASHP believes it would be confusing and counterproductive to characterize such activities as pharmaceutical care. ASHP believes that clinical and product-related pharmacy activities are essential, however, and are as important as the actions of pharmacists interacting directly with patients.

Pharmaceutical educators must teach pharmaceutical care to students.[18] Providers of continuing education should help practicing pharmacists and other pharmacy personnel to understand pharmaceutical care. Students and pharmacists should be taught to conceptualize and execute responsible medication-related problem-solving on behalf of individual patients. Curricula should be designed to produce graduates with sufficient knowledge and skills to provide pharmaceutical care competently.[8,18] Initiatives are under way to bring about these changes.[8] Practicing pharmacists must commit their time as preceptors and their workplaces as teaching laboratories for the undergraduate and postgraduate education and training necessary to produce pharmacists who can provide pharmaceutical care.[8]

Research is needed to evaluate various methods and systems for the delivery of pharmaceutical care.

Pharmaceutical care represents an exciting new vision for pharmacy. ASHP hopes that all pharmacists in all practice settings share in this vision and that the pharmaceutical care concept will serve as a stimulus for them to work toward transforming the profession to actualize that vision.

References

1. Brodie DC. Is pharmaceutical education prepared to lead its profession? The Ninth Annual Rho Chi Lecture. *Rep Rho Chi.* 1973; 39:6–12.

2. Brodie DC, Parish PA, Poston JW. Societal needs for drugs and drug-related services. *Am J Pharm Educ.* 1980; 44:276–8.

3. Hepler CD, Strand LM. Opportunities and responsibilities in pharmaceutical care. *Am J Hosp Pharm.* 1990; 47:533–43.

4. Penna RP. Pharmaceutical care: pharmacy's mission for the 1990s. *Am J Hosp Pharm.* 1990; 47:543–9.

5. Pierpaoli PG, Hethcox JM. Pharmaceutical care: new management and leadership imperatives. *Top Hosp Pharm Manage.* 1992; 12:1–18.

6. Oddis JA. Report of the House of Delegates: June 3 and 5, 1991. *Am J Hosp Pharm.* 1991; 48:1739–48.

7. American Pharmaceutical Association. An APhA white paper on the role of the pharmacist in comprehensive medication use management; the delivery of pharmaceutical care. Washington, DC: American Pharmaceutical Association; 1992 Mar.

8. Commission to Implement Change in Pharmaceutical Education. A position paper. Entry-level education in pharmacy: a commitment to change. *AACP News.* 1991; Nov (Suppl):14

9. Oddis JA. Report of the House of Delegates: June 1 and 3, 1992. *Am J Hosp Pharm.* 1992; 49:1962–73.

10. Gouveia WA. Measuring and managing patient outcomes. *Am J Hosp Pharm.* 1992; 49:2157–8.

11. MacKeigan LD, Pathak DS. Overview of health-related quality-of-life measures. *Am J Hosp Pharm.* 1992; 49:2236–45.

12. Galinsky RE, Nickman NA. Pharmacists and the mandate of pharmaceutical care. *DICP Ann Pharmacother.* 1991; 21:431–4.

13. Angaran DM. Quality assurance to quality improvement: measuring and monitoring pharmaceutical care. *Am J Hosp Pharm.* 1991; 48:1901–7.

14. Hepler CD. Pharmaceutical care and specialty practice. *Pharmacotherapy.* 1993; 13:64S–9S.

15. Zellmer WA. Expressing the mission of pharmacy practice. *Am J Hosp Pharm.* 1991; 48:1195. Editorial.

16. Smith WE, Benderev K. Levels of pharmaceutical care: a theoretical model. *Am J Hosp Pharm.* 1991; 48:540–6.

17. Strand LM, Cipole RJ, Morley PC, et al. Levels of pharmaceutical care: a needs-based approach. *Am J Hosp Pharm.* 1991; 48:547–50.

18. O'Neil EH. Health professions education for the future: schools in service to the nation. San Francisco, CA: Pew Health Profession Commission; 1993.

Approved by the ASHP Board of Directors, April 21, 1993, and by the ASHP House of Delegates, June 9, 1993. Developed by the ASHP Council on Professional Affairs.

The bibliographic citation for this document is as follows: American Society of Hospital Pharmacists. ASHP statement on pharmaceutical care. *Am J Hosp Pharm.* 1993; 50:1720–3.

ASHP Statement on Principles for Including Medications and Pharmaceutical Care in Health Care Systems

Introduction

The United States government, individual state governments, and private health care systems are moving toward reforming the way that they provide health care to their citizens or beneficiaries. As they do so, policy makers must improve their medication-use systems to address problems of access, quality, and cost of medicines and pharmaceutical care services. This document offers principles for achieving maximum value from the services of the nation's pharmacists.

Although pharmaceuticals and pharmaceutical care are among the most cost-effective methods of health care available, there is evidence that the public is not currently realizing the full potential benefit from these resources. Illnesses related to improper medication use are costing the health care systems in the United States billions of dollars per year in patient morbidity and mortality. Pharmacists are prepared and eager to help other health providers and patients prevent and resolve medication-related problems, and health care systems should facilitate and take advantage of pharmacists' expertise.

These principles are offered to guide health policy makers in their deliberations concerning the inclusion of medications and pharmacists' services in health care systems.

Principles

Principle I. Health care systems must make medications available to patients and provide for pharmaceutical care, which encompasses pharmacists' health care services and health promotional activities that ensure that medications are used safely, effectively, and efficiently for optimal patient outcomes.

Principle II. Careful distinction must be made between policies that affect pharmacist reimbursement and policies that affect pharmacist compensation. Health care systems must reimburse pharmacists for the medications they provide patients (including the costs of drug products, the costs associated with dispensing, and related administrative costs). Health care systems also must compensate pharmacists for the services and care that they provide to patients, which result in improved medication use and which may not necessarily be associated with dispensing.

Principle III. Patients differ in their needs for pharmaceutical care services. The method of compensating pharmacists for their services must recognize the value of the different levels and types of services that pharmacists provide to patients based on pharmacists' professional assessments of patients' needs.

Principle IV. Pharmacists must be enabled and encouraged to use their professional expertise in making medication-related judgments in collaboration with patients and health care colleagues. Health care systems must not erect barriers to pharmacists' exercising professional judgments; nor should health care systems prescribe specific services or therapies for defined types of patients.

Principle V. Pharmacists should have access to relevant patient information to support their professional judgments and activities. Pharmacists should be encouraged and permitted to make additions to medical records for the purpose of adding their findings, conclusions, and recommendations. Pharmacists will respect the confidential nature of all patient information.

Principle VI. Health care systems must be designed to enable, foster, and facilitate communication and collaboration among pharmacists and other care providers to ensure proper coordination of patients' medication therapies.

Principle VII. Quality assessment and assurance programs related to individual patient care should be implemented at local levels through collaborative efforts of health care practitioners rather than through centralized bureaucracies. Quality assessment and assurance procedures for medication use (such as pharmacy and therapeutics committees, formulary systems, drug-use evaluation programs, and patient outcomes analyses) are most effective when the professionals who care for covered patients are involved in the design and implementation of the procedures. Moreover, such programs must recognize local variations in epidemiology, demography, and practice standards. Information related to quality assessment and assurance activities must be held in confidence by all parties.

Principle VIII. Demonstration projects and evaluation studies in the delivery of pharmaceutical care must be enabled, fostered, and implemented. New services, quality assessment and assurance techniques, and innovative medication delivery systems are needed to improve the access to and quality of medication therapy and pharmaceutical care while containing costs.

Principle IX. Health care policies that are intended to influence practices of those associated with pharmacy, such as the pharmaceutical industry or prescribers, should address those audiences directly rather than through policies that affect reimbursement, compensation, or other activities of pharmacists.

Approved by the ASHP Board of Directors, November 18, 1992, and by the ASHP House of Delegates, June 7, 1993. Developed by a committee of the Joint Commission of Pharmacy Practitioners and subsequently reviewed and approved by the ASHP Council on Legal and Public Affairs.

The bibliographic citation for this document is as follows: American Society of Hospital Pharmacists. ASHP statement on principles for including medications and pharmaceutical care in health care systems. *Am J Hosp Pharm.* 1993; 50:756–7.

ASHP Statement on the Role of the Pharmacist in Patient-Focused Care

Patient-focused care is a term applied to a range of site-specific multidisciplinary work designs ideally intended to improve patient care outcomes and patient satisfaction while also improving efficiency and reducing costs. Patient-focused care has primarily been implemented in hospitals, although it could be applied in integrated health care systems and other settings as well. The term arose because of the perception that hospital functions have traditionally been "department-focused" in order to optimize the scheduling and efficiency of compartmentalized service units. This department focus often results in complex logistical processes, communication problems, delays in patient care, idle time for some employees, and numerous hospital employees interacting with the patient. Patient-focused care typically reorients functions, task assignments, and schedules to the needs of the patient through the use of various techniques, including (1) work redesign to eliminate unnecessary steps and documentation; (2) organizational restructuring, including significant decentralization of high-volume patient care services; (3) interdisciplinary patient care work teams; (4) cross-utilization of staff to carry out work previously done by specialists and to minimize the number of different staff members having unnecessary contact with a single patient; and (5) case management using multidisciplinary clinical care plans.[1] These management tools (interdisciplinary patient care work teams and case management in particular) may also be implemented in specific work sites independent of any reference to patient-focused care. Some of these tools might also be used to facilitate positive change within a pharmacy independent of any organizationwide initiative.

Patient-focused care evolved primarily from a consulting firm study, which concluded that a significant percentage of dollars was spent by hospitals to cover the logistics associated with scheduling direct patient care, documenting that the care was given, and paying for "structural idle time," such as time spent by specialized department-based staff waiting for orders or requests for service.[2]

ASHP supports the concept of patient-focused care when it (1) is planned and implemented with pharmacists' involvement; (2) fosters the provision of pharmaceutical care[3]; and (3) is motivated by a goal of improved patient care. Some patient-focused care arrangements, however, do not meet these criteria and have been perceived as detriments to the provision of pharmaceutical care.

The effect of patient-focused care on pharmacy practice can vary substantially by site. From a broad perspective, the idealistic goals and approaches to patient-focused care can be quite compatible with pharmaceutical care and, in fact, may facilitate its implementation. The elimination of some time-consuming documentation, scheduling, and idle time and the decentralization of services to the patient care unit may help to overcome major obstacles to pharmaceutical care, including access to patients, access to patient-specific clinical information, and access to other health care professionals.

Conversely, patient-focused care can be implemented with a less favorable effect on the pharmacy. Cost control and staff reduction are sometimes the primary intended outcomes of patient-focused care initiatives. In the negative extreme, organizations may be forced to undergo radical staff reduction, reorganization, and cross-training of staff to the point of misapplication of valuable professional talent and curtailment of important professional services.

A central message of this ASHP Statement is that pharmacists should become involved early and assertively in all aspects of patient-focused care when it is initiated or contemplated for their work sites. In general, pharmacists who have established some success in the provision of pharmaceutical care before patient-focused care is begun seem more likely to be positioned well for full involvement and invitation into the planning of such projects. ASHP recommends that pharmacists review published literature on patient-focused care and that they consult with other pharmacists who have successfully adapted to patient-focused care and used it in furthering pharmaceutical care.

Some general ideas regarding pharmacists' participation in patient-focused care follow.

1. Patient-focused care should be designed and implemented in ways that enhance or expand the capacity of pharmacy staff members to provide pharmaceutical care.[1]

2. Patient-focused care should be designed and implemented in ways that foster the pharmacist's adherence to established standards of professional practice, prevention of drug misadventures, and fulfillment of legal responsibilities.[1]

3. Pharmacy staff members assigned to patient care teams must be philosophically committed to the concept of interdisciplinary patient care and be prepared to contribute to the work of the teams.[1]

4. Pharmacists should be involved in the development of clinical care plans that involve medication use.[1]

5. The prevention, detection, and resolution of drug-related problems should be a high-priority function of patient-care-team pharmacists.[1]

6. Pharmacy staff members assigned to a specific patient care team should be consistently available for that team so that the number of different staff members working on a specific team is minimized.[1]

7. Pharmacy managers should anticipate efforts to simplify the drug distribution process for most medication orders.[1] Pharmacists should be open to experimentation with medication-use system changes. However, they have a professional obligation to consider the patient-safety implications of prospective changes.

8. In planning for patient-focused care, the role of pharmacy technicians in patient-focused care teams should be addressed. Different roles may be appropriate with respect to cross-training and cross-utilization of technicians with advanced credentials (e.g., certification or graduation from an accredited training program).

9. In patient-focused-care decision-making, special diligence should be exerted to consider the systemwide implications (especially patient safety implications) of decisions about products and procedures.

10. Pharmacy staff members, including pharmacy techni-

cians, working on patient care teams may be asked to assume cross-functional roles.[1] Requisite preparation and documented credentials should be obtained by staff members who are not trained, educated, or experienced in performing a particular task. Clear documentation of the roles and duties should exist in position descriptions and organizational policies and procedures.

11. If nonpharmacy personnel are used to perform tasks traditionally carried out by pharmacy personnel, this must be accomplished without compromising patient safety or violating laws or regulations. Appropriate oversight by pharmacists must be provided.

12. In some patient-focused care arrangements, the use of automated dispensing devices may be viewed as a justification for staff reduction and cost control. These devices have the potential for misuse if the system does not provide for an adequate review of the medication order by a pharmacist before the medication is administered to the patient.

13. In patient-focused care, charting by exception is sometimes proposed as a work simplification measure. This is an approach to patients' medical records in which it is assumed that all ordered medications have been administered and that they have been administered according to medication orders *unless* a record to the contrary is made. The safety of such an arrangement is questionable. Substantial safeguards would have to be in place for it to be acceptable. Unless such safeguards can be devised, overt charting of all doses of medications administered is seen as a safer procedure.

14. Organizational re-engineering associated with patient-focused care can be applied to different levels in an organization. It may be applied, for example, primarily at the patient care level and result in the formation of multidisciplinary care teams of professionals and others in direct contact with patients. In some cases, it has been applied organizationwide. In some extraordinary cases, entire departments, departmental structures, and departmental directorships have been abolished. When pharmacists have input into such decisions, they are encouraged to consider carefully which pharmacy functions may be better (including more safely) accomplished centrally or on a decentralized basis.

15. Consultants experienced in implementing patient-focused care may present data and experiences from one contract site as an indication of what can be achieved in a subsequent contract site. This may be useful information, but pharmacists are encouraged to carefully analyze the accuracy and applicability of the information in their own sites.

Pharmacists should make every effort to educate consultants on the pharmaceutical care role of the pharmacist in health systems.

Recommendations for Additional Reading

Bellaire DR. Work restructuring overview and implications for pharmacists. *Top Hosp Pharm Manage.* 1994; 14(Apr):7–16.

DeCostro RA. Another new day: the life of a patient-focused care pharmacist. *Am J Health-Syst Pharm.* 1995; 52: 51–4.

Lathrop JP. Restructuring health care: the patient-focused paradigm. San Francisco: Jossey-Bass; 1993.

Lathrop JP. Patient-focused care from the consultant's viewpoint: we didn't plan it this way. *Am J Health-Syst Pharm.* 1995; 52:45–8.

Lindstrom CC, Borggren LR. Pharmaceutical services in restructured patient care: a view from the trenches. *Am J Health-Syst Pharm.* 1995; 52:49–51.

Mansur JM, Chamerlik SJ. New roles for pharmacy managers in patient-centered care. *Am J Health-Syst Pharm.* 1995; 52:54–8.

Mansur JM, Chamerlik SJ, Bohenek W et al. Involvement of a pharmacy department in a hospital's transition to patient-centered care. *Top Hosp Pharm Manage.* 1994; 14(Apr):36–45.

Shane R, Kwong MM. Providing patient-focused care while maintaining the pharmacy department's structure. *Am J Health-Syst Pharm.* 1995; 52:58–60.

Vogel DP. Patient-focused care. *Am J Hosp Pharm.* 1993; 50:2321–9.

References

1. Vogel DP. Patient-focused care. *Am J Hosp Pharm.* 1993; 50: 2321–9.

2. Lathrop JP. The patient-focused hospital. *Healthc Forum J.* 1991; 34(Jul–Aug):17–21.

3. American Society of Hospital Pharmacists. ASHP statement on pharmaceutical care. *Am J Hosp Pharm.* 1993; 50:1720–3.

Approved by the ASHP Board of Directors, April 26, 1995, and by the ASHP House of Delegates, June 5, 1995. Developed by the Council on Professional Affairs.

The bibliographic citation for this document is as follows: American Society of Health-System Pharmacists. ASHP statement on the role of the pharmacist in patient-focused care. *Am J Health-Syst Pharm.* 1995; 52:1808–10.

ASHP
Guidelines

ASHP Guidelines for Selecting Pharmaceutical Manufacturers and Suppliers

Pharmacists are responsible for selecting, from hundreds of manufacturers and suppliers of drugs, those that will enable them to fulfill an important obligation: ensuring that patients receive pharmaceuticals and related supplies of the highest quality and at the lowest cost. These guidelines are offered as an aid to the pharmacist in achieving this goal.

Obligations of the Supplier

Pharmacists may purchase with confidence the products of those suppliers meeting the criteria presented here. Other factors such as credit policies, delivery times, and the breadth of a supplier's product line also must be considered when selecting a supplier.

Technical Considerations

1. On request of the pharmacist (an instrument such as the ASHP Drug Product Information Request Form[a] is useful in this regard), the supplier should furnish
   a. Analytical control data.
   b. Sterility testing data.
   c. Bioavailability data.
   d. Bioequivalency data.
   e. Descriptions of testing procedures for raw materials and finished products.
   f. Any other information that may be indicative of the quality of a given finished drug product.
   Testing data developed by independent laboratories should be identified by the supplier. All information should be supplied at no charge.
2. There should be no history of recurring product recalls indicative of deficient quality control procedures.
3. The supplier should permit visits (during normal business hours) by the pharmacist to inspect its manufacturing and control procedures.
4. All drug products should conform to the requirements of *The United States Pharmacopeia–The National Formulary (USP–NF)* (the most recent edition) unless otherwise specified by the pharmacist. Items not recognized by *USP–NF* should meet the specifications set forth by the pharmacist.
5. To the extent possible, all products should be available in single unit or unit dose packages. These packages should conform to the "ASHP Technical Assistance Bulletin on Single Unit and Unit Dose Packages of Drugs."[1]
6. The name and address of the manufacturer of the final dosage form and the packager or distributor should be present on the product labeling.
7. Expiration dates should be clearly indicated on the package label and, unless stability properties warrant otherwise, should occur in January or July.
8. Therapeutic, biopharmaceutic, and toxicologic information should be available to the pharmacist on request. Toxicity information should be available around the clock.
9. Patient/staff educational materials that are important for proper use of the product should be routinely available.
10. On request, the supplier should furnish proof of any claims made with respect to the efficacy, safety, and superiority of its products.
11. On request, the supplier should furnish, at no charge, a reasonable quantity of its products to enable the pharmacist to evaluate the products' physical traits, including pharmaceutical elegance (appearance and absence of physical deterioration or flaws), packaging, and labeling.

Distribution Policies

1. Whenever possible, delivery of a drug product should be confined to a single lot number.
2. Unless otherwise specified or required by stability considerations, not less than a 12-month interval between a product's time of delivery and its expiration date should be present.
3. The supplier should accept for full credit (based on purchase price), without prior authorization, any unopened packages of goods returned within 12 months of the expiration date. Credits should be in cash or applied to the institution's account.
4. The supplier should ship all goods in a timely manner, freight prepaid, and enclose a packing list with each shipment. All items "out of stock" should be noted, and the anticipated availability of the item should be clearly indicated. There should be no extensive recurrence of back orders.
5. The supplier should warrant title to commodities supplied, warrant them to be free from defects and imperfections and fit for any rational use of the product, and indemnify and hold the purchaser harmless against any and all suits, claims, and expenses, including attorneys' fees, damages, and injuries or any claims by third parties relating to the products.

Marketing and Sales Policies

1. The supplier should not, without written consent, use the pharmacist's or his or her organization's name in any advertising or other promotional materials or activities.
2. The supplier should honor formulary decisions made by the organization's pharmacy and therapeutics committee, and the supplier's sales representatives should comply with the organization's regulations governing their activities.
3. The supplier should not offer cash, equipment, or merchandise to the organization or its staff as an inducement to purchase its products.
4. Discounts should be in cash or cash credit, not merchandise, and should be clearly indicated on invoices and bills rather than consisting of end-of-year rebates or similar discount practices.
5. In entering into a contract to supply goods, the supplier should guarantee to furnish, at the price specified, any minimum amount of products so stated. If the supplier is unable to meet the supply commitment, the supplier

should reimburse the organization for any excess costs incurred in obtaining the product from other sources. If, during the life of the contract, a price reduction occurs, the lower price should prevail.

6. All parties to the bidding process should respect the integrity of the process and the contracts awarded thereby.

Responsibilities of the Purchaser

It may be desirable to purchase drugs or other commodities on a competitive bid basis. The pharmacist should ensure that competitive bidding procedures conform to the guidelines below:

1. Invitations to bid should be mailed to the suppliers' home offices with copies to their local representatives (if any), unless suppliers specify otherwise.
2. Potential bidders should be given no less than 3 weeks to submit a bid.
3. The opening date for bids should be specified and honored by the purchaser.
4. The language of the invitation to bid should be clear and should indicate the person (and organization address and telephone number) the bidder should contact in the event of questions or problems. Specifications should be complete with respect to products, packagings, and quantities desired.
5. If bidding forms are used, they should contain adequate space for the bidder to enter the information requested.
6. The winning bidder should be notified in writing. Unsuccessful bidders may be informed of who won the award at what price, if they so request.
7. The quantities specified in the invitation to bid should be a reasonable estimate of requirements.
8. If the invitation to bid is offered on behalf of a group of purchasers, the individual members of the group should not engage in bidding procedures of their own and should purchase the goods in question from the winning bidder.

Reference

1. American Society of Hospital Pharmacists. ASHP technical assistance bulletin on single unit and unit dose packages of drugs. *Am J Hosp Pharm.* 1985; 42:378–9.

ᵃAvailable from ASHP, 7272 Wisconsin Avenue, Bethesda, MD 20814.

Approved by the ASHP Board of Directors, November 14, 1990. Revised by the ASHP Council on Professional Affairs. Supersedes previous versions approved November 17–18, 1983, and September 22, 1989.

The bibliographic citation for this document is as follows: American Society of Hospital Pharmacists. ASHP guidelines for selecting pharmaceutical manufacturers and suppliers. *Am J Hosp Pharm.* 1991; 48:523–4.

ASHP Guidelines on Pharmacist-Conducted Patient Education and Counseling

Purpose

Providing pharmaceutical care entails accepting responsibility for patients' pharmacotherapeutic outcomes. Pharmacists can contribute to positive outcomes by educating and counseling patients to prepare and motivate them to follow their pharmacotherapeutic regimens and monitoring plans. The purpose of this document is to help pharmacists provide effective patient education and counseling.

In working with individual patients, patient groups, families, and caregivers, pharmacists should approach education and counseling as interrelated activities. ASHP believes pharmacists should educate and counsel all patients to the extent possible, going beyond the minimum requirements of laws and regulations; simply offering to counsel is inconsistent with pharmacists' responsibilities. In pharmaceutical care, pharmacists should encourage patients to seek education and counseling and should eliminate barriers to providing it.

Pharmacists should also seek opportunities to participate in health-system patient-education programs and to support the educational efforts of other health care team members. Pharmacists should collaborate with other health care team members, as appropriate, to determine what specific information and counseling are required in each patient care situation. A coordinated effort among health care team members will enhance patients' adherence to pharmacotherapeutic regimens, monitoring of drug effects, and feedback to the health system.

ASHP believes these patient education and counseling guidelines are applicable in all practice settings—including acute inpatient care, ambulatory care, home care, and long-term care—whether these settings are associated with integrated health systems or managed care organizations or are freestanding. The guidelines may need to be adapted; for example, for use in telephone counseling or for counseling family members or caregivers instead of patients. Patient education and counseling usually occur at the time prescriptions are dispensed but may also be provided as a separate service. The techniques and the content should be adjusted to meet the specific needs of the patient and to comply with the policies and procedures of the practice setting. In health systems, other health care team members share in the responsibility to educate and counsel patients as specified in the patients' care plans.

Background

The human and economic consequences of inappropriate medication use have been the subject of professional, public, and congressional discourse for more than two decades.[1-5] Lack of sufficient knowledge about their health problems and medications is one cause of patients' nonadherence to their pharmacotherapeutic regimens and monitoring plans; without adequate knowledge, patients cannot be effective partners in managing their own care. The pharmacy profession has accepted responsibility for providing patient education and counseling in the context of pharmaceutical care to improve patient adherence and reduce medication-related problems.[6-9]

Concerns about improper medication use contributed to the provision in the Omnibus Budget Reconciliation Act of 1990 (OBRA '90) that mandated an offer to counsel Medicaid outpatients about prescription medications. Subsequently, states enacted legislation that generally extends the offer-to-counsel requirement to outpatients not covered by Medicaid. Future court cases may establish that pharmacists, in part because of changing laws, have a public duty to warn patients of adverse effects and potential interactions of medications. The result could be increased liability for pharmacists who fail to educate and counsel their patients or who do so incorrectly or incompletely.[10]

Pharmacists' Knowledge and Skills

In addition to a current knowledge of pharmacotherapy, pharmacists need to have the knowledge and skills to provide effective and accurate patient education and counseling. They should know about their patients' cultures, especially health and illness beliefs, attitudes, and practices. They should be aware of patients' feelings toward the health system and views of their own roles and responsibilities for decision-making and for managing their care.[11]

Effective, open-ended questioning and active listening are essential skills for obtaining information from and sharing information with patients. Pharmacists have to adapt messages to fit patients' language skills and primary languages, through the use of teaching aids, interpreters, or cultural guides if necessary. Pharmacists also need to observe and interpret the nonverbal messages (e.g., eye contact, facial expressions, body movements, vocal characteristics) patients give during education and counseling sessions.[12]

Assessing a patient's cognitive abilities, learning style, and sensory and physical status enables the pharmacist to adapt information and educational methods to meet the patient's needs. A patient may learn best by hearing spoken instructions; by seeing a diagram, picture, or model; or by directly handling medications and administration devices. A patient may lack the visual acuity to read labels on prescription containers, markings on syringes, or written handout material. A patient may be unable to hear oral instructions or may lack sufficient motor skills to open a child-resistant container.

In addition to assessing whether patients know *how* to use their medications, pharmacists should attempt to understand patients' attitudes and potential behaviors concerning medication use. The pharmacist needs to determine whether a patient is willing to use a medication and whether he or she intends to do so.[13,14]

Environment

Education and counseling should take place in an environment conducive to patient involvement, learning, and acceptance—one that supports pharmacists' efforts to establish caring relationships with patients. Individual patients, groups, families, or caregivers should perceive the counseling environment as comfortable, confidential, and safe.

Education and counseling are most effective when conducted in a room or space that ensures privacy and opportunity to engage in confidential communication. If such an isolated space is not available, a common area can be restructured to maximize visual and auditory privacy from other patients or staff. Patients, including those who are disabled, should have easy access and seating. Space and seating should be adequate for family members or caregivers. The design and placement of desks and counters should minimize barriers to communication. Distractions and interruptions should be few, so that patients and pharmacists can have each other's undivided attention.

The environment should be equipped with appropriate learning aids, e.g., graphics, anatomical models, medication administration devices, memory aids, written material, and audiovisual resources.

Pharmacist and Patient Roles

Pharmacists and patients bring to education and counseling sessions their own perceptions of their roles and responsibilities. For the experience to be effective, the pharmacist and patient need to come to a common understanding about their respective roles and responsibilities. It may be necessary to clarify for patients that pharmacists have an appropriate and important role in providing education and counseling. Patients should be encouraged to be active participants.

The pharmacist's role is to verify that patients have sufficient understanding, knowledge, and skill to follow their pharmacotherapeutic regimens and monitoring plans. Pharmacists should also seek ways to motivate patients to learn about their treatment and to be active partners in their care. Patients' role is to adhere to their pharmacotherapeutic regimens, monitor for drug effects, and report their experiences to pharmacists or other members of their health care teams.[12,15] Optimally, the patient's role should include seeking information and presenting concerns that may make adherence difficult.

Depending on the health system's policies and procedures, its use of protocols or clinical care plans, and its credentialing of providers, pharmacists may also have disease management roles and responsibilities for specified categories of patients. This expands pharmacists' relationships with patients and the content of education and counseling sessions.

Process Steps

Steps in the patient education and counseling process will vary according to the health system's policies and procedures, environment, and practice setting. Generally, the following steps are appropriate for patients receiving new medications or returning for refills[12–21]:

1. Establish caring relationships with patients as appropriate to the practice setting and stage in the patient's health care management. Introduce yourself as a pharmacist, explain the purpose and expected length of the sessions, and obtain the patient's agreement to participate. Determine the patient's primary spoken language.

2. Assess the patient's knowledge about his or her health problems and medications, physical and mental capability to use the medications appropriately, and attitude toward the health problems and medications. Ask

open-ended questions about each medication's purpose and what the patient expects, and ask the patient to describe or show how he or she will use the medication.

Patients returning for refill medications should be asked to describe or show how they have been using their medications. They should also be asked to describe any problems, concerns, or uncertainties they are experiencing with their medications.

3. Provide information orally and use visual aids or demonstrations to fill patients' gaps in knowledge and understanding. Open the medication containers to show patients the colors, sizes, shapes, and markings on oral solids. For oral liquids and injectables, show patients the dosage marks on measuring devices. Demonstrate the assembly and use of administration devices such as nasal and oral inhalers. As a supplement to face-to-face oral communication, provide written handouts to help the patient recall the information.

    If a patient is experiencing problems with his or her medications, gather appropriate data and assess the problems. Then adjust the pharmacotherapeutic regimens according to protocols or notify the prescribers.

4. Verify patients' knowledge and understanding of medication use. Ask patients to describe or show how they will use their medications and identify their effects. Observe patients' medication-use capability and accuracy and attitudes toward following their pharmacotherapeutic regimens and monitoring plans.

Content

The content of an education and counseling session may include the information listed below, as appropriate for each patient's pharmacotherapeutic regimen and monitoring plan.[8,9,20] The decision to discuss specific pharmacotherapeutic information with an individual patient must be based on the pharmacist's professional judgment.

1. The medication's trade name, generic name, common synonym, or other descriptive name(s) and, when appropriate, its therapeutic class and efficacy.
2. The medication's use and expected benefits and action. This may include whether the medication is intended to cure a disease, eliminate or reduce symptoms, arrest or slow the disease process, or prevent the disease or a symptom.
3. The medication's expected onset of action and what to do if the action does not occur.
4. The medication's route, dosage form, dosage, and administration schedule (including duration of therapy).
5. Directions for preparing and using or administering the medication. This may include adaptation to fit patients' lifestyles or work environments.
6. Action to be taken in case of a missed dose.
7. Precautions to be observed during the medication's use or administration and the medication's potential risks in relation to benefits. For injectable medications and administration devices, concern about latex allergy may be discussed.
8. Potential common and severe adverse effects that may occur, actions to prevent or minimize their occurrence, and actions to take if they occur, including notifying the prescriber, pharmacist, or other health care provider.

9. Techniques for self-monitoring of the pharmacotherapy.
10. Potential drug–drug (including nonprescription), drug–food, and drug–disease interactions or contraindications.
11. The medication's relationships to radiologic and laboratory procedures (e.g., timing of doses and potential interferences with interpretation of results).
12. Prescription refill authorizations and the process for obtaining refills.
13. Instructions for 24-hour access to a pharmacist.
14. Proper storage of the medication.
15. Proper disposal of contaminated or discontinued medications and used administration devices.
16. Any other information unique to an individual patient or medication.

These points are applicable to both prescription and nonprescription medications. Pharmacists should counsel patients in the proper selection of nonprescription medications.

Additional content may be appropriate when pharmacists have authorized responsibilities in collaborative disease management for specified categories of patients. Depending on the patient's disease management or clinical care plan, the following may be covered:

1. The disease state: whether it is acute or chronic and its prevention, transmission, progression, and recurrence.
2. Expected effects of the disease on the patient's normal daily living.
3. Recognition and monitoring of disease complications.

Documentation

Pharmacists should document education and counseling in patients' permanent medical records as consistent with the patients' care plans, the health system's policies and procedures, and applicable state and federal laws. When pharmacists do not have access to patients' medical records, education and counseling may be documented in the pharmacy's patient profiles, on the medication order or prescription form, or on a specially designed counseling record.

The pharmacist should record (1) that counseling was offered and was accepted and provided or refused and (2) the pharmacist's perceived level of the patient's understanding.[9] As appropriate, the content should be documented (for example, counseling about food–drug interactions). All documentation should be safeguarded to respect patient confidentiality and privacy and to comply with applicable state and federal laws.[10]

References

1. Smith MC. Social barriers to rational drug therapy. *Am J Hosp Pharm.* 1972; 29:121–7.
2. Priorities and approaches for improving prescription medicine use by older Americans. Washington, DC: National Council on Patient Information and Education; 1987.
3. Manasse HR Jr. Medication use in an imperfect world: drug misadventuring as an issue of public policy, part 1. *Am J Hosp Pharm.* 1989; 46:929–44.
4. Manasse HR Jr. Medication use in an imperfect world: drug misadventuring as an issue of public policy, part 2. *Am J Hosp Pharm.* 1989; 46:1141–52.
5. Johnson JA, Bootman JL. Drug-related morbidity and mortality: a cost-of-illness model. *Arch Intern Med.* 1995; 155:1949–56.
6. Summary of the final report of the Scope of Pharmacy Practice Project. *Am J Hosp Pharm.* 1994; 51:2179–82.
7. Hepler CD, Strand LM. Opportunities and responsibilities in pharmaceutical care. *Am J Hosp Pharm.* 1990; 47:533–42.
8. Hatoum HT, Hutchinson RA, Lambert BL. OBRA 90: patient counseling—enhancing patient outcomes. *US Pharm.* 1993; 18(Jan):76–86.
9. OBRA '90: a practical guide to effecting pharmaceutical care. Washington, DC: American Pharmaceutical Association; 1994.
10. Lynn NJ, Kamm RE. Avoiding liability problems. *Am Pharm.* 1995; NS35(Dec):14–22.
11. Herrier RN, Boyce RW. Does counseling improve compliance? *Am Pharm.* 1995; NS35(Sep):11–2.
12. Foster SL, Smith EB, Seybold MR. Advanced counseling techniques: integrating assessment and intervention. *Am Pharm.* 1995; NS35(Oct):40–8.
13. Bond WS, Hussar DA. Detection methods and strategies for improving medication compliance. *Am J Hosp Pharm.* 1991; 48:1978–88.
14. Felkey BG. Adherence screening and monitoring. *Am Pharm.* 1995; NS35(Jul):42–51.
15. Herrier RN, Boyce RW. Establishing an active patient partnership. *Am Pharm.* 1995; NS35(Apr):48–57.
16. Boyce RW, Herrier RN, Gardner M. Pharmacist-patient consultation program, unit I: an interactive approach to verify patient understanding. New York: Pfizer Inc.; 1991.
17. Pharmacist-patient consultation program, unit II: counseling patients in challenging situations. New York: Pfizer Inc.; 1993.
18. Pharmacist-patient consultation program, unit III: counseling to enhance compliance. New York: Pfizer Inc.; 1995.
19. Boyce RW, Herrier RN. Obtaining and using patient data. *Am Pharm.* 1991; NS31(Jul):65–70.
20. Herrier RN, Boyce RW. Communicating risk to patients. *Am Pharm.* 1995; NS35(Jun):12–4.
21. APhA special report: medication administration problem solving in ambulatory care. Washington, DC: American Pharmaceutical Association; 1994.

Approved by the ASHP Board of Directors, November 11, 1996. Revised by the ASHP Council on Professional Affairs. Supersedes the ASHP Statement on the Pharmacist's Role in Patient-Education Programs dated June 3, 1991, and ASHP Guidelines on Pharmacist-Conducted Patient Counseling dated November 18, 1992.

The bibliographic citation for this document is as follows: American Society of Health-System Pharmacists. ASHP Guidelines on Pharmacist-Conducted Patient Education and Counseling. *Am J Health-Syst Pharm.* 1997; 54:431–4.

ASHP Guidelines: Minimum Standard for Pharmacies in Hospitals

Pharmacists work closely with other health practitioners to meet the needs of the public. The various societal needs for pharmaceutical care require that pharmacies provide a wide array of organized services. The primary purpose of this document is to serve as a guide for the provision of pharmaceutical services in hospitals; however, certain elements may be applicable to other health care settings. These Guidelines should also be useful in evaluating the scope and quality of these services.

As providers of pharmaceutical care, pharmacists are concerned with the outcomes of their services and not just the provision of these services. The elements of a pharmacy program that are critical to overall successful performance in a hospital include (1) leadership and practice management, (2) drug information and education, (3) activities to ensure rational medication therapy, (4) drug distribution and control, (5) facilities, and (6) participation in drug therapy research. Collectively, these elements represent a minimum level of practice that all hospital pharmacy departments must strive to provide on a consistent basis. While the scope of pharmaceutical services will likely vary from site to site, depending upon the needs of the patients served, these elements are inextricably linked to outcomes. Hence, failure to provide any of these services may compromise the overall quality of pharmaceutical care.

These Guidelines outline the minimum requirements for pharmaceutical services in hospitals. The reader is encouraged to review the ASHP practice standards referenced throughout this document for a more detailed description of the components of these services.

Standard I:
Leadership and Practice Management

Effective leadership and practice management skills are necessary for the delivery of pharmaceutical services in a manner consistent with the hospital's and patients' needs as well as continuous improvement in patient care outcomes. Pharmaceutical service management must focus on the pharmacist's responsibility to provide pharmaceutical care and to develop an organizational structure to support that mission.

The director of the pharmacy shall be responsible for (1) setting the short- and long-term goals of the pharmacy based on the needs of the patients served, the specific needs of the hospital (and any health system of which the hospital may be a component), and developments and trends in health care and hospital pharmacy practice, (2) developing plans and schedules for achieving these goals, (3) directing the implementation of the plans and the day-to-day activities associated with them, (4) determining whether the goals and schedule are being met, and (5) instituting corrective actions where necessary. The director of the pharmacy, in carrying out the aforementioned tasks, shall employ an adequate number of competent, qualified personnel. A part-time director of the pharmacy has the same basic obligations and responsibilities as a full-time director.

- **Education and training, director.** The pharmacy shall be managed by a professionally competent, legally qualified pharmacist. The director of the pharmacy service must be thoroughly knowledgeable about hospital pharmacy practice and management. He or she should have completed a pharmacy residency program accredited by the American Society of Health-System Pharmacists.[1] An advanced management degree (e.g., M.B.A., M.H.A., M.S.) is desirable.

- **Pharmacy mission.** The pharmacy shall have a written mission statement that, at a minimum, reflects both patient care and operational responsibilities. Other aspects of the mission may be appropriate as well, for example, educational and research responsibilities in the case of teaching and research hospitals. The statement shall be consistent with the mission of the hospital (and health system of which the hospital may be a component). The mission should be understood by every employee and other participant (e.g., students and residents) in the pharmacy's activities.

- **Support personnel.** Sufficient support personnel (pharmacy technicians, clerical, secretarial) shall be employed to facilitate the implementation of pharmaceutical care. Pharmacy technicians should be certified by the Pharmacy Technician Certification Board and should have completed an accredited training program. Appropriate supervisory controls must be maintained and documented.

- **Work schedules and assignments.** The director of the pharmacy shall ensure that work schedules, procedures, and assignments optimize the use of personnel and resources.

- **Education and training.** All personnel must possess the education and training needed to fulfill their responsibilities. All personnel must participate in relevant continuing-education programs and activities as necessary to maintain or enhance their competence.[2]

- **Recruitment and selection of personnel.** Personnel must be recruited and selected on the basis of job-related qualifications and prior performance.

- **Orientation of personnel.** There must be an established procedure for orienting new personnel to the pharmacy, the hospital, and their respective positions.[3]

- **Performance evaluation.** Procedures for the routine evaluation of the performance of pharmacy personnel shall exist.

- **Position descriptions.** Areas of responsibility within the pharmacy shall be clearly defined. Written position descriptions for all categories of pharmacy personnel must exist and must be revised as necessary.

- **Operations manual.** An operations manual governing pharmacy functions (e.g., administrative, operational, and clinical) shall exist. It should include long-term goals for the pharmacy. The manual must be revised when necessary to reflect changes in procedures, organization, and objectives. All personnel should be familiar with the contents of the manual. Appropriate mechanisms to ensure compliance with the policies and procedures should be established.

- **Drug expenditures.** Policies and procedures for managing drug expenditures shall exist. They should address such methods as competitive bidding, group purchasing, utilization-review programs, and cost-effective patient services.[4]

- **Workload and financial performance.** A process shall exist to routinely monitor workload and financial performance. This process should provide for the determination and analysis of hospital and system-wide costs of medication therapy. A pharmacist should be an integral part of the hospital's financial management team.
- **Committee involvement.** A pharmacist should be a member of and actively participate in those committees responsible for establishing medication-related policies and procedures as well as those committees responsible for the provision of patient care.
- **Quality assessment and improvement.** There shall be an ongoing, systematic program for quality assessment and improvement of the pharmacy and medication-use process. This program should be integrated with the hospital's or health system's quality assessment and quality improvement activities. Quality improvement activities related to the distribution, administration, and use of medications shall be routinely performed. Feedback to appropriate individuals about the quality achieved shall be provided.
- **24-Hour pharmaceutical services.** Adequate hours of operation for the provision of needed pharmaceutical services must be maintained; 24-hour pharmaceutical services should be provided if possible. Twenty-four-hour pharmaceutical services should exist in *all* hospitals with clinical programs that require intensive medication therapy (e.g., transplant programs, open-heart surgery programs, and neonatal intensive care units). When 24-hour pharmacy service is not feasible, a pharmacist must be available on an on-call basis.
- **After-hours pharmacy access.** In the absence of 24-hour pharmaceutical services, access to a limited supply of medications should be available to authorized nonpharmacists for use in carrying out urgent medication orders. The list of medications to be accessible and the policies and procedures to be used (including subsequent review of all activity by a pharmacist) shall be developed by the pharmacy and therapeutics (P&T) committee (or its equivalent). Items for such access should be chosen with safety in mind, limiting wherever possible medications, quantities, dosage forms, and container sizes that might endanger patients. Routine after-hours access to the pharmacy by nonpharmacists (e.g., nurses) for access to medications is strongly discouraged; this practice should be minimized and eliminated to the fullest extent possible. The use of well-designed night cabinets, after-hours medication carts, and other methods precludes the need for nonpharmacists to enter the pharmacy.[5] For emergency situations in which nonpharmacist access is necessary, policies and procedures should exist for safe access to medications by persons who receive telephone authorization from an on-call pharmacist.
- **Practice standards and guidelines.** The practice standards and guidelines of the American Society of Health-System Pharmacists and the Joint Commission on Accreditation of Healthcare Organizations (JCAHO) or other appropriate accrediting body should

be viewed as applicable, and the hospital should strive to meet these standards regardless of the particular financial and organizational arrangements by which pharmaceutical services are provided to the facility and its patients.

- **Laws and regulations.** Applicable laws and regulations must be met and relevant documentation of compliance must be maintained (e.g., records, material safety data sheets, copies of state board regulations).
- **Patient confidentiality.** The pharmacist shall respect and protect patient confidentiality by safeguarding access to computer databases and reports containing patient information. Patient information should be shared only with authorized health professionals and others authorized within the hospital or health system as needed for the care of patients.

Standard II:
Drug information and Education

The pharmacist shall provide patient-specific drug information and accurate and comprehensive information about drugs to other pharmacists, other health professionals, and patients as appropriate.

Up-to-date drug information shall be available, including current periodicals and recent editions of textbooks in appropriate pharmaceutical and biomedical subject areas. Electronic information is desirable. This information may be provided in conjunction with medical libraries and other available resources. Appropriate drug information resources shall be readily accessible to pharmacists located in patient care areas. No medication should be administered to a patient unless medical and nursing personnel have received adequate information about, and are familiar with, its therapeutic use, potential adverse effects, and dosage.

- **Drug information requests.** Responses to general and patient-specific drug information requests shall be provided in an accurate and timely manner. A process shall exist to assess and ensure the quality of responses to requests.
- **Medication-therapy monographs.** Medication-therapy monographs for medications under consideration for formulary addition or deletion shall be available. These monographs should be based on an analytical review of pertinent literature. Each monograph shall include a comparative therapeutic and economic assessment of each medication proposed for addition.
- **Patient education.** Pharmacists should be available for and actively participate in patient education. Pharmacists must help to ensure that all patients are given adequate information (including information on ethical issues, if any) about the medications they receive. Patient education activities shall be coordinated with the nursing, medical, and other clinical staff as needed.[6]
- **Dissemination of drug information.** Pharmacists should keep the hospital's staff informed about the use of medications on an ongoing basis through appropriate publications, presentations, and programs. Pharmacists should ensure timely dissemination of drug product information (e.g., recall notices, labeling changes).

Standard III:
Optimizing Medication Therapy

An important aspect of pharmaceutical care is optimizing medication use. This must include processes designed to ensure the safe and effective use of medications and increase the probability of desired patient outcomes. The pharmacist, in concert with the medical and nursing staff, must develop policies and procedures for ensuring the quality of medication therapy.

- *Medical record documentation.* Clinical actions and recommendations by pharmacists that are designed to ensure safe and effective use of medications and that have a potential effect on patient outcomes should be documented in patients' medical records.[7]
- *Medication histories.* Pharmacists should prepare or have immediate access to comprehensive medication histories for each patient's medical record or other databases (e.g., medication profile), or both. A pharmacist-conducted medication history for each patient is desirable.
- *Medication orders.* All prescribers' medication orders (except in emergency situations) must be reviewed for appropriateness by a pharmacist before the first dose is dispensed. Any questions regarding the order must be resolved with the prescriber at this time, and a written notation of these discussions must be made in the patient's medical record or pharmacy copy of the prescriber's order. Information concerning changes must be communicated to the appropriate health professional.
- *Medication-therapy monitoring.* Medication-therapy monitoring shall be conducted for appropriate patients and medication use. Medication-therapy monitoring includes an assessment of
  a. The therapeutic appropriateness of the patient's medication regimen.
  b. Therapeutic duplication in the patient's medication regimen.
  c. The appropriateness of the route and method of administration of the medication.
  d. The degree of patient compliance with the prescribed medication regimen.
  e. Medication–medication, medication–food, medication–laboratory test, and medication–disease interactions.
  f. Clinical and pharmacokinetic laboratory data to evaluate the efficacy of medication therapy and to anticipate toxicity and adverse effects.
  g. Physical signs and clinical symptoms relevant to the patient's medication therapy.
- *Therapeutic purpose.* Prescribers should be encouraged to routinely communicate the condition being treated or the therapeutic purpose of medications with all prescription and medication orders.
- *Pharmacist consultations.* Pharmacists should provide oral and written consultations to other health professionals regarding medication-therapy selection and management.
- *Medication-use evaluation.* An ongoing medication-use evaluation program shall exist to ensure that medications are used appropriately, safely, and effectively.[8]
- *Medication-use policy development.* The pharmacist shall be a member of the P&T committee, the institutional review board, and the infection control, patient care, medication-use evaluation, and other committees that make decisions concerning medication use.
- *Documentation of pharmaceutical care and outcomes.* The pharmacy shall have an ongoing process for consistent documentation (and reporting to medical staff, administrators, and others) of pharmaceutical care and patient outcomes from medication therapy and other pharmacy actions.
- *Continuity of care.* The pharmacist shall routinely contribute to processes ensuring that each patient's pharmaceutical care is maintained regardless of transitions that occur across different care settings (for example, among different components of a health system or between inpatient and community pharmacies or home care services).
- *Work redesign initiatives.* The pharmacist must be involved in work redesign initiatives such as patient-focused care, where they exist. These efforts should be such that pharmaceutical care is enhanced and supported.
- *Clinical care plans.* Pharmacists must be involved in the development of clinical care plans involving medication therapy.
- *Microbial resistance.* Policies and procedures addressing microbial resistance to anti-infectives shall exist. Pharmacists should review laboratory reports of microbial sensitivities and advise prescribers if microbial resistance is noted.
- *Medication-therapy decisions.* The pharmacist's prerogatives to initiate, monitor, and modify medication therapy for individual patients, consistent with laws, regulations, and hospital policy, shall be clearly delineated and approved by the P&T committee (or comparable body).
- *Immunization programs.* The pharmacy shall participate in the development of hospital policies and procedures concerning preventive and postexposure immunization programs for patients and hospital employees.[9]
- *Substance-abuse programs.* The pharmacy shall assist in the development of and participate in hospital substance-abuse prevention and employee assistance programs, where they exist.

Standard IV:
Medication Distribution and Control

The pharmacy shall be responsible for the procurement, distribution, and control of *all* drug products used in the hospital (including medication-related devices and pharmaceutical diagnostics) for inpatient and ambulatory patients.[10] Policies and procedures governing these functions shall be developed by the pharmacy with input from other appropriate hospital staff and committees.

- *Medication orders.* All patient medication orders shall be contained in the patient's medical record. A direct copy of the prescriber's order, either hard copy or prescriber-entered electronic transmission (preferred method), shall be received by the pharmacist. Order-transmittal safeguards should be used to ensure the security of the prescriber's order. All medication orders shall be reviewed by a pharmacist and assessed in relation to a medication profile before administration, unless an established procedure exists for the use of an approved list of medications for specific treatment circumstances and emergencies. A system shall exist to ensure that medication orders are not inappropriately continued.

- *Formulary.* A formulary of approved medications shall be maintained by the pharmacy.[11]
- *Prescribing.* Medications shall be prescribed by individuals who have been granted appropriate clinical privileges in the hospital and are legally permitted to order medications. The pharmacy shall advocate and foster practitioners' conformance with standardized, approved terminology and abbreviations to be used throughout the hospital when prescribing medications.
- *Medication administration.* Only personnel who are authorized by the hospital and appropriately trained shall be permitted to administer medications to a patient. This may include pharmacists and other pharmacy personnel.
- *Extemporaneous compounding.* Drug formulations, dosage forms, strengths, and packaging that are not available commercially but are needed for patient care shall be prepared by appropriately trained personnel in accordance with applicable practice standards and regulations (e.g., FDA, state board of pharmacy). Adequate quality assurance procedures shall exist for these operations.[12]
- *Sterile products.* All sterile medications shall be prepared and labeled in a suitable environment by appropriately trained personnel. Quality assurance procedures for the preparation of sterile products shall exist.[13]
- *Unit dose packaging.* Whenever possible, medications shall be available for inpatient use in single-unit packages and in a ready-to-administer form. Manipulation of medications before administration (e.g., withdrawal of doses from multidose containers, labeling containers) by final users should be minimized.[14]
- *Medication storage.* Medications shall be stored and prepared under proper conditions of sanitation, temperature, light, moisture, ventilation, segregation, and security to ensure medication integrity and personnel safety.
- *Adverse drug reactions.* An ongoing program for monitoring, reporting, and preventing adverse drug reactions shall be developed.[15]
- *Medication errors.* Pharmacists, with physicians and other appropriate hospital personnel, shall establish policies and procedures with respect to medication-error prevention and reporting.[5] Ongoing monitoring and review of medication errors with corresponding appropriate action should be maintained.
- *Drug product recalls.* A written procedure shall exist for the handling of a drug product recall. There should be an established process for removing from use any drugs or devices subjected to a recall.
- *Patient's own medications.* Drug products and related devices brought into the hospital by patients shall be identified by pharmacy and documented in the patient's medical record if the medications are to be used during hospitalization. They shall be administered only pursuant to a prescriber's order and according to hospital policies and procedures.
- *Vendors' representatives.* Written policies governing the activities of representatives of vendors of drug products (including related supplies and devices) within the hospital shall exist.[16]

- *Samples.* The use of medication samples shall be eliminated to the extent possible. However, if samples are permitted, the pharmacy must control these products to ensure proper storage, maintenance of records, and product integrity.
- *Manufacturers and suppliers.* Criteria for selecting drug product manufacturers and suppliers shall be established by the pharmacy to ensure high quality of drug products.[17]
- *Cytotoxic and hazardous drug products.* Policies and procedures for storage, handling, and disposal of cytotoxic and other hazardous drug products shall exist.[18]
- *Controlled substances.* Accountability procedures shall exist to ensure control of the distribution and use of controlled substances and other medications with a potential for abuse.[19]
- *Nondrug substances.* The pharmacy shall seek and obtain documented authorization from appropriate medical staff and hospital committees for the pharmacologic use of any chemical substance that has never received FDA approval for any drug use. Documentation must exist to ensure that appropriate risk management measures (e.g., obtaining informed consent) have been taken.
- *Medication storage area inspections.* All stocks of medications shall be inspected routinely to ensure the absence of outdated, unusable, or mislabeled products. Storage conditions that would foster medication deterioration and storage arrangements that might contribute to medication errors also must be assessed, documented, and corrected.
- *Floor stock.* Floor stocks of medications generally shall be limited to medications for emergency use and routinely used safe items (e.g., mouthwash, antiseptic solutions). The potential for medication errors and adverse effects must be considered for every medication allowed as floor stock.
- *Disaster services.* A procedure shall exist for providing pharmaceutical services in case of disaster.
- *Medical emergencies.* The pharmacy shall participate in hospital decisions about emergency medication kits and the role of pharmacists in medical emergencies.
- *Drug delivery systems, administration devices, and automated dispensing machines.* Pharmacists shall provide leadership and advice in organizational and clinical decisions regarding drug delivery systems, administration devices, and automated dispensing machines and should participate in the evaluation, use, and monitoring of these systems and devices.[20] The potential for medication errors associated with such systems and devices must be thoroughly evaluated.

Standard V: Facilities, Equipment, and Information Resources

To ensure optimal operational performance and quality patient care, adequate space, equipment, and supplies shall be available for all professional and administrative functions relating to medication use. These resources must be located in areas that facilitate the provision of services to patients, nurses, prescribers, and other health care providers and must be integrated with the hospital's communication and delivery or transportation systems. Facilities shall be constructed, arranged, and equipped to promote safe and efficient work and to avoid damage to or deterioration of drug products.

- *Medication storage.* Facilities shall exist to enable the storage and preparation of medications under proper conditions of sanitation, temperature, light, moisture, ventilation, segregation, and security to ensure medication integrity and personnel safety throughout the hospital.

- *Packaging and compounding.* Designated space and equipment for packaging and compounding drug products and preparing sterile products shall exist. There shall be a suitable work environment that promotes orderliness and efficiency and minimizes potential for contamination of products.[13,14]

- *Cytotoxic and hazardous drug products.* Special precautions, equipment, and training for storage, handling, and disposal of cytotoxic and other hazardous drug products shall exist to ensure the safety of personnel, patients, and visitors.[18]

- *Drug information.* Adequate space, resources, and information-handling and communication technology shall be available to facilitate the provision of drug information.

- *Consultation space.* In outpatient dispensing areas, a private area for pharmacist–patient consultations shall be available to enhance patients' knowledge and compliance with prescribed medication regimens.

- *Office and meeting space.* Office and meeting areas shall be available for administrative, educational, and training activities.

- *Automation.* Automated mechanical systems and software may be useful in promoting accurate and efficient medication ordering and preparation, drug distribution, and clinical monitoring, provided they are safely used and do not hinder the pharmacist's review of (and opportunity to intervene in) medication orders before the administration of first doses. An interface with a comprehensive pharmacy computer system is encouraged. Pharmacy personnel must supervise the stocking of medications in dispensing machines.

- *Record maintenance.* Adequate space shall exist for maintaining and storing records (e.g., equipment maintenance, controlled substances inventory, material safety data sheets) to ensure compliance with laws, regulations, accreditation requirements, and sound management techniques. Appropriate licenses, permits, and tax stamps shall be present. Equipment shall be adequately maintained and certified in accordance with applicable practice standards, laws, and regulations. There shall be documentation of equipment maintenance and certification.

- *Computerized systems.* Computer resources should be used to support secretarial functions, maintain patient medication profile records, perform necessary patient billing procedures, manage drug product inventories, and interface with other available computerized systems to obtain patient-specific clinical information for medication therapy monitoring and other clinical functions and to facilitate the continuity of care to and from other care settings.

Standard VI: Research

The pharmacist should initiate, participate in, and support medical and pharmaceutical research appropriate to the goals, objectives, and resources of the specific hospital.[21]

- *Policies and procedures.* The pharmacist shall ensure that policies and procedures for the safe and proper use of investigational drugs are established and followed.[22]

- *Distribution and control.* The pharmacy shall be responsible for overseeing the distribution and control of all investigational drugs. Investigational drugs shall be approved for use by an institutional review board and shall be dispensed and administered to consenting patients according to an approved protocol.[22]

- *Institutional review board.* A pharmacist shall be included on the hospital's institutional review board.

- *Drug information.* The pharmacist shall have access to information on all investigational studies and similar research projects involving medications and medication-related devices used in the hospital. The pharmacist shall provide pertinent written information (to the extent known) about the safe and proper use of investigational drugs, including possible adverse effects and adverse drug reactions to nurses, pharmacists, physicians, and other health care professionals called upon to administer, dispense, and prescribe these medications.

References

1. American Society of Hospital Pharmacists. ASHP residency accreditation regulations and standards on definitions of pharmacy residencies and fellowships. *Am J Hosp Pharm.* 1987; 44:1142–4.

2. American Society of Hospital Pharmacists. ASHP statement on continuing education. *Am J Hosp Pharm.* 1990; 47:1855.

3. American Society of Hospital Pharmacists. ASHP technical assistance bulletin on the recruitment, selection, and retention of pharmacy personnel. *Am J Hosp Pharm.* 1994; 51:1811–5.

4. American Society of Hospital Pharmacists. ASHP technical assistance bulletin on assessing cost-containment strategies for pharmacies in organized healthcare settings. *Am J Hosp Pharm.* 1992; 49:155–60.

5. American Society of Hospital Pharmacists. ASHP guidelines on preventing medication errors in hospitals. *Am J Hosp Pharm.* 1993; 50:305–14.

6. American Society of Hospital Pharmacists. ASHP statement on the pharmacist's role in patient education programs. *Am J Hosp Pharm.* 1991; 48:1780.

7. American Society of Hospital Pharmacists. ASHP guidelines for obtaining authorization for documenting pharmaceutical care in patient medical records. *Am J Hosp Pharm.* 1989; 46:338–9.

8. American Society of Hospital Pharmacists. ASHP guidelines on the pharmacist's role in drug-use evaluation. *Am J Hosp Pharm.* 1988; 45:385–6.

9. American Society of Hospital Pharmacists. ASHP technical assistance bulletin on the pharmacist's role in immunization. *Am J Hosp Pharm.* 1993; 50:501–5.

10. American Society of Hospital Pharmacists. ASHP statement on the pharmacist's responsibility for distribution and control of drug products. *Am J Hosp Pharm.* 1995; 52:747.

11. American Society of Hospital Pharmacists. ASHP statement on the formulary system. *Am J Hosp Pharm.* 1983; 40:1384–5.

12. American Society of Hospital Pharmacists. ASHP

technical assistance bulletin on compounding nonsterile products in pharmacies. *Am J Hosp Pharm.* 1994; 51:1441–8.

13. American Society of Hospital Pharmacists. ASHP technical assistance bulletin on quality assurance for pharmacy-prepared sterile products.*Am J Hosp Pharm.* 1993; 50:2386–98.

14. American Society of Hospital Pharmacists. ASHP technical assistance bulletin on single unit and unit dose packages of drugs. *Am J Hosp Pharm.* 1985; 42:378–9.

15. American Society of Hospital Pharmacists. ASHP guidelines on adverse drug reaction monitoring and reporting. *Am J Health-Syst Pharm.* 1995; 52:417–9.

16. American Society of Hospital Pharmacists. ASHP guidelines for pharmacists on the activities of vendors' representatives in organized health care systems.*Am J Hosp Pharm.* 1994; 51:520–1.

17. American Society of Hospital Pharmacists. ASHP guidelines for selecting pharmaceutical manufacturers and suppliers. *Am J Hosp Pharm.* 1991; 48:523–4.

18. American Society of Hospital Pharmacists. ASHP technical assistance bulletin on handling cytotoxic and hazardous drugs. *Am J Hosp Pharm.* 1990; 47: 1033–49.

19. American Society of Hospital Pharmacists. ASHP technical assistance bulletin on use of controlled substances in organized health-care settings. *Am J Hosp Pharm.* 1993; 50:489–501.

20. American Society of Hospital Pharmacists. ASHP statement on the pharmacist's role with respect to drug delivery systems and administration devices. *Am J Hosp Pharm.* 1993; 50:1724–5.

21. American Society of Hospital Pharmacists. ASHP guidelines for the use of investigational drugs in organized health-care settings. *Am J Hosp Pharm.* 1991; 48:315–9.

22. American Society of Hospital Pharmacists. ASHP statement on pharmaceutical research in organized health-care settings.*Am J Hosp Pharm.* 1991; 48:1781.

Approved by the ASHP Board of Directors, September 22, 1995. Revised by the ASHP Council on Professional Affairs. Supersedes an earlier version dated November 14–15, 1984.

The bibliographic citation for this document is as follows: American Society of Health-System Pharmacists. ASHP guidelines: minimum standard for pharmacies in hospitals.*Am J Health-Syst Pharm.* 1995; 52:2711–7.

ASHP Guidelines for Pharmaceutical Research in Organized Health-Care Settings

The promotion of research in the health and pharmaceutical sciences and in pharmaceutical services is a purpose of the American Society of Hospital Pharmacists, as stated in its Charter.[1] In keeping with this purpose, pharmacists in organized health-care settings should understand the (1) basic need for research and systematic problem solving in pharmacy practice; (2) fundamental scientific approach; (3) basic components of a research plan; (4) process of documenting and reporting findings; and (5) responsibilities of investigators with respect to patients, employers, grantors, and science in general.

In its purest form, scientific research is the systematic, controlled, empirical, and critical investigation of hypothetical propositions (theories) about presumed relationships among natural phenomena.[2] Aspects of the research process (e.g., problem definition, systematic data gathering, interpretation, and reporting), however, are also applicable to resolving specific practice problems. Independent, intraprofessional, and interdisciplinary collaborative research and problem solving are encouraged.

Need

Since pharmacy is based on the theories of the pharmaceutical, medical, and social sciences, pharmacy's advancement is linked to advancement in those sciences. Scientific inquiry, through formal research and systematic problem solving, leads to an expansion of knowledge and thus to advancement. Both research and systematic problem solving in organized health-care settings are needed for developing knowledge in pharmaceutics and drug therapy and for evaluation, modification, and justification of specific practices. Therefore, an understanding of the research process is important to pharmacists in such settings.

Primary areas for research by pharmacists in organized health-care settings are those in which pharmacists possess special expertise or unique knowledge. These areas include drug therapy, pharmaceutics, bioavailability, pharmacy practice administration, sociobehavioral aspects of pharmaceutical service systems, and application of information handling and computer technology to pharmacy practice.

The Scientific Approach

Aspects of the scientific approach may be applied to formal research and systematic problem solving. The scientific approach consists of four basic steps:

1. *Problem—Obstacle—Idea.*[3] The scientist experiences an obstacle to understanding or curiosity as to why something is as it is. The scientist's first step is to express the idea in some reasonably manageable form, even if it is ill defined and tentative.
2. *Hypothesis.* The scientist looks back on experience for possible solutions—personal experience, the literature, and contacts with other scientists. A tentative proposition (hypothesis) is formulated about the relationship between two or more variables in the problem; for example, "If such and such occurs, then so and so results."

3. *Reasoning—Deduction.* The scientist deduces the consequences of the formulated hypothesis. The scientist may find that the deductions reveal a new problem that is quite different from the original one. On the other hand, deductions may lead to the conclusion that the problem cannot be solved with existing technical tools. Such reasoning can help lead to wider, more basic, and more significant problems as well as to more narrow (testable) implications of the original hypothesis.
4. *Observation—Test—Experiment.* If the problem has been well stated, the hypotheses have been adequately formulated, and the implications of the hypotheses have been carefully deduced, the next step is to test the relationships expressed by the hypotheses, that is, the relationships among the variables. All testing is for one purpose: putting the relationships among the variables to an empirical test. It is not the hypotheses that are tested but the deduced implications of the hypotheses. On the basis of the research evidence, each hypothesis is either accepted or rejected.

Components of a Research Plan

Formal research frequently requires the development of a written plan (protocol or proposal). In funded research, the plan may take the form of a grant application. A typical plan might include

1. A problem statement.
2. A review of available literature on the subject.
3. The objectives for the project, including the hypotheses and the to-be-tested relationships among variables.
4. A description of the methodology to be used.
5. A description of statistical analyses to be applied to the data collected.
6. A budget and time frame for the project (where applicable).
7. The expected applicability of the research findings.

Documentation and Reporting

The structure of a research report is similar to the structure of a research plan. A typical outline is as follows:

1. Problem.
   a. Theories, hypotheses, and definitions.
   b. Previous research: the literature.
2. Methodology.
   a. Sample and sampling method.
   b. Experimental procedures and instrumentation.
   c. Measurement of variables.
   d. Statistical methods of analysis.
   e. Pretesting and pilot studies.
3. Results, interpretation, and conclusions.

The statement of the problem sets the general stage for the reader and may be in question form. A common practice is to state the broader, general problem and then to state the hypotheses, both general and specific. All important variables should be defined, both in general and in operational terms, giving a justification for the definitions used, if needed.

The general and research literature related to the problem is discussed to explain the theoretical rationale of the problem, to tell the reader what research has and has not been carried out on the problem, and to show that this particular investigation has not been conducted before (except in the case of validating research).

The methodology section should meticulously describe what was done so as to enable another investigator to reproduce the research, reanalyze the data, and arrive at unambiguous conclusions about the adequacy of the methods. This section should tell what samples were used, how they were selected, and why they were selected. The means of measurement of the variables should be described. The data analysis methods should be outlined and justified. Where pilot studies and pretesting were used, they should be described.

Results and data should be condensed and expressed in concise form. Limitations and weaknesses of the study should be discussed. The question of whether the data support the hypotheses must be foremost in the mind of the report writer. Everything written should relate the results and data to the problem and the hypotheses.

Investigators' Responsibilities

Investigators bear a general responsibility to be scientifically objective in their research inquiries, conclusions, and reports. They bear a responsibility for being methodical and meticulous in the gathering of research data. They also bear both a fiduciary and a reporting responsibility to employers and grantors. In general, employee investigators are at least partially responsible to their employer organizations in the choice of research topics. Research funded from sources outside an investigator's organization may impose additional contractual obligations on the investigator and the organization.

In research involving patients, investigators are responsible for protecting patients from harm while the patients are participating in the research. All research involving patients should be reviewed and approved, before initiation, by an institutional review board. Written, informed consent should be obtained from every patient participating in each research project.[4] Meticulous recordkeeping is required regarding the clinical experience of patients participating in research projects.

Employee investigators bear responsibility for helping their organizations differentiate true, objective research from product marketing trials and promotions that may purport to be research projects. Grants for bona fide research typically bear a direct cost-recovery relationship to projects and typically involve the direct transfer of grant funds from grantors to the employee investigator's employer organization. Specific institutional policies vary widely, but employee investigators can generally better fulfill their fiduciary responsibilities when funds are not distributed directly from grantors to investigators. In keeping with their fiduciary responsibilities and their responsibility to be scientifically objective, investigators should be wary of arrangements in which prospective grantors offer inducements of value (gifts, trips, experiences, publicity, publications, etc.) to investigators, institutions, or patients before, during, or after the completion of proposed projects.

Investigators should make legitimate efforts to document publicly the findings of research in scientific, objectively refereed publications.

References

1. American Society of Hospital Pharmacists. Governing documents of the American Society of Hospital Pharmacists. Bethesda, MD: American Society of Hospital Pharmacists; 1984.
2. Kerlinger F. Foundations of behavioral research. New York: Holt, Rinehart and Winston; 1964:13.
3. Dewey J. How we think. Boston: Heath; 1933:106–18, as adapted to the scientific framework by Kerlinger, op cit., p 13–5.
4. American Society of Hospital Pharmacists. ASHP guidelines for the use of investigational drugs in institutions. *Am J Hosp Pharm*. 1983; 40:449–51.

Approved by the ASHP Board of Directors, September 30, 1988. Developed by the Council on Professional Affairs. Supersedes the "ASHP Guidelines for Scientific Research in Institutional Pharmacy" approved on November 15, 1977.

The bibliographic citation for this document is as follows: American Society of Hospital Pharmacists. ASHP guidelines for pharmaceutical research in organized health-care settings. *Am J Hosp Pharm*. 1989; 46:129–30.

ASHP Guidelines for Obtaining Authorization for Documenting Pharmaceutical Care in Patient Medical Records

Pharmaceutical care is an important component of the overall therapy of many patients in organized health-care settings. Actions by pharmacists that are designed to ensure safe and effective use of drugs and that have a potential effect on patient outcomes should be documented in patients' medical records.[1] In organized health-care settings, the authority to make entries in medical records is granted by the organization in accordance with organizational and, usually, medical staff policies.

The following steps are recommended for obtaining authorization:

1. Identify, within the organization, the specific organizational and medical staff committees whose recommendations or decisions will be required to establish authority for pharmacists to make medical record entries. Determine the necessary sequence of these approvals. Committees typically involved are the pharmacy and therapeutics (P&T) committee, the executive committee of the medical staff, a quality-assurance committee, and a medical records committee.

2. Determine the existing organizational and medical staff policies regarding authority for medical record entries. These policies may provide specific guidance on how to proceed in particular organizations.

3. Identify other nonphysician and nonnursing care providers in the organization who have been granted such authority. Consult with them regarding the process used to establish the authority.

4. Determine the accepted method and format for submitting a proposal to obtain authority. In some organizations, a written proposal may be required. If so, determine the desired format (length, style, and necessary supporting justification). An oral presentation to, or a meeting with, the deciding bodies may be required. If so, determine the extent of remarks and supporting materials desired by these bodies.

5. Draft a written plan describing
   a. Examples of information to be documented in medical records.
   b. The location within the medical record where entries will be made and any special format or forms proposed. The creation of new medical record forms may require review and approval by specific organizational or medical staff committees.

6. Review the plan with the chairperson of the P&T committee, the director of nursing, the director of medical records, and representatives of the organization's administration. The organization's risk management office and legal counsel also should be advised and consulted.

7. Seek the endorsement and recommendation of the P&T committee.

8. In appropriate sequence, seek the endorsement or decision of any other committees necessary for ultimate approval. Monitor the proposal's course through the various committees and offer assistance, as required, to each chairperson to clarify information or provide any necessary supplementary materials.

9. When the final approving body grants the authority, facilitate (or directly handle, as appropriate) communication of the new policy to those affected in the organization (e.g., nursing, medical staff, quality-assurance staff, and medical records department).

Examples of information a pharmacist may need to document in the patient medical record include, but are not limited to

1. A summary of the patient's medication history on admission.

2. Oral and written consultations provided to other health-care professionals regarding the patient's drug therapy selection and management.

3. Physicians' verbal orders received directly by the pharmacist.

4. Clarifications of drug orders.

5. Adjustments made in the patient's drug dosage, dose frequency, dosage form, and route of administration.

6. Drugs, including investigational drugs, administered.

7. Potential drug-related problems that warrant surveillance.

8. Drug therapy monitoring findings, including:
   a. Therapeutic appropriateness of the patient's drug regimen, including the route and method of administration.
   b. Therapeutic duplication in the patient's drug regimen.
   c. Degree of patient compliance with the prescribed drug regimen.
   d. Actual and potential drug–drug, drug–food, drug–laboratory data, and drug–disease interactions.
   e. Clinical and pharmacokinetic laboratory data pertinent to the patient's drug regimen.
   f. Actual and potential drug toxicity and adverse effects.
   g. Physical signs and clinical symptoms relevant to the patient's drug therapy.

9. Drug-related patient education and counseling provided.

Reference

1. American Society of Hospital Pharmacists. ASHP statement on the pharmacist's clinical role in organized health-care settings. *Am J Hosp Pharm.* 1988; 45:890–1.

Approved by the ASHP Board of Directors, November 16, 1988. Developed by the ASHP Council on Professional Affairs. Supersedes an earlier version approved by the ASHP Board of Directors, November 16–17, 1978.

The bibliographic citation for this document is as follows: American Society of Hospital Pharmacists. ASHP guidelines for obtaining authorization for documenting pharmaceutical care in patient medical records. *Am J Hosp Pharm.* 1989; 46:338–9.

ASHP Guidelines for the Use of Investigational Drugs in Organized Health-Care Settings

Hospitals and other organized health-care settings, the primary centers for clinical studies using investigational drugs,[a] must ensure that policies and procedures for the safe use of these drugs are established and followed. This document is designed to help develop these policies and procedures and evaluate those currently in use.

Basic Principles

Procedures for the use of investigational drugs should be based on these basic principles:[b]

1. An organization that is the setting for investigational drug studies must ensure that such studies contain adequate safeguards for itself, its staff, the scientific integrity of the study, and, especially, the patient. There must be written policies and procedures for the approval, management, and control of investigational drug studies including compassionate use medications, agents approved for use under a treatment protocol for investigational new drugs (treatment IND), and Phase IV investigational drugs. All involved staff must be fully informed about, and comply with, these policies and procedures.

2. All investigational drug studies must meet accepted ethical, legal, and scientific standards and be conducted by appropriately qualified investigators.

3. All patients who participate in investigational drug studies must freely consent, usually in writing, to treatment with the drugs. This consent must be obtained from the patient or the patient's legally authorized representative before treatment is begun, and only after accurate and complete information about the study objectives and the risks and benefits associated with the study drugs has been provided.[c] No unreasonable inducements (i.e., excessive coercion or undue influence) should be offered to patients to encourage their participation in the study.

Guidelines for Organized Health-Care Settings

The following recommendations will serve as a guide to the development of investigational drug policies and procedures in keeping with the aforementioned basic principles:

1. As required by federal regulation, clinical research performed in institutions and other settings must be reviewed and approved by an institutional review board (IRB), often titled a "Committee on Human Investigations" or "Clinical Research Committee." This committee must evaluate each proposed clinical research study in terms of its compliance with recognized ethical, legal, and scientific standards. No clinical study may be initiated unless approved, in writing, by the committee. Oral approval may be granted in emergency situations, but emergency use must be reported to the IRB within a specified number of days; subsequent use is subject to full IRB review. Treatment

IND protocols are also subject to IRB review and approval, unless the drugs are needed for emergency use or the protocol has an FDA-approved waiver from IRB requirements.

   The committee must also monitor approved studies to ensure that they are carried out appropriately and reassess each protocol at least annually. In the event that an existing protocol is disapproved by the IRB, organizational policies and procedures should provide guidance on the conversion of patients to other therapies. The director of pharmacy, investigational drug pharmacist, or the director's designee should be a member of the IRB and be consulted by the committee whenever drug studies are reviewed.

2. Investigational drugs must be used only under the supervision of the principal investigator or authorized coinvestigators, all of whom must be members of the professional staff. The determination of qualifications for investigators is the responsibility of the sponsor and the IRB. Properly qualified pharmacists may serve as principal investigators or coinvestigators.

3. The principal investigator is responsible for obtaining the informed consent of the patient to participate in the study. The informed consent process must conform to current federal and state regulations. Approval of the consent document by the IRB is required. Review by legal counsel may be desirable also. The following items must be addressed, either in the consent document or in its accompanying oral explanation by the investigator:

    a. A fair representation of the nature and purpose of the study, the expected benefits, and the foreseeable risks or discomfort involved. The name and telephone number of the principal investigator and person(s) to contact for answers to questions about the study or drug should be provided. Any compensation or treatment that will be furnished in the event of injury should be described. Any costs for which the patient will be held responsible should be described.

    b. A balanced description of the alternative treatments available, including their respective risks and benefits.

    c. A general description of study procedures, identification of any procedures that are experimental, and expected length of therapy with the drug.

    d. A statement to the effect that (1) participation is voluntary, (2) the patient may withdraw from the study at any time, (3) refusal to participate or withdrawal from the study will involve no penalty or loss of benefits to which the subject is otherwise entitled, and (4) the principal investigator may remove the patient from the study if circumstances warrant.

    e. The name of the drug(s), name and signature of the patient (or the patient's legally authorized representative), name and signature of the principal investigator or coinvestigator, and name and signature of a witness.

f. A statement of who will have access to any study records that contain patient identifiers, including monitoring personnel from the study sponsor or Food and Drug Administration (FDA) who may inspect the records to assess compliance with the study protocol and all regulations.

The consent form should be as detailed as is practical, minimizing the amount of information that must be presented orally. For non-English-speaking patients, the consent form should be in the patient's own language when feasible, or adequate interpretation should be provided. The patient (or his or her representative) must have adequate time to read the consent form before signing it and should receive a copy of the signed form. The patient should retain a copy of the consent form. Additional copies of the consent form should be kept on file as required by the sponsor, the IRB, and the individual organization.

4. The principal investigator is responsible for the proper maintenance of case report forms and all other records required in the study by the site, drug sponsor, or FDA.

5. The organization's drug use control system must contain the following elements with respect to investigational drugs:

a. Drugs must be properly packaged in accordance with all applicable standards and regulations (e.g., FDA, *USP–NF*, and the Poison Prevention Packaging Act).

b. Drugs must be labeled properly so as to ensure their safe use by the nursing staff and patient (see Item 4 under "Guidelines for Pharmacists").

c. There must be a mechanism to ensure that sufficient supplies of the drugs are always available for the duration of the study.

d. A mechanism must be in place to allow the pharmacist or other designated health-care provider to break the blinding code and reveal the identity of the study drug to other health-care professionals in a medical emergency.

e. Nurses, pharmacists, and physicians called on to administer or dispense investigational drugs should have adequate written information about their (1) pharmacology (particularly adverse effects); (2) storage requirements; (3) method of dose preparation, administration, and disposal of unused drugs; (4) precautions to be taken, including handling recommendations; (5) authorized prescribers; (6) patient monitoring guidelines; and (7) any other material pertinent to the safe and proper use of the drugs. These health-care providers also should be informed about the overall study objectives and procedures, and a complete copy of the protocol should be available for reference.

f. Bulk supplies of the drug must be properly stored and adequately secured. When practical, all bulk supplies should be stored in the pharmacy department. When bulk supplies are stored outside of the pharmacy, methods used by the investigator responsible for such drugs should be audited by the pharmacy to ensure that the storage, dispensing, accountability, and security of the investigational drugs are in compliance with federal and state regulations and standards used by the pharmacy.

g. There must be a method to ensure that only authorized practitioners prescribe the drug and that all patients who receive it have provided the necessary consent.

h. Records of the amounts of drug received from the sponsor and of its disposition (amounts dispensed to patients, returned to sponsor, etc.) must be maintained. These records should be retained as required by regulation. Generally, records should be maintained for 2 years following the date of an approved new drug application (NDA) for the indication that is being investigated or, if the application is not approved or no application is filed, for 2 years after the investigation is discontinued and FDA is notified.

i. If the patient is to receive the drug at another facility, suitable arrangements for its transfer must be made. Sufficient information for safe use of the drug (see Item e), including a copy of the patient's signed consent form, the study protocol, and a copy of the IRB approval letter, must accompany the drug. The facility to which the drug is transferred should have written procedures governing the proper handling of investigational drugs.

j. The institution's records on investigational drug studies should be designed so that various descriptive reports (e.g., the names of all drugs under study and the names of those patients who have received a given drug) may be generated conveniently and expeditiously.

The drug control responsibilities previously described should be assigned to the pharmacy department.[1,2] In addition, pharmacists may serve as principal investigators or coinvestigators, and pharmacists may be able to assist in protocol development, drug procurement, preparation of codes for blinded studies, patient education and monitoring, education of nursing and other personnel, data collection and analysis, and special dosage form and packaging development.

Guidelines for Pharmacists

The pharmacist is responsible for ensuring that procedures for the control of investigational drug use, as previously described, are developed and implemented. Suggestions to accomplish this follow, although each facility must develop procedures specific to its own needs and organization.

1. A copy of the IRB-approved research protocol and investigator's brochure or drug data sheet, or both, should be kept in the pharmacy.

2. Using the protocol and additional information (if needed) supplied by the principal investigator, the pharmacy should prepare an investigational drug data sheet that concisely summarizes for the medical, nursing, and pharmacy staffs information pertinent to use of the drug. This communication should contain, at the minimum

a. Drug designation and common synonym(s).

b. Dosage form(s) and strength(s).

c. Usual dosage range, including dosage schedule and route of administration.

d. Indications.

e. Expected therapeutic effect.

f. Expected and potential adverse effects, including symptoms of toxicity and their treatment.

g. Contraindications.

h. Storage requirements.

i. Instructions for dosage preparation and administration, including stability and handling guidelines.

j. Instructions for disposition of unused doses.

k. Names and telephone numbers of principal and authorized coinvestigators.

l. Drug interactions, if known.

The drug data sheet should be reviewed by the principal investigator and the pharmacy and therapeutics committee. Copies should be distributed to the appropriate pharmacy staff and all patient-care units where the drug will be used. It is the responsibility of the involved staff to become familiar with the information in these data sheets.

3. When practical, investigational drug supplies should be stored in the pharmacy. When investigational drug supplies are stored outside the pharmacy, methods used by the investigator responsible for such drugs should be audited by the pharmacy to ensure that the storage, dispensing, accountability, and security of the investigational drug comply with federal and state regulations and standards used by the pharmacy.

The pharmacy should maintain a perpetual inventory record for drugs stored in the pharmacy. This record should contain the drug's name; dosage form and strength; lot number; expiration date; name, address, and telephone number of the sponsor; protocol number; and any other information needed for ordering the drug. It should provide for recording data on the disposition of the drug (amounts received, amounts transferred or wasted, amounts dispensed, dates, patient names or codes, and names of prescribers), the amount currently on hand, the minimum reorder level, and the recorder's initials. The inventory record should also reflect drug dosages that were dispensed but not administered and were returned to the pharmacy.

4. The dispensing of investigational drugs should be integrated with the rest of the drug distribution and control system, including, but not limited to, packaging, labeling, order review, profile maintenance, delivery, and quality-assurance procedures. However, prescription labels for investigational drugs should be distinguishable from other labels by an appropriate legend (e.g., "investigational drug"). There must be a method to verify that a valid, signed consent form has been received from the patient before the initial supply of drug is dispensed. The drug must be dispensed only on the order of an authorized investigator.

5. Patient education and monitoring of therapy (including adverse drug reaction monitoring) are two clinical functions that are particularly important and applicable to investigational drugs. These functions should be provided in a coordinated fashion by the pharmacy and nursing staffs and the authorized investigator(s).

6. At the conclusion of the study, the pharmacy should return, transfer, or dispose of all unused drugs according to the specific instructions provided by the sponsor.

7. The pharmacy should prepare an annual or semiannual descriptive summary of investigational drug use. This summary should include the number of drug studies in progress and a list of all drugs studied during the previous period.

8. Drug costs and other expenses associated with investigational drug studies (e.g., costs of recordkeeping and drug administration) should be properly allocated and reimbursed. Policies and procedures should address the role of the department of pharmacy in billing patients and third-party payers for investigational services, ancillary goods, and investigational drug agents.

Elaboration on these guidelines and further information on investigational drug studies may be found in the ASHP publication *Pharmacy-Coordinated Investigational Drug Services.*[3]

Guidelines for the Pharmaceutical Industry

The pharmaceutical company, or any study sponsor, that supports the use of investigational drugs in institutions should receive reliable and valid data. The following recommendations will serve as a guide to the pharmaceutical industry or other study sponsors to ensure that investigational drug use is managed appropriately and that studies are conducted effectively, efficiently, and safely.

1. Drugs must be properly packaged in accordance with all applicable standards and regulations (e.g., FDA, *USP–NF*, and the Poison Prevention Packaging Act).

2. Drugs must be properly labeled in accordance with applicable regulations (federal and state) and standards (e.g., ASHP). If possible, ample space should be left on the drug container for further labeling by the pharmacist. Expiration dates and lot numbers should also be noted on the label.

3. A 24-hour telephone number should be available to study personnel, including the principal investigator and the department of pharmacy. In the event of an emergency, information should be available pertaining to (1) adverse effects and their treatment; (2) emergency protocol management and dosing and administration guidelines; (3) the ability to break a "blinded code" to determine the treatment regimen; and (4) the mechanism of procuring an emergency supply of medication, as in the case of compassionate use drugs.

4. Company representatives should be designated to handle routine requests, such as for additional forms and resupply of investigational drugs. If possible, a direct phone line or fax should be available to expedite requests.

5. Investigational drugs should be shipped to the principal investigator in care of the department of pharmacy, with a designated person in the pharmacy responsible for requesting supplies of investigational drugs. The following information regarding procurement should also be supplied to the department of pharmacy:

a. Name and telephone number of the sponsor's study monitor or field representative.

b. Estimated time for fulfillment of orders.

c. Limits on quantities that can be ordered.

d. Special ordering instructions.

e. How the order is to be shipped (e.g., specific package shipping firms).

f.   Disposition of invoice or drug receipt form once drug is received.

6.   The following information should be supplied to the department of pharmacy, preferably in a readily retrievable, standardized format:

a.   Storage conditions required before and after preparation.

b.   Amounts and types of diluents for reconstitution and administration and the resulting final concentration of active drug.

c.   Stability of the prepared (i.e., ready-to-administer, reconstituted, or diluted) product.

d.   Compatibility with other products.

e.   Light sensitivity.

f.   Filtration needs.

g.   Expiration dates.

h.   Special instructions for preparation and administration.

i.   Acceptable and recommended routes and methods of administration, including rates.

j.   Adverse effects on or during administration (e.g., pain, phlebitis, and nausea) and their avoidance or treatment.

k.   Usual dosage regimens and highest dose tested.

l.   Contraindications.

m.   Drug interactions, if known.

n.   Special precautions for storage, handling, and disposal of the drugs, including cytotoxic and hazardous drugs. For all hazardous drugs, the department of pharmacy must be supplied with material safety data sheets.

o.   Mechanism of action/pharmacology.

p.   Pharmacokinetic characteristics.

q.   Criteria for patient exclusion.

7.   If all unused drugs are to be returned to the sponsor, information regarding storage and return handling procedures should be provided to the pharmacy. Drugs that are contaminated, outdated, or otherwise unsuitable should be returned to the sponsor or destroyed according to the institution's policies and procedures. These options should be agreed on beforehand by the sponsor and the pharmacy.

8.   Additional educational materials for use in informing pharmacists, physicians, and nurses about the investigational drug and research protocol should be available in the pharmacy.

9.   A complete copy of the research protocol and drug information sheet should be supplied to the pharmacy department.

10. An appropriate allotment of research funds should be designated to the pharmacy department for

a.   Personnel.

b.   Storage facilities.

c.   Equipment.

d.   Ancillary products, such as diluents and solutions.

e.   Forms and miscellaneous clerical materials.

f.   Computer and other data processing costs.

g.   Other expenses attributable to the pharmacy's involvement in the study.

h.   Apportioned pharmacy overhead costs.

11. Sponsors should respond to requests for information from departments of pharmacy involved in treating one or a few patients without formal research approval. This may occur, for example, when a principal investigator wishes to treat a patient hospitalized (e.g., in an emergency) at a facility other than his or her principal practice site.

12. Sponsors should consult with pharmacy departments, physicians, and others involved in their investigational drug studies for information when marketing approval for an investigational drug is sought. Because of their experience with the agent, these practitioners can supply valuable suggestions for labeling, packaging, palatability, routes of administration, and other dosage form characteristics, as well as information regarding patient monitoring and education.

13. The aforementioned guidelines would also apply to Phase IV investigational drugs.

14. A pharmaceutical company that sponsors an investigational drug study should provide final closure details within 6 months of trial completion. This includes prompt notification of closure, directions for drug disposition, and final audits of all study records.

References

1.   Accreditation manual for hospitals. Vol. 1: Standards. Oakbrook Terrace, IL: Joint Commission on Accreditation of Healthcare Organizations; 1990.

2.   American Society of Hospital Pharmacists. ASHP guidelines: minimum standard for pharmacies in institutions. *Am J Hosp Pharm.* 1985; 42:372–5.

3.   Stolar MH, ed. Pharmacy-coordinated investigational drug services. Revised ed. Bethesda, MD: American Society of Hospital Pharmacists; 1986.

[a]In this document, investigational drugs are defined as those that are being considered for but have not as yet received marketing approval by the Food and Drug Administration for human use and those drugs that have FDA approval for at least one indication but are being studied as research medications for new indications, new routes of administration, or new dosage forms.

[b]The principles and procedures described here are applicable to all clinical drug studies, not just those involving investigational drugs.

[c]In certain emergency situations, prior consent may be waived.

Approved by the ASHP Board of Directors, November 14, 1990. Revised by the ASHP Council on Professional Affairs. Supersedes previous versions approved December 12, 1978, and November 18, 1982.

The bibliographic citation for this document is as follows: American Society of Hospital Pharmacists. ASHP guidelines for the use of investigational drugs in organized health-care settings. *Am J Hosp Pharm.* 1991; 48:315–9.

ASHP Guidelines for Implementing and Obtaining Compensation for Clinical Services by Pharmacists

For some time, pharmacies in organized health-care settings have been moving from a product-centered structure to a more patient-oriented clinical practice. Clinical pharmacy services or patient-oriented pharmaceutical services are now a recognized and necessary component of health care. However, new trends in reimbursement, such as prospective pricing and capitation payments, provide different incentives for hospitals—to manage in terms of product lines instead of patient services.

In such a financial environment, it is essential that the value of any nonproduct-centered service be well documented and that the service be cost-justifiable. Pharmacists planning to initiate new clinical services may have to meet certain administrative requirements, including the following: (1) to provide an accurate accounting of all of the resources required; (2) to delineate the costs of the service and its effect on patient outcomes; (3) to obtain approval from the institution's administration and medical staff for provision of the service on a routine basis; and (4) to identify an appropriate mechanism for patient charging and for obtaining reimbursement or payment[a] from the third-party payer.

Generally, third-party payers do not have formal policies that prohibit their reimbursing and paying providers for clinical pharmacy services. However, payment is predicated on acceptance and endorsement of the service by the involved administrative and medical staffs and by the third-party payer's formal review and approval of the benefit coverage (and, in the case of patients covered by private insurance plans, by the provision of the service as a covered benefit of their plan). Approval of reimbursement for clinical services, however, varies from area to area and from carrier to carrier.

This document presents a set of general guidelines for use in obtaining administrative support and subsequent reimbursement or payment for a new pharmaceutical service. Often, many steps of the process may be omitted. For example, it should not be necessary to conduct a preliminary trial of a widely accepted, though not universally adopted, service (such as use of patient medication profiles). However, a careful review of the literature may be necessary for documenting the direct impact of the new service on expenses and determining whether or not the proposed new service will generate a revenue surplus. With fixed reimbursement, hospital administrators are unlikely to approve any new service unless its benefits are fully documented and unless its result is an overall savings.

When clinical pharmacy services are initially established in the hospital, they should be viewed as an important component of the drug use continuum, not as a separate entity. After establishment of the initial clinical services at the hospital, the approach to obtaining additional clinical services should focus on patient audit results and on the approval of the pharmacy and therapeutics (P&T) committee.

These guidelines are written for use by pharmacy directors in hospitals. However, they can be adapted for use in other situations (e.g., by a pharmacist providing services as part of a medical group practice or a health maintenance organization).

The guidelines are as follows:

1. Prepare, for the provider's administration, a written proposal for short-term (e.g., 3 months) implementation of the proposed service. The proposal should include the following elements:
   a. A clear, concise description of the service.
   b. The rationale for the service, including published references if available.
   c. Written support for the service by the P&T committee and other appropriate parties (e.g., infections committee, department of nursing, and applicable medical services).
   d. The expected benefits of the service to patients and the institution in terms of costs and quality of care, as measured by indices such as decrease in length of stay, decrease in incidence of therapeutic failures, decrease in duration of therapy, and decrease in drug expenditures. *This is the most important section of the document; for the proposal to receive administration approval, the available information and calculations must prove that the benefits exceed the costs of providing the service.*
   e. Estimated startup and operating expenses and revenue[b] of the service, plus its personnel, equipment, and material requirements.
2. Obtain the administration's formal approval of the implementation project.
3. Initiate the project, keeping complete records of all expenses, outputs (e.g., the number of patient consultations), and personnel hours devoted to it. In addition to the indices listed in Item 1d, the following elements should be documented: changes in length of stay, costs of treatment, and changes in levels of personnel productivity. This information will be needed to develop charges for the service and to obtain reimbursement or payment.
4. On completion of the project, prepare a report of its implementation for the administration. This report should focus on fiscal and workload data, including total pharmacy cost per patient, service unit, or diagnosis-related group, and a suggested charge based on these data. Information on acceptance of the program by patients and staff should be included when possible. This report should also project the manpower and financial resources needed to perform the service as a routine pharmacy function.
5. Obtain formal approval from administration to implement the service on an institutionwide basis.
6. Assist the institution's administration and financial manager in developing the information needed to include the costs of the service in its compensation agreements with third-party carriers. To obtain compensation, certain administrative requirements (such as formal approval of the service by the P&T committee) may have to be met.
7. Regularly evaluate the objectives and impact of the new program or service, based on changes in payment

mechanisms, and prepare annual updates on these clinical pharmacy services. For example, it will become important to report annual cost savings or decreased readmissions over a baseline figure.

---

[a]Generally, payment refers to prospective compensation, and reimbursement refers to retrospective compensation.

[b]In cooperation with the provider's fiscal offices, and depending on the acceptance of the service within the health-care system, the pharmacy department should determine whether payment for the service can or should be received.

Approved by the ASHP Board of Directors, April 25, 1985. Developed by the ASHP Council on Administrative Affairs. Supersedes the "ASHP Guidelines for Implementing and Obtaining Reimbursement for Clinical Pharmaceutical Services," approved November 13–14, 1980.

The bibliographic citation for this document is as follows: American Society of Hospital Pharmacists. ASHP guidelines for implementing and obtaining compensation for clinical services by pharmacists. *Am J Hosp Pharm.* 1985; 42:1581–2.

ASHP Guidelines on Medication-Use Evaluation

Medication-use evaluation (MUE) is a performance improvement method that focuses on evaluating and improving medication-use processes with the goal of optimal patient outcomes. MUE may be applied to a medication or therapeutic class, disease state or condition, a medication-use process (prescribing, preparing and dispensing, administering, and monitoring), or specific outcomes.[1] Further, it may be applied in and among the various practice settings of organized health systems.

MUE encompasses the goals and objectives of drug-use evaluation (DUE) in its broadest application, with an emphasis on improving patient outcomes. Use of "MUE," rather than "DUE,"[2] emphasizes the need for a more multifaceted approach to improving medication use. MUE has a common goal with the pharmaceutical care it supports: to improve an individual patient's quality of life through achievement of predefined, medication-related therapeutic outcomes.[3,4] Through its focus on the system of medication use, the MUE process helps to identify actual and potential medication-related problems, resolve actual medication-related problems, and prevent potential medication-related problems that could interfere with achieving optimum outcomes from medication therapy.

In organized health systems, MUE must be conducted as an organizationally authorized program or process that is proactive, criteria based, designed and managed by an interdisciplinary team, and systematically carried out. It is conducted as a collaborative effort of prescribers, pharmacists, nurses, administrators, and other health care professionals on behalf of their patients.

MUE Objectives

Some typical objectives of MUE include

- Promoting optimal medication therapy.
- Preventing medication-related problems.
- Evaluating the effectiveness of medication therapy.
- Improving patient safety.
- Establishing interdisciplinary consensus on medication-use processes.
- Stimulating improvements in medication-use processes.
- Stimulating standardization in medication-use processes.
- Enhancing opportunities, through standardization, to assess the value of innovative medication-use practices from both patient-outcome and resource-utilization perspectives.
- Minimizing procedural variations that contribute to suboptimal outcomes of medication use.
- Identifying areas in which further information and education for health care professionals may be needed.
- Minimizing costs of medication therapy. These costs may be only partly related to the direct cost of medications themselves. When medications are selected and managed optimally from the outset, the costs of complications and wasted resources are minimized, and overall costs are decreased.
- Meeting or exceeding internal and external quality standards (e.g., professional practice standards, accreditation standards, or government laws and regulations).

Steps of the MUE Process

While the specific approach varies with the practice setting and patient population being served, the following common steps occur in the ongoing MUE process:

- Establish organizational authority for the MUE process and identify responsible individuals and groups.
- Develop screening mechanisms (indicators) for comprehensive surveillance of the medication-use system.
- Set priorities for in-depth analysis of important aspects of medication use.
- Inform health care professionals (and others as necessary) in the practice setting(s) about the objectives and expected benefits of the MUE process.
- Establish criteria, guidelines, treatment protocols, and standards of care for specific medications and medication-use processes. These should be based on sound scientific evidence from the medical and pharmaceutical literature.
- Educate health care professionals to promote the use of criteria, guidelines, treatment protocols, and standards of care.
- Establish mechanisms for timely communication among health care professionals.
- Initiate the use of MUE criteria, guidelines, treatment protocols, and standards of care in the medication-use process.
- Collect data and evaluate care.
- Develop and implement plans for improvement of the medication-use process based on MUE findings (if indicated).
- Assess the effectiveness of actions taken, and document improvements.
- Incorporate improvements into criteria, guidelines, treatment protocols, and standards of care, when indicated.
- Repeat the cycle of planning, evaluating, and taking action for ongoing improvement in medication-use processes.
- Regularly assess the effectiveness of the MUE process itself and make needed improvements.

Selecting Medications and Medication-Use Processes for Evaluation

Medications or medication-use processes should be selected for evaluation for one or more of the following reasons:

1. The medication is known or suspected to cause adverse reactions, or it interacts with another medication, food, or diagnostic procedure in a way that presents a significant health risk.
2. The medication is used in the treatment of patients who may be at high risk for adverse reactions.
3. The medication-use process affects a large number of patients or the medication is frequently prescribed.
4. The medication or medication-use process is a critical component of care for a specific disease, condition, or procedure.

5. The medication is potentially toxic or causes discomfort at normal doses.
6. The medication is most effective when used in a specific way.
7. The medication is under consideration for formulary retention, addition, or deletion.
8. The medication or medication-use process is one for which suboptimal use would have a negative effect on patient outcomes or system costs.
9. Use of the medication is expensive.

Indicators Suggesting a Need for MUE Analysis

Certain events (indicators) serve as "flags" of potential opportunities to improve medication use. Some are

- Adverse medication events, including medication errors, preventable adverse drug reactions, and toxicity.
- Signs of treatment failures, such as unexpected readmissions and bacterial resistance to anti-infective therapy.
- Pharmacist interventions to improve medication therapy, categorized by medication and type of intervention.
- Nonformulary medications used or requested.
- Patient dissatisfaction or deterioration in quality of life.

Roles and Responsibilities in the MUE Process

The roles of individual health care professionals in MUE may vary according to practice setting, organizational goals, and available resources. The organizational body (e.g., quality management committee, pharmacy and therapeutics committee) responsible for the MUE process should have, at a minimum, prescriber, pharmacist, nurse, and administrator representation. Other health care professionals should contribute their unique perspectives when the evaluation and improvement process addresses their areas of expertise and responsibility. Temporary working groups may be used for specific improvement efforts.

Pharmacist's Responsibilities in MUE

Pharmacists, by virtue of their expertise and their mission of ensuring proper medication use, should exert leadership and work collaboratively with other members of the health care team in the ongoing process of medication-use evaluation and improvement.[5] Responsibilities of pharmacists in the MUE process include

- Developing an operational plan for MUE programs and processes that are consistent with the health system's overall goals and resource capabilities.
- Working collaboratively with prescribers and others to develop criteria for specific medications and to design effective medication-use processes.
- Reviewing individual medication orders against medication-use criteria and consulting with prescribers and others in the process as needed.
- Managing MUE programs and processes.
- Collecting, analyzing, and evaluating patient-specific data to identify, resolve, and prevent medication-related problems.

- Interpreting and reporting MUE findings and recommending changes in medication-use processes.
- Providing information and education based on MUE findings.

Resources

Some resources helpful in designing and managing an MUE process are listed here.

- The primary professional literature and up-to-date reference texts are key resources necessary for the development of MUE criteria. In general, local consensus should be based on medical and pharmaceutical literature recommendations.
- Published criteria, such as found in *AJHP* and ASHP's *Criteria for Drug Use Evaluation* (volumes 1–4), provide medication-specific criteria that may be adapted for local use.
- Computer software programs, including proprietary programs designed specifically for MUE functions, may be helpful in managing data and reporting.
- External standards-setting bodies, such as the Joint Commission on Accreditation of Healthcare Organizations, publish medication-use indicators that can help to identify portions of the medication-use system that require improvement.

Follow-up Actions in an MUE Process

The MUE process itself should be reviewed regularly to identify opportunities for its improvement. The success of an MUE process should be assessed in terms of improved patient outcomes. Medication-use system changes that evolve from MUE findings should be developed by the departments and medical services with responsibility for providing care, rather than solely through a committee having oversight for MUE (e.g., a pharmacy and therapeutics committee). Typical follow-up actions based on MUE findings include contact with individual prescribers and other health care professionals, information and education (newsletters, seminars, clinical care guidelines) for health care professionals, changes in medication-use systems, and changes in medication-therapy monitoring processes. MUE should be conducted as an ongoing interdisciplinary and collaborative improvement process. Punitive reactions to quality concerns are often counterproductive. It is important to communicate and commend positive achievements (care that meets or exceeds expectations) and improvements.

Pitfalls

Some common pitfalls to avoid in performing MUE activities include the following[6]:

1. Lack of authority. An MUE process that does not involve the medical staff is likely to be ineffective. Authoritative medical staff support and formal organizational recognition of the MUE process are necessary.
2. Lack of organization. Without a clear definition of the roles and responsibilities of individuals involved (e.g., who will develop criteria, who will communicate with other departments, who will collect and summarize data, and who will evaluate data), an MUE process may not succeed.

3. Poor communication. Everyone affected by the MUE process should understand its importance to the health system, its goals, and its procedures. The pharmacist should manage the MUE process and have the responsibility and authority to ensure timely communication among all professionals involved in the medication-use process. Criteria for medication use should be communicated to all affected professionals prior to the evaluation of care. MUE activity should be a standing agenda item for appropriate quality-of-care committees responsible for aspects of medication use.

4. Poor documentation. MUE activities should be well documented, including summaries of MUE actions with respect to individual medication orders and the findings and conclusions from collective evaluations. Documentation should address recommendations made and follow-up actions.

5. Lack of involvement. The MUE process is not a one-person task, nor is it the responsibility of a single department or professional group. Medication-use criteria should be developed through an interdisciplinary consensus process. Lack of administrative support can severely limit the effectiveness of MUE. The benefits of MUE should be conveyed in terms of improving patient outcomes and minimizing health-system costs.

6. Lack of follow-through. A one-time study or evaluation independent of the overall MUE process will have limited success in improving patient outcomes. The effectiveness of initial actions must be assessed and the action plan adjusted if necessary. It is important not to lose sight of the improvement goals.

7. Evaluation methodology that impedes patient care. Data collection should not consume so much time that patient care activities suffer. Interventions that can improve care for an individual patient should not be withheld because of the sampling technique or evaluation methodology.

8. Lack of readily retrievable data and information management. Existing data capabilities need to be assessed and maximum benefit obtained from available computerized information management resources. Deficiencies in information gathering and analysis should be identified and priorities for upgrading information support established.

References

1. Nadzam DM. Development of medication-use indicators by the Joint Commission on Accreditation of Healthcare Organizations. *Am J Hosp Pharm.* 1991; 48:1925–30.

2. American Society of Hospital Pharmacists. ASHP guidelines on the pharmacist's role in drug-use evaluation. *Am J Hosp Pharm.* 1988; 45:385–6.

3. Hepler CD, Strand LM. Opportunities and responsibilities in pharmaceutical care. *Am J Hosp Pharm.* 1990; 47:533–43.

4. American Society of Hospital Pharmacists. ASHP statement on pharmaceutical care. *Am J Hosp Pharm.* 1993; 30:1720–3.

5. Angaran DM. Quality assurance to quality improvement: measuring and monitoring pharmaceutical care. *Am J Hosp Pharm.* 1991; 48:1901–7.

6. Todd MW. Drug use evaluation. In: Brown TR, ed. Handbook of institutional pharmacy practice. 3rd ed. Bethesda, MD: American Society of Hospital Pharmacists; 1992.

Approved by the ASHP Board of Directors, April 24, 1996. Developed by the ASHP Council on Professional Affairs. Supersedes the ASHP Guidelines on the Pharmacist's Role in Drug-Use Evaluation, dated November 19, 1987.

The bibliographic citation for this document is as follows: American Society of Health-System Pharmacists. ASHP guidelines on medication-use evaluation. *Am J Health-Syst Pharm.* 1996; 53:1953–5.

ASHP Guidelines on Pharmaceutical Services for Ambulatory Patients

This document is a guide to the provision of pharmaceutical services to ambulatory patients. These guidelines are intended for use by all pharmacists, including those practicing in hospitals, clinics, managed care settings, mail service pharmacies, community pharmacies, and ambulatory care centers and those serving patients in nursing homes and other extended-care settings in an ambulatory care prescription-dispensing manner.

Ambulatory care pharmaceutical operations and services occur in a broad spectrum of settings, from freestanding pharmacies to institutions such as hospitals. Because this document is intended to be as broadly applicable as possible, terms such as *director, pharmacist, medical staff, nursing staff, department, pharmacy and therapeutics committee,* and *organization* are used in their broadest senses. Because of differences in settings and organizational complexity, some aspects of the document may be more applicable in certain settings than others. The principles underlying the statements in this document are intended to be sufficiently clear that pharmacists in various settings can adapt the ideas for application in their own work sites.

Administration

All services must be directed by a professionally competent, legally qualified pharmacist. The director should be thoroughly knowledgeable about and have experience in ambulatory care pharmacy practice and management. Preferably, the director should have completed an accredited ambulatory care pharmacy practice residency or have had equivalent experience. The director should be assisted by such other pharmacists and staff as required by the scope and volume of activity. The director should be responsible for

1. Setting long- and short-range goals of the pharmacy or the ambulatory care service.
2. Developing plans and schedules for achieving these goals.
3. Supervising the implementation and execution of the plan.
4. Determining whether the goals are being met and making the appropriate operational changes as necessary.
5. Preparing periodic qualitative and quantitative reports with respect to achievement of the goals.

The director is responsible for promulgating policies and procedures pertaining to personnel assigned to ambulatory care pharmaceutical services. Written position descriptions should exist for all positions. The roles, limits of authority, and supervisory procedures for supportive personnel should be clearly defined and in writing. Scheduled periodic performance evaluations should occur for all personnel. Written policies and procedures should exist for

1. The recruitment, hiring, orientation, discipline, and discharge of all personnel.

2. Ensuring that all personnel have or receive the education, training, and experience required for their assigned duties; provisions should be made as required for staff development and continuing education.
3. Establishing and maintaining staff work schedules that meet the needs of patients served by the organization.

If the pharmacy is a site for the education and training of pharmacy undergraduate or graduate students, residents, or fellows, the director should be responsible for all operational and patient care actions of such "students." In the case of residents, the director should serve as the program director or preceptor.

In sites with multiple pharmacies, a pharmacist in charge should be designated for each separate location.

The director is responsible for

1. Promulgating policies and procedures with respect to all production, dispensing, and service operations.
2. The ongoing monitoring of the quality of the products and services of the pharmacy.
3. Financial management of the pharmacy, including the preparation of budgets and financial analyses and reports.
4. Ensuring the pharmacy's compliance with applicable standards (e.g., accreditation standards) and local, state, and federal laws and regulations.
5. The application of automated data processing systems as they pertain to the operation and services of the pharmacy.
6. Committee participation to interface with the medical and nursing staffs and other departments as applicable.
7. The establishment of agreements with outside pharmacies and pharmacists for the provision of ambulatory care pharmaceutical services to patients of the organization.

Facilities and Equipment

The pharmacy should be located in an area that facilitates the provision of services to patients. Space and equipment in an amount and type to provide for the professional and administrative functions of the pharmacy and to provide for secure and environmentally controlled storage and preparation of drugs should exist. Designated spaces and equipment suitable for packaging, labeling, and compounding drugs and preparing injectable drugs should exist.

There should be private areas for pharmacist–patient consultations. There should be adequate space and resources for the provision of drug information. There should be adequate data processing resources to maintain patient medication profile records, to perform necessary patient billing procedures, to manage drug inventories, and, preferably, to interface with other available computerized systems for the purpose of obtaining patient-specific clinical information necessary to perform drug therapy monitoring and other clinical functions. There should be a convenient waiting area for patients.

Drug Order Processing

All dispensing functions must be performed by or under the supervision of a pharmacist.

The pharmacist should develop familiarity with the prescribing practices of the individual prescribers who typically prescribe for patients served by the pharmacy.

The pharmacist should interact with prescribers to exert a positive influence on prescribing. Interaction should occur not only when prescribing incongruities are encountered but also when a more optimal regimen may be available. Prescribing should be influenced by direct individual interaction and through broad interventions. Examples of broad interventions include educational programs, drug information publications, formulary systems, pharmacy and therapeutics (P&T) committee policies, and drug use evaluation programs.

Drugs should be administered and dispensed to ambulatory patients only on the oral or written order of authorized prescribers. Mechanisms should exist for the pharmacist to review original written (or direct copies of original written) drug orders before dispensing drugs. Transcribed drug orders prepared by nonpharmacists are not acceptable. Oral drug orders should be accepted only by a pharmacist.

The clinical appropriateness of the choice of drug and its dosage, route of administration, and amount should be reviewed by the pharmacist. Patients' medication histories should be obtained and assessed, including the use of prescription and nonprescription drugs. The patient's current and previous diseases (and previous treatments used for them), concurrent drugs, allergies and the potential for toxicity, drug interactions, and adverse drug reactions should be reviewed. Any duplication of drugs and any potential drug–drug, drug–food, or drug–laboratory test interactions should be assessed for clinical significance and dealt with appropriately. Pharmacokinetic data, including serum drug level information, should be used as appropriate in the review process.

Medication profiles must be maintained for all patients. The pharmacist must monitor profiles for indications of drug abuse, misuse, or noncompliance. Any problems encountered should be resolved by the pharmacist.

When legally permissible, the pharmacist should make medication histories and medication profile information available to other health-care providers responsible for the patient's care.

The pharmacists should have ready access to the patient's medical "chart" information. The pharmacist should have chart notation privileges and should document oral communications in the chart and in his or her files.

The pharmacist should be an integral part of any program involving home drug administration. The pharmacist should be involved in evaluating potential home health-care patients to determine whether they are capable of safely and effectively participating in the home administration of drugs.

The pharmacist should prepare, in a timely and accurate manner, those drug formulations, strengths, dosage forms, and packages prescribed, including those that are not commercially available but are needed in the care of patients. The pharmacist should assess the physical and chemical compatibility of substances to be compounded and select packaging materials for preserving the integrity, cleanliness, and potency of compounded and noncompounded drugs. Adequate quality-assurance procedures should exist in compounding operations.

Pharmacy personnel should prepare all injectable drugs to be administered to ambulatory and home care patients, except in emergencies.

Appropriate checking and quality-assurance procedures must be used to ensure the accuracy of all drug products and drug preparation and dispensing processes. Activities of supportive personnel must be supervised by a pharmacist.

The pharmacist must take an active role in direct drug therapy management.

Drugs dispensed must be completely and correctly labeled and packaged in accordance with all applicable regulations and accepted standards of practice. When feasible, it is desirable for drugs to be dispensed in unopened manufacturers' packages. Whenever possible, drugs should be supplied in tamper-evident packaging.

At a minimum, containers of drugs dispensed to ambulatory patients must bear the following information:

1. Name, address, and telephone number of the pharmacy.
2. Date of dispensing.
3. Serial number of the prescription.
4. Patient's full name.
5. Name of the drug (generic name, unless the number of generic ingredients, e.g., in a combination product, precludes listing them).
6. Directions to the patient for use of the drug.
7. Name of prescriber.
8. Precautionary information.
9. Initials (or name) of the responsible pharmacist.

Other information that may be required by applicable state and federal requirements must appear as well.

Patient Education. The pharmacist must routinely provide consultation appropriate for the individual patient.

The pharmacist should ensure that the patient receives and understands all information required for the proper use of the drug. Directions for use should be clearly expressed. Supplementary written information (e.g., patient information leaflets and auxiliary labels on containers) should be provided as necessary to reinforce oral communication.

The pharmacy should maintain appropriate information resources and develop mechanisms for transmitting information to patients.

The pharmacy should maintain a body of pharmaceutical literature containing current primary, secondary, and tertiary literature sources. Scientific and professional practice journals in pharmacy and medicine should be directly available or readily accessible in a timely enough manner to enable clinical decisionmaking on behalf of immediate patients.

Reference texts should be current and provide detailed information in at least the following areas: drug action, drug side effects, adverse drug effects, doses, drugs of choice, efficacy, formulations, incompatibilities, identifications (foreign and American), indications, interactions, laws and regulations, pharmacology, nonprescription drugs, pathophysiology, pharmacokinetics, and toxicology.

Appropriate to the patient population served, information for pharmacists and educational materials for patients should be available on such topics as

1. Hypertension.
2. Cardiovascular disease.

3. Diabetes.
4. Hypercholesterolemia.
5. Nutrition.
6. Physical fitness.
7. Smoking cessation.
8. Substance abuse.
9. Arthritis.
10. Asthma and chronic obstructive pulmonary disease.
11. Seizure disorders.
12. Common household poisoning and treatment.
13. Sexually transmitted diseases.

Using suitable oral, written, or audiovisual communication techniques, the pharmacist must inform, educate, and counsel patients (or their representatives or caregivers) as appropriate about the following items for each medication dispensed:

1. Name (trade name, generic name, common synonym, or other descriptive name).
2. Intended use and expected action.
3. Route, dosage form, dosage, and administration schedule.
4. Special directions for preparation.
5. Special directions for administration.
6. Precautions to be observed during administration.
7. Common adverse effects that may be encountered, including their avoidance and actions required if they occur.
8. Techniques for self-monitoring of drug therapy.
9. Proper storage.
10. Potential drug–drug or drug–food interactions or other therapeutic contraindications.
11. Prescription refill information.
12. Action to be taken in the event of a missed dose.
13. Any other information peculiar to the specific patient or drug.

These points are applicable to both prescription and nonprescription drugs. In addition, pharmacists should counsel patients as appropriate in the proper selection of nonprescription drugs as well as when and whether they should be used.

The patient must be monitored for adverse effects and therapeutic outcome at each encounter. Laboratory tests to assess therapeutic outcome and minimize or detect adverse effects should be recommended at the appropriate times.

Adverse drug reactions must be reported to drug manufacturers, appropriate agencies, and organizational committees.

The pharmacy must maintain prescription records on file for the appropriate time period in compliance with state and federal requirements. Computer systems for prescription records must be secure against unauthorized entry.

Dispensing by Prescribers. Since drugs are potentially hazardous and patients may lack the knowledge necessary to use most drugs safely and effectively without professional advice, certain fundamental protections should be available to all patients when drugs are dispensed to them. Among these protections are the following:

• Professional assessment of the patient's complete medication history, including the use of prescription and nonprescription drugs.

• Professional assessment of the clinical appropriateness of each drug prescribed (and its dose and dosage regimen) in light of the patient's medication history, current and previous diseases, concurrent drugs, allergies and the potential for toxicity, drug interactions, and adverse drug reactions.

• Professional assessment of the physical and chemical compatibility of substances to be compounded.

• Accurate and appropriate selection and timely preparation and compounding of drug products for dispensing.

• Selection of packaging materials suitable for each drug's intended use and for preserving each drug's integrity, cleanliness, and potency.

• Provision of accurate, understandable, and legally complete and correct labeling for each drug.

• Appropriate counseling and education for the patient regarding each drug's use and its potential adverse effects at the time of dispensing and thereafter, as needed.

• Maintenance of patient-specific drug use records and accountability records of all drugs dispensed.

These protections should be routinely and readily available to all patients. Any circumstance under which these protections must be diminished should be exceptional and temporary.

These pharmaceutical functions, including dispensing, should be performed by or under the supervision of licensed individuals with professional and clinical pharmaceutical expertise.

Prescribers and pharmacists should collaborate professionally in prescribing and dispensing activities to provide an informational check-and-balance system that will minimize errors and optimize rational drug therapy.

Both prescribing and dispensing of drugs should be performed in a circumstance free of potential financial conflict of interest on the part of both the prescriber and the dispenser. A potential for financial conflict of interest is pronounced when the same individual performs both the prescribing and the dispensing functions.

Given the above, arrangements in which prescribers routinely perform pharmaceutical functions, including dispensing, potentially deprive patients of certain fundamental protections and are, therefore, undesirable.

In exceptional circumstances (e.g., when access to a pharmacist is not feasible for the patient), prescribers may have to dispense. When they do so, they are performing pharmaceutical functions and they must comply with all relevant laws and standards governing pharmaceutical functions. They should personally perform the dispensing; the action must not be delegated.

Other Operational Guidelines

The pharmacist should be responsible for establishing the pharmacy's hours of operation in keeping with patients' needs.

The pharmacy should maintain an up-to-date formulary of drug products approved by the medical staff. The drugs to be included in the formulary should be selected by the medical staff, e.g., through a P&T committee or its equivalent. The pharmacist must be responsible for establishing specifications for drug products and for selecting their sources of supply.

The pharmacist must be responsible for the procurement, distribution, and control of all drugs for ambulatory patients.

The pharmacist should participate in the evaluation, selection, distribution, and control of all drug administration devices used for patients. The pharmacist should ensure that patients receive instruction in the proper use of such devices.

The pharmacist should be responsible for drug-product problem reporting and drug administration device defect reporting. All defects should be reported to the products' manufacturers, the United States Pharmacopeial Convention, Inc., and the Food and Drug Administration.

Adequate security must be maintained to prevent drug theft. Only authorized personnel should be allowed in pharmacies, drug storerooms, or other areas where drugs are stored.

Policies for the distribution and security of prescription order forms should exist.

An accountability system for controlled substances that meets all applicable governmental requirements must be maintained.

Policies and procedures should exist for the removal from use of any drugs subjected to a product recall. Provisions should exist for contacting patients to whom recalled drugs may have been previously dispensed.

The pharmacist must establish policies and procedures for handling hazardous drugs.

Stocks of drugs held in nonpharmacy areas (e.g., nursing station, clinic, or physician's office) for direct administration to ambulatory patients should be minimal. To the extent possible, such stocks should be limited to emergency drugs. All drug storage areas must be routinely inspected to ensure that no expired or unusable items are present and that all items are properly labeled and stored.

The pharmacist must be responsible for supplying and checking for expired drugs and drug supplies in emergency carts or kits.

The pharmacist should be responsible for policies and procedures pertaining to the use of investigational drugs (if used). The pharmacist should be responsible for storing, packaging, labeling, and distributing investigational drugs and maintaining inventory records. The pharmacy should be the designated shipment destination of all investigational drugs shipped by sponsors to investigators. The pharmacist should be responsible for the provision of drug administration information about these drugs to personnel administering the drugs.

To the extent possible, the use of drug samples should be prohibited. A written policy and procedure on the use of samples that is approved by the medical staff should exist.

Written procedures should exist for the provision of drugs and pharmaceutical services in the event of a disaster.

Written policies and procedures governing the activities of drug manufacturers' sales representatives should exist. These policies and procedures should be made known to sales representatives.

The pharmacist providing pharmaceutical care to ambulatory patients is responsible for obtaining timely professional continuing education pertinent to the care and services he or she provides.[1]

Reference

1. American Society of Hospital Pharmacists. ASHP statement on continuing education. *Am J Hosp Pharm.* 1990; 47:1855.

Approved by the ASHP Board of Directors, November 14, 1990. Developed by the ASHP Council on Professional Affairs. Supersedes the "ASHP Statement on the Provision of Pharmaceutical Services in Ambulatory Care Settings," approved March 20, 1980, and April 21, 1980, and the "ASHP Guidelines: Minimum Standard for Ambulatory Care Pharmaceutical Services," approved November 19, 1981.

The bibliographic citation for this document is as follows: American Society of Hospital Pharmacists. ASHP guidelines on pharmaceutical services for ambulatory patients. *Am J Hosp Pharm.* 1991; 48: 311–5.

ASHP Guidelines on Adverse Drug Reaction Monitoring and Reporting

Pharmacists in organized health care systems should develop comprehensive, ongoing programs for monitoring and reporting adverse drug reactions (ADRs).[1] It is the pharmacist's responsibility and professional obligation to report any suspected ADRs. ADR-monitoring and reporting programs encourage ADR surveillance, facilitate ADR documentation, promote the reporting of ADRs, provide a mechanism for monitoring the safety of drug use in high-risk patient populations, and stimulate the education of health professionals regarding potential ADRs. A comprehensive, ongoing ADR program should include mechanisms for monitoring, detecting, evaluating, documenting, and reporting ADRs as well as intervening and providing educational feedback to prescribers, other health care professionals, and patients. Additionally, ADR programs should focus on identifying problems leading to ADRs, planning for positive changes, and measuring the results of these changes. Positive outcomes resulting from an ADR program should be emphasized to support program growth and development.

ASHP does not suggest that there is a predictable rate of incidence or severity of ADRs. The number and severity of ADRs reported in a given organization or setting would vary with the organization's size, type, patient mix, drugs used, and the ADR definition used.

Definitions

ASHP defines a significant ADR as any unexpected, unintended, undesired, or excessive response to a drug that

1. Requires discontinuing the drug (therapeutic or diagnostic),
2. Requires changing the drug therapy,
3. Requires modifying the dose (except for minor dosage adjustments),
4. Necessitates admission to a hospital,
5. Prolongs stay in a health care facility,
6. Necessitates supportive treatment,
7. Significantly complicates diagnosis,
8. Negatively affects prognosis, or
9. Results in temporary or permanent harm, disability, or death.

Consistent with this definition, an *allergic reaction* (an immunologic hypersensitivity, occurring as the result of unusual sensitivity to a drug) and an *idiosyncratic reaction* (an abnormal susceptibility to a drug that is peculiar to the individual) are also considered ADRs.

Several other definitions of ADRs exist, including those of the World Health Organization (WHO),[2] Karch and Lasagna,[3] and the Food and Drug Administration (FDA).[4]

WHO: "Any response to a drug which is noxious and unintended, and which occurs at doses normally used in man for prophylaxis, diagnosis, or therapy of disease, or for the modification of physiological function."

Karch and Lasagna: "Any response to a drug that is noxious and unintended, and that occurs at doses used in humans for prophylaxis, diagnosis, or therapy, excluding failure to accomplish the intended purpose."

FDA: For reporting purposes, FDA categorizes a *serious adverse event* (events relating to drugs or devices) as one in which "the patient outcome is death, life-threatening (real risk of dying), hospitalization (initial or prolonged), disability (significant, persistent, or permanent), congenital anomaly, or required intervention to prevent permanent impairment or damage."

For perspective, it may be helpful to note events that are not classified as ADRs. A *side effect* is defined by ASHP as an expected, well-known reaction resulting in little or no change in patient management (e.g., drowsiness or dry mouth due to administration of certain antihistamines or nausea associated with the use of antineoplastics). ASHP further defines a side effect as an effect with a predictable frequency and an effect whose intensity and occurrence are related to the size of the dose. Additionally, drug withdrawal, drug-abuse syndromes, accidental poisoning, and drug-overdose complications should not be defined as ADRs.

While individual health care organizations may need to apply ADR surveillance to different degrees for different groups of patients, ASHP believes it would be greatly beneficial if a common definition of ADRs were used in all settings to facilitate reporting, collective surveillance, and ADR-trend research.

Program Features

A comprehensive ADR-monitoring and reporting program should be an integral part of an organization's overall drug-use system. An ADR-monitoring and reporting program should include the following features:

1. The program should establish
    a. An ongoing and concurrent (during drug therapy) surveillance system based on the reporting of suspected ADRs by pharmacists, physicians, nurses, or patients.[5]
    b. A prospective (before drug therapy) surveillance system for high-risk drugs or patients with a high risk for ADRs.
    c. A concurrent surveillance system for monitoring alerting orders. Alerting orders include the use of "tracer" drugs that are used to treat common ADRs (e.g., orders for immediate doses of antihistamines, epinephrine, and corticosteroids), abrupt discontinuation or decreases in dosage of a drug, or stat orders for laboratory assessment of therapeutic drug levels.[6,7]
2. Prescribers, caregivers, and patients should be notified regarding suspected ADRs.
3. Information regarding suspected ADRs should be reported to the pharmacy for complete data collection and analysis, including the patient's name, the patient's medical and medication history, a description of the

suspected ADR, the temporal sequence of the event, any remedial treatment required, and sequelae.

4. High-risk patients should be identified and monitored. High-risk patients include but are not limited to pediatric patients, geriatric patients, patients with organ failure (e.g., hepatic or renal failure), and patients receiving multiple drugs.[6]

5. Drugs likely to cause ADRs ("high-risk" drugs) should be identified, and their use should be monitored. Examples of drugs that may be considered as high risk include aminoglycosides, amphotericin, antineoplastics, corticosteroids, digoxin, heparin, lidocaine, phenytoin, theophylline, thrombolytic agents, and warfarin.[6]

6. The cause(s) of each suspected ADR should be evaluated on the basis of the patient's medical and medication history, the circumstances of the adverse event, the results of dechallenge and rechallenge (if any), alternative etiologies, and a literature review.

7. A method for assigning the probability of a reported or suspected ADR (e.g., confirmed or definite, likely, possible, and unlikely) should be developed to categorize each ADR. Algorithms[8–10] may be useful in establishing the causes of suspected ADRs. Subjective questions and the professional judgment of a pharmacist can be used as additional tools to determine the probability of an ADR. Questions might include the following:

    a. Was there a temporal relationship between the onset of drug therapy and the adverse reaction?
    b. Was there a dechallenge; i.e., did the signs and symptoms of the adverse reaction subside when the drug was withdrawn?
    c. Can signs and symptoms of the adverse reaction be explained by the patient's disease state?
    d. Were there any laboratory tests that provide evidence for the reaction being an ADR?
    e. What was the patient's previous general experience with the drug?
    f. Did symptoms return when the agent was readministered?

8. A method for ranking ADRs by severity should be established.[11]

9. A description of each suspected ADR and the outcomes from the event should be documented in the patient's medical record.

10. Serious or unexpected ADRs should be reported to the Food and Drug Administration (FDA) or the drug's manufacturer (or both).[a]

11. All ADR reports should be reviewed and evaluated by a designated multidisciplinary committee (e.g., a pharmacy and therapeutics committee).

12. ADR-report information should be disseminated to health care professional staff members for educational purposes. Good topics for medical staff education include preventing ADRs and appropriate and effective care for patients who experience ADRs. Educational programs can be conducted as morning "report" discussions, newsletters, "grand rounds" presentations, algorithms for treatment, and multidisciplinary reviews of drug-use evaluations. Patient confidentiality should be preserved.

13. In settings where it is possible, a pharmacy-coordinated ADR team or committee, consisting of a physician, nurse, quality improvement leader, an adminis-

trator, and a pharmacist is recommended.[12–15] The team should be charged with adopting a definition for the organization, promoting awareness of the consequences of ADRs, establishing mechanisms for identifying and reporting ADRs, reviewing ADR patterns or trends, and developing preventive and corrective interventions.

14. Continuous monitoring of patient outcomes and patterns of ADRs is imperative. Findings from an ADR-monitoring and reporting program should be incorporated into the organization's ongoing quality improvement activities. The process should include the following:

    a. Feedback to all appropriate health care staff,
    b. Continuous monitoring for trends, clusters, or significant individual ADRs,
    c. Educational efforts for prevention of ADRs, and
    d. Evaluation of prescribing patterns, patient monitoring practices, patient outcomes, and the ADR program's effect on overall and individual patient outcomes.

An overall goal of the ADR process should be the achievement of positive patient outcomes.

Benefits

An ongoing ADR-monitoring and reporting program can provide benefits to the organization, pharmacists, other health care professionals, and patients. These benefits include (but are not limited to) the following:

1. Providing an indirect measure of the quality of pharmaceutical care through identification of preventable ADRs and anticipatory surveillance for high-risk drugs or patients.

2. Complementing organizational risk-management activities and efforts to minimize liability.

3. Assessing the safety of drug therapies, especially recently approved drugs.

4. Measuring ADR incidence.

5. Educating health care professionals and patients about drug effects and increasing their level of awareness regarding ADRs.

6. Providing quality-assurance screening findings for use in drug-use evaluation programs.

7. Measuring the economic impact of ADR prevention as manifested through reduced hospitalization, optimal and economical drug use, and minimized organizational liability.

Role of the Pharmacist

Pharmacists should exert leadership in the development, maintenance, and ongoing evaluation of ADR programs. They should obtain formal endorsement or approval of such programs through appropriate committees (e.g., a pharmacy and therapeutics committee and the executive committee of the medical staff) and the organization's administration. In settings where applicable, input into the design of the program should be obtained from the medical staff, nursing staff, quality improvement staff, medical records department, and risk managers.[8,16–18] The pharmacist should facilitate

1. Analysis of each reported ADR,

2. Identification of drugs and patients at high risk for being involved in ADRs,

3. The development of policies and procedures for the ADR-monitoring and reporting program,

4. A description of the responsibilities and interactions of pharmacists, physicians, nurses, risk managers, and other health professionals in the ADR program,

5. Use of the ADR program for educational purposes,

6. Development, maintenance, and evaluation of ADR records within the organization,

7. The organizational dissemination and use of information obtained through the ADR program,

8. Reporting of serious ADRs to the FDA or the manufacturer (or both), and

9. Publication and presentation of important ADRs to the medical community.

Direct patient care roles for pharmacists should include patient counseling on ADRs, identification and documentation in the patient's medical record of high-risk patients, monitoring to ensure that serum drug concentrations remain within acceptable therapeutic ranges, and adjusting doses in appropriate patients (e.g., patients with impaired renal or hepatic function).

References

1. American Society of Hospital Pharmacists. ASHP technical assistance bulletin on hospital drug distribution and control. *Am J Hosp Pharm.* 1980; 37:1097–103.

2. Requirements for adverse reaction reporting. Geneva, Switzerland: World Health Organization; 1975.

3. Karch FE, Lasagna L. Adverse drug reactions—a critical review. *JAMA.* 1975; 234:1236–41.

4. Kessler DA. Introducing MedWatch, using FDA form 3500, a new approach to reporting medication and device adverse effects and product problems. *JAMA.* 1993; 269:2765–8.

5. Prosser TR, Kamysz PL. Multidisciplinary adverse drug reaction surveillance program. *Am J Hosp Pharm.* 1990; 47:1334–9.

6. Koch KE. Adverse drug reactions. In: Brown TR, ed. Handbook of institutional pharmacy practice. 3rd ed. Bethesda, MD: American Society of Hospital Pharmacists; 1992.

7. Koch KE. Use of standard screening procedures to identify adverse drug reactions. *Am J Hosp Pharm.* 1990; 47:1314–20.

8. Karch FE, Lasagna L. Toward the operational identification of adverse drug reactions. *Clin Pharmacol Ther.* 1977; 21:247–54.

9. Kramer MS, Leventhal JM, Hutchinson TA, et al. An algorithm for the operational assessment of adverse drug reactions. I. Background, description, and instructions for use. *JAMA.* 1979; 242:623–32.

10. Naranjo CA, Busto U, Sellers EM, et al. A method for estimating the probability of adverse drug reactions. *Clin Pharmacol Ther.* 1981; 30:239–45.

11. Hartwig SC, Siegel J, Schneider PJ. Preventability and severity assessment in reporting adverse drug reactions. *Am J Hosp Pharm.* 1992; 49:2229–32.

12. Accreditation Manual for Hospitals. Chicago: Joint Commission on Accreditation of Healthcare Organizations; 1989:121, 180.

13. Keith MR, Bellanger-McCleery RA, Fuchs JE. Multidisciplinary program for detecting and evaluating adverse drug reactions. *Am J Hosp Pharm.* 1989; 46:1809–12.

14. Kimelblatt BJ, Young SH, Heywood PM, et al. Improved reporting of adverse drug reactions. *Am J Hosp Pharm.* 1988; 45:1086–9.

15. Nelson RW, Shane R. Developing an adverse drug reaction reporting program. *Am J Hosp Pharm.* 1983; 40:445–6.

16. Swanson KM, Landry JP, Anderson RP. Pharmacy-coordinated, multidisciplinary adverse drug reaction program. *Top Hosp Pharm Manage.* 1992; 12(Jul):49–59.

17. Flowers P, Dzierba S, Baker O. A continuous quality improvement team approach to adverse drug reaction reporting. *Top Hosp Pharm Manage.* 1992; 12(Jul): 60–7.

18. Guharoy SR. A pharmacy-coordinated, multidisciplinary approach for successful implementation of an adverse drug reaction reporting program. *Top Hosp Pharm Manage.* 1992; 12(Jul):68–74.

---

[a]To report an adverse drug event to the FDA, use the MedWatch program. Reports can be mailed (MedWatch, 5600 Fishers Lane, Rockville, MD 20852-9787), faxed (800-FDA-0178), called in (800-FDA-1088), or reported by modem (800-FDA-7737). An easy-to-use FDA form 3500 can be used. This form should be available from a pharmacy.

Approved by the ASHP Board of Directors, November 16, 1994. Revised by the ASHP Council on Professional Affairs. Supersedes a previous version dated November 16, 1988.

The bibliographic citation for this document is as follows: American Society of Health-System Pharmacists. ASHP guidelines on adverse drug reaction monitoring and reporting. *Am J Health-Syst Pharm.* 1995; 52:417–9.

ASHP Guidelines on Pharmacists' Relationships with Industry

In the practice of their profession, pharmacists should be guided only by the consideration of patient care. Pharmacists should neither accept nor retain anything of value that has the potential to affect materially their ability to exercise judgments solely in the interests of patients. A useful criterion in determining acceptable activities and relationships is this: Would the pharmacist be willing to have these relationships generally known? Notwithstanding this responsibility, pharmacists may benefit from guidance in their relationships with industry. To this end, the following suggestions are offered.

Gifts and Hospitality

Gifts, hospitality, or subsidies offered to pharmacists by industry should not be accepted if acceptance might influence, or appear to others to influence, the objectivity of clinical judgment or drug product selection and procurement.

Continuing Education

Providers of continuing education that accept industry funding for programs should develop and enforce policies to maintain complete control of program content.

Subsidies to underwrite the costs of continuing-education conferences, professional meetings, or staff development programs can contribute to the improvement of patient care and are permissible. Payments to defray the costs of a conference should not be accepted directly or indirectly from industry by pharmacists attending the conference or program. Contributions to special or educational funds for staff development are permissible as long as the selection of staff members who will receive the funds is made by the department of pharmacy.

It is appropriate for faculty at conferences or meetings to accept reasonable honoraria and reimbursement for reasonable travel, lodging, and meal expenses. However, direct subsidies from industry should not be accepted to pay the costs of travel, lodging, or other personal expenses of pharmacists attending conferences or meetings, nor should subsidies be accepted to compensate for the pharmacists' time.

Scholarships or other special funds to permit pharmacy students, residents, and fellows to attend carefully selected educational conferences may be permissible as long as the selection of students, residents, or fellows who will receive the funds is made by the academic or training institution.

Consultants and Advisory Arrangements

Consultants who provide genuine services for industry may receive reasonable compensation and accept reimbursement for travel, lodging, and meal expenses. Token consulting or advisory arrangements cannot be used to justify compensating pharmacists for their time, travel, lodging, and other out-of-pocket expenses.

Clinical Research

Pharmacists who participate in practice-based research of pharmaceuticals, devices, or other programs should conduct their activities in accord with basic precepts of accepted scientific methodology. Practice-based drug studies that are, in effect, promotional schemes to entice the use of a product or program are unacceptable.

Disclosure of Information

To avoid conflicts of interest or appearances of impropriety, pharmacists should disclose consultant or speaker arrangements or substantial personal financial holdings with companies under consideration for formulary inclusion or related decisions. To inform audiences fully, speakers and authors should disclose, when pertinent, consultant or speaker and research funding arrangements with companies.

Additional Issues

The advice in this document is noninclusive and is not intended to limit the legitimate exchange of prudent scientific information.

Approved by the ASHP Board of Directors, November 20, 1991. Developed by the ASHP Council on Legal and Public Affairs.

The language used in many of the guidance issues contained in this document was adapted, with permission, from documents developed by the American Medical Association (*JAMA*. 1991; 265:501) and the American College of Physicians (*Ann Intern Med*. 1990; 112:624–6).

The bibliographic citation for this document is as follows: American Society of Hospital Pharmacists. ASHP guidelines on pharmacists' relationships with industry. *Am J Hosp Pharm*. 1992; 49:154.

ASHP Guidelines on
Formulary System Management

Preamble

The purposes of these guidelines are to

- Provide an outline of recommended techniques and processes for formulary system management.
- Define terms associated with formulary system management.
- Provide guidance and direction to pharmacists on how to apply the concepts of formulary system management within the context of the "ASHP Statement on the Formulary System."[1]
- Describe the pharmacist's responsibility and leadership role, in partnership with the medical staff, in the management of the formulary system.

The formulary system, as defined in the "ASHP Statement on the Formulary System," is a method for evaluating and selecting suitable drug products for the formulary of an organized health-care setting.[1] Formulary system management is the application of various techniques to ensure high quality and cost-effective drug therapy through the formulary system.

The formulary of an organized health-care setting (e.g., a given hospital, managed care, or home-care operation) is a list of drugs (and associated information) that are considered by the professional staff in that setting to be the most useful in patient care.[1]

Development, maintenance, and approval of the formulary are the responsibilities of the pharmacy and therapeutics (P&T) committee, or its equivalent, which exists as a committee of the medical staff.[2] These responsibilities include oversight of the procedures used to carry out these formulary functions. The information a formulary should contain and the way a formulary should be organized are described in the "ASHP Technical Assistance Bulletin on Drug Formularies."[3]

Three key elements are important for the establishment and maintenance of a credible formulary. They are

1. A collaborative work relationship among health-care professionals, such as occurs in an organized health-care setting.
2. A defined medical staff (or physician-provider network) that practices within that health-care setting.
3. An interdisciplinary P&T committee as a committee of the medical staff.

Principles of
Formulary System Management

The purpose for ongoing management of the formulary system is to optimize patient care through rational selection and use of drugs and drug products within the health-care setting. Pharmacists play a primary role in assessing the relative safety and efficacy of pharmaceuticals nominated for addition to or deletion from the formulary. Through the application of techniques of formulary system management and through reevaluation and improvement of these techniques as necessary, the effectiveness of the formulary system is continuously assessed, resulting in quality improvement of the overall drug use process. Both therapeutic outcomes and costs related to the drug use process can thus be optimized.

Prescriber acceptance of the formulary management process is essential to effect quality improvements through formulary system management. Pharmacists play a key leadership role in fostering this acceptance by clarifying and supporting the goals and processes of formulary system management. Restated, the goal of formulary system management should be sound therapeutics. To achieve this goal successfully, prescribers should be actively involved in developing the techniques used to manage the formulary system. Communication and understanding among pharmacists, prescribers, other health-care providers, and the P&T committee members should be timely and routine. Pharmacists should ensure that a balanced presentation of drug information is provided to prescribers.

Techniques of formulary system management fall into three general categories: (1) drug use evaluation, (2) formulary maintenance, and (3) drug product selection.

Drug Use Evaluation

Drug use evaluation is an ongoing, structured, organizationally authorized process designed to ensure that drugs are used appropriately, safely, and effectively. A well-designed drug use evaluation program applies continuous quality improvement methods to the drug use process. Drug use evaluation should be a part of the hospital's overall quality-assurance program.[4] The role and responsibilities of pharmacists in drug use evaluation are identified in the "ASHP Guidelines on the Pharmacist's Role in Drug Use Evaluation."[5] Drug use evaluation is a quality-assurance activity, but it may also be considered a formulary system management technique. The P&T committee should be involved in the drug use evaluation process.

Effective drug use evaluation begins with drug use criteria or treatment guidelines approved by the P&T committee on behalf of the medical staff. Drug use evaluation should measure and compare the outcomes of patients whose treatment did, or did not, comply with approved criteria or guidelines. Based on this comparative information, criteria or guidelines can be revised, compliance can be encouraged, educational programs can be initiated, or changes can be made to the formulary system. Drug use evaluation programs should include provisions for periodic review of all components of the system.

Drug Use Criteria. In cases where a drug poses potential efficacy, toxicity, or utilization problems for the health-care setting, criteria may be established by the P&T committee to promote appropriate use. Drug use criteria are approved guidelines regarding how, or under what conditions, a drug is recommended for use. Preliminary drug use criteria should be developed at the time that a drug is proposed for addition to the formulary. Drug use criteria should be updated as needed over time. There are three general types of criteria:

diagnosis criteria, prescriber criteria, and drug-specific criteria. Criteria of any type can be used independently or in combination.

Diagnosis criteria identify indications that constitute acceptable uses for a formulary drug within the health-care setting. Protocols, if any, for restricting the use of a formulary drug to specific diagnoses or medical conditions should be established by the P&T committee. For instance, a particular colony-stimulating factor might be approved for use only as an adjunct to cancer chemotherapy. Use of this drug for other indications would then fall outside the approved diagnosis criteria.

Prescriber criteria identify prescribers approved to use specific formulary drugs or drug classes. Examples include limiting the use of specific injectable antibiotics to infectious disease specialists or establishing cardiologists or emergency room physicians as the only approved prescribers for thrombolytic drugs.

Drug-specific criteria identify approved doses, frequency of administration, duration of therapy, or other aspects that are specific to the use of a formulary drug. An example would be limiting the dosing of a long-acting injectable antibiotic to once every 24 hours. More frequent dosing regimens might require approval by an infectious disease specialist.

Treatment Guidelines. Treatment guidelines are similar to drug use criteria, except that treatment guidelines focus on disease-based drug therapy. Whereas drug use criteria relate to a specific drug, treatment guidelines outline a recommended therapeutic approach to specific diseases. This approach generally identifies the use of several different drugs, depending on disease severity or specific patient characteristics. A treatment guideline, for example, may outline a recommended approach to treating community-acquired pneumonia, reflux esophagitis, or otitis media, or it may list drugs to be used in bone marrow transplantation.

Treatment guidelines are typically developed and approved by P&T committees for high risk, high volume, or problem-prone diseases encountered in the health-care setting.

Formulary Maintenance

Formulary maintenance techniques include

- Therapeutic drug class review.
- Processes by which drug products are added to or deleted from the formulary.
- Use of nonformulary drugs in unique patient situations.

To be effective in improving the drug use process, pharmacists and medical staff must work collaboratively. The pharmacist should assume responsibility and a leadership role in the development and presentation of information required by the P&T committee for decisionmaking. The medical staff must understand and support the processes by which these techniques are applied, as well as participate in the development and review of information.

Therapeutic Drug Class Review. It is useful for the P&T committee to review the use and therapeutic effects of several classes of drug products every year. Examples of drug classes suitable for review are nonsteroidal anti-inflam-

matory agents, injectable cephalosporins, antihistamines, β-blockers, and neuromuscular blockers. These reviews can be prompted by criteria set by the P&T committee itself. For example, based on the number of adverse drug reaction reports, new information in the medical literature, or drug class expenditures, the committee can determine which classes of formulary drugs are worthy of reassessment.

The goal is to identify preferred agents based on effectiveness, toxicity, or cost differences within the same class. It is important that appropriate medical staff input, outside the committee, be solicited during these reviews. Outcomes of therapeutic class reviews can include development of new drug use criteria, new treatment guidelines, or changes to the formulary.

Formulary Addition or Deletion. To strengthen the ability of the P&T committee to make sound decisions on changes to the formulary, it is recommended that there be an approved policy and procedure for requesting changes to the formulary. This process typically involves submission of a request to the P&T committee by pharmacists or members of the medical staff.[2]

Consideration of a drug for addition to the formulary should include a review of an evaluation report (monograph) prepared by the pharmacy. A recommendation on how to prepare and organize an evaluation report can be found in the "ASHP Technical Assistance Bulletin on the Evaluation of Drugs for Formularies."[6] In addition to monograph information, an impact statement describing the effects of the proposed change on the quality and cost of patient care and drug therapy should accompany each request for addition to or deletion from the formulary.

The use of predetermined decision-reassessment dates is advised (e.g., the drug is placed on the formulary for a 6-month evaluation) to allow the committee to review the actual impact of certain formulary decisions. Reassessment dates are especially useful in situations where the expected impact of the formulary decision on the quality or cost of drug therapy may be significant or uncertain.

Use of Nonformulary Drugs. In general, only formulary drugs are endorsed as appropriate for *routine* use within the organized health-care setting. The underlying principle for the existence of a process for approval of nonformulary drugs is that individual or unique patient needs can exist that may not be satisfied by the use of formulary drugs.

There should be an approved policy and procedure for obtaining approval for use of nonformulary drugs. This process should include the generation of information on the use of nonformulary drugs to enable the P&T committee to review trends in nonformulary drug use, which may influence formulary addition or deletion decisions. There should also be a process in place for obtaining nonformulary drugs in a timely manner.

In managed care settings, the decision to approve the use of nonformulary drugs is separate from the decision to grant payment coverage for a drug. Coverage decisions are governed by the patient's contract with a specific health plan.

Drug Product Selection

Pharmacists and prescribers must understand the concept of therapeutic equivalence to ensure proper application of generic substitution and therapeutic interchange principles.

Pharmacists should assume a leadership role in drug product selection by proposing opportunities for drug product selection. This includes evaluation and assessment of bioequivalence data; storage, dispensing, and administration characteristics; cost; and other relevant product information. Pharmacists must also ensure that products of adequate quality are procured.

The application of generic substitution and therapeutic interchange principles may result in a drug product being dispensed to the patient that is different from the product originally prescribed. To ensure high quality drug therapy, therapeutic equivalence between the product dispensed and that prescribed must be ensured.

Therapeutic Equivalence. The 1991 edition of the *Approved Drug Products with Therapeutic Equivalence Evaluations* (FDA Orange Book) describes therapeutic equivalence as a guideline to assist in drug substitution between chemically identical products.[7] Both generic substitution and therapeutic interchange, however, should be safe and effective if the therapeutic equivalence of products to be exchanged has been established. For the purpose of this document, drugs are considered therapeutically equivalent if they can be expected to produce essentially the same therapeutic outcome and toxicity.

The use of therapeutically equivalent products can contribute to improvement in the drug use process by maintaining a high quality of drug therapy in the most cost-effective manner.

Generic Substitution. For the purpose of this document, generic substitution is defined as the substitution of drug products that contain the same active ingredient(s) and are chemically identical in strength, concentration, dosage form, and route of administration to the drug product prescribed (i.e., these are "pharmaceutical equivalents" as defined in the FDA Orange Book[7]). These products can also be termed "generic equivalents." Logically, these products should display therapeutic equivalence.

The key word in this definition is "identical." For example, the substitution of one brand of propranolol tablets for another represents the application of generic substitution if the strength of the active ingredients and the dosage form are identical. To ensure quality patient care, the two propranolol products must also be shown to achieve therapeutic equivalence as defined above. The substitution of purified pork insulin for human insulin is not generic substitution, because the products are not chemically identical. However, the interchangeability of these products may be acceptable under the principle of therapeutic interchange (discussed below), provided that therapeutic equivalence can be ensured.

Prescribers have the prerogative to override a generic substitution. In some cases, a patient preference may negate an otherwise acceptable generic substitution. The P&T committee is responsible for determining which drugs are acceptable for generic substitution and for developing guidelines for pharmacists who carry out this formulary system management activity. Typically, pharmacists determine which products are purchased and dispensed as generic substitutes. In most health-care settings, prescribers prospectively authorize generic substitution during their credentialing process. Notification of generic substitution is generally not provided to the prescriber at the time that a generic equivalent is dispensed.

Therapeutic Interchange. Therapeutic interchange is defined, for the purpose of this document, as the interchange of various therapeutically equivalent drug products by pharmacists under arrangements between pharmacist(s) and authorized prescriber(s) who have previously established and jointly agreed on conditions for interchanges.

Therapeutic interchange occurs pursuant to development of agreements between pharmacists and prescribers and implies that there is appropriate and timely communication between them. Therapeutic interchange agreements can vary from simple understandings to complex protocols. For example, a therapeutic interchange agreement permitting interchange between cephradine and cephalexin may be a simple arrangement; the dose and dosage form of the two drugs are equivalent, and the drugs typically can be interchanged in the treatment of any disease for which the drugs are indicated. A therapeutic interchange arrangement that permits the interchangeability of different colony-stimulating factors in treating a specific diagnosis pursuant to specific protocols might be more complex. In either case, the P&T committee acts on behalf of the medical staff to develop and approve these arrangements.

The approval of a therapeutic interchange arrangement is typically a separate decision by a P&T committee, unrelated to adding or deleting drugs from the formulary. In some settings, all drugs that may be therapeutically interchanged are acceptable to the formulary, and the pharmacy is authorized to purchase and dispense the most cost-effective products. In other settings, certain drug products are deemed interchangeable, but the P&T committee designates a preferred product and approves it for formulary addition. Then the other equivalent drugs or products are deleted from the formulary.

To remain effective over time, therapeutic interchange decisions should be routinely reviewed and revised as appropriate. Therapeutic interchange may not be appropriate for all patients. Professional judgment must be exercised by the pharmacist and the prescriber. Consultation with the prescriber and the patient may be necessary. Prescribers have the prerogative to override a therapeutic interchange. In some cases, a patient preference may negate an otherwise acceptable therapeutic interchange.

Pharmacists should strive for consistency of product use to avoid unnecessary switching of products dispensed to patients. When a change is made, the pharmacist should ensure that appropriate monitoring and followup are undertaken to identify and prevent any unexpected or untoward patient response. The pharmacist should provide appropriate notification and educational materials to prescribers, patients, and other health-care providers as needed regarding therapeutic interchange decisions.

References

1.   American Society of Hospital Pharmacists. ASHP statement on the formulary system. *Am J Hosp Pharm.* 1983; 40:1384–5.

2.   American Society of Hospital Pharmacists. ASHP statement on the pharmacy and therapeutics committee. *Am J Hosp Pharm.* 1984; 41:1621.

3.   American Society of Hospital Pharmacists. ASHP technical assistance bulletin on drug formularies. *Am J Hosp Pharm.* 1991; 48:791–3.

4.   Joint Commission on Accreditation of Healthcare Organizations. Accreditation manual for hospitals. Chi-

cago: Joint Commission on Accreditation of Healthcare Organizations; 1992:140.

5. American Society of Hospital Pharmacists. ASHP guidelines on the pharmacist's role in drug-use evaluation. *Am J Hosp Pharm.* 1988; 45:385–6.

6. American Society of Hospital Pharmacists. ASHP technical assistance bulletin on the evaluation of drugs for formularies. *Am J Hosp Pharm.* 1988; 45:386–7.

7. U.S. Department of Health and Human Services. Approved drug products with therapeutic equivalence evaluations. 11th ed. Washington, DC: U.S. Government Printing Office; 1991:1–3.

Approved by the ASHP Board of Directors, November 20, 1991. Developed by the ASHP Council on Professional Affairs. Marvin A. Chamberlain developed the initial draft for council review.

The bibliographic citation for this document is as follows: American Society of Hospital Pharmacists. ASHP guidelines on formulary system management. *Am J Hosp Pharm.* 1992; 49:648–52.

ASHP Guidelines on Preventing Medication Errors in Hospitals

The goal of drug therapy is the achievement of defined therapeutic outcomes that improve a patient's quality of life while minimizing patient risk.[1] There are inherent risks, both known and unknown, associated with the therapeutic use of drugs (prescription and nonprescription) and drug administration devices. The incidents or hazards that result from such risk have been defined as drug misadventuring, which includes both adverse drug reactions (ADRs) and medication errors.[2] This document addresses medication errors—episodes in drug misadventuring that should be preventable through effective systems controls involving pharmacists, physicians and other prescribers, nurses, risk management personnel, legal counsel, administrators, patients, and others in the organizational setting, as well as regulatory agencies and the pharmaceutical industry.

This document suggests medication error prevention approaches that should be considered in the development of organizational systems and discusses methods of managing medication errors once they have occurred. These guidelines are primarily intended to apply to the inpatient hospital setting because of the special collaborative processes established in the setting [e.g., formulary system, pharmacy and therapeutics (P&T) committee, and opportunity for increased interaction among health-care providers].

Recommendations for practice settings other than hospitals are beyond the scope of this document, although many of the ideas and principles may be applicable.

Medication errors compromise patient confidence in the health-care system and increase health-care costs. The problems and sources of medication errors are multidisciplinary and multifactorial. Errors occur from lack of knowledge, substandard performance and mental lapses, or defects or failures in systems.[3,4] Medication errors may be committed by both experienced and inexperienced staff, including pharmacists, physicians, nurses, supportive personnel (e.g., pharmacy technicians), students, clerical staff (e.g., ward clerks), administrators, pharmaceutical manufacturers, patients and their caregivers, and others. The incidence of medication errors is indeterminate; valid comparisons of different studies on medication errors are extremely difficult because of differences in variables, measurements, populations, and methods.[2]

Many medication errors are probably undetected. The outcome(s) or clinical significance of many medication errors may be minimal, with few or no consequences that adversely affect a patient. Tragically, however, some medication errors result in serious patient morbidity or mortality.[3] Thus, medication errors must not be taken lightly, and effective systems for ordering, dispensing, and administering medications should be established with safeguards to prevent the occurrence of errors. These systems should involve adequately trained and supervised personnel, adequate communications, reasonable workloads, effective drug handling systems, multiple procedural and final product checks by separate individuals, quality management, and adequate facilities, equipment, and supplies.

The pharmacist's mission is to help ensure that patients make the best use of medications.[5] This applies to all drugs used by inpatients or ambulatory patients, including oral or injectable products, radiopharmaceuticals, radiopaque contrast media, anesthetic gases, blood-fraction drugs, dialysis fluids, respiratory therapy agents, investigational drugs, drug samples, drugs brought into the hospital setting by patients, and other chemical or biological substances administered to patients to evoke a pharmacological response.[6]

Through a systems-oriented approach, the pharmacist should lead collaborative, multidisciplinary efforts to prevent, detect, and resolve drug-related problems that can result in patient harm.[1] An understanding of the risk factors associated with medication errors should enable improved monitoring of patients and medications associated with increased risk for serious errors and should enable the development of organizational systems designed to minimize risk.[7] The pharmacist should participate in appropriate organizational committees and work with physicians, nurses, administrators, and others to examine and improve systems to ensure that medication processes are safe.

Types of Medication Errors

Medication errors include prescribing errors, dispensing errors, medication administration errors, and patient compliance errors. Specific types of medication errors are categorized in Table 1, based on a compilation of the literature.[3,7–18]

A *potential error* is a mistake in prescribing, dispensing, or planned medication administration that is detected and corrected through intervention (by another health-care provider or patient) before actual medication administration. Potential errors should be reviewed and tabulated as separate events from errors of occurrence (errors that actually reach patients) to identify opportunities to correct problems in the medication use system even before they occur. Detection of potential errors should be a component of the hospital's routine quality improvement process. Documentation of instances in which an individual has prevented the occurrence of a medication error will help identify system weaknesses and will reinforce the importance of multiple checks in the medication use system.

Recommendations for Preventing Medication Errors

Organizational systems for ordering, dispensing, and administering medications should be designed to minimize error. Medication errors may involve process breakdowns in more than one aspect of a system. This section provides recommendations to the management staff (general and departmental) of hospitals, as well as to individual prescribers, pharmacists, nurses, patients, pharmaceutical manufacturers, and others.

Organizational and Departmental Recommendations. Organizational policies and procedures should be established to prevent medication errors. Development of the policies and procedures should involve multiple departments, including pharmacy, medicine, nursing, risk management, legal counsel, and organizational administration. The following recommendations are offered for organizational

Table 1.
Types of Medication Errors[3,7-18,a]

Type	Definition
Prescribing error	Incorrect drug selection (based on indications, contraindications, known allergies, existing drug therapy, and other factors), dose, dosage form, quantity, route, concentration, rate of administration, or instructions for use of a drug product ordered or authorized by physician (or other legitimate prescriber); illegible prescriptions or medication orders that lead to errors that reach the patient
Omission error[b]	The failure to administer an ordered dose to a patient before the next scheduled dose, if any
Wrong time error	Administration of medication outside a predefined time interval from its scheduled administration time (this interval should be established by each individual health care facility)
Unauthorized drug error[c]	Administration to the patient of medication not authorized by a legitimate prescriber for the patient
Improper dose error[d]	Administration to the patient of a dose that is greater than or less than the amount ordered by the prescriber or administration of duplicate doses to the patient, i.e., one or more dosage units in addition to those that were ordered
Wrong dosage-form error[e]	Administration to the patient of a drug product in a different dosage form than ordered by the prescriber
Wrong drug-preparation error[f]	Drug product incorrectly formulated or manipulated before administration
Wrong administration-technique error[g]	Inappropriate procedure or improper technique in the administration of a drug
Deteriorated drug error[h]	Administration of a drug that has expired or for which the physical or chemical dosage form integrity has been compromised
Monitoring error	Failure to review a prescribed regimen for appropriateness and detection of problems, or failure to use appropriate clinical or laboratory data for adequate assessment of patient response to prescribed therapy
Compliance error	Inappropriate patient behavior regarding adherence to a prescribed medication regimen
Other medication error	Any medication error that does not fall into one of the above predefined categories

[a] The categories may not be mutually exclusive because of the multidisciplinary and multifactorial nature of medication errors.

[b] Assumes no prescribing error. Excluded would be (1) a patient's refusal to take the medication or (2) a decision not to administer the dose because of recognized contraindications. If an explanation for the omission is apparent (e.g., patient was away from nursing unit for tests or medication was not available), that reason should be documented in the appropriate records.

[c] This would include, for example, a wrong drug, a dose given to the wrong patient, unordered drugs, and doses given outside a stated set of clinical guidelines or protocols.

[d] Excluded would be (1) allowable deviations based on preset ranges established by individual health care organizations in consideration of measuring devices routinely provided to those who administer drugs to patients (e.g., not administering a dose based on a patient's measured temperature or blood glucose level) or other factors such as conversion of doses expressed in the apothecary system to the metric system and (2) topical dosage forms for which medication orders are not expressed quantitatively.

[e] Excluded would be accepted protocols (established by the pharmacy and therapeutics committee or its equivalent) that authorize pharmacists to dispense alternate dosage forms for patients with special needs (e.g., liquid formulations for patients with nasogastric tubes or those who have difficulty swallowing), as allowed by state regulations

[f] This would include, for example, incorrect dilution or reconstitution, mixing drugs that are physically or chemically incompatible, and inadequate product packaging.

[g] This would include doses administered (1) via the wrong route (different from the route prescribed), (2) via the correct route but at the wrong site (e.g., left eye instead of right), and (3) at the wrong rate of administration.

[h] This would include, for example, administration of expired drugs and improperly stored drugs.

management and clinical staff:[3,8,11-14,16,19-29]

1. Using the principles of the formulary system, the P&T committee (or its equivalent)—composed of pharmacists, physicians, nurses, and other health professionals—should be responsible for formulating policies regarding the evaluation, selection, and therapeutic use of drugs in organized health-care settings.

2. Care and consideration must be given in hiring and assigning personnel involved in medication ordering, preparation, dispensing, administration, and patient education. Policies and procedures should be developed that ensure adequate personnel selection, training, supervision, and evaluation. This would include the need to ensure proper interviewing, orientation, evaluation of competency, supervision, and opportunities for continuing professional and technical education.

3. Sufficient personnel must be available to perform tasks adequately. Policies and procedures should ensure that reasonable workload levels and working hours are established and rarely exceeded.

4. Suitable work environments should exist for the preparation of drug products. Potential error sources within the work environment, such as frequent interruptions, should be identified and minimized.

5. Lines of authority and areas of responsibility within the hospital should be clearly defined for medication ordering, dispensing, and administration. The system should ensure adequate written and oral communications among personnel involved in the medication use process to optimize therapeutic appropriateness and to enable medications to be prescribed, dispensed, and administered in a timely fashion. All systems should provide for review and verification of the prescriber's original order (except in emergency situations) before a drug product is dispensed by a pharmacist. Any necessary clarifications or changes in a medication order must be resolved with the prescriber before a medication is administered to the patient. Written documentation of such consultations should be made in the patient's medical record or other appropriate record. Nursing staff should be informed of any changes made in the medication order. Changes required to correct incorrect orders should be regarded as potential errors, assuming the changes occurred in time to prevent the error from reaching the patient.

6. There should be an ongoing, systematic program of quality improvement and peer review with respect to the safe use of medications. A formal drug use evalu-

ation (DUE) program, developed and conducted through collaborative efforts among medicine, pharmacy, and nursing, should be integrated and coordinated with the overall hospital quality improvement program. To prevent medication errors, a portion of the DUE program should focus on monitoring the appropriate use of any drugs associated with a high frequency of adverse events, including specific drug classes (such as antimicrobials, antineoplastic agents, and cardiovascular drugs) and injectable dosage forms (e.g., potassium products, narcotic substances, heparin, lidocaine, procainamide, magnesium sulfate, and insulin). The quality improvement program should include a system for monitoring, reviewing, and reporting medication errors to assist in identifying and eliminating causes of errors (system breakdowns) and preventing their recurrence. Table 2 lists common causes of medication errors, i.e., areas where there may be system breakdowns.

7. Pharmacists and others responsible for processing drug orders should have routine access to appropriate clinical information about patients (including medication, allergy, and hypersensitivity profiles; diagnoses; pregnancy status; and laboratory values) to help evaluate the appropriateness of medication orders.

8. Pharmacists should maintain medication profiles for all patients, both inpatients and ambulatory patients, who receive care at the hospital. This profile should include adequate information to allow monitoring of medication histories, allergies, diagnoses, potential drug interactions and ADRs, duplicate drug therapies, pertinent laboratory data, and other information.

9. The pharmacy department must be responsible for the procurement, distribution, and control of all drugs used within the organization. Adequate hours for the provision of pharmaceutical services must be maintained; 24-hour pharmaceutical service is strongly recommended in hospital settings. In the absence of 24-hour pharmaceutical service, access to a limited supply of medications should be available to authorized nonpharmacists for use in initiating urgent medication orders. The list of medications to be supplied and the policies and procedures to be used (including subsequent review of all activity by a pharmacist) should be developed by the P&T committee (or its equivalent). Items should be chosen with safety in mind, limiting wherever possible medications, quantities, dosage forms, and container sizes that might endanger patients. The use of well-designed night

cabinets, after-hours drug carts, and other methods would preclude the need for non-pharmacists to enter the pharmacy. Access to the pharmacy by non-pharmacists (e.g., nurses) for removal of doses is strongly discouraged; this practice should be minimized and eliminated to the fullest extent possible. When 24-hour pharmacy service is not feasible, a pharmacist must be available on an "on-call" basis.

10. The pharmacy manager (or designee), with the assistance of the P&T committee (or its equivalent) and the department of nursing, should develop comprehensive policies and procedures that provide for efficient and safe distribution of all medications and related supplies to patients. For safety, the recommended method of distribution within the organized health-care setting is the unit dose drug distribution and control system.

11. Except in emergency situations, all sterile and nonsterile drug products should be dispensed from the pharmacy department for individual patients. The storage of nonemergency floor stock medications on the nursing units or in patient-care areas should be minimized. Particular caution should be exercised with respect to drug products that have commonly been involved in serious medication errors or whose margin of safety is narrow, such as concentrated forms of drug products that are intended to be diluted into larger volumes (e.g., concentrated lidocaine and potassium chloride for injection concentrate). All drug storage areas should be routinely inspected by pharmacy personnel to ensure adequate product integrity and appropriate packaging, labeling, and storage. It is important that drug products and other products for external use be stored separately from drug products for internal use.

12. The pharmacy director and staff must ensure that all drug products used in the organizational setting are of high quality and integrity. This would include, for example, (1) selecting multisource products supported by adequate bioavailability data and adequate product packaging and labeling, (2) maintaining an unexpired product inventory, and (3) keeping abreast of compendial requirements.

13. The use of a patient's own or "home" medications should be avoided to the fullest extent possible. Use of such medications should be allowed only if there is a need for the patient to receive the therapy, the drug product is not obtainable by the pharmacy, and no alternative therapy can be prescribed. If such medications are used, the prescribing physician must write an appropriate order in the patient's medical record. Before use, a pharmacist should inspect and identify the medication. If there are any unresolved questions with respect to product identity or integrity, the medication must not be used.

14. All discontinued or unused drugs should be returned to the department of pharmacy immediately on discontinuation or at patient discharge. Discharged patients must not be given unlabeled drug products to take home, unless they are labeled for outpatient use by the pharmacy in accordance with state and federal regulations. Discharged patients should be counseled about use of any medications to be used after discharge.

15. It is recommended that there be computerized pharmacy systems in place that enable automated checking for doses, duplicate therapies, allergies, drug interac-

Table 2.
Common Causes of Medication Errors

Ambiguous strength designation on labels or in packaging
Drug product nomenclature (look-alike or sound-alike names, use of lettered or numbered prefixes and suffixes in drug names)
Equipment failure or malfunction
Illegible handwriting
Improper transcription
Inaccurate dosage calculation
Inadequately trained personnel
Inappropriate abbreviations used in prescribing
Labeling errors
Excessive workload
Lapses in individual performance
Medication unavailable

tions, and other aspects of use. Where possible, the use of technological innovations such as bar coding is recommended to help identify patients, products, and care providers. Pharmacy-generated medication administration records or labels are recommended to assist nurses in interpreting and documenting medication activities.

16. Adequate drug information resources should be available for all health-care providers involved in the drug use process.

17. Standard drug administration times should be established for the hospital by the P&T committee (or its equivalent), with input from the departments of nursing and pharmacy. Policies and procedures should allow for deviations from the standard times when necessary. Further, standard drug concentrations and dosage charts should be developed to minimize the need for dosage calculations by staff.

18. The P&T committee (or its equivalent) should develop a list of standard abbreviations approved for use in medication ordering. There should be efforts to prohibit or discourage the use of other abbreviations in medication ordering.

19. A review mechanism should be established through the P&T committee specifying those responsible for data collection and evaluation of medication error reports. The review group should investigate causes of errors and develop programs for decreasing their occurrence. The review group should be composed of representatives from pharmacy, nursing, medicine, quality assurance, staff education, risk management, and legal counsel.

20. The pharmacy department, in conjunction with nursing, risk management, and the medical staff, should conduct ongoing educational programs to discuss medication errors, their causes, and methods to prevent their occurrence. Such programs might involve seminars, newsletters, or other methods of information dissemination.

Recommendations for Prescribers. Prescribing is an early point at which medication errors can arise. It has been estimated that 1% of hospitalized patients suffer adverse events as the result of medical mismanagement[30] and that drug-related complications are the most common type of adverse event.[7] The following recommendations for preventing medication errors are suggested for physicians and other prescribers:[3,7,11–16,31]

1. To determine appropriate drug therapy, prescribers should stay abreast of the current state of knowledge through literature review, consultation with pharmacists, consultation with other physicians, participation in continuing professional education programs, and other means. It is especially crucial to seek information when prescribing for conditions and diseases not typically experienced in the prescriber's practice.

2. Prescribers should evaluate the patient's total status and review all existing drug therapy before prescribing new or additional medications to ascertain possible antagonistic or complementary drug interactions. To evaluate and optimize patient response to prescribed drug therapy, appropriate monitoring of clinical signs and symptoms and of relevant laboratory data is necessary.

3. In hospitals, prescribers should be familiar with the medication ordering system (e.g., the formulary system, participation in DUE programs, allowable delegation of authority, procedures to alert nurses and others to new drug orders that need to be processed, standard medication administration times, and approved abbreviations).

4. Drug orders should be complete. They should include patient name, generic drug name, trademarked name (if a specific product is required), route and site of administration, dosage form, dose, strength, quantity, frequency of administration, and prescriber's name. In some cases, a dilution, rate, and time of administration should be specified. The desired therapeutic outcome for each drug should be expressed when the drug is prescribed. Prescribers should review all drug orders for accuracy and legibility immediately after they have prescribed them.

5. Care should be taken to ensure that the intent of medication orders is clear and unambiguous. Prescribers should

    a. Write out instructions rather than using nonstandard or ambiguous abbreviations. For example, write "daily" rather than "q.d.," which could be misinterpreted as q.i.d. (causing a drug to be given four times a day instead of once) or as o.d. (for right eye).

    b. Do not use vague instructions, such as "take as directed," because specific instructions can help differentiate among intended drugs.

    c. Specify exact dosage strengths (such as milligrams) rather than dosage form units (such as one tablet or one vial). An exception would be combination drug products, for which the number of dosage form units should be specified.

    d. Prescribe by standard nomenclature, using the drug's generic name (United States Adopted Name or USAN), official name, or trademarked name (if deemed medically necessary). Avoid the following: locally coined names (e.g., Dr. Doe's syrup); chemical names [e.g., 6-mercaptopurine (instead of mercaptopurine) could result in a sixfold overdose if misinterpreted]; unestablished abbreviated drug names (e.g., "AZT" could stand for zidovudine, azathioprine, or aztreonam); acronyms; and apothecary or chemical symbols.

    e. Always use a leading zero before a decimal expression of less than one (e.g., 0.5 ml). Conversely, a terminal zero should never be used (e.g., 5.0 ml), since failure to see the decimal could result in a 10-fold overdose. When possible, avoid the use of decimals (e.g., prescribe 500 mg instead of 0.5 g).

    f. Spell out the word "units" (e.g., 10 units regular insulin) rather than writing "u," which could be misinterpreted as a zero.

    g. Use the metric system.

6. Written drug or prescription orders (including signatures) should be legible. Prescribers with poor handwriting should print or type medication or prescription orders if direct order entry capabilities for computerized systems are unavailable. A handwritten order

should be completely readable (not merely recognizable through familiarity). An illegible handwritten order should be regarded as a potential error. If it leads to an error of occurrence (that is, the error actually reaches the patient), it should be regarded as a prescribing error.

7. Verbal drug or prescription orders (that is, orders that are orally communicated) should be reserved only for those situations in which it is impossible or impractical for the prescriber to write the order or enter it in the computer. The prescriber should dictate verbal orders slowly, clearly, and articulately to avoid confusion. Special caution is urged in the prescribing of drug dosages in the teens (e.g., a 15-mEq dose of potassium chloride could be misheard as a 50-mEq dose). The order should be read back to the prescriber by the recipient (i.e., the nurse or pharmacist, according to institutional policies). When read back, the drug name should be spelled to the prescriber and, when directions are repeated, no abbreviations should be used (e.g., say "three times daily" rather than "t.i.d."). A written copy of the verbal order should be placed in the patient's medical record and later confirmed by the prescriber in accordance with applicable state regulations and hospital policies.

8. When possible, drugs should be prescribed for administration by the oral route rather than by injection.

9. When possible, the prescriber should talk with the patient or caregiver to explain the medication prescribed and any special precautions or observations that might be indicated, including any allergic or hypersensitivity reactions that might occur.

10. Prescribers should follow up and periodically evaluate the need for continued drug therapy for individual patients.

11. Instructions with respect to "hold" orders for medications should be clear.

Recommendations for Pharmacists. The pharmacist is expected to play a pivotal role in preventing medication misuse. The value of pharmacists' interventions to prevent medication errors that would have resulted from inappropriate prescribing has been documented.[7,32,33] Ideally, the pharmacist should collaborate with the prescriber in developing, implementing, and monitoring a therapeutic plan to produce defined therapeutic outcomes for the patient.[1] It is also vital that the pharmacist devote careful attention to dispensing processes to ensure that errors are not introduced at that point in the medication process. The following recommendations are suggested for pharmacists:[3,4,8–10,14,16,18–20,28,29]

1. Pharmacists should participate in drug therapy monitoring (including the following, when indicated: the assessment of therapeutic appropriateness, medication administration appropriateness, and possible duplicate therapies; review for possible interactions; and evaluation of pertinent clinical and laboratory data) and DUE activities to help achieve safe, effective, and rational use of drugs.

2. To recommend and recognize appropriate drug therapy, pharmacists should stay abreast of the current state of knowledge through familiarity with literature, consultation with colleagues and other health-care providers, participation in continuing professional education programs, and other means.

3. Pharmacists should make themselves available to prescribers and nurses to offer information and advice about therapeutic drug regimens and the correct use of medications.

4. Pharmacists should be familiar with the medication ordering system and drug distribution policies and procedures established for the organizational setting to provide for the safe distribution of all medications and related supplies to inpatients and ambulatory patients. In particular, pharmacists should be familiar with all elements that are designed into the system to prevent or detect errors. Actions by any staff that would (even unintentionally) defeat or compromise those elements should serve as "alerts" to the pharmacist that safety may be affected. Any necessary followup action (e.g., education or reeducation of staff) should ensue promptly. Policies and procedures to be followed for "hold" orders should be clear and understood by pharmacy, medical, and nursing staffs.

5. Pharmacists should never assume or guess the intent of confusing medication orders. If there are any questions, the prescriber should be contacted prior to dispensing.

6. When preparing drugs, pharmacists should maintain orderliness and cleanliness in the work area and perform one procedure at a time with as few interruptions as possible.

7. Before dispensing a medication in nonemergency situations, the pharmacist should review an original copy of the written medication order. The pharmacist should ensure that all work performed by supportive personnel or through the use of automated devices is checked by manual or technological means. All processes must conform with applicable state and federal laws and regulations. Pharmacists should participate in, at a minimum, a self-checking process in reading prescriptions, labeling (drug or ingredients and pharmacist-generated labeling), and dosage calculations. For high risk drug products, when possible, all work should be checked by a second individual (preferably, another pharmacist). Pharmacists must make certain that the following are accurate: drug, labeling, packaging, quantity, dose, and instructions.

8. Pharmacists should dispense medications in ready-to-administer dosage forms whenever possible. The unit dose system is strongly recommended as the preferred method of drug distribution. The need for nurses to manipulate drugs (e.g., measure, repackage, and calculate) prior to their administration should be minimized.

9. Pharmacists should review the use of auxiliary labels and use the labels prudently when it is clear that such use may prevent errors (e.g., "shake well," "for external use only," and "not for injection").

10. Pharmacists should ensure that medications are delivered to the patient-care area in a timely fashion after receipt of orders, according to hospital policies and procedures. If medication doses are not delivered or if therapy is delayed for any reason pending resolution of a detected problem (e.g., allergy or contraindications), the pharmacist should notify the nursing staff of the delay and the reason.

11. Pharmacists should observe how medications are actually being used in patient-care areas to ensure that dispensing and storage procedures are followed and to

assist nurses in optimizing patient safety.

12. Pharmacy staff should review medications that are returned to the department. Such review processes may reveal system breakdowns or problems that resulted in medication errors (e.g., omitted doses and unauthorized drugs).

13. When dispensing medications to ambulatory patients (e.g., at discharge), pharmacists should counsel patients or caregivers and verify that they understand why a medication was prescribed and dispensed, its intended use, any special precautions that might be observed, and other needed information. For inpatients, pharmacists should make their services available to counsel patients, families, or other caregivers when appropriate.

14. Pharmacists should preview and provide advice on the content and design of preprinted medication order forms or sheets if they are used.

15. Pharmacists should maintain records sufficient to enable identification of patients receiving an erroneous product.

Recommendations for Nurses. By virtue of their direct patient-care activities and administration of medications to patients, nurses—perhaps more than any other health-care providers—are in an excellent position to detect and report medication errors. Nurses often serve as the final point in the checks-and-balances triad (physicians and other prescribers, pharmacists, and nurses) for the medication use process; thus, they play an important role in risk reduction. The following recommendations for preventing medication administration errors are suggested:[3,14,16,17,34]

1. Nurses who practice in organized health-care settings should be familiar with the medication ordering and use system (e.g., participation in DUE activities, order processing, and standard medication administration times).

2. Nurses should review patients' medications with respect to desired patient outcomes, therapeutic duplications, and possible drug interactions. Adequate drug information (including information on medication administration and product compatibilities) should be obtained from pharmacists, nurses, other health-care providers, the literature, and other means when there are questions. There should be appropriate followup communication with the prescriber when this is indicated.

3. All drug orders should be verified before medication administration. Nurses should carefully review original medication orders before administration of the first dose and compare them with medications dispensed. Transcriptions of orders should be avoided to the extent possible and should be recognized as prime opportunities for errors. Doses should not be administered unless the meaning of the original order is clear and unambiguous and there are no questions with respect to the correctness of the prescribed regimen. Nurses should check the identity and integrity (e.g., expiration date and general appearance) of the medications dispensed before administering them. When there are discrepancies, the nurse should contact the pharmacy department and determine the appropriate action.

4. Patient identity should be verified before the administration of each prescribed dose. When appropriate, the patient should be observed after administration of the drug product to ensure that the doses were administered as prescribed and have the intended effect.

5. All doses should be administered at scheduled times unless there are questions or problems to be resolved. Medication doses should not be removed from packaging or labeling until immediately before administration. The administration of medication should be documented as soon as it is completed.

6. When standard drug concentrations or dosage charts are not available, dosage calculations, flow rates, and other mathematical calculations should be checked by a second individual (e.g., another nurse or a pharmacist).

7. The drug distribution system should not be circumvented by "borrowing" medications from one patient (or another hospital area) to give to a different patient or by stockpiling unused medications. If there are apparent missing doses, it is important that the pharmacy be contacted for explanation or correction. There may be an important reason why the dose was not sent to the patient-care area (e.g., allergy, contraindication, and questionable dose), and resolution of the potential question or problem may be pending.

8. If there are questions when a large volume or number of dosage units (e.g., more than two tablets, capsules, vials, or ampuls) is needed for a single patient dose, the medication order should be verified. Consult with the pharmacist and prescriber as appropriate.

9. All personnel using medication administration devices (e.g., infusion pumps) should understand their operation and the opportunities for error that might occur with the use of such devices.

10. Nurses should talk with patients or caregivers to ascertain that they understand the use of their medications and any special precautions or observations that might be indicated. Any counseling needed should be provided before the first dose is administered, when possible.

11. When a patient objects to or questions whether a particular drug should be administered, the nurse should listen, answer questions, and (if appropriate) double check the medication order and product dispensed before administering it to ensure that no preventable error is made (e.g., wrong patient, wrong route, and dose already administered). If a patient refuses to take a prescribed medication, that decision should be documented in the appropriate patient records.

Recommendations for Patients and Personal Caregivers. Patients (or their authorized caregivers or designees) have the right to know about all aspects of their care, including drug therapy. When patient status allows, health-care providers should encourage patients to take an active role in their drug use by questioning and learning about their treatment regimens. Generally, if patients are more knowledgeable, anxieties about the uncertainty of treatments can be alleviated and errors in treatment may be prevented. The following suggestions are offered to help patients whose health status allows, and their caregivers, make the best use of medications:[3]

1. Patients should inform appropriate direct health-care providers (e.g., physicians, nurses, and pharmacists) about all known symptoms, allergies, sensitivities, and

current medication use. Patients should communicate their actual self-medication practices, even if they differ from the prescribed directions.

2. Patients should feel free to ask questions about any procedures and treatments received.

3. Patients should learn the names of the drug products that are prescribed and administered to them, as well as dosage strengths and schedules. It is suggested that patients keep a personal list of all drug therapy, including prescribed drugs, nonprescription drugs, home remedies, and medical foods. Patients should also maintain lists of medications that they cannot take and the reasons why. This information should be shared with health-care providers. Patients should be assertive in communicating with health-care providers when anything seems incorrect or different from the norm.

4. After counseling from an authorized health-care provider about the appropriateness of the medication, patients should take all medications as directed.

Recommendations for Pharmaceutical Manufacturers and Approval Organizations.

Poor designs with respect to drug product packaging and labeling, as well as selection of inappropriate or confusing nomenclature, have been identified as factors that contribute to serious medication errors by practitioners.[4,35-37] Pharmaceutical manufacturers and approval agencies should be responsive to efforts of practitioners to minimize errors. The following guidelines are recommended for the pharmaceutical industry and regulatory authorities:[3,4,16,38]

1. Drug manufacturers and the Food and Drug Administration are urged to involve pharmacists, nurses, and physicians in decisions about drug names, labeling, and packaging.

2. Look-alike or sound-alike trademarked names and generic names should be avoided.

3. Similar proprietary appearances of packaging and labeling should be avoided, because look-alike products contribute to medication errors.

4. The use of lettered or numbered prefixes and suffixes in trademarked names is generally discouraged. Lettered prefixes or suffixes could be mistaken for instructions or strength. Commonly used medical abbreviations should never be used in trademarked names (e.g., "HS" could stand for half-strength or a bedtime dose). Numbers as part of trademarked names could be mistaken for quantities to be administered. Coined abbreviations that could be misinterpreted (e.g., MTX, U, and HCTZ) should not be used in trademarked names.

5. Special instructions should be highlighted on labeling, such as the need for dilution before administration.

6. The most prominent items on the product label should be information in the best interest of safety (e.g., product name and strength). Less prominence should be given to company names or logos.

7. Drug manufacturers are encouraged to make dosage forms available commercially in unit dose and unit-of-dispensing containers, as well as bulk packaging, to facilitate their appropriate use in all practice settings.

8. Drug manufacturers must communicate with health-care providers (i.e., pharmacists, physicians, and nurses) when changes are made in product formulations or dosage forms.

Monitoring and Managing Medication Errors

Monitoring Medication Errors.

Ongoing quality improvement programs for monitoring medication errors are needed. The difficulty in detecting errors has long been recognized as one of the barriers to studying the problem effectively.[39] Medication errors should be identified and documented and their causes studied in order to develop systems that minimize recurrence.[3,4,7,10,11,14,16,22,40] Several error monitoring techniques exist (e.g., anonymous self-reports, incident reports, critical incident technique, and disguised observation technique) and may be applied as appropriate to determine the rates of errors.[9,40,41] There are differences in the validity of data obtained by the various error monitoring techniques or combined techniques. Program managers should determine the best method for use in their organizations in consideration of utility, feasibility, and cost. Monitoring programs for medication errors should consider the following risk factors:[6,10,11,22,40,41]

1. Work shift (higher error rates typically occur during the day shift).

2. Inexperienced and inadequately trained staff.

3. Medical service (e.g., special needs for certain patient populations, including geriatrics, pediatrics, and oncology).

4. Increased number or quantity of medications per patient.

5. Environmental factors (lighting, noise, and frequent interruptions).

6. Staff workload and fatigue.

7. Poor communication among health-care providers.

8. Dosage form (e.g., injectable drugs are associated with more serious errors).

9. Type of distribution system (unit dose distribution is preferred; floor stock should be minimized).

10. Improper drug storage.

11. Extent of measurements or calculations required.

12. Confusing drug product nomenclature, packaging, or labeling.

13. Drug category (e.g., antimicrobials).

14. Poor handwriting.

15. Verbal (orally communicated) orders.

16. Lack of effective policies and procedures.

17. Poorly functioning oversight committees.

Managing Medication Errors.

Medication errors result from problematic processes, but the outcomes of medication errors could range from minimal (or no) patient risk to life-threatening risk. Classification of the potential seriousness and clinical significance of detected medication errors should be based on predefined criteria established by the P&T committee (or its equivalent). The error classification should be based on the original order, standard medication dispensing and administration procedures, dosage forms available, acceptable deviation ranges, potential for adverse consequences and patient harm, and other factors.[6,32,41]

Classification of medication errors should allow for better management of followup activities upon medication error detection. A simple classification of medication errors is the following: (1) clinically significant (includes potentially fatal or severe, potentially serious, and potentially significant errors) or (2) minor.[7,33] Hartwig, Denger, and Schneider defined seven medication error severity levels, as follows:[41]

Level 0—Nonmedication error occurred (potential errors would be classified here).

Level 1—An error occurred that did not result in patient harm.

Level 2—An error occurred that resulted in the need for increased patient monitoring but no change in vital signs and no patient harm.

Level 3—An error occurred that resulted in the need for increased patient monitoring with a change in vital signs but no ultimate patient harm, or any error that resulted in the need for increased laboratory monitoring.

Level 4—An error occurred that resulted in the need for treatment with another drug or an increased length of stay or that affected patient participation in an investigational drug study.[a]

Level 5—An error occurred that resulted in permanent patient harm.

Level 6—An error occurred that resulted in patient death.

Medication error classifications could also be based on probability and severity scales analogous to those used in ADR reporting programs.[42,43]

Determination of the causes of medication errors should be coupled with assessment of the severity of the error. While quality management processes should include programs to decrease the incidence of all medication errors, effort should be concentrated on eliminating the causes of errors associated with greater levels of severity. There should be established mechanisms for tracking drugs or drug classes that are involved in medication errors. Correlations between errors and the method of drug distribution should also be reviewed (e.g., unit dose, floor stock, or bulk medications; premixed or extemporaneously compounded products; and oral or injectable products). These processes will help identify system problems and stimulate changes to minimize the recurrence of errors.

Quality improvement programs should provide guidance for patient support, staff counseling and education, and risk management processes when a medication error is detected. Incident reporting policies and procedures and appropriate counseling, education, and intervention programs should be established in all hospitals. Risk management processes for medication errors should include pharmacists, physicians, and nurses, in addition to risk management specialists, legal counsel, and others as appropriate. The following actions are recommended upon error detection:[3,7,10,11,16,17,27,43]

1. Any necessary corrective and supportive therapy should be provided to the patient.
2. The error should be documented and reported immediately after discovery, in accordance with written procedures. For clinically significant errors, an immediate oral notice should be provided to physicians, nurses, and pharmacy managers. A written medication error report should follow promptly.
3. For clinically significant errors, fact gathering and investigation should be initiated immediately. Facts that should be determined and documented include what happened, where the incident occurred, why the incident occurred, how the incident occurred, and who was involved. Appropriate product evidence (e.g., packaging and labeling) should be retrieved and retained for future reference until causative factors are eliminated or resolved.
4. Reports of clinically significant errors and the associated corrective activities should be reviewed by the supervisor and department head of the area(s) involved, the appropriate organizational administrator, the organizational safety committee (or its equivalent), and legal counsel (as appropriate).
5. When appropriate, the supervisor and the staff members who were involved in the error should confer on how the error occurred and how its recurrence can be prevented. Medication errors often result from problems in systems rather than exclusively from staff performance or environmental factors;[2,3,44] thus, error reports should not be used for punitive purposes but to achieve correction or change.
6. Information gained from medication error reports and other means that demonstrates continued failure of individual professionals to avoid preventable medication errors should serve as an effective management and educational tool in staff development or, if necessary, modification of job functions or staff disciplinary action.
7. Supervisors, department managers, and appropriate committees should periodically review error reports and determine causes of errors and develop actions to prevent their recurrence (e.g., conduct organizational staff education, alter staff levels, revise policies and procedures, or change facilities, equipment, or supplies).
8. Medication errors should be reported to a national monitoring program so that the shared experiences of pharmacists, nurses, physicians, and patients can contribute to improved patient safety and to the development of valuable educational services for the prevention of future errors. Reports of medication errors can be made by telephone to the United States Pharmacopeial Convention, Inc. (USP) Medication Errors Reporting Program (1-800-23ERROR). Reports can be submitted to USP on a confidential basis if the reporter so chooses. Other reporting programs may also be in existence or under development. Reporting programs are intended to track trends and inform practitioners, regulators, and the pharmaceutical industry of potential product and system hazards that have a documented association with medication errors.

References

1. Hepler CD, Strand LM. Opportunities and responsibilities in pharmaceutical care. *Am J Hosp Pharm.* 1990; 47:533–43.
2. Manasse HR Jr. Medication use in an imperfect world: drug misadventuring as an issue of public policy, part 1. *Am J Hosp Pharm.* 1989; 46:929–44.
3. Davis NM, Cohen MR. Medication errors: causes and prevention. Huntingdon Valley, PA: Neil M. Davis Associates; 1981.
4. Zellmer WA. Preventing medication errors. *Am J Hosp Pharm.* 1990; 47:1755–6. Editorial.
5. Zellmer WA. ASHP plans for the future. *Am J Hosp Pharm.* 1986; 43:1921. Editorial.
6. American Society of Hospital Pharmacists. ASHP statement on the pharmacist's responsibility for distri-

bution and control of drugs. *Am J Hosp Pharm.* 1991; 48:1782.

7. Lesar RS, Briceland LL, Delcoure K, et al. Medication prescribing errors in a teaching hospital. *JAMA.* 1990; 263:2329–34.

8. American Society of Hospital Pharmacists. ASHP technical assistance bulletin on hospital drug distribution and control. *Am J Hosp Pharm.* 1980; 37:1097–103.

9. Allan EL, Barker KN. Fundamentals of medication error research. *Am J Hosp Pharm.* 1990; 47:555–71.

10. Betz RP, Levy HB. An interdisciplinary method of classifying and monitoring medication errors. *Am J Hosp Pharm.* 1985; 42:1724–32.

11. Leape LL, Brennan TA, Laird N, et al. The nature of adverse events in hospitalized patients—results of the Harvard medical practice study II. *N Engl J Med.* 1991; 324:377–84.

12. Ingrim NB, Hokanson JA, Guernsey BG, et al. Physician noncompliance with prescription-writing requirements. *Am J Hosp Pharm.* 1983; 40:414–7.

13. Anderson RD. The physician's contribution to hospital medication errors. *Am J Hosp Pharm.* 1971; 28:18–25.

14. Cooper JW. Consulting to long-term care patients. In: Brown TR, Smith MC, eds. Handbook of institutional pharmacy practice. 2nd ed. Baltimore, MD: Williams & Wilkins; 1986:649–61.

15. Bedell SE, Dertz DC, Leeman D, et al. Incidence and characteristics of preventable iatrogenic cardiac arrest. *JAMA.* 1991; 265:2815–20.

16. Fuqua RA, Stevens KR. What we know about medication errors: a literature review. *J Nurs Qual Assur.* 1988; 3:1–17.

17. Intravenous Nurses Society. Intravenous nursing standards of practice. *J Intraven Nurs.* 1990; 13(Apr):Suppl.

18. American Society of Hospital Pharmacists. ASHP statement on the pharmacist's clinical role in organized health care settings. *Am J Hosp Pharm.* 1989; 46:2345–6.

19. American Society of Hospital Pharmacists. ASHP guidelines on the pharmacist's role in drug-use evaluation. *Am J Hosp Pharm.* 1988; 45:385–6.

20. American Society of Hospital Pharmacists. ASHP guidelines: minimum standard for pharmacies in institutions. *Am J Hosp Pharm.* 1985; 42:372–5.

21. American Society of Hospital Pharmacists. ASHP guidelines for obtaining authorization for documenting pharmaceutical care in patient medical records. *Am J Hosp Pharm.* 1989; 46:338–9.

22. Barker KN, Pearson RE. Medication distribution systems. In: Brown TR, Smith MC, eds. Handbook of institutional pharmacy practice. 2nd ed. Baltimore, MD: Williams & Wilkins; 1986:325–51.

23. Cohen MR, Davis NM. Assuring safe use of parenteral dosage forms in hospitals. *Hosp Pharm.* 1990; 25:913–5. Editorial.

24. American Society of Hospital Pharmacists. ASHP statement on the pharmacy and therapeutics committee. *Am J Hosp Pharm.* 1992; 49:2008–9.

25. Barker KN, Pearson RE, Hepler CD, et al. Effect of an automated bedside dispensing machine on medication errors. *Am J Hosp Pharm.* 1984; 41:1352–8.

26. American Society of Hospital Pharmacists. ASHP guidelines for selecting pharmaceutical manufacturers and suppliers. *Am J Hosp Pharm.* 1991; 48:523–4.

27. Joint Commission on Accreditation of Healthcare Organizations. 1992 Accreditation manual for hospitals, vol. 1: standards. Oakbrook Terrace, IL: Joint Commission on Accreditation of Healthcare Organizations; 1991.

28. American Society of Hospital Pharmacists. ASHP guidelines on pharmacist-conducted patient counseling. *Am J Hosp Pharm.* 1984; 41:331.

29. American Society of Hospital Pharmacists. ASHP statement on unit dose drug distribution. *Am J Hosp Pharm.* 1989; 46:2346.

30. Brennan TA, Leape LL, Laird NM, et al. Incidence of adverse events and negligence in hospitalized patients—results of the Harvard medical practice study I. *N Engl J Med.* 1991; 324:370–6.

31. American Society of Hospital Pharmacists. Medication errors: a closer look (videocassette). Bethesda, MD: American Society of Hospital Pharmacists; 1988. 20 min.

32. Folli HL, Poole RL, Benitz WE, et al. Medication error prevention by clinical pharmacists in two children's hospitals. *Pediatrics.* 1987; 19:718–22.

33. Blum KV, Abel SA, Urbanski CJ, et al. Medication error prevention by pharmacists. *Am J Hosp Pharm.* 1988; 45:1902–3.

34. American Society of Hospital Pharmacists and American Nurses Association. ASHP and ANA guidelines for collaboration of pharmacists and nurses in institutional care settings. *Am J Hosp Pharm.* 1980; 37:253–4.

35. Derewicz HJ. Color-coded packaging and medication errors. *Am J Hosp Pharm.* 1978; 35:1344–6. Letter.

36. Myers CE. Color-coding of drug product labels and packages. *Am J Hosp Pharm.* 1988; 45:1660.

37. Clifton GD, Record KE. Color coding of multisource products should be standardized or eliminated. *Am J Hosp Pharm.* 1988; 45:1066. Letter.

38. Proceedings of the 41st annual session of the ASHP House of Delegates. Report of the House of Delegates. *Am J Hosp Pharm.* 1990; 47:1807–17.

39. Barker KN, McConnell WE. The problems of detecting medication errors in hospitals. *Am J Hosp Pharm.* 1962; 19:361–9.

40. McClure ML. Human error—a professional dilemma. *J Prof Nurs.* 1991; 7:207.

41. Hartwig SC, Denger SD, Schneider PJ. A severity-indexed, incident-report based medication-error reporting program. *Am J Hosp Pharm.* 1991; 48:2611–6.

42. Maliekal J, Thornton J. A description of a successful computerized adverse drug reaction tracking program. *Hosp Formul.* 1990; 25:436–42.

43. Miwa LJ, Fandall RJ. Adverse drug reaction program using pharmacist and nurse monitors. *Hosp Formul.* 1986:1140–6.

44. Anderson ER Jr. Disciplinary action after a serious medication error. *Am J Hosp Pharm.* 1987; 44:2690, 2692.

---

aThe mention of investigational drugs in the definition of level 4 errors (and nowhere else in the levels) may lead some to believe that any error involving an investigational drug should automatically be classified as a level 4 error. However, in discussing this issue at its September 1992 meeting, the ASHP Council on Professional Affairs noted that it is the effect on the patient (for a medication of any type) that really should determine what level of error is involved.

Approved by the ASHP Board of Directors, June 23, 1993, reaffirming the version approved November 18, 1992. Developed by the ASHP Council on Professional Affairs.

The bibliographic citation for this document is as follows: American Society of Hospital Pharmacists. ASHP guidelines on preventing medication errors in hospitals. *Am J Hosp Pharm*. 1993; 50:305–14.

ASHP Guidelines on the Pharmacist's Role in Home Care

The purpose of these guidelines is to define the role of the pharmacist in providing pharmaceutical care to patients in the home. (For brevity, the term "home" is used throughout this document. The guidance offered, however, should be understood to be applicable to any place of residence in which the care described is provided.) Broadly defined, home-care services include all health-related products and services provided to a patient at home. They range from personal care, respite care, and shopping assistance to high technology medical care such as dialysis and infusion therapy.[1] For the purposes of these guidelines, home care refers to the provision of pharmaceutical products and clinical monitoring to patients in the home including, but not limited to, home infusion therapy and other injectable drug therapy and enteral nutrition therapy. These guidelines apply to the pharmacist's role in providing home care and are not intended to apply to home health services that do not involve the provision of pharmacy services.

Home-care services are provided by a variety of organizations including hospitals, community pharmacies, home health agencies, and specialized home infusion companies. These guidelines apply to the provision of home-care services by pharmacists practicing in all health-care settings. It should be noted that different aspects of home care may be provided by different organizations. When services are shared among providers, pharmacists have a professional responsibility to ensure that all patient-care responsibilities are defined, understood, agreed on, and documented in advance by all providers.

Initial Patient Assessment

The pharmacist should ensure that each patient referred for home care is assessed for appropriateness on the basis of formal, predetermined admission criteria, including the following:

- Patient, family, and caregiver agreement with services being provided in the home.
- Ability and willingness of the patient or caregiver to be trained to administer medications properly.
- Home environment conducive to the provision of home-care services (e.g., electricity, running water, and cleanliness).
- Reasonable geographical access to the patient by the home-care provider.
- Psychosocial and family support (e.g., caregiver counseling, financial assistance and counseling, and suitable family environment).
- Ongoing prescriber involvement in the assessment and treatment of the patient.
- Medical condition and prescribed medication therapy suitable for home-care services and prognosis with clearly defined outcome goals.
- Appropriate indication, dose, route, and method of administration of medications.
- Appropriate laboratory tests for monitoring patient response to medications ordered.

Before the start of home-care services, patients should be informed of their rights and responsibilities. These should be explained in detail and given to the patient, family member, or other caregiver in writing.

When the first dose of medication is to be given in the home, the pharmacist should use clinical judgment in determining, in conjunction with the prescriber, home-care nurse, and patient or caregiver, whether home administration of the first dose is appropriate. Policies and procedures should define parameters to be used in making this decision and precautions necessary when first doses are administered in the home (e.g., emergency medications, monitoring and observation, and presence of health-care professional).[2]

Once a patient is accepted for home-care service but before the initiation of therapy, the pharmacist should assess the patient's current status and develop a thorough patient database in order to provide a basis for ongoing drug therapy monitoring and an evaluation tool for measuring patient outcomes.

The complete patient database should be documented in the patient's home-care record. This database should include, at a minimum:

- Patient's name, address, telephone number, and date of birth.
- Person to contact in the event of an emergency and contact information.
- Patient's height, weight, and sex.
- All diagnoses.
- Location and type of intravenous access, when necessary.
- Laboratory test results.
- Pertinent medical history and physical findings.
- Drug-related problem list.
- Accurate history of allergies.
- Initial and ongoing pharmaceutical assessment.
- Detailed medication profile including all medications (prescription and nonprescription), home remedies, and investigational and nontraditional therapies that the patient is receiving.
- Prescriber's name, address, telephone number, and any other pertinent information (e.g., Drug Enforcement Administration number).
- Other agencies and individuals involved in the patient's care and directions for contacting them.
- Medication history.
- Goals and expected duration of therapy.
- Desired outcome indicators.
- Patient education provided.
- Any functional limitations of the patient.
- Any pertinent social history or findings (e.g., alcohol consumption and tobacco use).

In obtaining this information, the pharmacist may use the past medical record; laboratory test results; direct communication with the patient, nurse, and prescriber; and direct observation. When the pharmacist cannot directly observe the patient, the patient's home-care nurse may provide the results of direct observation and physical assessment. If a shared service agreement exists among multiple providers, the pharmacist should ensure that this agreement specifies the responsibilities of each provider for obtaining and sharing pertinent patient information.

Patient Education, Training, and Counseling

The pharmacist is responsible for ensuring that the patient or caregiver receives appropriate education, training, and counseling regarding the patient's drug therapy. Other health-care professionals may be involved. A home-care pharmacist should be readily accessible in the event that questions or problems arise. Professional judgment should be employed in determining what information should be included in patient education and training. The following should be considered:

- Description of drug therapy including drug, dose, dosing interval, and duration of therapy.
- Goals of drug therapy.
- Importance of compliance in following the therapy plan.
- Proper aseptic technique.
- Proper care of the catheter and catheter site.
- Proper administration of medications.
- Inspection of medications, containers, and supplies before use.
- Equipment use, maintenance, and troubleshooting.
- Home inventory maintenance and procedures for securing additional supplies and medications when needed.
- Potential adverse effects, drug–drug interactions, and drug–nutrient interactions and their management.
- Special precautions for the preparation, storage, handling, and disposal of the drug, supplies, and biomedical waste.
- Information on contacting health-care providers involved in the patient's care.
- Emergency procedures.

Guidelines on patient counseling and education are available elsewhere.[3,4] Patient counseling and education should be performed in accordance with applicable state regulations and documented in the patient's home-care record.

Product, Device, and Ancillary Supply Selection

The pharmacist, in collaboration with other health-care professionals and the patient, is responsible for the selection of infusion devices, ancillary drugs (e.g., heparin flush and 0.9% sodium chloride), and ancillary supplies (e.g., dressing kits, syringes, and administration sets). Pharmacists should be thoroughly trained and knowledgeable in the selection and use of these devices, drugs, and supplies. Factors involved in the selection of devices and ancillary supplies may include the following:

- Stability and compatibility of prescribed medication(s) in infusion device reservoirs.
- Ability of an infusion device to accommodate the appropriate volume of medication and diluent and to deliver the prescribed dose at the appropriate rate.

- Ability of patient or caregiver to learn to operate an infusion device.
- Potential for patient complications and noncompliance.
- Patient convenience.
- Nursing or caregiver experience with therapy and selected devices.
- Prescriber preference.
- Cost considerations.
- Safety features of infusion devices.

The home-care pharmacist, in consultation with the prescriber, should determine when emergency medications and supplies (e.g., anaphylaxis kits) should be dispensed to home-care patients. When standing orders for ancillary drugs or supplies or standardized treatment protocols are used, the pharmacist should review each protocol to determine its appropriateness for the patient. Information on the selection of infusion devices and catheters is available elsewhere.[5–7]

Development of Pharmaceutical Care Plans

The pharmacist, in collaboration with the patient or caregiver and other health-care professionals, is responsible for developing an appropriate pharmaceutical care plan for each patient. The pharmaceutical care plan should be developed as part of the patient's overall care plan. The pharmaceutical care plan should be based on information obtained from the initial pharmacy assessment and other relevant information obtained from the nurse, prescriber, patient, and caregiver. At a minimum, the pharmaceutical care plan should include the following:[8]

- Actual or potential drug therapy problems and their proposed solutions.
- Desired outcomes of drug therapy provided.
- A monitoring plan specifying objective and subjective parameters (e.g., vital signs, laboratory tests, physical findings, and patient response) for monitoring outcomes and drug therapy-related problems (e.g., toxicity, adverse reactions, and noncompliance).
- Frequency for proactive monitoring of the above parameters.

The pharmaceutical care plan should be developed at the initiation of therapy and reviewed and updated on a regular basis. The degree of detail of the pharmaceutical care plan should be based on the complexity of drug therapy and the patient. The Joint Commission on Accreditation of Healthcare Organizations *Accreditation Manual for Home Care* includes examples of pharmaceutical care plans for various therapies.[9]

The pharmacist is responsible for communicating the pharmaceutical care plan to other health-care professionals involved in the care of the patient and regularly communicating any updates as they occur. The pharmaceutical care plan and updates should be a part of the patient's home-care record.

Patient Clinical Monitoring

The pharmacist is responsible for ongoing clinical monitoring of the patient's drug therapy according to the pharmaceutical care plan developed and for appropriately documenting and communicating the results of all monitoring activities to other health-care professionals involved in the patient's care. The pharmacist is also responsible for ensuring that relevant information is obtained from the patient, caregiver, and other health-care professionals and documenting this information in the patient's home-care record. Pharmacists may wish to develop clinical monitoring protocols, in collaboration with prescribers and others, for various therapies. In most home-care practice sites, the pharmacist is responsible for obtaining the medication order from the prescriber. Pharmacists may receive laboratory results before other health-care providers. In such cases, the pharmacist is responsible for communicating the laboratory test results to the prescriber and other health-care providers. The pharmacist should provide an interpretive analysis of the information and recommendations for dose adjustments, continuation, or discontinuation of drug therapy. The pharmacist should ensure that sufficient laboratory test results are readily available for monitoring the patient's therapy. In shared service arrangements, clinical monitoring responsibilities should be delineated.

Effective Communication with Prescribers, Nurses, and Other Health-Care Personnel

Effective communication among pharmacists, prescribers, nurses, and other health-care personnel is critical to the care of the patient. The pharmacist should ensure that effective channels of communication regarding the care of the patient are in place, including shared service arrangements (e.g., pain assessments and laboratory test data). Both oral and written communication methods may be used for communicating patient information. Confidentiality of patient information and pertinent federal and state regulations should be considered by the pharmacist. All relevant clinical communication should be documented in the patient's home-care record. It is recommended that personnel involved in the care of the patient (e.g., nurses, pharmacists, dietitians, delivery representatives, and reimbursement coordinators) meet regularly (e.g., weekly patient rounds) to discuss the clinical status of the patient and any operational issues related to the care of the patient.

The patient, family, caregiver, and all health-care personnel involved in the care of the patient should have access to a pharmacist 24 hours a day. Before transferring patient-care responsibilities, the pharmacist is responsible for providing a summary of all relevant clinical information to another pharmacist providing coverage for that patient (e.g., on-call pharmacist).

Direct Communication with Patient and Caregiver

The pharmacist providing home-care services should establish free and open channels of communication with the patient or caregiver. The pharmacist should contact the patient or caregiver as soon as the patient is accepted for service to

- Obtain information needed for the initial pharmacy assessment.
- Provide supplemental patient education and counseling as needed.

- Assess drug therapy compliance.
- Inform the patient how to contact the pharmacist when needed.
- Assess drug therapy problems [e.g., side effects, adverse drug reactions (ADRs), and noncompliance].

All patient contacts should be documented in the patient's home-care record.

Coordination of Drug Preparation, Delivery, Storage, and Administration

The pharmacist is responsible for ensuring the proper acquisition, compounding, dispensing, storage, delivery, and administration of all medications and related equipment and supplies. Compounding of sterile products should comply with applicable practice standards, accreditation standards, and pertinent state and federal regulations. If these services are being provided by another pharmacy, the pharmacist should have reasonable assurance that these standards are being met by the pharmacy providing the service. Pharmacists may administer medications to patients in the home setting unless prohibited by applicable statutes and regulations.

The pharmacist should ensure that the delivery of medications and supplies to the patient occurs in a timely manner to avoid inappropriate interruption in drug therapy. Further, the pharmacist should ensure that storage conditions during the delivery process and in the patient's home are consistent with the recommendations for storage of the product and expiration dating. The temperature of home refrigerators or freezers in which medications are stored should be within acceptable limits and should be monitored by the patient or caregiver regularly. The pharmacist should ensure that an adequate inventory of medications and ancillary supplies are available in the patient's home. It may be appropriate to provide additional inventory for unforeseen circumstances where extra doses or supplies may be required (e.g., wastage, breakage, and emergencies).

Employee and Patient Safety and Universal Precautions

A home-care organization is responsible for assisting in the education and training of employees, patients, family members, and caregivers in appropriate safety and universal precautions[9] as mandated by the Occupational Safety and Health Administration. The pharmacist should ensure that the home-care organization provides appropriate instruction and training for its employees and patients, including appropriate disposal and handling of medical waste, procedures for prevention and management of needle sticks, handling of cytotoxic and hazardous medications,[10,11] and Material Safety Data Sheets. The pharmacist should be a key resource in the development of such training programs. The pharmacist should assume an active role in the home-care organization's infection control activities.[12] For high risk patients, it may be advisable to consider using a system or device (e.g., needleless system) to minimize the potential for needle sticks.

Documentation in Home-Care Record

A home-care record should be developed and used for documenting the home-care services provided to each patient. Written organizational policies and procedures should address the security of home-care records and specify personnel who have the authority to review and make entries in home-care records. The confidentiality of patient information should be stressed to all personnel.

The pharmacist is responsible for documenting all pharmacy clinical activities in the patient's home-care record in a timely manner. To minimize duplication of information, general clinician-oriented forms are preferred over specific nursing, pharmacy, or other healthcare professional forms.

It may be advisable for organizations that provide multiple home-care services (e.g., pharmacy, nursing, and respiratory services) to use a single home-care record for documenting all clinical information regarding each patient. The home-care record should be accessible at all times to authorized personnel involved in the care of the patient.

ADR Reporting

The home-care pharmacist should assist in the development of a program for reporting and monitoring all adverse drug- and device-related events. Such activities should be consistent with the "ASHP Guidelines on Adverse Drug Reaction Monitoring and Reporting."[13] The pharmacist should ensure that the prescriber is notified promptly of any suspected ADR.

ADRs should serve as outcome indicators of quality, and the monitoring of ADRs should be a part of the organization's ongoing quality improvement program. To improve patient outcomes, relevant ADR trends should be integrated into staff development and inservice education programs for pharmacists and nurses. Serious ADRs should be reported promptly to the manufacturer or Food and Drug Administration.[14]

Participation in Clinical Trials in the Home

The pharmacist should play a key role in the development of policies and procedures for handling investigational drugs in the home-care setting. The "ASHP Guidelines for the Use of Investigational Drugs in Organized Health-Care Settings"[15] may be used as a guideline for the development of such policies and procedures.

When patient participation in an investigational drug study is initiated in the institutional setting or other setting before the patient's transfer to the home-care setting, it is important that the home-care pharmacist obtain and keep on file sufficient information about the investigational protocol and drugs. If an investigational drug is dispensed or administered by the home-care organization, a copy of the informed consent form signed by the patient should be placed in the patient's home-care record. The home-care pharmacist should review the protocol before the patient is admitted to the home-care service to determine whether treatment of the patient in the home is appropriate. When investigational drug inventories are maintained in the home-care pharmacy, the pharmacist is responsible for accurate recordkeeping. The pharmacist should be an active participant in coordinating and monitoring investigational drug studies in home care.

Participation in Quality Improvement Activities

Pharmacists and other members of the pharmacy staff (e.g., technicians) should be active participants in quality improvement activities in their organizations. A quality improvement program for home care should monitor patient satisfaction and outcomes. Aspects of care that may be monitored include the following:

- Unscheduled inpatient admissions.
- Unexpected discontinuation of infusion therapy.
- Interruption of infusion therapy.
- Development of infection(s).
- Reported adverse drug- and device-related reactions.
- Medication errors.
- Medication-related problems.

The quality improvement program should also include appropriate quality control measures for the compounding of sterile products and other activities.

Policies and Procedures

The home-care pharmacist should be an active participant in the development of organizational policies and procedures. The organization should maintain current policies and procedures on all aspects of patient care and quality assurance. Activities that should be addressed in policies and procedures include, but are not limited to, criteria for patient acceptance to home-care services, patient training and education, drug preparation and dispensing, equipment maintenance, quality control and quality assurance in sterile product compounding, infection control, and documentation in patients' home-care records.

Licensure and Accreditation

Pharmacies providing home-care services should be licensed by the state board of pharmacy and other appropriate regulatory agencies. Some states require special licensure for pharmacies preparing sterile products to be dispensed to outpatients. Pharmacists dispensing medications to patients who reside in other states may also be subject to applicable regulations in those states; additional licensure may be necessary. Accreditation of the organization by the Joint Commission or the Community Health Accreditation Program is recommended. The pharmacist should be knowledgeable of all applicable laws, regulations, and standards.

Continuing Education and Training

Pharmacists should receive training in the provision of home-care services. Pharmacists should participate in ongoing continuing-education activities as defined in the "ASHP Statement on Continuing Education"[16] to improve knowledge and skills related to home care. When appropriate, pharmacists should assist in training and education programs for other home health care personnel. Whenever possible, pharmacists should participate in the provision of student clerkship, externship, and internship training, as well as postgraduate residency training.

References

1. Pelham LD, Norwood MR. Home health care services. In: Brown TR, ed. Handbook of institutional pharmacy practice. 3rd ed. Bethesda, MD: American Society of Hospital Pharmacists; 1992:357–66.
2. McNulty TJ. Initiation of antimicrobial therapy in the home. *Am J Hosp Pharm*. 1993; 50:773–4.
3. American Society of Hospital Pharmacists. ASHP statement on the pharmacist's role in patient education programs. *Am J Hosp Pharm*. 1991; 48:1780.
4. American Society of Hospital Pharmacists. ASHP guidelines on pharmacist-conducted patient counseling. *Am J Hosp Pharm*. 1993; 50:505–6.
5. American Society of Hospital Pharmacists. ASHP statement on the pharmacist's role with respect to drug delivery systems and administration devices. *Am J Hosp Pharm*. 1993; 50:771–2.
6. Kwan J. High-technology i.v. infusion devices. *Am J Hosp Pharm*. 1991; 48(Suppl 1):S36–S51.
7. Bowles C, McKinnon BT. Selecting infusion devices. *Am J Hosp Pharm*. 1993; 50:1228–30.
8. Hepler CD, Strand LM. Opportunities and responsibilities in pharmaceutical care. *Am J Hosp Pharm*. 1990; 47:533–43.
9. Joint Commission on Accreditation of Healthcare Organizations. Accreditation manual for home care. Oakbrook Terrace, IL: Joint Commission on Accreditation of Healthcare Organizations; 1993.
10. American Society of Hospital Pharmacists. ASHP technical assistance bulletin on handling cytotoxic and hazardous drugs. *Am J Hosp Pharm*. 1990; 47:1033–49.
11. Schaffner A. Safety precautions in home chemotherapy. *Am J Nurs*. 1984; 84:346–7.
12. American Society of Hospital Pharmacists. ASHP statement on the pharmacist's role in infection control. *Am J Hosp Pharm*. 1986; 43:2006–8.
13. American Society of Hospital Pharmacists. ASHP guidelines on adverse drug reaction monitoring and reporting. *Am J Hosp Pharm*. 1989; 46:336–7.
14. Draft form for reporting suspect adverse events and product problems with medications and devices; notice. *Fed Regist*. 1993; 58:1168–73.
15. American Society of Hospital Pharmacists. ASHP guidelines for the use of investigational drugs in organized health-care settings. *Am J Hosp Pharm*. 1991; 48:315–9.
16. American Society of Hospital Pharmacists. ASHP statement on continuing education. *Am J Hosp Pharm*. 1990; 47:1855.

Approved by the ASHP Board of Directors, June 6, 1993. Developed by the ASHP Council on Professional Affairs.

The bibliographic citation for this document is as follows: American Society of Hospital Pharmacists. ASHP guidelines on the pharmacist's role in home care. *Am J Hosp Pharm*. 1993; 50:1940–4.

ASHP Guidelines for Pharmacists on the Activities of Vendors' Representatives in Organized Health Care Systems

For purposes of this document, vendors' representatives are defined as agents who promote products and provide information and services to health care providers on behalf of manufacturers and suppliers. The narrow focus of this document is on those vendors who serve and interact with settings with respect to drug products, drug-related devices, and other equipment, supplies, and services purchased by pharmacies.

Each individual setting should develop its own specific policies and procedures relating to the activities of vendors' representatives. Such policies and procedures should supplement and complement applicable federal, state, and local laws and regulations (for example, statutes that address prescription drug-product sampling). The ASHP Guidelines on Pharmacists' Relationships with Industry, the ASHP Guidelines for Selecting Pharmaceutical Manufacturers and Suppliers, and setting-specific conflict-of-interest policies may be helpful in the development of policies and procedures.[1,2] The policies and procedures should be developed by the setting's pharmacy and therapeutics committee (or equivalent body) and approved by higher authorities in the setting as required. Depending on the individual setting, policies and procedures may be useful in the following areas.

1. *A defined scope of applicability.* The vendors' representatives to which any policies and procedures apply should be defined by the individual setting. For example, if the policies and procedures are applicable only to drug-product vendors' representatives and not to those promoting medical–surgical supplies, packaging equipment, or drug administration devices, this should be clearly stated.

2. *Orientation of representatives.* In some individual settings, vendors' representatives receive an orientation packet upon their initial visit to the setting. Such a packet might contain a copy of the setting's policies and procedures, a medical staff directory, and the formulary. Some settings provide a formal orientation program that includes meeting key individuals and touring the setting.

3. *Directory.* In some individual settings, a file of current vendor-contact information is maintained in the pharmacy. A form for recording such information might include the following:
   - The vendor's name and address;
   - The name, address, telephone number, and answering service number (if any), and drug-product assignment (purview) of each representative;
   - The name, address, and telephone number of the representative's manager;
   - The names, telephone numbers, and emergency telephone numbers of the vendor's directors of distribution, sales, and product information (titles may vary); and
   - The names and telephone numbers of the vendor's medical director and research director (titles may vary).

4. *Availability of vendor-contact information to professionals in the setting.* In some individual settings, the pharmacy department provides the setting's professional staff with the information in item 3, upon request.

5. *Registration while on premises.* In some individual settings, vendors' representatives register with the pharmacy department or other designated department upon each visit to the setting. At such time, the vendors' representatives document the time, purpose, and location of their appointments. In many settings, during the registration process, the representative is provided with a dated name badge to be prominently worn along with the representative's current vendor-supplied name tag (if any).

6. *Locations permitted.* In some individual settings, restriction (if any) from patient care and pharmacy storage and work areas in the setting are specified in the policies and procedures. Meetings with professional staff are conducted in areas convenient to staff and generally in non-patient-care areas.

7. *Appointments and purposes.* In some individual settings, representatives are encouraged to schedule appointments with appropriate pharmacy department staff to
   - Provide information useful for product evaluation. Representatives might be asked to include balanced scientific literature (journal reprints, for example) on drug-product safety and efficacy, as well as documentation of likely cost benefits.
   - Provide timely information on the vendor's products and services.
   - Facilitate procurement and crediting transactions.
   - Obtain and provide information necessary to support the setting's formulary system.
   - Facilitate informational activities for the pharmacy staff and other health care professionals with respect to the vendor's products.

8. *Exhibits.* In some individual settings, the pharmacy department provides opportunities for vendors' representatives to distribute informational material by arranging for organized, scheduled exhibits. Policies and procedures about the times, places, content, and conduct of such events are established.

9. *Dissemination of promotional materials.* In some individual settings, there are policies and procedures about the dissemination (by vendors' representatives) of information on formulary and nonformulary products, including the designation of appropriate categories of recipients of the information (e.g., attending physicians, department chairmen, house staff physicians). Representatives may be asked to promptly provide the pharmacy department with copies of all informational and promotional materials disseminated in the setting. The Food and Drug Administration (FDA) prohibits

the advertising and promotion of drug products for uses not reflected in FDA-approved product labeling ("unlabeled uses").[3] Pharmacists and other health care professionals should be aware of these laws and regulations when evaluating the content of promotional materials.

10. *Samples.* In some individual settings, there are policies and procedures with respect to product samples. ASHP urges that the use of drug samples within the institution be eliminated to the extent possible.[4,5]

11. *Noncompliance.* In some individual settings, policies and procedures exist to address noncompliance with the policies and procedures by either vendors' representatives or professional staff.

Each setting should have policies and procedures concerning research to be conducted on its premises. Pharmacists and vendors' representatives should clearly differentiate research from sales and promotional activities, applying appropriate policies and procedures accordingly.[6] Generally, scientific research involving drug products is coordinated through research departments of product manufacturers rather than through sales and promotional representatives.

References

1. American Society of Hospital Pharmacists. ASHP guidelines on pharmacists' relationships with industry. *Am J Hosp Pharm.* 1992; 49:154.

2. American Society of Hospital Pharmacists. ASHP guidelines for selecting pharmaceutical manufacturers and suppliers. *Am J Hosp Pharm.* 1991; 48:523–4.

3. American Society of Hospital Pharmacists. ASHP statement on the use of medications for unlabeled uses. *Am J Hosp Pharm.* 1992; 49:927–8.

4. American Society of Hospital Pharmacists. ASHP guidelines: minimum standard for pharmacies in institutions. *Am J Hosp Pharm.* 1985; 42:372–5.

5. Greenberg RB. The Prescription Drug Marketing Act of 1987. *Am J Hosp Pharm.* 1988; 45:2118–26.

6. American Society of Hospital Pharmacists. ASHP guidelines for pharmaceutical research in organized health-care settings. *Am J Hosp Pharm.* 1989; 46:129–30.

Approved by the ASHP Board of Directors, November 17, 1993. Developed by the Council on Professional Affairs.

The bibliographic citation for this document is as follows: American Society of Hospital Pharmacists. ASHP guidelines for pharmacists on the activities of vendors' representatives in organized health care systems. *Am J Hosp Pharm.* 1994; 51:520–1.

ASHP Guidelines for Providing Pediatric Pharmaceutical Services in Organized Health Care Systems

Patient care consists of integrated domains of care, including medical care, nursing care, and pharmaceutical care. The provision of pharmaceutical care involves not only medication therapy but decisions about medication selection, dosages, routes and methods of administration, medication therapy monitoring, and the provision of medication-related information and counseling to individual patients.[1] The pediatric patient population poses some unique challenges to the pharmaceutical care provider in terms of these medication-related activities. These challenges include the lack of published information on the therapeutic uses and monitoring of drugs in pediatric patients; the lack of appropriate commercially available dosage forms and concentrations of many drugs for pediatric patients; and the resulting need to develop innovative ways of ensuring that the patient receives the drug in a manner that allows the intended therapeutic effect to be realized.[2] These guidelines are intended to assist pharmacists in meeting the special needs of the pediatric patient in any organized health care setting.

General Principles

The pharmacy service should be organized in accordance with the principles of good management. It should be under the direction of a pharmacist and be provided with sufficient physical facilities, personnel, and equipment to meet the pharmaceutical care needs of the pediatric population. Resources necessary for compounding and testing alternative doses and dosage forms of commercially available products are essential. The pharmacy should comply with all applicable federal, state, and local laws, codes, statutes, and regulations.[3] The setting should meet applicable accreditation criteria of the Joint Commission on Accreditation of Healthcare Organizations. Organizations such as the National Association of Children's Hospitals and Related Institutions, the American Academy of Pediatrics, and the Pediatric Pharmacy Administrative Group are useful sources of further information on pediatric health care services.

Orientation and Training Programs

Orientation, training, and staff development programs for pharmacists providing services to pediatric patients should emphasize dosage calculations, dosage-form selection appropriate to the patient's age and condition, and specialized drug preparation and administration techniques. Pharmacists should be familiar with the pharmacokinetic and pharmacodynamic changes that occur with age (e.g., in volume of distribution, protein binding, renal elimination, metabolism, muscle mass, and fluid requirements) and with disease-specific conditions that might affect drug choice or administration (e.g., short-gut syndrome, lactose intolerance). A sensitivity to the nature, frequency, and severity of medication-related errors in the pediatric population is important for all pharmacy personnel.[4]

Inpatient Services

A lack of availability of commercially prepared dosage forms, combined with the documented risk of calculation errors, requires the use of comprehensive unit dose drug distribution systems and intravenous (i.v.) admixture services for pediatric patients. Appropriate dosage standardization in both oral and parenteral drug distribution systems may facilitate the provision of these services.

Unit Dose System. The pediatric unit dose system must meet the original intent of these systems, which is to minimize errors and provide drugs to the patient care areas in ready-to-administer form. Multidose containers and stock medications should be avoided. An extemporaneous preparation service should facilitate the preparation and packaging of medications according to sound compounding principles.

I.V. Admixture Service. The drugs provided by the i.v. admixture service should include all i.v. push, i.v. minibag, intramuscular, and subcutaneous doses; large-volume injections; antineoplastic agents; parenteral nutrient fluids; ophthalmic products; peritoneal dialysis solutions; and irrigation fluids. Knowledge of pediatric fluid requirements and limitations, drug administration techniques and devices, and acceptable volumes for intramuscular injection is critical. Care should be taken when making dilutions to maximize concentrations of drug products (when safe to do so) for fluid-sensitive patients, as well as to minimize hyperosmolar solutions that might lead to destruction of vasculature or, in the neonate, intraventricular hemorrhage. Quality controls for both manually prepared and computer-driven preparation should exist to ensure that each product contains the ingredients ordered and that they are properly labeled. Knowledge of products that contain benzyl alcohol and the risks of this substance in neonates is essential in a pediatric i.v. admixture service.

The labels of all products should be evaluated for legibility, clarity of expression, and their potential for leading to a medication error.[5] Labels should include the drug name; the drug concentration; the route of administration; the expiration date or time; appropriate instructions for administration, additional preparation, and storage; and the lot number (if a batch-prepared product).[6]

Ambulatory Care Services

Ambulatory care pharmacy services should be attentive to the unique drug needs of the pediatric patient. These include the need for special dosage forms (e.g., liquids and chewable tablets), measuring devices, and detailed counseling on drug administration. When product stability is a problem, caregivers may have to be taught how to prepare an appropriate dosage form in the home. Consideration must be given to taste and the need for an extra prescription container to be taken to school or daycare. Children should be included whenever possible in discussions concerning their medications. In the ambulatory care setting, the pharmacist is well positioned to play a role in preventive health care, including poison prevention and immunization.[7]

Drug Information

Drug information services should provide the pharmacist practicing in the pediatric setting with information unique to the pediatric population. References should include pediatric medical texts and current information on pediatric dosages, extemporaneous formulations, drug compatibilities and stability, poison control, and drug effects during pregnancy and lactation. Drug information should be available in areas where decisions are being made about drug therapy. Literature supporting the use of drugs for unlabeled uses in pediatric patients should also be available.[8] Pharmacists should provide other health care professionals with information on new and investigational drugs, adverse effects of and contraindications to drug therapy, compatibility and stability information, dosage computations, pharmacokinetics, and drug interactions. This may be accomplished through educational presentations, seeing patients in conjunction with other caregivers ("rounding"), and printed materials (e.g., newsletters).

Therapeutic Drug Monitoring

Therapeutic drug monitoring enables assessment of therapeutic outcomes and recognition at the earliest moment of an undesirable response to a drug. Both desired and undesired effects should be documented. The person performing therapeutic drug monitoring should take into consideration the age-related differences in dosage when recommending or reviewing drug therapy.

Pharmacokinetic Services

For both oral and injectable drugs, pharmacokinetic services should ensure that the drug has been administered appropriately before samples are taken for the measurement of serum drug concentrations. The frequency and timing of sampling should also be monitored to avoid excessive and traumatic sampling in children. Knowledge of age-related differences in absorption, distribution, metabolism, and elimination is essential for the pharmacist who is involved in pharmacokinetic services for pediatric patients. The collection and publication of accurate pharmacokinetic data on the pediatric population are encouraged.

Patient and Caregiver Education

Pharmacists should counsel and educate patients and caregivers about their medications, including the purpose of each medication, dosage instructions, potential drug interactions, potential adverse effects, and any specific age-related issues (e.g., compounding and diluting techniques, measuring and administration instructions). Caregivers should be informed of any drug products for which crushing, chewing, dividing, or diluting should be avoided. Suggestions about masking the taste of an unpleasant medication should also be provided. Administration of products, including ophthalmics, otics, inhalers, and injectables, should be

demonstrated. The prevention of accidental ingestion of medications should also be emphasized. The benefits of educational programs are best realized when a cooperative multidisciplinary approach is used. Sharing of pertinent information by all participants is fundamental to the success of patient education services.[9]

Medication Errors

Systems for the recognition, documentation, and prevention of medication errors are essential for the pediatric population. Pharmacist participation in quality-improvement committees and the participation of pharmacists, nurses, physicians, and risk managers are important in minimizing medication errors in pediatric patients. The development and enforcement of policies and procedures for minimizing medication errors are essential. Pediatric patients are especially vulnerable to errors caused by mistakes in calculations. Pharmacists should recognize that since some commercially available products are available in strengths that can be potentially toxic to a pediatric patient, special scrutiny of these products is necessary.[5]

Adverse Drug Reactions

Pediatric patients frequently have the same kinds of adverse drug reactions that adults have, but adverse reactions in the pediatric population may be harder to recognize or of greater or lesser intensity. The lack of literature on newly introduced therapeutic agents makes it imperative to monitor experience with new drugs initially used in the pediatric population. Comprehensive adverse drug reaction monitoring and reporting programs are important in reducing the occurrence of these reactions in pediatric patients.[10]

Drug-Use Evaluation

Drug-use evaluation should be directed at drugs with a low therapeutic index that require extensive monitoring, those that are responsible for serious medication errors in the institution, and those that are found to be associated with high frequency of preventable adverse drug reactions. Cost-related issues may also become important in the evaluations, since many expensive drugs are not available in package sizes appropriate for the pediatric patient.

Research

Pediatric patients have long been recognized as "therapeutic orphans" because of a relative absence of therapeutic trials in this patient population. The reasons for this are numerous and include ethical issues, potential adverse publicity, possible litigation, methodological hurdles, and an inability to justify such studies for economic reasons. Nonetheless, the need for timely and effective research on medication safety, efficacy, and practical application in the pediatric population is compelling. The paucity of pediatric drug information, the impact of new drug delivery systems, the expansion of adult diseases (such as AIDS) into the pediatric population, and expanded applications of new and established therapeutic agents are all areas warranting additional research. The pediatric pharmacist can be directly involved in collaboration with other health care providers in conducting pediatric research. Examples of pediatric research topics include, but are not limited to, the following:

- Safety and efficacy of drug products in pediatric patients;
- Pharmacokinetics and pharmacodynamics of new medications;
- Stability, safety, and efficacy of extemporaneously compounded sterile and nonsterile drug products;
- Safety and efficacy of administration techniques;
- Comparative evaluations of medications addressing treatment regimens, outcomes of therapy, and their relative costs;
- Behavioral and socioeconomic compliance issues in pediatric pharmaceutical care; and
- New and existing pharmacy drug distribution systems and services for pediatric patients.

Examples of direct involvement include

- Serving as a member of an institutional review board,
- Maintenance, oversight, and dissemination of all information on investigational drug studies and comparative trials involving medications in the pediatric population; and
- Maintenance, coordination, and oversight of policies and procedures involving investigational drug studies and comparative trials involving medications in the pediatric population.

References

1. American Society of Hospital Pharmacists. ASHP statement on pharmaceutical care. *Am J Hosp Pharm.* 1993; 50:1720–3.
2. Pediatric Pharmacy Administration Group Committee on Pediatric Pharmacy Practice. Pediatric pharmacy practice guidelines. *Am J Hosp Pharm.* 1991; 48:2475–7.
3. American Society of Hospital Pharmacists. ASHP guidelines: minimum standard for pharmacies in institutions. *Am J Hosp Pharm.* 1985; 42:372–5.
4. Folli HL, Poole RL, Benitz WE, et al. Medication error prevention by clinical pharmacists in two children's hospitals. *Pediatrics.* 1987; 79:718–22.
5. American Society of Hospital Pharmacists. ASHP guidelines on preventing medication errors in hospitals. *Am J Hosp Pharm.* 1993; 50:305–14.
6. American Society of Hospital Pharmacists. ASHP technical assistance bulletin on single unit and unit dose packages of drugs. *Am J Hosp Pharm.* 1985; 42:378–9.
7. American Society of Hospital Pharmacists. ASHP technical assistance bulletin on the pharmacist's role in immunization. *Am J Hosp Pharm.* 1993; 50:501–5.
8. American Society of Hospital Pharmacists. ASHP statement on the use of medications for unlabeled uses. *Am J Hosp Pharm.* 1992; 49:2006–8.
9. American Society of Hospital Pharmacists. ASHP guidelines on pharmacist-conducted patient counseling. *Am J Hosp Pharm.* 1993; 50:505–6.
10. American Society of Hospital Pharmacists. ASHP guidelines on adverse drug reaction monitoring and reporting. *Am J Hosp Pharm.* 1989; 46:336–7.

Approved by the ASHP Board of Directors, April 27, 1994. Developed by the ASHP Council on Professional Affairs.

The bibliographic citation for this document is as follows: American Society of Hospital Pharmacists. ASHP guidelines for providing pediatric pharmaceutical services in organized health care systems. *Am J Hosp Pharm.* 1994; 51:1690–2.

ASHP Guidelines on Pharmaceutical Services in Correctional Facilities

Introduction

Pharmaceutical services in correctional facilities encompass many aspects of community, hospital, and consultant pharmacy practice. These guidelines are intended to address some of the unique aspects of pharmacy practice and services in correctional facilities. Some correctional facilities may not require, or be able to obtain, the services of a pharmacist. However, the concepts, principles, and recommendations contained in this standard are applicable to all correctional facilities, regardless of size or type. Thus, the part-time pharmacy director or consultant pharmacist has the same basic obligations and responsibilities as his or her full-time counterpart in larger settings. This document should serve as a guide for the provision of pharmaceutical services in correctional institutions.

Administration

Pharmaceutical services are an integral part of health care provided in correctional institutions. The pharmacist is usually responsible for multiple tasks ranging from the management of the pharmacy to the direct provision of services to inmate-patients. Two primary management responsibilities pertain to human and fiscal resources.

Personnel[1]

- Sufficient support personnel should be available to maximize the use of pharmacists in tasks requiring professional judgment. Appropriate supervisory controls for support personnel should be maintained. The use of pharmacy technicians graduated from ASHP-accredited pharmacy technician training programs is recommended. Pharmacy technicians should be certified by the Pharmacy Technician Certification Board.
- All personnel should possess the education and training needed to carry out their responsibilities. The competence of all staff may be enhanced through relevant continuing education. Credentialing of eligible staff as Certified Correctional Health Professionals through the National Commission on Correctional Health Care is recommended.
- A pharmacist should be available, at a minimum, on a consulting basis; the pharmacist should visit each facility no less than monthly. If the only pharmaceutical services provided are those of a consultant pharmacist, the consultant pharmacist should assume the role of pharmacy director.
- If the pharmacist is an employee of a contract vendor, he or she should be designated as the pharmacy director and assume the associated obligations and responsibilities.
- Health care services should be available to inmate-patients 24 hours a day. Pharmacist services should also be available, at least on an "on call" basis.
- Other pertinent guidelines of the American Society of Health-System Pharmacists, the National Commission

on Correctional Health Care, and the American Correctional Association should be followed, and requirements set by federal, state, and local laws and regulations with respect to personnel should be met.

Fiscal Resources

Pharmacists serving correctional institutions should strive to manage expenses while providing optimal care to the inmate-patients. The pharmacist should

- Work with the administrators of the correctional institution to establish a budget for the operation of the pharmacy.
- Consider factors unique to each institution for the development of the budget (e.g., total inmate capacity, average daily inmate population, demographics of the inmate population).
- Make allowances for the disproportionate amount of chronic communicable disease in the prison population and the regional variability of diseases.
- Apply the ASHP Technical Assistance Bulletin on Assessing Cost-Containment Strategies for Pharmacies in Organized Health-Care Settings, as appropriate.[2]

Policies and Procedures

A policies and procedures manual specifically written to address aspects of pharmacy practice in the correctional facility should exist.

- All policies and procedures should conform to federal, state, and local laws and regulations.
- The pharmacy director should be familiar with the Standards for Health Services promulgated by the National Commission on Correctional Health Care and the standards of the American Correctional Association.
- The pharmacy director should be familiar with the constitutional rights of inmate-patients, current literature about inmates' rights, and court rulings affecting the practice of correctional health care in general and correctional pharmacy in particular. Attention to these concepts should be reflected in the manual.
- The pharmacy director should be familiar with current literature, laws, and regulations governing confidentiality, consent, and other areas of correctional health care that diverge from more traditional standards of pharmacy practice. Attention to these should be reflected in the manual.
- Transportation of inmate-patients' medications within and among facilities should be addressed.
- Security of drug products, entry into the pharmacy during the absence of a pharmacist, use of night cabinets, emergency supplies of medications, and disaster services should be addressed.
- Policies and procedures on the pharmacy's role in preparing lethal injections for capital punishment should exist.

Administrative Reports

Administrative reports generated by the pharmacy department will vary from facility to facility depending on the level of pharmaceutical services provided. Reports should include

- The amounts and cost of drugs and services furnished
- Destruction of unusable or outdated medications
- Inventory value and quantities
- Records of formal meetings with administrators, physicians, nurses, and other staff and any changes implemented as a result of those meetings
- Minutes of pharmacy and therapeutics committee meetings
- Medication administration records
- Reports of quality-control and quality-improvement activities
- Reports generated as required by applicable state laws regulating the practice of pharmacy. (While often not specifically written for the practice of correctional pharmacy, these laws are nonetheless usually pertinent to pharmacy practice within the correctional setting.)

Facilities

The pharmacy should be located within or in an area contiguous to the space provided for other health care services. Facilities should be adequate to accommodate appropriate security of all drug products, especially controlled substances.[3]

Purchasing, Distribution, and Control of Medications

Purchasing, distribution, and control of medications are essential elements of any pharmacy operation. Adequate methods to ensure that these responsibilities are met should exist.[4]

Purchasing

- The pharmacy director should be responsible for choosing the sources from which to obtain drug products.
- The pharmacy director should ensure that all medications meet applicable legal requirements. Guidance on the obligations of drug product suppliers and purchasers appears in the ASHP Guidelines for Selecting Pharmaceutical Manufacturers and Suppliers.[5]
- The pharmacy director should ensure that medications purchased from sources other than manufacturers or wholesalers (e.g., other pharmacies, contract providers) meet all applicable legal requirements. All suppliers should be able, at the request of the pharmacy director, to provide data on the quality of products.
- To the extent possible, all drug products should be contained in single-unit or unit dose packages.

Distribution

The pharmacist is responsible for the distribution and control of all drug products (including diagnostics and drug-related devices).

- A unit dose drug distribution and control system is recommended.

- The system employed should focus on patient safety and result in a minimal incidence of medication errors and adverse drug reactions. Ongoing processes for the monitoring and reporting of adverse drug reactions and the detection and prevention of medication errors should exist.
- The system employed should be cost-effective.
- The system employed should foster drug-control and drug-use monitoring.
- The system employed should foster patient compliance, recovery of drugs because of expired orders, and ultimate destruction of all unusable and outdated medications.
- Inmates should not be used in the distribution process.
- Patient confidentiality should be ensured in the distribution process (e.g., patients receiving medications for the treatment of AIDS).

Drug Storage

- The pharmacy director should ensure the proper security of medications stored in each location.
- The pharmacy director should ensure that drug products are stored in accordance with manufacturer or USP requirements.
- The pharmacy director should ensure that stored drug products are not expired.

Control

- A process for the recovery of medications dispensed to inmate-patients after the discontinuance of orders or in compliance with automatic stop orders should exist.
- A process for minimizing and eliminating unauthorized use of medications by anyone other than the intended patient (e.g., exchange of medications between inmates) should exist.
- A process for minimizing and eliminating pilferage should exist.
- A process for monitoring and preventing the dispensing of unusually large quantities of medications should exist.
- A process for preventing the dispensing of sufficient doses of any medication to enable potential suicide should exist. Individuals who are evaluated as high risks for suicide should be identified.
- A process for the security and dispensing of controlled substances should exist.
- The pharmacy director, in conjunction with the facility's medical staff and other responsible health authorities, should maintain policies and procedures for the routine review and renewal of medication orders and for any automatic discontinuance of orders.
- Access to patients' medication records should be limited to authorized personnel only. Complete access by the pharmacist should be ensured.
- A process for pharmacist review of medication orders to ensure patient safety and appropriateness of medication should exist. Medication orders (except in emergency situations) should be reviewed by the pharmacist before the first dose is dispensed.

Medication Administration

While medication administration is traditionally the responsibility of nurses, in the correctional setting some or all of this responsibility may be assigned to other personnel.

- The pharmacy director should be familiar with standards of the National Commission on Correctional Health Care with respect to medication administration by non-health-care personnel, and policies and procedures specifically addressing such administration should exist.
- The pharmacy director should participate in development of medication administration forms and ensure that all relevant information is incorporated into the forms.
- The pharmacy director should regularly educate all personnel involved in medication administration. These educational programs should include information on proper administration, indications, monitoring for adverse effects and allergic reactions, documentation, accountability, confidentiality, and the importance of compliance. Inmates who repeatedly refuse to take medications should be counseled by a pharmacist.
- Policies should be developed regarding the administration of medication to inmate-patients assigned to jobs or on work-release programs.
- Policies and procedures should be developed to ensure continuity of therapy upon release. Released inmates should have access to a limited supply of medications; either the drugs should be provided upon release or released inmates should have a prescription order transmitted to the pharmacy of their choice.

Documentation

- Medication administration records should be reviewed by the pharmacist at least monthly for proper documentation of medication administration.
- Review of the medication administration record should include assessments of documentation of medications administered, doses, frequency of administration, compliance, start and stop dates, and medication allergies.
- Pharmacist interventions should be documented in patients' medical records.
- The pharmacist should document refills in accordance with state laws and regulations.
- Policies and procedures should exist for documenting the transportation of medication among separate sites in correctional facilities, including accountability from pickup to drop off.
- A consistent pattern of refusal by an inmate-patient to take medication should be documented in the patient's medical record.
- Policies and procedures should exist for the proper documentation of the receipt, placement in inventory, dispensing, administration, and destruction of controlled substances.

Emergency Services

- A pharmacist should educate medical and correctional personnel on the proper use of medications stocked for emergency use.
- A pharmacist should be available on an on-call basis in case of emergencies.
- Policies and procedures for the use of emergency kits of medications in life-threatening situations should exist. These kits should be maintained by a pharmacist.

- The pharmacy director should maintain policies and procedures for accessibility of medications in case of riots or other emergency situations.
- The pharmacy director, in conjunction with the medical director or other responsible health authority and the correctional institution's administrator, should develop policies and the procedures that complement the standards of the National Commission on Correctional Health Care regarding emergency services.

Therapeutic Policies

- The pharmacy director should be a member of the pharmacy and therapeutics committee or its equivalent.
- A formulary should exist in accordance with the ASHP Statement on the Formulary System, the ASHP Guidelines on Formulary System Management, the ASHP Technical Assistance Bulletin on Drug Formularies, and the ASHP Technical Assistance Bulletin on the Evaluation of Drugs for Formularies.[6–9]
- Drug products selected for formulary inclusion should serve the needs of the inmate-patient population and at the same time be as cost-effective as possible. The pharmacy director should ensure that cost is not the only determinant for drug product selection.
- Procedures should exist for the provision of nonformulary medications when necessary.
- The pharmacy director should, in conjunction with the facility's medical staff, maintain policies and procedures for the use of investigational medications that ensure adherence to the rights of inmate-patients.
- The pharmacy director should, in conjunction with the facility's psychiatrist or medical director, maintain policies and procedures for the use of psychotropic medications.
- The pharmacy director should be familiar with laws and regulations governing the treatment of patients with AIDS and make appropriate procedural allowances for the treatment of these patients.
- The pharmacist should have input into decisions about infection control policies and procedures pertinent to medication use.

Quality Improvement

- The pharmacy director should encourage the development of and participate in an ongoing quality improvement process that includes drug-use evaluation and drug-regimen review.

Drug Information

- A program should exist for regular education of health care and pertinent non-health-care personnel with respect to medication use.
- An up-to-date resource library that includes current publications and those required by law and regulation should be maintained by the pharmacy.
- The pharmacist should provide drug consultations as required to nurses, physician assistants, physicians, and any others involved in initiating, executing, and monitoring medication therapy.
- The pharmacist should educate and counsel inmate-patients on the proper use of medications.

Research

- Policies and procedures for the use of investigational drugs within the correctional facility should exist. (Additional guidance on pertinent policies and procedures can be found in the ASHP Guidelines for the Use of Investigational Drugs in Organized Health-Care Settings.[10])
- The pharmacy director should adhere to the Federal Regulations on Medical Research in Correctional Facilities (45 C.F.R. 46, revised March 6, 1983) when devising policies and procedures for use of investigational drugs.
- Information on issues that affect pharmacy practice within the correctional environment (e.g., criminology, medical–legal issues, endemic patient population) should be maintained.

References

1. American Society of Hospital Pharmacists. ASHP guidelines: minimum standard for pharmacies in institutions. *Am J Hosp Pharm.* 1985; 42:372–5.
2. American Society of Hospital Pharmacists. ASHP technical assistance bulletin on assessing cost-containment strategies for pharmacies in organized health-care settings. *Am J Hosp Pharm.* 1992; 49:155–60.
3. American Society of Hospital Pharmacists. ASHP technical assistance bulletin on use of controlled substances in organized health-care settings. *Am J Hosp Pharm.* 1993; 50:489–501.
4. American Society of Hospital Pharmacists. ASHP technical assistance bulletin on drug distribution and control. *Am J Hosp Pharm.* 1980; 37:1097–103.
5. American Society of Hospital Pharmacists. ASHP guidelines for selecting pharmaceutical manufacturers and suppliers. *Am J Hosp Pharm.* 1991; 48:523–4.
6. American Society of Hospital Pharmacists. ASHP guidelines on formulary system management. *Am J Hosp Pharm.* 1992; 49:648–52.
7. American Society of Hospital Pharmacists. ASHP technical assistance bulletin on drug formularies. *Am J Hosp Pharm.* 1991; 48:791–3.
8. American Society of Hospital Pharmacists. ASHP technical assistance bulletin on the evaluation of drugs for formularies. *Am J Hosp Pharm.* 1988; 45:386–7.
9. American Society of Hospital Pharmacists. ASHP statement on the formulary system. *Am J Hosp Pharm.* 1983; 1384–5.
10. American Society of Hospital Pharmacists. ASHP guidelines for the use of investigational drugs in organized health-care settings. *Am J Hosp Pharm.* 1991; 48:315–9

Approved by the ASHP Board of Directors, April 26, 1995. Developed by the Council on Professional Affairs. Drafted for council review by Ronald L. Rideman.

The bibliographic citation for this document is as follows: American Society of Health-System Pharmacists. ASHP guidelines on pharmaceutical services in correctional facilities. *Am J Health-Syst Pharm.* 1995; 52:1810–3.

ASHP Guidelines on a Standardized Method for Pharmaceutical Care

Need for a Standardized Method

The purpose of this document is to provide pharmacists with a standardized method for the provision of pharmaceutical care in component settings of organized health systems. Since the introduction of the pharmaceutical care concept[1] and the development of the ASHP Statement on Pharmaceutical Care,[2] considerable variation in pharmacists' provision of pharmaceutical care has been noted. ASHP believes pharmacists need a standardized method for providing pharmaceutical care.

This document describes a standardized method based on functions that all pharmacists should perform for individual patients in organized health systems. The use of this method would foster consistency in the provision of pharmaceutical care in all practice settings. It would support continuity of care both within a practice setting (e.g., among pharmacists on different work shifts caring for an acutely ill inpatient) and when a patient moves among practice settings (e.g., when an inpatient is discharged to home or ambulatory care). Further, a standardized method would establish consistent documentation so that patient-specific and medication-related information could be shared from pharmacist to pharmacist and among health professionals.

The need to identify the functions involved in pharmaceutical care and the critical skills necessary to provide it was discussed at the San Antonio consensus conference in 1993.[3] Functions for the provision of pharmaceutical care were identified by the practitioner task force of the Scope of Pharmacy Practice Project.[4] Those functions have been defined in more detail in the pharmacotherapy series of the ASHP Clinical Skills Program.[5–9]

These Guidelines are not specific to any practice setting. ASHP believes this standardized method can be used in acute care (hospitals), ambulatory care, home care, long-term care, and other practice settings. Functions can be tailored as appropriate for a given practice setting. It is recognized that the degree of standardization and tailoring appropriate for a given work site will depend on the practice environment, the organization of services (e.g., patient-focused or department-focused), working relationships with other health professionals, the health system's and patient's financial arrangements, and the health system's policies and procedures. ASHP believes the use of the systematic approaches encouraged by these guidelines will assist pharmacists in implementing and providing pharmaceutical care in their work sites.

Functions of Pharmaceutical Care

ASHP believes that a standardized method for the provision of pharmaceutical care should include the following:

- Collecting and organizing patient-specific information,
- Determining the presence of medication-therapy problems,
- Summarizing patients' health care needs,
- Specifying pharmacotherapeutic goals,
- Designing a pharmacotherapeutic regimen,
- Designing a monitoring plan,
- Developing a pharmacotherapeutic regimen and corresponding monitoring plan in collaboration with the patient and other health professionals,
- Initiating the pharmacotherapeutic regimen,
- Monitoring the effects of the pharmacotherapeutic regimen, and
- Redesigning the pharmacotherapeutic regimen and monitoring plan.

These major functions have been adapted, in part, from the pharmacotherapy series of the ASHP Clinical Skills Program and the final report of the ASHP Model for Pharmacy Practice Residency Learning Demonstration Project.

Collecting and Organizing Pertinent Patient-Specific Information. Information should be collected and used as a patient-specific database to prevent, detect, and resolve the patient's medication-related problems and to make appropriate medication-therapy recommendations. The database should include the following sections, each containing specific types of information to the extent that it is relevant to medication therapy:

Demographic
> Name
> Address
> Date of birth
> Sex
> Religion and religious affiliation
> Occupation

Administrative
> Physicians and prescribers
> Pharmacy
> Room/bed numbers
> Consent forms
> Patient identification number

Medical
> Weight and height
> Acute and chronic medical problems
> Current symptoms
> Vital signs and other monitoring information
> Allergies and intolerances
> Past medical history
> Laboratory information
> Diagnostic and surgical procedures

Medication therapy
> Prescribed medications
> Nonprescription medications
> Medications used prior to admission
> Home remedies and other types of health products used
> Medication regimen
> Compliance with therapy
> Medication allergies and intolerances
> Concerns or questions about therapy
> Assessment of understanding of therapy
> Pertinent health beliefs

Behavioral/lifestyle
> Diet
> Exercise/recreation
> Tobacco/alcohol/caffeine/other substance use or abuse
> Sexual history
> Personality type
> Daily activities

Social/economic
> Living arrangement
> Ethnic background
> Financial/insurance/health plan

Objective and subjective information should be obtained directly from patients (and family members, other caregivers, and other health professionals as needed). A physical assessment should be performed as needed. In addition, information can be obtained by reviewing the patient's health record and other information sources.

Information in the patient's health record should be understood, interpreted, and verified for accuracy before decisions are made about the patient's medication therapy. With access to the patient's health record comes the professional responsibility to safeguard the patient's rights to privacy and confidentiality. The Privacy Act of 1974,[10] professional practice policies,[11,12] and policies and procedures of organized health systems provide guidance for the pharmacist in judging the appropriate use of patient-specific information.

The patient (as well as family members, caregivers, and other members of the health care team as needed) should be interviewed. This is necessary for the pharmacist to establish a direct relationship with the patient, to understand the patient's needs and desired outcome, to obtain medication-related information, and to clarify and augment other available information. Pharmacists in many practice settings, including ambulatory care, may need to perform physical assessments to collect data for assessing and monitoring medication therapy.

Information, including clinical laboratory test results, gathered or developed by other members of the health care team may not be in the patient's health record. Therefore, to ensure that the patient information is current and complete, other sources should be checked. Other sources may include medication profiles from other pharmacies used by the patient.

Although it is ideal to have a comprehensive database for all patients, time and staffing limitations may necessitate choices regarding the quantity of information and the number of patients to follow. Choices could be determined by the health system's policies and procedures, by clinical care plans, or by disease management criteria in the patient's third-party health plan.

Systems for recording patient-specific data will vary, depending on pharmacists' preferences and practice settings. Electronic documentation is recommended. Some information may already be in the patient's health record. Therefore, when authorized, the additional information gathered by the pharmacist should be recorded in the patient's health record so that it can be shared with other health professionals. Abstracted summaries and work sheets may also be useful.

Determining the Presence of Medication-Therapy Problems. Conclusions should be drawn from the integration of medication-, disease-, laboratory test-, and patient-specific information. The patient's database should be assessed for any of the following medication-therapy problems:

- Medications with no medical indication,
- Medical conditions for which there is no medication prescribed,
- Medications prescribed inappropriately for a particular medical condition,
- Inappropriate medication dose, dosage form, schedule, route of administration, or method of administration,
- Therapeutic duplication,
- Prescribing of medications to which the patient is allergic,
- Actual and potential adverse drug events,
- Actual and potential clinically significant drug–drug, drug–disease, drug–nutrient, and drug–laboratory test interactions,
- Interference with medical therapy by social or recreational drug use,
- Failure to receive the full benefit of prescribed medication therapy,
- Problems arising from the financial impact of medication therapy on the patient,
- Lack of understanding of the medication therapy by the patient, and
- Failure of the patient to adhere to the medication regimen.

The relative importance of problems must be assessed on the basis of specific characteristics of the patient or the medication. Checklists, work sheets, and other methods may be used to determine and document the presence of medication-therapy problems. The method should be proactive and should be used consistently from patient to patient.

Summarizing Patients' Health Care Needs. The patient's overall needs and desired outcomes and other health professionals' assessments, goals, and therapy plans should be considered in determining and documenting the medication-related elements of care that are needed to improve or prevent deterioration of the patient's health or well-being.

Specifying Pharmacotherapeutic Goals. Pharmacotherapeutic goals should reflect the integration of medication-, disease-, laboratory test-, and patient-specific information, as well as ethical and quality-of-life considerations. The goals should be realistic and consistent with goals specified by the patient and other members of the patient's health care team. The therapy should be designed to achieve definite medication-related outcomes and improve the patient's quality of life.

Designing a Pharmacotherapeutic Regimen. The regimen should meet the pharmacotherapeutic goals established with the patient and reflect the integration of medication-, disease-, laboratory test-, and patient-specific information; ethical and quality-of-life considerations; and pharmacoeconomic principles. It should comply with the health system's medication-use policies, such as clinical care plans and disease management plans. The regimen should be designed for optimal medication use within both the health system's and the patient's capabilities and financial resources.

Designing a Monitoring Plan for the Pharmacotherapeutic Regimen. The monitoring plan should effectively evaluate achievement of the patient-specific pharmacotherapeutic goals and detect real and potential adverse effects. Measurable, observable parameters should be determined for each goal. Endpoints should be established for assessing whether the goal has been achieved. The needs of the patient, characteristics of the medication, needs of other health care team members, and policies and procedures of the health care setting will influence the monitoring plan.

Developing a Pharmacotherapeutic Regimen and Corresponding Monitoring Plan. The regimen and plan developed in collaboration with the patient and other health professionals should be systematic and logical and should represent a consensus among the patient, prescriber, and pharmacist. The approach selected should be based on consideration of the type of practice setting, its policies and procedures, practice standards, and good professional relations with the prescriber and patient. The regimen and monitoring plan should be documented in the patient's health record to ensure that all members of the health care team have this information.

Initiating the Pharmacotherapeutic Regimen. Depending on the regimen and plan, the pharmacist could, as appropriate, implement all or portions of the pharmacotherapeutic regimen. Actions should comply with the health system's policies and procedures (e.g., prescribing protocols) and correspond to the regimen and plan. Orders for medications, laboratory tests, and other interventions should be clear and concise. All actions should be documented in the patient's health record.

Monitoring the Effects of the Pharmacotherapeutic Regimen. Data collected according to the monitoring plan should be sufficient, reliable, and valid so that judgments can be made about the effects of the pharmacotherapeutic regimen. Changes in patient status, condition, medication therapy, or nonmedication therapy since the monitoring plan was developed should be considered. Missing or additional data should be identified. Achievement of the desired endpoints should be assessed for each parameter in the monitoring plan. A judgment should be made about whether the pharmacotherapeutic goals were met. Before the pharmacotherapeutic regimen is adjusted, the cause for failure to achieve any of the pharmacotherapeutic goals should be determined.

Redesigning the Pharmacotherapeutic Regimen and Monitoring Plan. Decisions to change the regimen and plan should be based on the patient's outcome. When clinical circumstances permit, one aspect of the regimen at a time should be changed and reassessed. Recommendations for pharmacotherapeutic changes should be documented in the same manner used to document the original recommendations.

Pharmacist's Responsibility

An essential element of pharmaceutical care is that the pharmacist accepts responsibility for the patient's pharmacotherapeutic outcomes. The same commitment that is applied to designing the pharmacotherapeutic regimen and monitoring plan for the patient should be applied to its implementation. The provision of pharmaceutical care requires monitoring the regimen's effects, revising the regimen as the patient's condition changes, documenting the results, and assuming responsibility for the pharmacotherapeutic effects.

References

1. Hepler CD, Strand LM. Opportunities and responsibilities in pharmaceutical care. *Am J Hosp Pharm.* 1990; 47:533–43.
2. American Society of Hospital Pharmacists. ASHP statement on pharmaceutical care. *Am J Hosp Pharm.* 1993; 50:1720–3.
3. Implementing pharmaceutical care. Proceedings of an invitational conference conducted by the American Society of Hospital Pharmacists and the ASHP Research Foundation. *Am J Hosp Pharm.* 1993; 50: 1585–656.
4. Summary of the final report of the Scope of Pharmacy Practice Project. *Am J Hosp Pharm.* 1994; 51:2179–82.
5. Shepherd MF. Clinical skills program pharmacotherapy series module 1. Reviewing patient medical charts. Bethesda, MD: American Society of Hospital Pharmacists; 1992.
6. Mason N, Shimp LA. Clinical skills program pharmacotherapy series module 2. Building a pharmacist's patient data base. Bethesda, MD: American Society of Hospital Pharmacists; 1993.
7. Mason N, Shimp LA. Clinical skills program—module 3. Constructing a patient's drug therapy problem list. Bethesda, MD: American Society of Hospital Pharmacists; 1993.
8. Jones WN, Campbell S. Clinical skills program pharmacotherapy series module 4. Designing and recommending a pharmacist's care plan. Bethesda, MD: American Society of Hospital Pharmacists; 1994.
9. Frye CB. Clinical skills program pharmacotherapy series module 5. Monitoring the pharmacist's care plan. Bethesda, MD: American Society of Hospital Pharmacists; 1994.
10. PL 93-579. 5 U.S.C.A. 552a (88 Stat. 1896).
11. ASHP guidelines for obtaining authorization for documenting pharmaceutical care in patient medical records. *Am J Hosp Pharm.* 1989; 46:338–9.
12. Principles of practice for pharmaceutical care. Washington, DC: American Pharmaceutical Association; 1995.

Approved by the ASHP Board of Directors, April 24, 1996. Developed by the ASHP Council on Professional Affairs.

The bibliographic citation for this document is as follows: American Society of Health-System Pharmacists. ASHP guidelines on a standardized method for pharmaceutical care. *Am J Health-Syst Pharm.* 1996; 53:1713–6.

ASHP Guidelines on the Provision of Medication Information by Pharmacists

Definition of Terms and Basic Concepts

The provision of medication information is among the fundamental professional responsibilities of pharmacists in health systems. The primary focus of this Guidelines document is to help pharmacists in various practice settings develop a systematic approach to providing medication information. Medication information may be patient specific, as an integral part of pharmaceutical care, or population based, to aid in making decisions and evaluating medication use for groups of patients (e.g., medication evaluation for formulary changes, medication-use evaluations). The goal of providing carefully evaluated, literature-supported evidence to justify specific medication-use practices should be to enhance the quality of patient care and improve patient outcomes. To be an effective provider of medication information, the pharmacist must be able to[1]

1. Perceive and evaluate the medication information needs of patients and families, health care professionals, and other personnel, and
2. Use a systematic approach to address medication information needs by effectively searching, retrieving, and evaluating the literature and appropriately communicating and applying the information to the patient care situation.

Medication Information Activities

A variety of medication information activities may be provided, depending on the particular practice setting and need. The following activities, which are often performed in an organized health care setting, are enhanced by using a systematic approach to meeting medication information needs[2-5]:

1. Providing medication information to patients and families, health care professionals, and other personnel.
2. Establishing and maintaining a formulary based on scientific evidence of efficacy and safety, cost, and patient factors.
3. Developing and participating in efforts to prevent medication misadventuring, including adverse drug event and medication error reporting and analysis programs.
4. Developing methods of changing patient and provider behaviors to support optimal medication use.
5. Publishing newsletters to educate patients, families, and health care professionals on medication use.
6. Educating providers about medication-related policies and procedures.
7. Coordinating programs to support population-based medication practices (e.g., development of medication-use evaluation criteria and pharmacotherapeutic guidelines).
8. Coordinating investigational drug services.
9. Providing continuing-education services to the health care professional staff.
10. Educating pharmacy students and residents.
11. Applying health economic and outcome analysis.
12. Developing and maintaining an active research program.

An individual pharmacist may have full or partial responsibility for all or some of these activities. For example, preparing drug monographs for pharmacy and therapeutics committees was once considered almost exclusively the responsibility of the drug information center or drug information specialist. As pharmacy practice has evolved, the expertise and knowledge base of individual pharmacy practitioners have been integrated into this process. The pharmacist may prepare the monograph or, if a medication is adopted for use, may assist in designing the medication use evaluation (MUE) criteria, collecting data, or educating health care professionals on appropriate use. Any of these activities may contribute to a larger medication policy management program coordinated by a medication information center or specialist. As pharmacists in various organized health care settings have become more involved in providing pharmaceutical care, their activities have become less distributive and more information based, requiring a higher level of competence by all pharmacists in meeting medication information needs.

Systematic Method for Responding to Medication Information Needs

The provision of medication information can be initiated by the pharmacist or requested by other health care professionals, patients and their family members, or the general public. The process is similar, regardless of how a medication information question is generated (e.g., by the pharmacist or by another health professional) or the context in which the information will be used (e.g., in a newsletter or for solving a patient-specific problem). The pharmacist must not only accumulate and organize the literature but also objectively evaluate and apply the information from the literature to a particular patient or situation.[6-8] Consideration should be given to the ethical and legal aspects of responding to medication information requests.[9,10] A systematic method can be outlined as follows:

1. To probe for information and develop a response with the appropriate perspective, consider the education and professional or experiential background of the requester.
2. Identify needs by asking probing questions of the patient, family members, or health care professional or by examining the medical record to identify the true question. This helps in optimizing the search process and assessing the urgency for a response.
3. Classify requests as patient-specific or not and by type of question (e.g., product availability, adverse drug event, compatibility, compounding/formulation, dosage/administration, drug interaction, identification, pharmacokinetics, therapeutic use/efficacy, safety in pregnancy and nursing, toxicity and poisoning) to aid in assessing the situation and selecting resources.

4. Obtain more complete background information, including patient data, if applicable, to individualize the response to meet the patient's, family's, or health care professional's needs.

5. Perform a systematic search of the literature by making appropriate selections from the primary, secondary, and tertiary literature and other types of resources as necessary.

6. Evaluate, interpret, and combine information from the several sources. Other information needs should be anticipated as a result of the information provided.

7. Provide a response by written or oral consultation, or both, as needed by the requester and appropriate to the situation. The information, its urgency, and its purpose may influence the method of response.

8. Perform a follow-up assessment to determine the utility of the information provided and outcomes for the patient (patient-specific request) or changes in medication-use practices and behaviors.

9. Document the request, information sources, response, and follow-up as appropriate for the request and the practice setting.

Resources

It is the responsibility of the pharmacist to ensure that up-to-date resources, including representative primary, secondary, and tertiary literature, are available to assist in answering a variety of types of medication information requests. Pharmacists should be familiar with not only the components of the literature (e.g., primary) but also the features of individual resources in each component; this makes searching more efficient so that time can be used optimally in analyzing, applying, and communicating the information. The drug information modules of the ASHP Clinical Skills Program[6–8] describe the strengths and weaknesses of the different literature components and list frequently used resources and the types of information included in each publication. The following should be considered in purchasing literature resources:

1. Attributes of the literature (e.g., frequency of update, qualifications and affiliations of authors, year of publication, type of information, organization of material, type of medium, and cost).

2. Practice setting of the pharmacist (e.g., type of facility and needs of individuals within the environment).

3. Literature currently available and readily accessible.

4. Funds allocated for literature purchases.

The volume and sophistication of medication information, as well as the demand for it, are increasing, and human memory has limitations. Consideration should be given to using computers as a tool in the decision-making process. There are several areas in which computers can be valuable in the provision of medication information.[11] Databases are available for information management, retrieval, and communication. Information management databases include software for MUE, documentation of questions and responses, and preparation of reports of adverse drug events. Information retrieval sources include bibliographic databases (e.g., International Pharmaceutical Abstracts, Iowa Drug Information Service, MEDLINE) and full-text databases (e.g., Drug Information Fulltext).[12,13] Textbooks (e.g.,

AHFS Drug Information) and journals can also be accessed through computer technology. Some information is available through electronic bulletin boards (e.g., PharmNet) and the Internet.[14–16] Computerized medical records can also be a valuable tool in assessing either individual patient needs or population-based needs.

Documentation and Quality Assessment

Individual practicing pharmacists should base their documentation of medication information requests and responses on the type and purpose of the request and the subsequent use of the documentation. For patient-specific medication information, requests and responses could be documented in the patient's medical record. Documentation may also be considered necessary for quality assessment and other performance improvement and management activities.

Documentation of medication information requests and responses should include, as appropriate for the purposes of the documentation, the following:

1. Date and time received.
2. Requester's name, address, method of contact (e.g., telephone or beeper number), and category (e.g., health care discipline, patient, public).
3. Person assessing medication information needs.
4. Method of delivery (e.g., telephone, personal visit, mail).
5. Classification of request.
6. Question asked.
7. Patient-specific information obtained.
8. Response provided.
9. References used.
10. Date and time answered.
11. Person responding to request.
12. Estimated time in preparation and for communication.
13. Materials sent to requesters.
14. Outcome measures suggested (e.g., impact on patient care, improvements in medication use, and requester satisfaction).

Responses to requests for medication information should be accurate, complete, and timely for maximal clinical usefulness and to establish credibility for pharmacist-provided information. Quality assessment of responses should be included in the medication information process; this could be selective for certain types of patient-specific requests, random by numbers of requests or for certain time periods, or on some other basis appropriate to meet the needs of the health system.

Keeping Current

It is the responsibility of the pharmacist to keep abreast of advancements both in the tools that can be used to systematically address information requests and in the information itself regarding pharmacotherapeutic or other issues affecting the practice of pharmacy.

References

1. Troutman WG. Consensus-derived objectives for drug information education. *Drug Inf J.* 1994; 28:791–6.
2. Rosenberg JM, Ruentes RJ, Starr CH, et al. Pharmacist-operated drug information centers in the United

States. *Am J Health Syst-Pharm*. 1995; 52:991–6.

3. ASHP supplemental standard and learning objectives for residency training in drug information practice. In: Practice standards of ASHP 1994–95. Hicks WE, ed. Bethesda, MD: American Society of Hospital Pharmacists; 1994.

4. American Society of Hospital Pharmacists. ASHP accreditation standard for residency in pharmacy practice (with an emphasis on pharmaceutical care). *Am J Hosp Pharm*. 1992; 49:146–53.

5. American Society of Hospital Pharmacists. ASHP statement on the pharmacist's clinical role in organized health care settings. *Am J Hosp Pharm*. 1989; 46:2345–6.

6. Galt KA. Clinical skills program drug information series, module 1. Analyzing and recording a drug information request. Bethesda, MD: American Society of Hospital Pharmacists; 1994.

7. Smith GH, Norton LL, Ferrill MJ. Clinical skills program drug information series, module 2. Evaluating drug literature. Bethesda, MD: American Society of Health-System Pharmacists; 1995.

8. Galt KA, Calis KA, Turcasso NM. Clinical skills program drug information series, module 3. Responding to a drug information request. Bethesda, MD: American Society of Health-System Pharmacists; 1995.

9. Kelly WN, Krause EC, Krowinski WJ, et al. National survey of ethical issues presented to drug information centers. *Am J Hosp Pharm*. 1990; 47:2245–50.

10. Arnold RM, Nissen JC, Campbell NA. Ethical issues in a drug information center. *Drug Intell Clin Pharm*. 1987; 21:1008–11.

11. Dasta JF, Greer ML, Speedie SM. Computers in health care: overview and bibliography. *Ann Pharmacother*. 1992; 26:109–17.

12. Hoffman T. The ninth annual medical hardware and software buyers' guide. *MD Comput*. 1992; 9: 359–500.

13. Baker DE, Smith G, Abate MA. Selected topics in drug information access and practice: an update. *Ann Pharmacother*. 1994; 28:1389–94.

14. Gora-Harper ML. Value of pharmacy-related bulletin board services as a drug information resource. *J Pharm Technol*. 1995; 11:95–8.

15. Glowniak JV, Bushway MK. Computer networks as a medical resource. *JAMA*. 1994; 271:1934–9.

16. McKinney WP, Barnas GP, Golub RM. The medical applications of the Internet: information resources for research, education and patient care. *J Gen Intern Med*. 1994; 9:627–34.

Approved by the ASHP Board of Directors, April 24, 1996. Developed by the ASHP Council on Professional Affairs.

The bibliographic citation for this document is as follows: American Society of Health-System Pharmacists. ASHP guidelines on the provision of medication information by pharmacists. *Am J Health-Syst Pharm*. 1996; 53:1843–5.

ASHP Guidelines on the Pharmacist's Role in the Development of Clinical Care Plans

Purpose

Providing clinically appropriate and cost-effective care that results in the best patient outcomes is an accepted goal of pharmacy and health systems. The emergence of managed care and other market-driven health care reforms have stimulated the development of coordinated, standardized methods for optimizing both outcomes and resource utilization.

ASHP suggests the term clinical care plan (CCP) to describe a general method of using predetermined, time-staged actions for managing the care of patients who have clearly defined diagnoses or require certain procedures. ASHP believes CCPs are applicable to the management of patients moving among health systems' multiple levels of care and practice settings. Because pharmacotherapy is often a necessary component of CCPs, pharmacists should be involved. By participating and taking leadership roles in the development and use of CCPs, pharmacists can contribute to cost-effective patient care and help to establish health care team collaboration in the provision of pharmaceutical care. This is consistent with efforts by the Joint Commission on Accreditation of Healthcare Organizations to promote team approaches to patient care and performance improvement.

ASHP believes pharmacists should be proactive in the development of CCPs for their health systems. The purposes of this document are to describe pharmacists' role in the development and use of CCPs and to help pharmacists plan their involvement. Involvement in the early stages of CCP development is desirable; however, CCP development in any particular health system is cyclical, and pharmacists and pharmacy departments should seek opportunities to become involved at any step in the cycle.

Background

Pharmacists should focus on incorporating in the development and use of CCPs contemporary pharmaceutical care principles (e.g., pharmacoeconomics, formulary management) and activities and services (e.g., assessing medication orders, developing pharmacotherapeutic regimens and monitoring plans, educating and counseling patients, calculating pharmacokinetic doses, managing anticoagulation therapy, conducting medication-use evaluations [MUEs], developing preprinted order forms).[1-3] Pharmacists should perform the following functions in a typical CCP: oversee the selection of medications by using an evidence-based approach, develop the criteria for medication selection or dose, and monitor for drug efficacy and adverse effects.

CCPs derive from the industrial engineering concept of critical paths.[4] The term critical pathways has evolved with health care applications of this concept, originally associated with inpatient acute care and primarily used by nursing. Other terms for CCPs include care guides, clinical pathways, and CareMaps.[5] CCPs have evolved to include continuous quality improvement (CQI) concepts.[6] Once the disease or procedure is selected for CCP development, a multidisciplinary team analyzes its current management

(including variances, costs, and outcomes), evaluates the scientific literature, and develops a plan of care. The planned actions for each discipline on the health care team are mapped on a time line for the specific disease or procedure.[7]

CCPs and similar tools are being developed in many facilities.[8-14] Pharmacists should not only become involved in inpatient acute care CCPs but also form alliances with ambulatory care, home care, and long-term care pharmacists and other health care providers to foster the provision of seamless pharmaceutical care.

Pharmacist Involvement

These guidelines suggest actions to prepare pharmacists and pharmacy departments for involvement in the development of CCPs and their use in varying levels of care and practice settings. The applicability of these actions and ideas will depend on a pharmacist's or pharmacy department's current level of involvement in patient care and in CCP development and use.

Preparing for a Role in CCP Development. Pharmacists should learn about their health system's approach to CCP development and assess their personal capabilities and readiness to become involved. They should

1. Review the health system's current strategic plan to learn the role played by CCPs.
2. Educate the pharmacy staff on the purposes and processes of CCP development and the contents of CCPs. The patient care decisions required in CCPs demand clinical knowledge, and the pharmacotherapy involved should be based on evidence in the scientific literature. An effective contributor to the CCP process needs to use CQI, group process, teamwork, negotiation, and administrative skills.
3. Discuss CCP experiences with pharmacy colleagues within and outside your health system. Create a forum within your health system for continual dialogue about CCPs; for example, make CCPs a regular agenda item for the pharmacy and therapeutics (P&T) committee and other multidisciplinary clinical meetings and departmental staff meetings.
4. Monitor the literature of pharmacy, nursing, quality management, health systems, health care, and management for ideas on the development and implementation of CCPs.
5. Identify opportunities for contributing, through the provision of pharmaceutical care, to the health system's patient care delivery and improvement efforts.

Initiating Involvement. Pharmacists should begin their involvement in the CCP process in ways most appropriate to their health system's structure, culture, practice settings, and policies and procedures. This may vary substantially from one health system to another, but pharmacists generally should

1. Develop relationships with nursing, medical, dietary, laboratory, quality management, and other personnel

through routine meetings, nursing and medical forums, and other multidisciplinary opportunities. These relationships should be used to promote the contributions that pharmacists can make to collaborative team approaches to patient care.

2. Support or initiate the implementation of a multidisciplinary committee for CCP development and oversight. Ensure that the P&T committee is represented on the oversight committee.

3. Seek the appointment of pharmacists to the health system's CCP oversight committee and development teams. The pharmacy department should support the use of CCPs as an effective way to integrate and align services, processes, and costs.

4. Identify a consistent process for selecting the most appropriate pharmacists to participate on the various CCP development teams.

5. Offer to accept staff or leadership roles; for example, assist with or consult on literature evaluation for the health system's CCP development teams.

6. Ensure the ongoing involvement of the P&T committee in the CCP process. The P&T committee could facilitate the process by

   - Reviewing and endorsing the pharmacotherapy proposed for inclusion in each CCP.
   - Maintaining a pharmacotherapy database to facilitate CCP updates when new medications and pharmacotherapeutic alternatives become available.
   - Providing expert information on medications and pharmacotherapy.
   - Establishing a standing P&T subcommittee or liaison position that would assist CCP development teams. The subcommittee or liaison would have the opportunity to educate the CCP team about the formulary process, the MUE process, the appropriate use of restricted medications, and other critical medication-use issues.
   - Publishing the health system's CCP experiences in the P&T committee newsletter.

7. Emphasize pharmacists' responsibility for implementing CCP steps that involve medication distribution, pharmacotherapeutic regimens and monitoring, and patient education and counseling.

8. Initiate, after appropriate approvals, the development of the pharmacotherapy components of CCPs.

9. Offer to evaluate and adapt the pharmacotherapeutic components of existing protocols and guidelines for CCPs under development.

10. Develop patient education and counseling materials for the pharmacotherapeutic components of the CCPs.

11. Advocate the development of preprinted medication orders (hard copy or electronic) for the CCP.

Maintaining Involvement. Pharmacists' continued involvement will depend on their ability to demonstrate their contributions to patient care delivery and improvement efforts to the CCP oversight committee and development teams and to the health system's administration. To accomplish this, pharmacists can

1. Obtain CCPs from other institutions as examples of and frameworks for mapping care. These should not, however, be adopted directly, because acceptance and use are much higher when CCPs are developed or adapted by the users.

2. Incorporate CCPs into the pharmacy department's culture by building responsibilities and performance expectations for CCP development and use into pharmacists' job descriptions.

3. Identify and train pharmacy staff on their roles and responsibilities for implementing the pharmaceutical care components of CCPs.

4. Provide objective clinical input that is based on scientific evidence, not on anecdotal preference.

5. Oversee CCP development to ensure consistency of terminology (e.g., generic drug names, decimal and unit usage), rational medication use, and appropriate monitoring. This could be done by the P&T committee or by a pharmacist who coordinates and reviews the pharmacotherapy efforts of all CCPs.

6. Maintain good working relationships with CCP development teams. The pharmacist member should be confident, assertive, cooperative, and an effective communicator.

7. Maintain or develop clinical and health care management skills through continual self-education.

Contributing to the CQI Aspects of CCPs. The pharmacist should ensure that the pharmaceutical care actions of the CCP contribute to achieving patient satisfaction, desired clinical outcomes, and financial goals by doing the following:

1. Monitor literature for best practice results and compare these with the health system's experience.

2. Ensure that an internal system of CCP tracking and therapeutic review allows for the rapid insertion of new, more effective therapies into the CCP.

3. Assist in the development of patient satisfaction surveys.

4. Monitor the results of the CCPs and use them to perform MUEs.[15] Since patients enrolled in CCPs are receiving predetermined pharmacotherapeutic regimens and monitoring, this is an excellent opportunity to perform disease- and outcome-oriented MUEs. Review the variances and outcomes from the CCP and determine the pharmacotherapy effect on them; use this analysis to modify the CCP. *Note: The pharmacotherapy component must be specific enough (e.g., medication and dose) that its influence on the outcomes can be determined with confidence.*

Ensuring "Fluidity" of a CCP from One Level of Care or Practice Setting to Another. ASHP suggests that integration of the organizational components providing care, as well as their disease-specific clinical activities, be included in the CCP process. To provide continuity of care, the CCP should specify referral patterns among the levels of care and practice settings. To accomplish this, pharmacists can

1. Ensure that members of all organizational components are included in the development of the CCP, as appropriate for the particular disease or procedure. These might include personnel in the helicopter or ambulance, the operating room, the intensive care unit, the stepdown unit, the general nursing unit, the rehabilitation unit, the long-term care facility, the ambulatory care clinic, and home care.

2. Develop relationships with key managed care partners by

- Inviting pharmacist members of managed care partners to participate in the CCP development process.
- Exchanging CCPs with the managed care partners.
- Creating work teams to ensure continuity.

3. Organize interdisciplinary sharing of information (e.g., recent laboratory results) and documentation that all health care providers would find useful.

4. Develop a plan to communicate and monitor both internal and external CCPs so that pharmacists have a full understanding of the CCP process and can assess, reassess, and adjust the CCP as necessary when new therapeutic modalities emerge. Optimize this by using electronic and Internet technology to
- Rapidly insert new pharmacotherapies into CCPs where appropriate.
- Evaluate what pharmacotherapies are in which CCPs, to ensure consistency in medication management.

5. Initiate dialogue among the patient's pharmacists to ensure continuity of the individual patient's CCP. For example, upon admission, the hospital pharmacist, if necessary and with the patient's permission, should contact the patient's community pharmacist(s) to obtain information. This would include an accurate medication history (prescription and nonprescription products and home remedies), history of adverse drug reactions or allergies, patient attitudes and medication-taking behaviors (adherence, health beliefs, social and cultural issues), and any self-monitoring the patient uses. *Note: This does not obviate the requirement for the pharmacist to establish a relationship with the patient and to obtain information directly.*

Upon discharge (following local policies and procedures and with the patient's permission) the hospital pharmacist should prepare a discharge summary and forward it to the community or home care pharmacist, physician, and other relevant health care providers (e.g., the home care nurse). This discharge summary should include the patient's chief complaint, history of present illness (including hospital course), medications on admission and discharge, aspects of patient education and counseling, monitoring plan (including patient self-monitoring, and plan for long-term monitoring of the patient's pharmacotherapeutic regimen), and the name of a person to contact with questions.

The CCP Process

A health system should use a CCP process that will meet its needs within its own structure, culture, practice settings, and policies and procedures. The following example of a CCP process[4] incorporates CQI concepts.

1. **Select Diagnoses and Procedures.** The usual criteria for selection of diagnoses and procedures include high cost, high volume, and high risk. Inpatient acute care-based CCPs can be developed for common or specialized diagnoses (e.g., myocardial infarction) or procedures (e.g., transurethral prostatectomy or coronary-artery bypass grafting). Ambulatory care-based CCPs should focus on diagnoses that are commonly encountered (e.g., diabetes mellitus), are likely to cause changes in health status (e.g., uncontrolled asthma), or involve complicated pharmacotherapeutic

regimens (e.g., AIDS). The criteria for selection should be developed with input from administrative and clinical leaders to ensure acceptance and should be based on scientific evidence.

2. **Appoint a Development Team.** The development team should include key health care providers from all organizational components involved in the CCP. *Note: Although insurance carriers and managed care providers may not have representatives on the development team, their protocols or guidelines should be evaluated by the team for inclusion in the CCP.*

3. **Conduct a Search of the Scientific Literature.** A literature search conducted early in the process will help to identify measures for assessing current processes and outcomes and will ensure an evidence-based approach to the CCP.

4. **Document Current Process and Outcomes.** The current processes, costs, variances, and outcomes need to be documented, usually through retrospective chart review and benchmarking. The benchmarking process may be internal or external to the health system. Depending on the health system's resources, benchmarking may rely on retrospective chart review or may also use computerized databases that compare physicians' resource use, health system costs, and outcomes for specific diagnosis-related groups. This step identifies the health-system's best practice, which is then compared with published clinical practice guidelines, preferably consensus based (e.g., guidelines from the Agency for Health Care Policy and Research or the American Heart Association). The team developing the CCP should use an evidence-based approach to identify, discuss, and resolve the gaps between practice guidelines and their current practice.

5. **Develop the CCP (Including Patient-Education Material and Measures of Conformance and Outcomes).** The multidisciplinary, standardized development of the CCP ensures integration of care and elimination of duplication and oversights.
   a. *The CCP*
   - Define the specific goals or measurable outcomes of the CCP (e.g., decreased length of stay, decreased ventilator time, decreased pain scores, early ambulation).
   - Select the focus areas or categories of actions essential to achieving the goals or outcomes. To ensure consistency and continuity, these focus areas are usually standardized for all CCPs developed within a health system; examples of focus areas are treatments, medications, and patient education and counseling.
   - Determine the appropriate time frame. This will vary according to the disease or procedure being addressed and the practice setting (e.g., emergency room, ambulatory care clinic, acute care hospital). The time frame may be specified in minutes, hours, days, or phases.
   - Insert the activity for the focus area under the appropriate time frame (e.g., "pharmacist provides medication-use education and counseling on discharge day").
   b. *Patient education*
   - Modify the CCP, using lay terms in the patient's primary language, to educate the

patient about activities to be performed, time frames, and expected outcomes. In some practice settings, the patient may be an active partner in CCP decision-making and implementation.

   c. *Monitoring*
- Identify measures of conformance and variance so that the CCP and the resulting outcomes can be continually improved. Variances are deviations from the CCP that may be positive or negative, avoidable or unavoidable. Sources of variances include patient responses to medications, physician decisions, and system breakdowns.

   d. *Documentation*
- Develop a single, multidisciplinary work sheet or other tool that describes the CCP's actions and time frames and provides cells for documenting that actions were performed.[7]

6. ***Obtain Approval of the CCP and Educate Participants.*** To ensure global acceptance among all health care provider groups, the CCP should be approved by appropriate committees, especially those of the medical staff. P&T committee review of pharmacotherapeutic issues associated with the CCP should occur early enough in the CCP development process that therapeutic concerns can be effectively evaluated as they arise, rather than at the end of the process when they could necessitate an extensive rework by the CCP development team.

After approval, all health care team members involved in the care of the patients affected by the CCP should be educated about the outcomes, specific actions and time frames, and professional responsibilities required by the CCP.

7. ***Implement the CCP.*** After the necessary education and training, the CCP is available for patient enrollment and use. The actions and resources required for implementation should be discussed and agreed upon during CCP development. Staff members should be designated to identify patients suitable for the CCP and to guide their enrollment and the CCP's use. When patients are enrolled in a CCP, they are assigned to a health care team whose members have specific responsibilities for actions and time frames.

8. ***Determine Whether Results Are Acceptable.*** Results should support the original goals of the CCP. Analysis of the results and variances, as well as new information (new indications for medications) and technologies (new pharmacotherapy) that become available, provides data for continuous improvement of the CCP.

Pharmacist's Responsibility

Involvement in the CCP process is an opportunity for pharmacists to apply contemporary pharmaceutical care processes and services in a more collaborative way. Most health systems are implementing the CCP process in ways that are appropriate to their own environment, structure, culture, practice settings, and policies and procedures. Since pharmacists possess the knowledge and skills to enhance the CCP process and help achieve its purposes of cost containment, improved quality of care, and desired patient outcomes, they should become involved in the CCP processes in their health systems.

References

1. American Society of Hospital Pharmacists. ASHP statement on pharmaceutical care. *Am J Hosp Pharm.* 1993; 50:1720–3.
2. Joint Commission of Pharmacy Practitioners. Principles for including medications and pharmaceutical care in health care systems. *Am J Hosp Pharm.* 1993; 50:1726–7.
3. American Society of Health-System Pharmacists. ASHP guidelines on a standardized method for pharmaceutical care. *Am J Health-Syst Pharm.* 1996; 53: 1713–6.
4. Coffey RJ, Richards JS, Remmert CS, et al. An introduction to critical paths. *Qual Manag Health Care.* 1992; 1(1):45–54.
5. Lumsdon K, Hagland M. Mapping care. *Hosp Health Netw.* 1993; 67(20):34–40.
6. Jaggers LD. Differentiation of critical pathways from other health care management tools. *Am J Health-Syst Pharm.* 1996; 53:311–3.
7. Kirk JK, Michael KA, Markowsky SJ, et al. Critical pathways: the time is here for pharmacist involvement. *Pharmacotherapy.* 1996; 16:723–33.
8. Koch KE. Opportunities for pharmaceutical care with critical pathways. *Top Hosp Pharm Manage.* 1995; 14(4):1–7.
9. Stevenson LL. Critical pathway experience at Sarasota Memorial Hospital. *Am J Health-Syst Pharm.* 1995; 52:1071–3.
10. Gousse GC, Rousseau MR. Critical pathways at Hartford Hospital. *Am J Health-Syst Pharm.* 1995; 52: 1060–3.
11. Shane R, Vinson B. Use of critical pathways and indicators in pharmacy practice. *Top Hosp Pharm Manage.* 1995; 14(4):55–67.
12. Gouveia WA, Massaro FJ. Critical pathway experience at New England Medical Center. *Am J Health-Syst Pharm.* 1995; 52:1068–70.
13. Saltiel E. Critical pathway experience at Cedars-Sinai Medical Center. *Am J Health-Syst Pharm.* 1995; 52:1063–8.
14. Nelson SP. Critical pathways at University of Iowa Hospitals and Clinics. *Am J Health-Syst Pharm.* 1995; 52:1058–60.
15. American Society of Health-System Pharmacists. ASHP guidelines on medication-use evaluation. *Am J Health-Syst Pharm.* 1996; 53:1953–5.

Approved by the ASHP Board of Directors, November 16, 1996. Developed by the ASHP Council on Professional Affairs.

The bibliographic citation for this document is as follows: American Society of Health-System Pharmacists. ASHP Guidelines on the Pharmacist's Role in the Development of Clinical Care Plans. *Am J Health-Syst Pharm.* 1997; 54:314–8.

ASHP
Technical Assistance Bulletins

ASHP Technical Assistance Bulletin on Hospital Drug Distribution and Control

Drug control (of which drug distribution is an important part) is among the pharmacist's most important responsibilities. Therefore, adequate methods to assure that these responsibilities are met must be developed and implemented. These guidelines will assist the pharmacist in preparing drug control procedures for all medication-related activities. The guidelines are based on the premise that the pharmacy is responsible for the procurement, distribution, and control of *all* drugs used within the institution. In a sense, the entire hospital is the pharmacy, and the pharmacy service is simply a functional service extending throughout the institution's physical and organizational structures.

It should be noted that, although this document is directed toward hospitals, much of it is relevant to other types of health-care facilities.

Pharmacy Policies, Procedures, and Communications

Policy and Procedure Manuals.[1] The effectiveness of the drug control system depends on adherence to policies (broad, general statements of philosophy) and procedures (detailed guidelines for implementing policy). The importance of an up-to-date policy and procedure manual for drug control cannot be overestimated. All pharmacy staff must be familiar with the manual; it is an important part of orientation for new staff and crucial to the pharmacy's internal communication mechanism. In addition, preparing written policies and procedures requires a thorough analysis of control operations; this review might go undone otherwise.

Drug control begins with the setting of policy. The authority to enforce drug control policy and procedures must come from the administration of the institution, with the endorsement of the medical staff, via the pharmacy and therapeutics (P&T) committee and/or other appropriate committee(s). Because the drug control system interfaces with numerous departments and professions, the P&T committee should be the focal point for communications relating to drug control in the institution. The pharmacist, with the cooperation of the P&T committee, should develop media such as newsletters, bulletins, and seminars to communicate with persons functioning within the framework of the control system.

Inservice Training and Education. Intra- and interdepartmental education and training programs are important to the effective implementation of policies and procedures and the institution's drug control system in general. They are part of effective communication and help establish and maintain professional relationships among the pharmacy staff and between it and other hospital departments. Drug control policies and procedures should be included in the pharmacy's educational programs.

Standards, Laws, and Regulations

The pharmacist must be aware of and comply with the laws, regulations, and standards governing the profession. Many of these standards and regulations deal with aspects of drug control. Among the agencies and organizations affecting institutional pharmacy practice are those described below.

Regulatory Agencies and Organizations. The U.S. government, through its Food and Drug Administration (FDA), is responsible for implementing and enforcing the federal Food, Drug, and Cosmetic Act. The FDA is responsible for the control and prevention of misbranding and of adulteration of food, drugs, and cosmetics moving in interstate commerce. The FDA also sets label requirements for food, drugs, and cosmetics; sets standards for investigational drug studies and for marketing of new drug products; and compiles data on adverse drug reactions.

The U.S. Department of the Treasury influences pharmacy operation by regulating the use of tax-free alcohol through the Bureau of Alcohol, Tobacco and Firearms. The U.S. Department of Justice affects pharmacy practice through its Drug Enforcement Agency (DEA) by enforcing the Controlled Substances Act of 1970 and other federal laws and regulations for controlled drugs.

Another federal agency, the Health Care Financing Administration, has established Conditions of Participation for hospitals and skilled nursing facilities to assist these institutions to qualify for reimbursement under the health insurance program for the aged (Medicare) and for Medicaid.

The state board of pharmacy is the agency of state government responsible for regulating pharmacy practice within the state. Practitioners, institutions, and community pharmacies must obtain licenses from the board to practice pharmacy or provide pharmacy services in the state. State boards of pharmacy promulgate numerous regulations pertaining to drug dispensing and control. (In some states, the state board of health licenses the hospital pharmacy separately or through a license that includes all departments of the hospital.)

Standards and guidelines for pharmaceutical services have been established by the Joint Commission on Accreditation of Hospitals (JCAH)[2] and the American Society of Hospital Pharmacists (ASHP).[3] The United States Pharmacopeial Convention also promulgates certain pharmacy practice procedures as well as official standards for drugs and drug testing. Professional practice guidelines and standards generally do not have the force of law but rather are intended to assist pharmacists in achieving the highest level of practice. They may, however, be employed in legal proceedings as evidence of what constitutes acceptable practice as determined by the profession itself.

In some instances, both federal and state laws may deal with a specific activity; in such cases, the more stringent law will apply.

The Medication System

Procurement: Drug Selection, Purchasing Authority, Responsibility, and Control.[4–6] The selection of pharmaceuticals is a basic and extremely important professional function of the hospital pharmacist who is charged with making decisions regarding products, quantities, product specifications, and sources of supply. It is the pharmacist's obligation to establish and maintain standards assuring the quality, proper storage, control, and safe use of all pharmaceuticals and related supplies (e.g., fluid administration sets); this responsibility must not be delegated to another individual. Although the actual purchasing of drugs and supplies may be performed by a nonpharmacist, the setting of quality standards and specifications requires professional knowledge and judgment and must be performed only by the pharmacist.

Economic and therapeutic considerations make it necessary for hospitals to have a well-controlled, continuously updated formulary. It is the pharmacist's responsibility to develop and maintain adequate product specifications to aid in the purchase of drugs and related supplies under the formulary system. The *USP–NF* is a good base for drug product specifications; there also should be criteria to evaluate the acceptability of manufacturers and distributors. In establishing the formulary, the P&T committee recommends guidelines for drug selection. However, when his knowledge indicates, the pharmacist must have the authority to reject a particular drug product or supplier.

Although the pharmacist has the authority to select a brand or source of supply, he must make economic considerations subordinate to those of quality. Competitive bid purchasing is an important method for achieving a proper balance between quality and cost when two or more acceptable suppliers market a particular product meeting the pharmacist's specifications. In selecting a vendor, the pharmacist must consider price, terms, shipping times, dependability, quality of service, returned goods policy, and packaging; however, prime importance always must be placed on drug quality and the manufacturer's reputation. It should be noted that the pharmacist is responsible for the quality of all drugs dispensed by the pharmacy.

Records. The pharmacist must establish and maintain adequate recordkeeping systems. Various records must be retained (and be retrievable) by the pharmacy because of governmental regulations; some are advisable for legal protection, others are needed for JCAH accreditation, and still others are necessary for sound management (evaluation of productivity, workloads, and expenses and assessment of departmental growth and progress) of the pharmacy department. Records must be retained for at least the length of time prescribed by law (where such requirements apply).

It is important that the pharmacist study federal, state, and local laws to become familiar with their requirements for permits, tax stamps, storage of alcohol and controlled substances, records, and reports.

Among the records needed in the drug distribution and control system are

- Controlled substances inventory and dispensing records.
- Records of medication orders and their processing.
- Manufacturing and packaging production records.
- Pharmacy workload records.
- Purchase and inventory records.
- Records of equipment maintenance.
- Records of results and actions taken in quality-assurance and drug audit programs.

Receiving Drugs. Receiving control should be under the auspices of a responsible individual, and the pharmacist must ensure that records and forms provide proper control upon receipt of drugs. Complete accountability from purchase order initiation to drug administration must be provided.

Personnel involved in the purchase, receipt, and control of drugs should be well trained in their responsibilities and duties and must understand the serious nature of drugs. All nonprofessional personnel employed by the pharmacy should be selected and supervised by the pharmacist.

Delivery of drugs directly to the pharmacy or other pharmacy receiving area is highly desirable; it should be considered mandatory for controlled drugs. Orders for controlled substances must be checked against the official order blank (when applicable) and against hospital purchase order forms. All drugs should be placed into stock promptly upon receipt, and controlled substances must be directly transferred to safes or other secure areas.

Drug Storage and Inventory Control. Storage is an important aspect of the total drug control system. Proper environmental control (i.e., proper temperature, light, humidity, conditions of sanitation, ventilation, and segregation) must be maintained wherever drugs and supplies are stored in the institution. Storage areas must be secure; fixtures and equipment used to store drugs should be constructed so that drugs are accessible only to designated and authorized personnel. Such personnel must be carefully selected and supervised. Safety also is an important factor, and proper consideration should be given to the safe storage of poisons and flammable compounds. Externals should be stored separately from internal medications. Medications stored in a refrigerator containing items other than drugs should be kept in a secured, separate compartment.

Proper control is important wherever medications are kept, whether in general storage in the institution or the pharmacy or patient-care areas (including satellite pharmacies, nursing units, clinics, emergency rooms, operating rooms, recovery rooms, and treatment rooms). Expiration dates of perishable drugs must be considered in all of these locations, and stock must be rotated as required. A method to detect and properly dispose of outdated, deteriorated, recalled, or obsolete drugs and supplies should be established. This should include monthly audits of all medication storage areas in the institution. (The results of these audits should be documented in writing.)

Since the pharmacist must justify and account for the expenditure of pharmacy funds, he must maintain an adequate inventory management system. Such a system should enable the pharmacist to analyze and interpret prescribing trends and their economic impacts and appropriately minimize inventory levels. It is essential that a system to indicate subminimum inventory levels be developed to avoid "outages," along with procedures to procure emergency supplies of drugs when necessary.

In-House Manufacturing, Bulk Compounding, Packaging, and Labeling.[7,8] As with commercially marketed drug products, those produced by the pharmacy must be accurate in identity, strength, purity, and quality. Therefore, there must be adequate process and finished product controls for all manufacturing/bulk compounding and packaging operations. Written master formulas and batch records (including product test results) must be maintained. All technical personnel must be adequately trained and supervised.

Packaging and labeling operations must have controls sufficient to prevent product/package/label mixups. A lot number to identify each finished product with its production and control history must be assigned to each batch.

The Good Manufacturing Practices of the FDA is a useful model for developing a comprehensive control system.

The pharmacist is encouraged to prepare those drug dosage forms, strengths, and packagings that are needed for optimal drug therapy but that are commercially unavailable. Adequate attention must be given to the stability, palatability, packaging, and labeling requirements of these products.

Medication Distribution (Unit Dose System).[9–11] Medication distribution is the responsibility of the pharmacy. The pharmacist, with the assistance of the P&T committee and the department of nursing, must develop comprehensive policies and procedures that provide for the safe distribution of all medications and related supplies to inpatients and outpatients.

For reasons of safety and economy, the preferred method to distribute drugs in institutions is the *unit dose* system. Although the unit dose system may differ in form depending on the specific needs, resources, and characteristics of each institution, four elements are common to all: (1) medications are contained in, and administered from, single unit or unit dose packages; (2) medications are dispensed in ready-to-administer form to the extent possible; (3) for most medications, not more than a 24-hour supply of doses is provided to or available at the patient-care area at any time; and (4) a patient medication profile is concurrently maintained in the pharmacy for each patient. Floor stocks of drugs are minimized and limited to drugs for emergency use and routinely used "safe" items such as mouthwash and antiseptic solutions.

(1) Physician's drug order: writing the order. Medications should be given (with certain specified exceptions) only on the *written* order of a qualified physician or other authorized prescriber. Allowable exceptions to this rule (i.e., telephone or verbal orders) should be put in written form immediately and the prescriber should countersign the nurse's or pharmacist's signed record of these orders within 48 (preferably 24) hours. Only a pharmacist or registered nurse should accept such orders. Provision should be made to place physician's orders in the patient's chart, and a method for sending this information to the pharmacy should be developed.

Prescribers should specify the date and time medication orders are written.

Medication orders should be written legibly in ink and should include

- Patient's name and location (unless clearly indicated on the order sheet).
- Name (generic) of medication.
- Dosage expressed in the metric system, except in instances where dosage must be expressed otherwise (i.e., units, etc.).
- Frequency of administration.
- Route of administration.
- Signature of the physician.
- Date and hour the order was written.

Any abbreviations used in medication orders should be agreed to and jointly adopted by the medical, nursing, pharmacy, and medical records staff of the institution.

Any questions arising from a medication order, including the interpretation of an illegible order, should be referred to the ordering physician by the pharmacist. It is desirable for the pharmacist to make (appropriate) entries in the patient's medical chart pertinent to the patient's drug therapy. (Proper authorization for this must be obtained.[12]) Also, a duplicate record of the entry can be maintained in the pharmacy profile.

In computerized patient data systems, each prescriber should be assigned a unique identifier; this number should be included in all medication orders. Unauthorized personnel should not be able to gain access to the system.

(2) Physician's drug order: medication order sheets. The pharmacist (except in emergency situations) must receive the physician's original order or a direct copy of the order before the drug is dispensed. This permits the pharmacist to resolve questions or problems with drug orders before the drug is dispensed and administered. It also eliminates errors which may arise when drug orders are transcribed onto another form for use by the pharmacy. Several methods by which the pharmacy may receive physicians' original orders or direct copies are

1. Self-copying order forms. The physician's order form is designed to make a direct copy (carbon or NCR) which is sent to the pharmacy. This method provides the pharmacist with a duplicate copy of the order and does not require special equipment. There are two basic formats:
   a. Orders for medications included among treatment orders. Use of this form allows the physician to continue writing his orders on the chart as he has been accustomed in the past, leaving all other details to hospital personnel.
   b. Medication orders separated from other treatment orders on the order form. The separation of drug orders makes it easier for the pharmacist to review the order sheet.
2. Electromechanical. Copying machines or similar devices may be used to produce an exact copy of the physician's order. Provision should be made to transmit physicians' orders to the pharmacy in the event of mechanical failure.
3. Computerized. Computer systems, in which the physician enters orders into a computer which then stores and prints out the orders in the pharmacy or elsewhere, are used in some institutions. Any such system should provide for the pharmacist's verification of any drug orders entered into the system by anyone other than an authorized prescriber.

(3) Physician's drug order: time limits and changes. Medication orders should be reviewed automatically when the patient goes to the delivery room, operating room, or a different service. In addition, a method to protect patients from indefinite, open-ended drug orders must be provided. This may be accomplished through one or more of the following: (1) routine monitoring of patients' drug therapy by a pharmacist; (2) drug class-specific, automatic stop-order policies covering those drug orders not specifying a number of doses or duration of therapy; and (3) automatic cancellation of all drug orders after a predetermined (by the P&T committee) time interval unless rewritten by the prescriber. Whatever the method used, it must protect the patient, as well as provide for a timely notification to the prescriber that the order will be stopped *before* such action takes place.

(4) Physician's drug order: receipt of order and drug profiles. A pharmacist must review and interpret every medication order and resolve any problems or uncertainties with it before the drug is entered into the dispensing system. This means that he must be satisfied that each questionable medication order is, in fact, acceptable. This may occur through study of the patient's medical record, research of the professional literature, or discussion with the prescriber or other medical, nursing, or pharmacy staff. Procedures to handle a drug order the pharmacist still believes is unacceptable (e.g., very high dose or a use beyond that contained in the package insert) should be prepared (and reviewed by the hospital's legal counsel). In general, the physician must be able to support the use of the drug in these situations. It is generally advisable for the pharmacist to document actions (e.g., verbal notice to the physician that a less toxic drug was available and should be used) relative to a questionable medication order on the pharmacy's patient medication profile form or other pharmacy document (not in the medical record).

Once the order has been approved, it is entered into the *patient's medication profile.* A medication profile must be maintained in the pharmacy for all inpatients and those outpatients routinely receiving care at the institution. (Note: Equivalent records also should be available at the patient-care unit.) This essential item, which is continuously updated, may be a written copy or computer maintained. It serves two purposes. First, it enables the pharmacist to become familiar with the patient's total drug regimen, enabling him to detect quickly potential interactions, unintended dosage changes, drug duplications and overlapping therapies, and drugs contraindicated because of patient allergies or other reasons. Second, it is required in unit dose systems in order for the individual medication doses to be scheduled, prepared, distributed, and administered on a timely basis. The profile information must be reviewed by the pharmacist *before* dispensing the patient's drug(s). (It also may be useful in retrospective review of drug use.)

Patient profile information should include

- Patient's full name, date hospitalized, age, sex, weight, hospital I.D. number, and provisional diagnosis or reason for admission (the format for this information will vary from one hospital to another).
- Laboratory test results.
- Other medical data relevant to the patient's drug therapy (e.g., information from drug history interviews).
- Sensitivities, allergies, and other significant contra-indications.
- Drug products dispensed, dates of original orders, strengths, dosage forms, quantities, dosage frequency or directions, and automatic stop dates.
- Intravenous therapy data (this information may be kept on a separate profile form, but there should be a method for the pharmacist to review both concomitantly).
- Blood products administered.
- Pharmacist's or technician's initials.
- Number of doses or amounts dispensed.
- Items relevant or related to the patient's drug therapy (e.g., blood products) not provided by the pharmacy.

(5) Physician's drug order: records. Appropriate records of each medication order and its processing in the pharmacy must be maintained. Such records must be retained in accordance with applicable state laws and regulations. Any changes or clarifications in the order should be written in the chart. The signature(s) or initials of the person(s) verifying the transcription of medication orders into the medication profile should be noted. A way should be provided to determine, for all doses dispensed, who prepared the dose, its date of dispensing, the source of the drug, and the person who checked it. Other information, such as the time of receipt of the order and management data (number of orders per patient day and the like) should be kept as desired. Medication profiles also may be useful for retrospective drug use review studies.

(6) Physician's drug order: special orders.[5,6,13,14] Special orders (i.e., "stat" and emergency orders and those for nonformulary drugs, investigational drugs, restricted use drugs, or controlled substances) should be processed according to specific written procedures meeting all applicable regulations and requirements.

(7) Physician's drug order: other considerations. The pharmacy, nursing, and medical staffs, through the P&T committee, should develop a schedule of standard drug administration times. The nurse should notify the pharmacist whenever it is necessary to deviate from the standard medication schedule.

A mechanism to continually inform the pharmacy of patient admissions, discharges, and transfers should be established.

(8) Intravenous admixture services.[15] The preparation of sterile products (e.g., intravenous admixtures, "piggybacks," and irrigations) is an important part of the drug control system. The pharmacy is responsible for assuring that all such products used in the institution are (1) therapeutically and pharmaceutically appropriate (i.e., are rational and free of incompatibilities or similar problems) to the patient; (2) free from microbial and pyrogenic contaminants; (3) free from unacceptable levels of particulate and other toxic contaminants; (4) correctly prepared (i.e., contain the correct amounts of the correct drugs); and (5) properly labeled, stored, and distributed. Centralizing all sterile compounding procedures within the pharmacy department is the best way to achieve these goals.

Parenteral admixtures and related solutions are subject to the same considerations presented in the preceding sections on "physician's drug order." However, their special characteristics (e.g., complex preparation or need for sterility assurance) also mandate certain additional requirements concerning their preparation, labeling, handling, and quality control. These are described in Reference 15.

It is important that the pharmacy is notified of any problems that arise within the institution pertaining to the use of intravenous drugs and fluids (infections, phlebitis, and product defects).

(9) Medication containers, labeling, and dispensing: stock containers. The pharmacist is responsible for labeling medication containers. Medication labels should be typed or machine printed. Labeling with pen or pencil and the use of adhesive tape or china marking pencils should be prohibited. A label should not be superimposed on another label. The label should be legible and free from erasures and strikeovers. It should be firmly affixed to the container. The labels for stock containers should be protected from chemical action or abrasion and bear the name, address, and telephone number of the hospital. Medication containers and labels should not be altered by anyone other than pharmacy personnel. Prescription labels should not be distributed outside the pharmacy. Accessory labels and statements (shake well, may not

be refilled, and the like) should be used as required. Any container to be used outside the institution should bear its name, address, and phone number.

Important labeling considerations are

1. The metric system should be given prominence on all labels when both metric and apothecary measurement units are given.
2. The names of all therapeutically active ingredients should be indicated in compound mixtures.
3. Labels for medications should indicate the amount of drug or drugs in each dosage unit (e.g., per 5 ml and per capsule).
4. Drugs and chemicals in forms intended for dilution or reconstitution should carry appropriate directions.
5. The expiration date of the contents, as well as proper storage conditions, should be clearly indicated.
6. The acceptable route(s) of administration should be indicated for parenteral medications.
7. Labels for large volume sterile solutions should permit visual inspection of the container contents.
8. Numbers, letters, coined names, unofficial synonyms, and abbreviations should not be used to identify medications, with the exception of approved letter or number codes for investigational drugs (or drugs being used in blinded clinical studies).
9. Containers presenting difficulty in labeling, such as small tubes, should be labeled with no less than the prescription serial number, name of drug, strength, and name of the patient. The container should then be placed in a larger carton bearing a label with all necessary information.
10. The label should conform to all applicable federal, state, and local laws and regulations.
11. Medication labels of stock containers and repackaged or prepackaged drugs should carry codes to identify the source and lot number of medication.
12. Nonproprietary name(s) should be given prominence over proprietary names.
13. Amount dispensed (e.g., number of tablets) should be indicated.
14. Drug strengths, volumes, and amounts should be given as recommended in References 11 and 16.

(10) Medication containers, labeling, and dispensing: inpatient medications.[11,16] Drug products should be as ready for administration to the patient as the current status of pharmaceutical technology permits. Inpatient medication containers and packages should conform to applicable *USP* requirements and the guidelines in References 11 and 16.

Inpatient self-care and "discharge" medications should be labeled as outpatient prescriptions (see below).

(11) Medication containers, labeling, and dispensing: outpatient medications.[17] Outpatient medications must be labeled in accordance with state board of pharmacy and federal regulations. As noted, medications given to patients as "discharge medication" must be labeled in the pharmacy (not by nursing personnel) as outpatient prescriptions.

The source of the medication and initials of the dispenser should be noted on the prescription form at the time of dispensing. If feasible, the lot number also should be recorded.

An identifying check system to ensure proper identification of outpatients should be established.

Outpatient prescriptions should be packaged in accor-

dance with the provisions of the Poison Prevention Packaging Act of 1970 and any regulations thereunder. They must also meet any applicable requirements of the *USP*.

Any special instructions to or procedures required of the patient relative to the drug's preparation, storage, and administration should be either a part of the label or accompany the medication container received by the patient. Counseling of the patient sufficient to ensure understanding and compliance (to the extent possible) with his medication regimen must be conducted. Nonprescription drugs, if used in the institution, should be labeled as any other medication.

(12) Delivery of medications. Couriers used to deliver medications should be reliable and carefully chosen.

Pneumatic tubes, dumbwaiters, medication carts, and the like should protect drug products from breakage and theft. In those institutions having automatic delivery equipment, such as a pneumatic tube system, provision must be made for an alternative delivery method in case of breakdown.

All parts of the transportation system must protect medications from pilferage. Locks and other security devices should be used where necessary. Procedures for the orderly transfer of medications to the nurse should be instituted; i.e., drug carts or pneumatic tube carriers should not arrive at the patient-care area without the nurse or her designee acknowledging their arrival.

Medications must always be properly secured. Storage areas and equipment should meet the requirements presented in other sections of these guidelines.

(13) Administration of medications. The institution should develop detailed written procedures governing medication administration. In doing so, the following guidelines should be considered:

1. All medications should be administered by appropriately trained and authorized personnel in accordance with the laws, regulations, and institutional policies governing drug administration. It is particularly important that there are written policies and procedures defining responsibility for starting parenteral infusions, administering all intravenous medications, and adding medications to flowing parenteral fluids. Procedures for drug administration by respiratory therapists and during emergency situations also should be established. Exceptions to any of these policies should be provided in writing.
2. All medications should be administered directly from the medication cart (or equivalent) at the patient's room. The use of unit dose packaged drugs eliminates the need for medication cups and cards (and their associated trays), and they should not be used. A medication should not be removed from the unit dose package until it is to be administered.
3. Medications prepared for administration but not used must be returned to the pharmacy.
4. Medications should be given as near the specified time as possible.
5. The patient for whom the medication is intended should be positively identified by checking the patient's identification band or hospital number or by other means as specified by hospital policy.
6. The person administering the medication should stay with the patient until the dose has been taken. Exceptions to this rule are specific medications which may be left at the patient's bedside upon the physician's written order for self-administration.

7. Parenteral medications that are not to be mixed together in a syringe should be given in different injection sites on the patient or separately injected into the administration site of the administration set of a compatible intravenous fluid.

8. The pharmacy should receive copies of all medication error reports or other medication-related incidents.

9. A system to assure that patients permitted to self-medicate do so correctly should be established.

(14) Return of unused medication. All medications that have not been administered to the patient must remain in the medication cart and be returned to the pharmacy. Only those medications returned in unopened sealed packages may be reissued. Medications returned by outpatients should not be reused. Procedures for crediting and returning drugs to stock should be instituted. A mechanism to reconcile doses not given with nursing and pharmacy records should be provided.

(15) Recording of medication administration. All administered, refused, or omitted medication doses should be recorded in the patient's medical record according to an established procedure. Disposition of doses should occur immediately after administering medications to each patient and before proceeding to the next patient. Information to be recorded should include the drug name, dose and route of administration, date and time of administration, and initials of the person administering the dose.

Drug Samples and Medical Sales Representatives.[18] The use of drug samples within the institution is strongly discouraged and should be eliminated to the extent possible. They should never be used for inpatients (unless, for some reason, no other source of supply is available to the pharmacy). Any samples used must be controlled and dispensed through the pharmacy.

Written regulations governing the activities of medical sales representatives within the institution should be established. Sales representatives should receive a copy of these rules and their activities should be monitored.

Investigational Drugs.[13] Policies and procedures governing the use and control of investigational drugs within the institution are necessary. Detailed procedural guidelines are given in Reference 13.

Radiopharmaceuticals. The basic principles of compounding, packaging, sterilizing, testing, and controlling drugs in institutions apply to radiopharmaceuticals. Therefore, even if the pharmacy department is not directly involved with the preparation and dispensing of these agents, the pharmacist must ensure that their use conforms to the drug control principles set forth in this document.

"Bring-In" Medications. The use of a patient's own medications within the hospital should be avoided to the extent possible. They should be used only if the drugs are not obtainable by the pharmacy. If they are used, the physician must write an appropriate order in the patient's medical chart. The drugs should be sent to the pharmacy for verification of their identity; if not identifiable, they must not be used. They should be dispensed as part of the unit dose system, not separate from it.

Drug Control in Operating and Recovery Rooms.[19] The institution's drug control system must extend to its operating room complex. The pharmacist should ensure that all drugs used within this area are properly ordered, stored, prepared, and accounted for.

Emergency Medication Supplies. A policy to supply emergency drugs when the pharmacist is off the premises or when there is insufficient time to get to the pharmacy should exist. Emergency drugs should be limited in number to include only those whose prompt use and immediate availability are generally regarded by physicians as essential in the proper treatment of sudden and unforeseen patient emergencies. The emergency drug supply should not be a source for normal "stat" or "p.r.n." drug orders. The medications included should be primarily for the treatment of cardiac arrest, circulatory collapse, allergic reactions, convulsions, and bronchospasm. The P&T committee should specify the drugs and supplies to be included in emergency stocks.

Emergency drug supplies should be inspected by pharmacy personnel on a routine basis to determine if contents have become outdated and are maintained at adequate levels. Emergency kits should have a seal which visually indicates when they have been opened. The expiration date of the kit should be clearly indicated.

Pharmacy Service When the Pharmacy Is Closed. Hospitals provide services to patients 24 hours a day. Pharmaceutical services are an integral part of the total care provided by the hospital, and the services of a pharmacist should be available at all times. Where around the clock operation of the pharmacy is not feasible, a pharmacist should be available on an "on call" basis. The use of "night cabinets" and drug dispensing by nonpharmacists should be minimized and eliminated wherever possible.

Drugs must not be dispensed to outpatients or hospital staff by anyone other than a pharmacist while the pharmacy is open. If it is necessary for nurses to obtain drugs when the pharmacy is closed and the pharmacist is unavailable, written procedures covering this practice should be developed. They generally should provide for a limited supply of the drugs most commonly needed in these situations; the drugs should be in proper single dose packages and a log should be kept of all doses removed. This log must contain the date and time the drugs were removed, a complete description of the drug product(s), name of the (authorized) nurse involved, and the patient's name.

Drugs should not be dispensed to emergency room patients by nonpharmacist personnel if the pharmacy is open. When no pharmacist is available, emergency room patients should receive drugs packaged, to the extent possible, in single unit packages; no more than a day's supply of doses should be dispensed. The use of an emergency room "formulary" is recommended.[20]

Adverse Drug Reactions. The medical, nursing, and pharmacy staffs must always be alert to the potential for, or presence of, adverse drug reactions. A written procedure to record clinically significant adverse drug reactions should be established. They should be reported to the FDA, the involved drug manufacturer, and the institution's P&T committee (or its equivalent). Adverse drug reaction reports should contain

- Patient's age, sex, and race.
- Description of the drug reaction and the suspected cause.

- Name of drug(s) suspected of causing the reaction.
- Administration route and dose.
- Name(s) of other drugs received by patient.
- Treatment of the reaction, if any.

These reports, along with other significant reports from the literature, should be reviewed and evaluated by the P&T committee. Steps necessary to minimize the incidence of adverse drug reactions in the facility should be taken.

Medication Errors. If a medication error is detected, the patient's physician must be informed immediately. A written report should be prepared describing any medication errors of clinical import observed in the prescribing, dispensing, or administration of a medication. This report, in accordance with hospital policy, should be prepared and sent to the appropriate hospital officials (including the pharmacy) within 24 hours.

These reports should be analyzed, and any necessary action taken, to minimize the possibility of recurrence of such errors. Properly utilized, these incident reports will help to assure optimum drug use control. Medication error reports should be reviewed periodically by the P&T committee. (It should be kept in mind that, in the absence of an organized, independent error detection system, most medication errors will go unnoticed.)

The following definitions of medication errors are suggested. A *medication error* is broadly defined as a dose of medication that deviates from the physician's order as written in the patient's chart or from standard hospital policy and procedures. Except for errors of omission, the medication dose must actually reach the patient; i.e., a wrong dose that is detected and corrected before administration to the patient is not a medication error. Prescribing errors (e.g., therapeutically inappropriate drugs or doses) are excluded from this definition.

Following are the nine categories of medication errors:

1. *Omission error*: the failure to administer an ordered dose. However, if the patient refuses to take the medication, no error has occurred. Likewise, if the dose is not administered because of recognized contraindications, no error has occurred.
2. *Unauthorized drug error*: administration to the patient of a medication dose not authorized for the patient. This category includes a dose given to the wrong patient, duplicate doses, administration of an unordered drug, and a dose given outside a stated set of clinical parameters (e.g., medication order to administer only if the patient's blood pressure falls below a predetermined level).
3. *Wrong dose error*: any dose that is the wrong number of preformed units (e.g., tablets) or any dose above or below the ordered dose by a predetermined amount (e.g., 20%). In the case of ointments, topical solutions, and sprays, an error occurs only if the medication order expresses the dosage quantitatively, e.g., 1 inch of ointment or two 1-second sprays.
4. *Wrong route error*: administration of a drug by a route other than that ordered by the physician. Also included are doses given via the correct route but at the wrong site (e.g., left eye instead of right).
5. *Wrong rate error*: administration of a drug at the wrong rate, the correct rate being that given in the physician's order or as established by hospital policy.

6. *Wrong dosage form error*: administration of a drug by the correct route but in a different dosage form than that specified or implied by the physician. Examples of this error type include use of an ophthalmic ointment when a solution was ordered. Purposeful alteration (e.g., crushing of a tablet) or substitution (e.g., substituting liquid for a tablet) of an oral dosage form to facilitate administration is generally not an error.
7. *Wrong time error*: administration of a dose of drug greater than ± X hours from its scheduled administration time, X being as set by hospital policy.
8. *Wrong preparation of a dose*: incorrect preparation of the medication dose. Examples are incorrect dilution or reconstitution, not shaking a suspension, using an expired drug, not keeping a light-sensitive drug protected from light, and mixing drugs that are physically/chemically incompatible.
9. *Incorrect administration technique*: situations when the drug is given via the correct route, site, and so forth, but improper technique is used. Examples are not using Z-track injection technique when indicated for a drug, incorrect instillation of an ophthalmic ointment, and incorrect use of an administration device.

Special Considerations Contributing to Drug Control

Pharmacy Personnel and Management.[21–24] Adequate numbers of competent personnel and a well-managed pharmacy are the keys to an effective drug control system. References 21–24 provide guidance on the competencies required of the pharmacy staff and on administrative requirements of a well-run pharmacy department.

Assuring Rational Drug Therapy: Clinical Services.[21,25] Maximizing rational drug use is an important part of the drug control system. Although all pharmacy services contribute to this goal in a sense, the provision of drug information to the institution's patients and staff and the pharmacy's clinical services are those that most directly contribute to rational drug therapy. They are, in fact, institutional pharmacists' most important contributions to patient care.

Facilities. Space and equipment requirements relative to drug storage have been discussed previously. In addition to these considerations, space and equipment must be sufficient to provide for safe and efficient drug preparation and distribution, patient education and consultation, drug information services, and proper management of the department.

Hospital Committees Important to Drug Control.[26,27] Several hospital committees deal with matters of drug control, and the pharmacist must actively participate in their activities. Among these committees (whose names may vary among institutions) are the P&T committee, infection control committee, use review committee, product evaluation committee, patient care committee, and the committee for protection of human subjects. Of particular importance to the drug control system are the formulary and drug use review (DUR) functions of the P&T committee (although DUR in many institutions may be under a use review or quality-assurance committee).

Drug Use Review.[28] Review of how drugs are prescribed and used is an important part of institutional quality-assurance and drug control systems. DUR programs may be performed retrospectively or, preferably, concurrently or prospectively. They may utilize patient outcomes or therapeutic processes as the basis for judgments about the appropriateness of drug prescribing and use. Depending on the review methodology, the pharmacist should be involved in

1. Preparing, in cooperation with the medical staff, drug use criteria and standards.
2. Obtaining quantitative data on drug use, i.e., information on the amounts and types of drugs used, prescribing patterns by medical service, type of patient, and so forth. These data will be useful in setting priorities for the review program. They also may serve as a measure of the effectiveness of DUR programs, assist in analyzing nosocomial infection and culture and sensitivity data, and help in preparing drug budgets.
3. Reviewing medication orders against the drug use criteria and standards.
4. Consulting with prescribers concerning the results of 3 above.
5. Participating in the followup activities of the review program, i.e., educational programs directed at prescribers, development of recommendations for the formulary, and changes in drug control procedures in response to the results of the review process.

It should be noted that the overall DUR program is a joint responsibility of the pharmacy and the organized medical staff; it is not unilaterally a pharmacy or medical staff function.

Quality Assurance for Pharmaceutical Services.[29] To ensure that the drug control system is functioning as intended, there should be a formalized method to (1) set precise objectives (in terms of outcome and process criteria and standards) for the system; (2) measure and verify the degree of compliance with these standards, i.e., the extent to which the objectives have been realized; and (3) eliminate any noncompliance situations. Such a *quality-assurance program* will be distinct from, though related to, the DUR activities of the department.

Drug Recalls. A written procedure to handle drug product recalls should be developed. Any such system should have the following elements:

1. Whenever feasible, notation of the drug manufacturer's name and drug lot number should appear on outpatient prescriptions, inpatient drug orders or profiles, packaging control records, and stock requisitions and their associated labels.
2. Review of these documents (prescriptions, drug orders, and so forth) to determine the recipients (patients and nursing stations) of the recalled lots. Optimally, this would be done by automated means.
3. In the case of product recalls of substantial clinical significance, a notice should go to the recipients that they have a recalled product. The course of action they should take should be included. In the case of outpatients, caution should be exercised not to cause undue alarm. The uninterrupted therapy of the patients must be assured; i.e., replacement of the recalled drugs generally will be required. The hospital's administra-

tion and nursing and medical staffs should be informed of any recalls having significant therapeutic implications. Some situations also may require notifying the physicians of patients receiving drugs that have been recalled.
4. Personal inspection of all patient-care areas should be made to determine if recalled products are present.
5. Quarantine of all recalled products obtained (marked "Quarantined—Do Not Use") until they are picked up by or returned to the manufacturer.
6. Maintenance of a written log of all recalls, the actions taken, and their results.

Computerization.[30] Many information handling tasks in the drug control system (e.g., collecting, recording, storing, retrieving, summarizing, transmitting, and displaying drug use information) may be done more efficiently by computers than by manual systems. Before the drug control system can be computerized, however, a comprehensive, thorough study of the existing manual system must be conducted. This study should identify the data flow within the system and define the functions to be done and their interrelationships. This information is then used as the basis to design or prospectively evaluate a computer system; any other considerations, such as those of the hospital accounting department, are subordinate.

The computer system must include adequate safeguards to maintain the confidentiality of patient records.

A backup system must be available to continue the computerized functions during equipment failure. All transactions occurring while the computer system is inoperable should be entered into the system as soon as possible.

Data on controlled substances must be readily retrievable in written form from the system.

Defective Drug Products, Equipment, and Supplies. The pharmacist should be notified of any defective drug products (or related supplies and equipment) encountered by the nursing or medical staffs. All drug product defects should be reported to the USP–FDA–ASHP Drug Product Defect Reporting Program.

Disposal of Hazardous Substances. Hazardous substances (e.g., toxic or flammable solvents and carcinogenic agents) must be disposed of properly in accordance with the requirements of the Environmental Protection Agency or other applicable regulations. The substances should not be poured indiscriminately down the drain or mixed in with the usual trash.

Unreconstituted vials or ampuls and unopened bottles of oral medications supplied by the National Cancer Institute (NCI) should be returned to the NCI's contract storage and distribution facility.

Other intact products should be returned to the original source for disposition.

Units of anticancer drugs no longer intact, such as reconstituted vials, opened ampuls, and bottles of oral medications, and any equipment (e.g., needles and syringes) used in their preparation require a degree of caution greater than with less toxic compounds to safeguard personnel from accidental exposure. The National Institutes of Health recommends that all such materials be segregated for special destruction procedures. The items should be kept in special containers marked *"Danger—Chemical Carcinogens."* Needles and syringes first should be rendered unusable and then placed in specially marked plastic bags. Care should be taken to prevent penetration and leakage of the bags. Excess liquids should be placed in sealed containers; the original vial is satisfactory. Disposal of all of the above materials should be by incineration to destroy organic material.

Alternate disposal for BCG vaccine products has been recommended by the Bureau of Biologics (BOB). The BOB suggests that all containers and equipment used with BCG vaccines be sterilized prior to disposal. Autoclaving at 121 °C for 30 minutes will sterilize the equipment.

At all steps in the handling of anticancer drugs and other hazardous substances, care should be taken to safeguard professional and support services personnel from accidental exposure to these agents.

References

1. Ginnow WK, King CM Jr. Revision and reorganization of a hospital pharmacy policy and procedure manual. *Am J Hosp Pharm.* 1978; 35:698–704.
2. Accreditation manual for hospitals 1980. Chicago: Joint Commission on Accreditation of Hospitals; 1979.
3. Publications, reprints and services. Washington, DC: American Society of Hospital Pharmacists; current edition.
4. American Society of Hospital Pharmacists. ASHP guidelines for selecting pharmaceutical manufacturers and distributors. *Am J Hosp Pharm.* 1976; 33:645–6.
5. American Society of Hospital Pharmacists. ASHP guidelines for hospital formularies. *Am J Hosp Pharm.* 1978; 35:326–8.
6. American Society of Hospital Pharmacists. ASHP statement of guiding principles on the operation of the hospital formulary system. *Am J Hosp Pharm.* 1964; 21:40–1.
7. American Society of Hospital Pharmacists. ASHP guidelines for repackaging oral solids and liquids in single unit and unit dose packages. *Am J Hosp Pharm.* 1979; 36:223–4.
8. 21 CFR Parts 210 and 211. Current good manufacturing practices in manufacturing, processing, packing or holding of drugs. April 1979.
9. Sourcebook on unit dose drug distribution systems. Washington, DC: American Society of Hospital Pharmacists; 1978.
10. American Society of Hospital Pharmacists. ASHP statement on unit dose drug distribution. *Am J Hosp Pharm.* 1975; 32:835.
11. American Society of Hospital Pharmacists. ASHP guidelines for single unit and unit dose packages of drugs. *Am J Hosp Pharm.* 1977; 34:613–4.
12. American Society of Hospital Pharmacists. ASHP guidelines for obtaining authorization for pharmacists' notations in the patient medical record. *Am J Hosp Pharm.* 1979; 36:222–3.
13. American Society of Hospital Pharmacists. ASHP guidelines for the use of investigational drugs in institutions. *Am J Hosp Pharm.* 1979; 36:221–2.
14. American Society of Hospital Pharmacists. ASHP guidelines for institutional use of controlled substances. *Am J Hosp Pharm.* 1974; 31:582–8.
15. Recommendations of the National Coordinating Committee on Large Volume Parenterals. Washington, DC: American Society of Hospital Pharmacists; 1980.
16. National Coordinating Committee on Large Volume Parenterals. Recommendations for the labeling of large volume parenterals. *Am J Hosp Pharm.* 1978; 35:49–51.
17. American Society of Hospital Pharmacists. ASHP guidelines on pharmacist-conducted patient counseling. *Am J Hosp Pharm.* 1976; 33:644–5.
18. Lipman AG, Mullen HF. Quality control of medical service representative activities in the hospital. *Am J Hosp Pharm.* 1974; 31:167–70.
19. Evans DM, Guenther AM, Keith TD, et al. Pharmacy practice in an operating room complex. *Am J Hosp Pharm.* 1979; 36:1342–7.
20. Mar DD, Hanan ZI, LaFontaine R. Improved emergency room medication distribution. *Am J Hosp Pharm.* 1978; 35:70–3.
21. American Society of Hospital Pharmacists. ASHP minimum standard for pharmacies in institutions. *Am J Hosp Pharm.* 1977; 34:1356–8.
22. American Society of Hospital Pharmacists. ASHP guidelines on the competencies required in institutional pharmacy practice. *Am J Hosp Pharm.* 1975; 32:917–9.
23. American Society of Hospital Pharmacists. ASHP training guidelines for hospital pharmacy supportive personnel. *Am J Hosp Pharm.* 1976; 33:646–8.
24. American Society of Hospital Pharmacists. ASHP competency standard for pharmacy supportive personnel in organized health care settings. *Am J Hosp Pharm.* 1978; 35:449–51.
25. American Society of Hospital Pharmacists. ASHP statement on clinical functions in institutional pharmacy practice. *Am J Hosp Pharm.* 1978; 35:813.
26. American Society of Hospital Pharmacists. ASHP statement on the pharmacy and therapeutics committee. *Am J Hosp Pharm.* 1978; 35:813–4.
27. American Society of Hospital Pharmacists. ASHP statement on the hospital pharmacist's role in infection control. *Am J Hosp Pharm.* 1978; 35:814–5.
28. Antibiotic use review and infection control: evaluating drug use through patient care audit. Chicago: InterQual, Inc.; 1978.
29. Model quality assurance program for hospital pharmacies, revised. Washington, DC: American Society of Hospital Pharmacists; 1980.
30. Sourcebook on computers in pharmacy. Washington, DC: American Society of Hospitals Pharmacists; 1978.

Developed by the ASHP Council on Professional Affairs. Approved by the ASHP Board of Directors, March 20, 1980. Revised November 1981.

This document contains numerous references to various official ASHP documents and other publications. Inclusion of the latter does not constitute endorsement of their content by the Society; they are, however, considered to be useful elaborations on certain subjects contained herein. To avoid redundancy with other ASHP documents, relevant references are cited in many sections of these guidelines. Most may be obtained from ASHP through its publications catalog. Copyright © 1980, American Society of Hospital Pharmacists, Inc. All rights reserved.

The bibliographic citation for this document is as follows: American Society of Hospital Pharmacists. ASHP technical assistance bulletin on hospital drug distribution and control. *Am J Hosp Pharm.* 1980; 37:1097–1103.

ASHP Technical Assistance Bulletin on Single Unit and Unit Dose Packages of Drugs

Drug packages must fulfill four basic functions:

1. Identify their contents completely and precisely.
2. Protect their contents from deleterious environmental effects (e.g., photodecomposition).
3. Protect their contents from deterioration due to handling (e.g., breakage and contamination).
4. Permit their contents to be used quickly, easily, and safely.

Modern drug distribution systems use single unit packages to a great extent and, in fact, such packages are central to the operation of unit dose systems, intravenous admixture services, and other important aspects of pharmacy practice. These guidelines have been prepared to assist pharmaceutical manufacturers and pharmacists in the development and production of single unit and unit dose packages, the use of which has been shown to have substantial benefits.

A *single unit* package is one that contains one discrete pharmaceutical dosage form, i.e., one tablet, one 2-ml volume of liquid, one 2-g mass of ointment, etc. A *unit dose* package is one that contains the particular dose of the drug ordered for the patient. A single unit package is also a *unit dose* or *single dose* package if it contains the particular dose of the drug ordered for the patient. A unit dose package could, for example, contain two tablets of a drug product.

General Considerations

Packaging Materials. Packaging materials (and the package itself) must possess the physical characteristics required to protect the contents from (as required) light, moisture, temperature, air, and handling. The material should not deteriorate during the shelf life of the contents. Packages should be of lightweight, nonbulky materials that do not produce toxic fumes when incinerated. Materials that may be recycled or are biodegradable, or both, are to be preferred over those that are not. Packaging materials should not absorb, adsorb, or otherwise deleteriously affect their contents. Information should be available to practitioners indicating the stability and compatibility of drugs with various packaging materials.

Shape and Form. Packages should be constructed so that they do not deteriorate with normal handling. They should be easy to open and use, and their use should require little or no special training or experience. Unless the package contains a drug to be added to a parenteral fluid or otherwise used in compounding a finished dosage form, it should allow the contents to be administered directly to the patient (or IPPB apparatus or fluid administration set) without any need for repackaging into another container or device (except for ampuls).

Label Copy. Current federal labeling requirements must be adhered to, with attention also given to the items at right. The desired copy and format are as follows:

**Nonproprietary Name
(and proprietary name if to be shown)
Dosage Form (if special or other than oral)
Strength
Strength of Dose and Total Contents Delivered
(e.g., number of tablets and their total dose)
Special Notes (e.g., refrigerate)
Expiration Date
Control Number**

1. *Nonproprietary and proprietary names.* The nonproprietary name and the strength should be the most prominent part of the package label. It is not necessary to include the proprietary name, if any, on the package. The name of the manufacturer or distributor should appear on the package. In addition, the name of the manufacturer of the finished dosage form should be included in the product labeling. The style of type should be chosen to provide maximum legibility, contrast, and permanence.

2. *Dosage form.* Special characteristics of the dosage form should be a part of the label, e.g., extended release. Packages should be labeled as to the route of administration if other than oral, e.g., topical use. In a package containing an injection, the acceptable injectable route(s) of administration should be stated on both outer and inner packages, i.e., both on the syringe unit and carton (if any).

3. *Strength.* Strength should be stated in accordance with terminology in the *American Hospital Formulary Service.* The metric system should be used, with dosage forms formulated to provide the rounded-off figures in the *USP* table of approximate equivalents and expressed in the smallest whole number. Micrograms should be used through 999, then milligrams through 999, then grams. Thus, 300 mg, *not* 5 gr, nor 325 mg, nor 0.3 g; 60 mg, *not* 1 gr, nor 0.06 g, nor 64.5 mg, nor 65 mg; 400 mcg, *not* 1/150 gr, nor 0.4 mg, nor 0.0004 g; ml (milliliters) should be used instead of cc (cubic centimeters).

4. *Strength of dose and total contents delivered.* The total contents and total dose of the package should be indicated. Thus, a unit dose package containing a 600-mg dose as two 300-mg tablets should be labeled "600 mg (as two 300-mg tablets)." Likewise, a 500-mg dose of a drug in a liquid containing 100 mg/ml should be labeled "Delivers 500 mg (as 5 ml of 100 mg/ml)."

5. *Special notes.* Special notes such as conditions of storage (e.g., refrigerate), preparation (e.g., shake well or moisten), and administration (e.g., not to be chewed) that are not obvious from the dosage form designation are to be included on the label.

6. *Expiration date.* The expiration date should be prominently visible on the package. If the contents must be reconstituted prior to use, the shelf life of the final product should be indicated. Unless stability data warrant otherwise, expiration dates should fall during

January and July to simplify recall procedures.

7. *Control number (lot number).* The control number should appear on the package.

Product Identification Codes. The use of product identification codes, appearing directly on the dosage form, is encouraged.

Evidence of Entry. The package should be so designed that it is evident, when the package is still intact, that it has never been entered or opened.

Specific Considerations

Oral Solids

1. *Blister package.* A blister package should
    a. Have an opaque and nonreflective backing (flat upper surface of package) for printing.
    b. Have a blister (dome or bubble) of a transparent material that is, preferably, flat bottomed.
    c. Be easily peelable.
    d. If it contains a controlled substance, be numbered sequentially for accountability purposes.
2. *Pouch package.* A pouch package should
    a. Have one side opaque and nonreflective for printing.
    b. Be easily deliverable, i.e., large tablets in large pouches, small tablets in small pouches.
    c. Tear from any point or from multiple locations.
    d. If it contains a controlled substance, be numbered sequentially for accountability purposes.
3. The packages should be such that contents can be delivered directly to the patient's mouth or hand.

Oral Liquids

1. The packages should be filled to deliver the labeled contents. It is recognized that overfilling will be necessary, depending on the shape of the container, the container material, and the formulation of the dosage form.
2. The label should state the contents as follows: Delivers _____mg (or g or mcg) in _____ml.
3. If reconstitution is required, the amount of vehicle to be added should be indicated. These directions may take the form of "fill to mark on container" in lieu of stating a specific volume.
4. Syringe-type containers for oral administration should not accept a needle and should be labeled "For Oral Use Only."
5. Containers should be designed to permit administration of contents directly from the package.

Injectables

1. The device should be appropriately calibrated in milliliters and scaled from the tip to the fill line. Calibrated space may be built into the device to permit addition of other drugs. The label should state the contents as follows: Delivers _____mg (or g or mcg) in _____ml.
2. An appropriate size needle may be an integral part of the device. The needle sheath should not be the plunger. The plunger should be mechanically stable in the barrel of the syringe.
3. The device should be of such a design that it is patient ready and assembly instructions are not necessary.
4. The sheath protecting the needle should be a nonpenetrable, preferably rigid material, to protect personnel from injury. The size of the needle should be indicated.
5. The device should be of such a design that easy and visible aspiration is possible. It should be as compact as possible and of such a size that it can be easily handled.

Parenteral Solutions and Additives

1. The approximate pH and osmolarity of parenteral solutions should be stated on the label. The amount of overfill also should be noted. Electrolyte solutions should be labeled in both mEq (or millimole) and mg concentrations. Solutions commonly labeled in terms of percent concentration, e.g., dextrose, should also be labeled in w/v terms.
2. Parenteral fluid container labels should be readable when hanging and when upright or in the normal manipulative position.
3. Drugs to be mixed with parenteral infusion solutions should be packaged into convenient sizes that minimize the need for solution transfers and other manipulations.
4. Partially filled piggyback-type containers should
    a. Be recappable with a tamperproof closure.
    b. Have a hanger.
    c. Have volume markings.
    d. Be designed to minimize the potential for contamination during use.
    e. Contain a partial vacuum for ease of reconstitution.
5. If an administration set is included with the container, it should be compatible with all large volume parenteral delivery systems.

Other Dosage Forms—Ophthalmics, Suppositories, Ointments, etc. Dosage forms other than those specifically discussed above should be adequately labeled to indicate their use and route of administration and should adhere to the above and other required package labeling and design criteria.

_____

Approved by the ASHP Board of Directors, November 14–15, 1984. Revised by the ASHP Council on Clinical Affairs. Supersedes the previous version, which was approved on March 31–April 1, 1977.

The bibliographic citation for this document is as follows: American Society of Hospital Pharmacists. ASHP technical assistance bulletin on single unit and unit dose packages of drugs. *Am J Hosp Pharm.* 1985; 42:378–9.

ASHP Technical Assistance Bulletin on Use of Controlled Substances in Organized Health-Care Settings

Introduction

Federal regulation of controlled substances was consolidated by the enactment of the Comprehensive Drug Abuse Prevention and Control Act of 1970 (21 USC 801 et seq.). Enforcement of the Act is generally administered by the Drug Enforcement Administration (DEA), created in 1973 as an arm of the Department of Justice. While the Food and Drug Administration (FDA) retains the authority to regulate specified habit-forming drugs, such substances may be subject to regulation by both FDA and DEA. DEA regulations dealing with narcotic drugs in treatment settings appear in Title 21, *Code of Federal Regulations*, Part 1300 to the end. FDA regulations can be found in Title 21, Part 291.

Despite the comprehensiveness of the Act, its amendments, and its regulations, questions remain concerning their application to the practice of pharmacy in hospitals, long-term care facilities, health maintenance organizations (HMOs), ambulatory care centers, licensed residential care facilities, and other institutional and home health care settings. ASHP originally approved guidelines to the regulations in 1973 in order to provide assistance to institutional pharmacists in interpreting the regulations.

The purpose of this Technical Assistance Bulletin is to provide an interpretation of present legal requirements that will assist in establishing acceptable professional practices under the Controlled Substances Act (CSA). The guidelines should be used in connection with the law and regulations. They are not intended as a substitute for knowledge of the law and regulations.

Just as with patient care, accountability is the responsibility of every discipline within an institution. However, ASHP also recognizes that the pharmacist has primary responsibility for the distribution of drugs throughout the institution, including control methods designed to ensure accountability of controlled substances. The pharmacist is responsible for assuming the leading role in the control of drugs that are subject to diversion and misuse.

In adopting the following guidelines, the requirements of the CSA have been interpreted to ensure compliance with the law while still allowing the organized health-care setting to promote high quality patient care in accordance with acceptable legal and professional standards. ASHP believes that these guidelines provide effective controls against diversion or misuse while ensuring that a proper level of professional attention to the needs of patients is maintained.

Research, laboratory procedures, and instructional uses are dealt with separately under their own heading. Methadone is also discussed separately in its own section.

A final word of caution is in order. Some state laws are more stringent than federal laws. Where this is the case, the stricter law also must be followed.

Definitions

The following selected definitions are derived from the CSA or regulations of federal agencies. The definitions are pre-sented here because they are critical to understanding the law or because of their effect on certain operative provisions of the law and its regulations. Most of the language contained in the definitions comes directly from the CSA or from DEA regulations. However, in certain instances, language has been added to assist in the understanding and application of the definitions.

1. ***Person.*** The term "person" is defined in the DEA regulations [21 CFR 1301.02(j)] but not in the CSA. It includes any individual, corporation, government or governmental subdivision or agency, business trust, partnership, association, or other legal entity. It would generally include a hospital but not the hospital pharmacy.

2. ***Agent.*** The term "agent" is defined in the CSA [CSA §102(3); 21 USC 802(3)] but not in the DEA regulations. It means an authorized person who acts on behalf of or at the direction of a manufacturer, distributor, or dispenser; such term does not include a common or contract carrier, public warehouseman, or employee of the carrier or warehouseman when acting in the usual and lawful course of the carrier's or warehouseman's business.

3. ***Pharmacist.*** The term "pharmacist" is defined in the DEA regulations [21 CFR 1304.02(g)] but not in the CSA. It means any individual licensed by a state to dispense controlled substances and also includes any other person (e.g., pharmacist intern) authorized by a state to dispense controlled substances under the supervision of a pharmacist licensed by that state.

4. ***Practitioner.*** The term "practitioner" is defined in the CSA [CSA §102(20); 21 USC 802(20)] but not in the DEA regulations. It means a physician, dentist, veterinarian, scientific investigator, pharmacy, hospital, or other person licensed, registered, or otherwise permitted, by the United States or the jurisdiction in which the practitioner practices or does research, to distribute, dispense, conduct research with respect to, administer, or use in teaching or chemical analysis, a controlled substance in the course of professional practice or research.

5. ***Individual Practitioner.*** The term "individual practitioner" is defined in the DEA regulations [21 CFR 1306.02(b)] but not in the CSA. It means a physician, dentist, veterinarian, or other individual licensed, registered, or otherwise permitted, by the United States or the jurisdiction in which he or she practices, to dispense a controlled substance in the course of professional practice. It does not include a pharmacist, pharmacy, or institutional practitioner.

6. ***Institutional Practitioner.*** The term "institutional practitioner" is defined in the DEA regulations [21 CFR 1306.02(c)] but not in the CSA. It means a hospital, intermediate care facility, skilled nursing facility, federally qualified or state-licensed HMO, or other entity (other than an individual) licensed, registered, or oth-

erwise permitted, by the United States or the jurisdiction in which it is located, to dispense a controlled substance in the course of professional practice. It does not include individual practitioners or a pharmacy.

7. *Dispense.* The term "dispense" is defined in the CSA [CSA §102(10); 21 USC 802(10)] but not in the DEA regulations. It means to deliver a controlled substance to an ultimate user or research subject by, or pursuant to the lawful order of, a practitioner, including the prescribing and administering of a controlled substance and the packaging, labeling, or compounding necessary to prepare the substance for delivery.

   Additionally, the term "dispenser," as defined in the CSA [CSA §102(10); 21 USC 802(10)] and the DEA regulations [21 CFR 1304.02(c)], means an individual practitioner, institutional practitioner, pharmacy, or pharmacist who dispenses a controlled substance.

8. *Administer.* The term "administer" is defined in the CSA [CSA §102(2); 21 USC 802(2)] but not in the DEA regulations. It means the direct application of a controlled substance to the body of a patient or research subject by either a practitioner (or in the practitioner's presence by the practitioner's authorized agent) or the patient or research subject at the direction and in the presence of the practitioner, whether such application be by injection, inhalation, ingestion, or any other route.

9. *Prescription.* The term "prescription" is defined in the DEA regulations [21 CFR 1306.02(f)] but not in the CSA. It means an order for medication that is dispensed to or for an ultimate user but does not include an order for medication that is dispensed for immediate administration to the ultimate user (e.g., an order to dispense a drug to an inpatient for immediate administration in a hospital is not a prescription). A medication order is not considered to be a prescription when it is dispensed from a pharmacy registered in the name of, and located at, an institution for an ultimate user who is a patient in the institution.

10. *Readily Retrievable.* The term "readily retrievable" is defined in the DEA regulations [21 CFR 1304.02(h)] but not in the CSA. It means that entries for controlled substances not maintained in separate written records are visually identifiable from other items appearing in the records (e.g., the use of asterisked or red-lined notations or, in the case of prescriptions, the letter "C" in red ink); or, where records are kept by automated data processing systems or other electronic or mechanized recordkeeping systems, the system possesses the capability to produce the controlled substance records in a reasonable time.

11. *Long-Term Care Facility.* The term "long-term care facility" is defined in the DEA regulations [21 CFR 1306.02(e)] but not in the CSA. It means a nursing home or a retirement care, mental care, or other facility or institution that provides extended health care to resident patients.

Registration

Persons Required to Register. Forms and fees. Every person who manufactures, distributes, dispenses, or conducts research with controlled substances, conducts narcotic maintenance or detoxification programs, or proposes to engage in any of these activities must obtain registration(s) unless exempted by law or DEA regulations. Dispensers may obtain registration for a period of up to 3 years, as determined by DEA. Manufacturers and distributors must obtain registration annually. Registration is accomplished by use of DEA Forms 224, 224a, 225, 225a, 363, and 363a, as required. The appropriate registration fee must be paid when the form is submitted to DEA. However, governmental registrants may claim exemption to the registration fee.

Types of Activities. Dispensing. Separate registration is required for dispensing. The hospital registration covers both inpatient and outpatient dispensing, unless outpatient dispensing is operated from a detached ambulatory care pharmacy.

Distribution. Separate registration is required for distribution of controlled substances to persons, other than employees or agents of the registrant, who will make final transfer to the ultimate user. If an institution regularly orders controlled substances for other facilities, it is in effect acting as a wholesaler and must register as a distributor.

An exception to the regulations allows for occasional distribution to other registrants without registration as a distributor, provided that the annual total number of dosage units of all controlled substances so distributed does not exceed 5% of the total number of dosage units of all controlled substances dispensed.

Place of Business. Separate registration is required for each principal place of business or professional practice. A principal place of business or practice is considered to be one general physical location. The hospital registration covers the entire institution. Separate registration is not required for satellite or decentralized pharmacy stations or outpatient pharmacies located onsite in the same institution. However, if the hospital has pharmacies that are physically removed from the main facility at different locations, each pharmacy may be required to register and obtain a separate DEA number depending on its distance from the main facility.

Contract pharmacy. A leased or contract pharmacy located on the premises of an existing DEA-registered hospital may operate under the hospital registration, provided that the hospital assumes full responsibility for the pharmacy operations and ensures full compliance with all applicable federal regulations governing the use of controlled substances. This would be permissible only if the hospital's responsibility for the operation is clearly set forth in the contract between the hospital and the contract pharmacy. Under these conditions, the pharmacy may perform all of the functions of a hospital pharmacy, including the dispensing of controlled substances pursuant to medication orders.

If the hospital does not wish to assume this responsibility, the contract pharmacy would be required to register with the DEA as a retail pharmacy, and a prescription would be required to dispense controlled substances to hospital patients.

A registered hospital is authorized to fill outpatient prescriptions without obtaining a retail pharmacy registration, provided that this practice is within its own use and allowed by state law. Outpatient "own use" includes the organized health-care setting's bona fide outpatients and its employees and medical staff and their families for their personal use. The same records as are required of a retail pharmacy must be maintained.

Pharmacy not onsite. Since registration is required for each principal place of business or professional practice where controlled substances are manufactured, distributed, or dispensed, a pharmacy not onsite at the institution must obtain a separate registration from the registration of the institution and must maintain all records required for a retail pharmacy.

Practitioners within Institution. Where the organized health-care setting is the registrant, its agents and employees are exempt from registration. The exemption permits institutional personnel to carry out functions of the institution with respect to controlled substances without being personally registered, provided that they are acting in the usual course of their business or employment. Thus, in this case, pharmacists do not need separate personal registration since DEA does not actually register pharmacists.

Additionally, a physician who practices only in a hospital that is itself registered with DEA as a practitioner need not apply for an additional personal registration. However, there are important limitations to the use of this exemption [21 CFR 1301.24(b)]. The employed physician (without a personal DEA registration) may not write prescriptions for controlled substances to be filled by

1. A pharmacy outside the hospital.
2. The hospital pharmacy if that pharmacy is itself registered as a practitioner.

The employed physician may administer or dispense controlled substances only while acting in the course of usual employment in the facility. (For application of this principle to unregistered interns, residents, or foreign-trained physicians, see the related subsection in the Prescriptions section of these guidelines.) State law determines for purposes of the CSA which agents or employees are authorized to have access to or responsibility for controlled substances. Institutions should have written policies that interpret state law and assign staff responsibility accordingly.

Termination of Registration.

1. The Administrator of DEA has authority under the CSA to suspend or revoke registration where the registrant
   a. Has materially falsified any application filed pursuant to or required by Title II or III of the CSA.
   b. Has been convicted of a felony under the CSA or of a felony under any other federal or state laws relating to controlled substances.
   c. Has had his or her state license or registration suspended, revoked, or denied and is no longer authorized by state law to manufacture, distribute, or dispense controlled substances, or has had the suspension, revocation, or denial of his or her registration recommended by competent state authority.

   The registration of a practitioner may now be denied if it is determined that such registration would be "inconsistent with the public interest." In determining the public interest, DEA may consider (1) the recommendations of the appropriate state licensing board or professional disciplinary authority, (2) the experience of the applicant in dispensing or conduct-

ing research with respect to controlled substances, (3) the applicant's conviction record under federal or state laws relating to the manufacture, distribution, or dispensing of controlled substances, (4) compliance with applicable state, federal, or local laws pertaining to controlled substances, and (5) such other conduct that may threaten the public health and safety.

These considerations, along with the three existing grounds noted above, also allow for the input of competent state authority recommending the suspension, revocation, or denial of a registration.

These factors expand DEA's authority to deal with problems of diversion at the practitioner level. Registrants have recourse to established administrative procedures under Section 1301.45 of the DEA regulations to ensure due process of law before suspension or revocation of registration.

2. The registration of any person is terminated if and when such person dies, ceases legal existence, discontinues business or professional practice, or changes his or her name or address as shown on the certificate of registration. The DEA must be promptly notified of the reason for termination. Where there is a change of name or address, the registrant is required to report this change.
3. Registration may not be assigned or transferred except in compliance with conditions designated in writing by DEA.

Records and Inventory

General. Every registrant under the Act must maintain, on a current basis, complete and accurate records of the receipt and disposition of all controlled substances. The records must include the following information for each controlled substance:

1. The name of the substance.
2. A description of each product in finished form (e.g., 10-mg tablet or 10-mg/ml concentration) and the number of units or volume of finished form in each commercial container (e.g., 100-tablet bottle or 3-ml vial).
3. The number of commercial containers of each such finished form received from other persons, including the date of receipt and number of containers in each shipment and the name, address, and registration number of the person from whom the containers were received.
4. The number of units or volume of products in finished form dispensed, including the name of the person to whom it was dispensed, the date of dispensing, the number of units or volume dispensed, and the written or typewritten name or initials of the individual who dispensed or administered the substance on behalf of the dispenser.
5. The number of units or volume of products in finished form of commercial containers disposed of in any other manner by the registrant, including the date of disposal and the quantity of the substance in finished form disposed.

All records must be kept for a 2-year period or longer if state or other laws mandate. Records of Schedule I or II substances must be maintained separately from all other records of the registrant; those records of substances listed in

Schedule III, IV, or V need not be kept separately, provided that the information is readily retrievable.

Inventory. To establish a starting point, the law requires a physical inventory of all controlled substances on the effective date of the Act or when the registrant first engages in business. A person registered to dispense controlled substances shall include in his or her inventory for each controlled substance in finished form the name and finished form of the substances (e.g., pentobarbital 100-mg tablets) and the number of containers and units per volume in each container. For substances that are damaged, outdated, awaiting disposal, being held for quality control, or maintained for extemporaneous compounding, the name, quantity, and reason for the continued maintenance of the substance are required. In determining units in an open commercial container, an exact count or measure of Schedule I or II drugs shall be made; an estimated count of Schedule III, IV, or V drugs shall be made unless the container holds more than 1000 tablets or capsules, in which case an exact count will be made.

An inventory must be taken every 2 years thereafter, on the date on which the initial inventory was taken, or on the registrant's regular physical inventory date, or on any other fixed date that does not vary by more than 6 months from the biennial date that would otherwise apply [21 CFR 1304.13]. For this biennial inventory and any other DEA-required inventories, the institution must record on that inventory record if it was taken at the beginning or end of that day's business and should note the name, initials, or signature of the person or persons taking that inventory. If the registrant elects to take the biennial inventory on his or her regular general physical inventory date or another fixed date, DEA must be notified of the election and of the date on which the biennial inventory will be taken.

The law specifically states that a perpetual inventory is not required. Nor does the law require periodic "audits." However, these procedures may be desirable in selected high risk areas or where diversion is suspected.

Records of Receipt. Order forms. To purchase substances in Schedule I or II, the law requires an official order form, DEA Form 222. After a substance purchased through Form 222 has been received, Copy 3 of the order form serves the requirement of a "separate" record and must be filed separately. No further record is needed. Order forms may be obtained only by registered persons. If the institutional pharmacist prepared and signed the registration application, he or she may obtain order forms on his or her own signature. If the institution's administrator signed the application for registration, the administrator should execute a power of attorney (to be retained on file) for DEA order forms to permit the pharmacist to obtain and execute order forms on his or her behalf. In a large institution, it may be desirable to designate more than one pharmacist on this power of attorney. The DEA regulations outline the form and substance of the power of attorney [21 CFR 1305.07].

The order form is prepared in triplicate. The purchaser submits Copy 1 and Copy 2 of the form to the supplier and retains Copy 3 in his or her own files to be used to record the quantity and the date on which the controlled substances are received. As stated above, the order forms must be maintained separately from all other records of the registrant.

The requirements for completing Form 222 are specifically stated in the DEA regulations. Pharmacists must take great care to ensure that they literally follow the directions listed on the back of the form for completing it. Additionally, care should be taken in actually completing the form because the regulation does not allow suppliers to fill an order if the form shows "any alteration, erasure, or change of any description" [21 CFR 1305.11(2)]. If an error is made when completing Form 222, all copies of the form should be voided and kept on file.

The regulations also note that a supplier, not a purchaser, may void an item on a DEA Form 222 [21 CFR 1305.15(a)]. Consequently, the supplier is the only individual who has the authority to indicate the cancellation on an order form.

DEA policy does not preclude generic substitution for products ordered on Form 222, provided that the name and National Drug Code (NDC) number of the actual product shipped is reflected on the form. Therefore, it would be acceptable to make a substitution provided that the customer (pharmacy) agrees to accept a generic rather than a brand name product, the generic product of a manufacturer rather than the one specified on the form, or a brand name product rather than a generic one. The purchaser (pharmacist) is not required to submit a new DEA Form 222 to accommodate such an order change.

Purchase orders, invoices, and other forms. Purchase orders, invoices, packing slips, and other business forms may serve as records of receipt for substances in Schedule III, IV, or V, if they are accurately reconciled against the drugs actually received. If noncontrolled substances are listed on the same business form, controlled substances should be made readily identifiable by use of a red line, asterisk, or some other annotation to meet the requirement that the records be readily retrievable. An alternative to using business forms as the record of receipt is the maintenance of a log book or inventory card system. However, in order to meet the retrievability requirements of the regulations, a single system (not both) should be used.

Computer records. If a computer or other automated data processing equipment is used, separate written records as described above are not required for controlled substances in any schedule, provided that (1) DEA order forms are maintained in accordance with DEA regulations, (2) specific information in the data bank can be retrieved within a reasonable period of time, and (3) such information is retained for a period of 2 years and includes all of the information required by DEA as described earlier in this section under the General subheading.

Patient Records. Administration records. The basic records of disposition within the institution are patient medical records. Medical records contain physicians' original drug orders authorizing the dispensing and administration of medications. It is not necessary for the physician to sign and write his or her DEA registration number on each order for a controlled substance. However, the physician's registration number and signature should be kept on file in the pharmacy. If it is not on file in the pharmacy, the physician should enter the number in the medical record.

If the prescriber is an unregistered intern, resident, or foreign-trained physician in the employ of the facility, he or she may use the institution's registration number in lieu of individual registration. To write outpatient prescription orders for controlled substances, he or she must be assigned a suffix code in addition to the institution's number. (See the related subsection in the section on Prescriptions.)

The medical record also contains nurses' entries indicating that drugs were administered to patients. This information may be contained in the nursing notes, in the progress notes, or on a medication treatment form.

Working solely from the medical record can be burdensome, especially with respect to reconciliation of medications issued and those administered. In addition, records for Schedule II substances must be maintained separately and those for Schedule III, IV, or V substances must be readily retrievable. Hence, it is desirable to maintain a derivative record from the medical record; such a record can be used for control purposes, with minimum interference to patient care. Adequate accountability does not require the use of any specific system or form. One type of effective and convenient-to-maintain record is a medication administration record (MAR). Variations of this record that achieve the same purpose may also be used. This record constitutes a separate section in the patient's chart, apart from the physicians' progress notes and nurses' notes.

For recordkeeping purposes, the MAR has a number of advantages. Most institutions already use, in one form or another, an MAR that contains the necessary information for patient-care purposes. Use of this record for control purposes eliminates the need to rewrite the same information on another record form, resulting in a significant savings of nursing and pharmacy time. If diversion does occur, the chances of discovery are increased because all clinical personnel are using the same records in caring for patients.

A second method of recordkeeping is a derivative record maintained by computer. Records of disposition used to provide information for computers or other automated data processing equipment need not conform to any particular format, provided that all required information (previously listed) is put into the system. The system must be designed so that records of Schedule II controlled substances can be retrieved separately from Schedule III, IV, and V records. As with other recordkeeping systems, computer records of disposition may be reconciled by comparing the quantities of controlled substances used and remaining against the quantities received.

A third form of record that could be used is the "certificate of disposition" or "proof of use" sheet. The same basic information is necessary as with other methods. Each time a dose of a controlled substance is administered, institutional personnel are required to make an entry on a manual form or in an automated control system. All controlled substances recorded as administered are reconciled against the physical inventory. One difficulty with this system is that these records do not contain the physicians' drug orders, complicating verification that drugs administered were in fact ordered. Patient charts are primary care records and are in constant use by physicians, nurses, pharmacists, and other personnel. Manual proof of use sheets are not used as often and, in fact, may not be used for many days for some seldom used drugs. Thus, falsification of proof of use sheets may go undetected for longer periods of time than with primary patient records such as the MAR. Automated systems with provisions for additional levels of security and control can improve this type of record. DEA generally does not consider patient profiles to be acceptable documents for recordkeeping since required information is often not included.

Outpatient dispensing. Prescriptions for outpatients (see related section under Prescriptions) must be filed separately if for substances in Schedule I or II. Prescriptions for Schedule III, IV, or V substances may be kept with other prescriptions if they are stamped in red ink, in the lower right corner, with a letter "C" that is no smaller than 1 inch high [21 CFR 1304.04(h)(2)].

Transfers between pharmacies. The transfer of original prescription information for Schedule III–V controlled substances for the purpose of refill dispensing is permissible (if allowed under existing state or other applicable law) between pharmacies on a one-time basis provided that

1. The transfer is communicated directly between two licensed pharmacists.
2. The transferring pharmacist records "void" on the invalidated prescription and records the name, address, and DEA number of the pharmacy to which it was transferred, the name of the pharmacist receiving the information, the date of the transfer, and the pharmacist transferring the information.
3. The receiving pharmacist writes the following on the face of the prescription: the word "transfer"; the date of issuance of the original prescription; the original number of refills authorized; the date of original dispensing; the number of valid refills remaining; the date of the last refill; the name, address, DEA number, and original prescription number of the pharmacy from which it was transferred; and the name of the transferring pharmacist.
4. Both pharmacies maintain the required records for 2 years from the date of the last refill.
5. Pharmacies electronically accessing the same prescription record satisfy all information requirements of a manual mode of prescription transferral.

Waste and disposal. Controlled substances may be disposed of other than by administration to a patient. An ampul might be dropped and broken, the patient might refuse a dose of medication, the medication might become contaminated or decomposed, or the prescriber might cancel an order. Whenever possible, all such medications should be returned to the pharmacy for final disposition.

Each organized health-care setting should develop a policy to be followed when any quantity of controlled substances must be discarded as wastage. Pharmacies providing injectable drugs to patients receiving home care should develop a policy on appropriate waste and disposal of unused narcotics. In developing these policies, pharmacists should consult with their state board of pharmacy and the DEA's Special Agent in Charge (SAC) within the region. State and local regulations should be consulted, as jurisdictions differ on requirements within various types of institutions. Policies should contain provisions for a second signature to witness the destruction of any controlled substance. Authority to witness destruction of a controlled substance should be limited to those individuals who are given authority within the institution to administer or dispense controlled substances.

The DEA regulations require that a registrant who desires or is required to dispose of controlled substances in his or her possession must request authority and disposal instructions from the SAC of the DEA office in the area where the registrant is located. If an institution is registered only as a dispenser of controlled substances and is not required to make periodic reports to DEA, then the request for disposal is made on DEA Form 41. The registrant must list the controlled substances for disposal and submit the form, in triplicate, to the SAC. The SAC shall authorize disposal by

1. Transferral to a person registered under the Act and authorized to possess the substance.
2. Delivery to an agent of the DEA or to the nearest office of DEA.
3. Destruction in the presence of an agent of DEA or other authorized person.
4. Other means determined by the SAC that ensure that the controlled substance does not become available to unauthorized persons.

The general method of disposal is incineration. Furthermore, DEA allows other reasonable types of disposal as long as the registrant receives approval of the disposal procedure from the SAC. However, flushing is no longer an appropriate method of disposal for controlled substances because of changes in the guidelines of the Environmental Protection Agency.

In lieu of disposal by DEA, authority has been granted for disposal of unwanted, outdated, controlled substances to agents of the individual states' narcotics control authorities and professional licensing board inspectors or investigators. In terms of disposal without a witness, DEA policy does not make a distinction between partially used controlled substances and other controlled substance waste. Partially used controlled substances should also be destroyed in accordance with DEA regulations. The local DEA office or state board of pharmacy should be contacted to determine if the state in which the institution is located performs these destructions. Contact the local DEA office to determine the conditions under which this can be done and the details for carrying out such disposal.

If the institution is required to dispose of controlled substances regularly, personnel may file a written request with the SAC to authorize the institution to dispose of those substances without prior authorization on the condition that records are maintained of such disposals and periodic reports are filed with DEA summarizing those disposals. Conditions may be placed on the disposal, such as the method of destruction and the frequency and details of the periodic reports. These requirements do not affect or alter any procedures established by the state in which the institution is registered. To ensure that the institution is in compliance with state laws and regulations regarding disposal, the registrant should also contact the appropriate state regulatory board before proceeding.

Additionally, in selected situations, the DEA may authorize more than one disposal annually without the presence of a witness from the DEA. Requests from an individual practitioner to destroy controlled substances in addition to the authorized annual disposal are handled on a case-by-case basis. Registrants must complete a legible Form DEA-41 listing all drugs to be destroyed and submit it to the nearest DEA office, with a letter requesting permission to destroy the drugs. The letter must be received by the DEA at least 2 weeks before the proposed destruction.

Prescriptions

General. Substances in Schedule II, III, or IV (and, in some states, V) may be dispensed or administered only pursuant to a written or oral prescription from a prescribing individual practitioner or pursuant to an order for medication made by an individual practitioner that is dispensed for immediate administration to the ultimate user. All such orders, or direct copies thereof, should be received and interpreted by the pharmacist before administration. The practitioner's order is the keystone to any control system. Without it, the entire system is rendered useless since counterfeit administration records could be entered as the means for diverting controlled substances. Administration of emergency medications from floor stock or emergency supplies should be provided for in written policies and procedures. In a small facility without onsite pharmaceutical services, all controlled substances must be dispensed pursuant to prescriptions.

Outpatients. Controlled substances may not be dispensed to outpatients for home use unless all of the prescription and labeling requirements of the law are met. Prescriptions for controlled substances in all schedules must include the name and strength of the drug to be dispensed, the dosage form, quantity prescribed, directions for use, the name and address of the patient, and the name, address, and registration number of the prescriber. Further, they must be dated as of, and signed on, the day they are issued [21 CFR 1306.05(a)].

For injectable products administered in the home, the prescription should include the concentration, rate of administration, and route of administration. If the medication is to be administered through patient-controlled analgesia devices, then other pertinent variables (e.g., dose, amount and frequency of bolus doses, and lockout period) should be included on the prescription.

Dispensing of Prescriptions. A prescription for controlled substances may be dispensed by a pharmacist acting in the usual course of his or her professional practice. The pharmacist must be employed in either a registered institution or a registered retail pharmacy.

Schedules II, III, IV, and V. Requirement of prescription. A pharmacist may dispense a controlled substance listed in Schedule II only pursuant to a written prescription signed by the prescribing individual practitioner. An exception occurs in an emergency situation [21 CFR 1306.11(d)]. Then, a pharmacist may dispense a controlled substance listed in Schedule II upon oral authorization provided that

1. The quantity prescribed and dispensed is limited to the amount needed to treat the patient during the emergency period.
2. The prescription is immediately reduced to writing by the pharmacist and contains all information required except for the signature of the prescriber.
3. The pharmacist makes a reasonable effort to determine that the oral authorization came from a registered individual practitioner. This may include a call to the prescriber using the telephone number listed in an appropriate directory or other good faith efforts to establish identity.
4. The prescribing individual practitioner delivers or mails a written prescription to the pharmacist within 72 hours. The phrase "Authorization for Emergency Dispensing" and the date of the oral order should be written on the prescription. Upon receipt, the pharmacist should attach the written prescription to the oral emergency prescription. If a written prescription is not received, the pharmacist should notify the nearest

office of the DEA or risk forfeiture of the authority to dispense without a written prescription conferred by the regulations [21 CFR 1306.11(d)].

Controlled substances listed in Schedules III–V, however, may be dispensed pursuant to either a written prescription or a telephoned order. An original prescription for a Schedule III or IV controlled substance received via the telephone may be entered directly into the computer system, provided that the computer system provides the necessary documentation required by law. A hard copy record may be required; it may be provided by the computer system.

Refills. Refills of prescriptions for Schedule II controlled substances are prohibited, except as stated below, but partial filling is permitted if the pharmacist is initially unable to supply the full quantity called for in a written or emergency oral prescription and a notation is made of the quantity supplied on the face of the written prescription. However, the remaining portion may be filled only within the 72-hour period. If the remaining portion is not filled within the 72-hour period, the pharmacist must notify the prescribing individual practitioner. No further quantity may be supplied beyond 72 hours without a new prescription.

Partial filling. A prescription for a Schedule II controlled substance written for a patient in a long-term care facility or for a patient with a medical diagnosis documenting a terminal illness may be filled in partial quantities [21 CFR 1306.13]. If there is any question whether a patient may be classified as having a terminal illness, the pharmacist must contact the prescribing practitioner before partially filling the prescription. The pharmacist must record on the prescription whether the patient is terminally ill or a patient in a long-term care facility.

For each partial filling, the dispensing pharmacist shall record on the prescription (or on another appropriate record, uniformly maintained and readily retrievable) the date of the partial filling, the quantity dispensed, the remaining quantity authorized to be dispensed, and the identification of the dispensing pharmacist. Schedule II prescriptions for patients in a long-term care facility or patients with a medical diagnosis documenting a terminal illness shall be valid for a period not to exceed 60 days from the issue date unless earlier terminated by the discontinuance of the medication. Information pertaining to current Schedule II prescriptions for patients in a long-term care facility or for patients with a medical diagnosis documenting a terminal illness may be maintained in a computerized system if this system has the capability to permit

1. Output (display or printout of the original prescription number).
2. Date of issue.
3. Identification of individual prescribing practitioner.
4. Identification of patient.
5. Address of the long-term care facility or address of the institution or residence of the patient.
6. Identification of medication authorized (including dosage form, strength, and quantity).
7. Listing of the partial fillings and quantities that have been dispensed under each prescription.
8. Identification of the prescribing pharmacist.

Refills for Schedule III or IV controlled substances may not be made more than 6 months after the date of issue and may not be refilled more than five times.

Refills for Schedule III–V controlled substances may be made only if expressly authorized by the prescribing individual practitioner on the prescription. Each refilling of a prescription shall be entered on the prescription or on another appropriate document. The practitioner may authorize additional refills of Schedule III or IV controlled substances on the original prescription through an oral refill authorization transmitted to the pharmacist if the total quantity authorized, including the amount of the original prescription, does not exceed five refills or extend beyond 6 months from the date of issue of the original prescription. The practitioner must execute a new and separate prescription for any additional quantities beyond the five-refill, 6-month limitation.

Interns, Residents, or Foreign-Trained Physicians. Interns, residents, or foreign-trained physicians on the institution's staff who do not have their own registration numbers may use the number of the institution plus a suffix code assigned to each by the institution.

The use of the institution's registration in lieu of personal registration is contingent on the practitioner being authorized under the law of the jurisdiction to prescribe, dispense, or administer drugs. The institution must also verify the practitioner's status under local law.

The practitioner must be authorized by the institution to use its number to dispense or prescribe, and the practitioner's activities must be within the scope of employment and in the usual course of professional practice.

A current list of the internal suffix codes must be kept by the institution and made available to other registrants and law enforcement agencies upon request for the purpose of verifying authority to prescribe. The list must identify each practitioner with the appropriate individual suffix code.

Labeling

Intrahospital Distribution. Controlled substances, as with all medications, must be properly labeled before distribution within the institution. In this manner, nursing personnel should know what items need identification in charting. In addition to the usual identifying information, the controlled status of such products may be indicated on the label by the use of a symbol or color code.

Outpatient Dispensing. The labeling for all schedules of controlled substances dispensed to outpatients must contain the date of filling, the pharmacy's name and address, the serial number of the prescription, names of patient and prescriber, directions for use, and the statement "Caution: Federal Law prohibits transfer of this drug to any person other than the patient for whom it was prescribed."

Where injectable drugs are used in the home and dosages may change frequently, each department of pharmacy should develop policies and procedures for reprogramming pumps, notifying caregivers of changes, and documenting dosage changes.

Offsite Pharmacy Services. The DEA regulations provide an exception to the labeling requirements in cases where controlled substances are prescribed for administration to an institutionalized patient and dispensed from a separately registered pharmacy serving the institution [21 CFR 1306.14 and 1306.24]. The controlled substance must not be in the possession of the patient, appropriate safeguards and records must be maintained, and the labeling system used must be adequate to identify the supplier, the product, and the patient and to set forth proper directions for use. No more than a 7-day supply of Schedule II controlled substances or, in the case of Schedules III and IV, no more than a 34-day supply or 100 dosage units, whichever is less, may be dispensed at one time under this labeling system.

Automated Systems. An automated distribution system can be used to assist in inventory control of controlled substances, but conformance with state and federal regulations must be ensured.

According to current DEA policy, automated data processing systems may be used to produce a backup record of the original, hard copy prescription. However, the original, hard copy prescription must be maintained even after entry into the computerized system. As such, prescriptions for Schedule II controlled substances could be entered into a computerized system as a backup record; however, the original, hard copy prescription must serve as the primary record of the prescription. The same would apply to a Schedule V controlled substance in states that require a prescription. However, in states that allow the purchase of a Schedule V controlled substance without a prescription, applicable state record-keeping requirements apply.

An automated data processing system may be used for the storage and retrieval of original and refill information for prescription orders for Schedule III and IV controlled substances. The conditions listed below for such a system are most applicable to outpatient prescriptions. A hospital order for medication is not a prescription and, therefore, is not required to meet requirements of that particular format [21 CFR 1306.02(f)]. However, all records must meet the requirements for accountability of the controlled substances dispensed or administered by institutional personnel. Additionally, the hospital records must be maintained in a readily retrievable manner [21 CFR 1304.03]. Automated data processing systems must meet the following requirements:

1. Any such computerized system must provide on-line retrieval (via display or hard copy printout) of original prescription order information. This shall include the original prescription number; date of issuance of the original prescription order by the practitioner; name and address of the patient; name, address, and DEA registration number of the practitioner; name, strength, dosage form, and quantity of the controlled substance prescribed (and quantity dispensed if different from the quantity prescribed); total number of refills authorized by the prescribing practitioner; and name or initials of the dispensing pharmacist. A unique numeric identifier (such as an NDC number) may be used in place of the name, strength, and dosage form. When requested by an authorized official, the information must be provided by name, strength, and dosage form.

2. At the end of each month, a record shall be generated that documents all original prescriptions and refills of Schedule III and IV controlled substances dispensed during that month. This record must segregate the original and refill information for Schedule III and IV controlled substance prescriptions from other prescriptions in the same data system. This record shall include the prescription number, date of issuance, name and address of the patient, name and address and DEA number of the practitioner, initials of the dis-

pensing pharmacist, and name, strength, dosage form, and quantity of the controlled substance prescribed. The quantity dispensed must be listed if different from the quantity prescribed. The monthly printouts must be provided upon request from an authorized official.

3. Accuracy and completeness of the original and refill information entered into an automated system must be verified each time by the individual pharmacist who fills an original prescription or refill order for a Schedule III or IV controlled substance (i.e., a thorough check of the data screen before the actual entry into the database). The system must be designed to protect against unauthorized access to and use of the automated system and associated data and must be able to identify the pharmacist filling the original prescription or refill. Such protection shall be accomplished as follows:

    a. Each authorized pharmacist shall be assigned a unique access code to be entered before each and every original prescription, refill order, or edit of data. The knowledge of assigned access codes and the ability to change, delete, or add them shall be strictly limited to a few individuals (e.g., pharmacy director, manager, or corporate security officer).

    b. Any such computerized system shall have the capability to produce a printout for the current month's original and refill data for Schedule III and IV controlled substance prescriptions. Such a printout must include all of the information required for the monthly printouts. The printout must be produced upon request of an authorized official.

    c. In the event that a pharmacy using such a computerized system experiences system downtime, the pharmacy must have an auxiliary procedure that will be used for documentation of original and refill prescriptions of Schedule III and IV controlled substances.

    d. A backup copy of original prescriptions and refill information must be made daily for that day's transactions. The backup copy can be stored on electronic media in lieu of a printed copy. The copy must be stored on an entirely separate storage medium distinct from the operating medium normally used and must be kept for 2 years after the transaction date.

Security

General. Only personnel authorized by written policies of the institution may have access to medication storage areas and supplies.

Central Storage Areas. Controlled substances in the pharmacy or other central storage areas should be stored in a securely locked, substantially constructed cabinet, vault, closet, or similar enclosure. As an alternative, controlled substances, except Schedule I drugs, may be dispersed throughout the stock of noncontrolled substances in such a manner as to obstruct theft or diversion. Controlled substances of any schedule that require refrigeration should be stored in a refrigerator within the locked storage room where other controlled substances are maintained, or within a lock box that has been secured to the inside of the refrigerator within the nursing station, or in a locked refrigerator in the pharmacy or nursing station.

Other Hospital Areas. *Nursing units.* When controlled substances kept as floor stock are stored on nursing units for extended periods of time, they should be in a securely locked, substantially constructed storage unit.

Carts. Medication carts containing controlled substances should be locked if they are used for storage or left unattended at nursing units.

Surgical, delivery, or special procedure areas. Increased emphasis should be placed on management of wasted narcotics (e.g., unused portions of syringes or ampuls) in these areas because they are frequently sources of higher amounts of diversion. There are a number of solutions for the control and security of controlled substances routinely used in these areas. Security in these areas may include the following:

1. Use the same physical security as at nurses' stations for floor stock and the same beginning and end of shift inventories; use the same type of record of administration as used for floor stock. (Record identifies drug, physician or anesthetist, date, adequate patient identification, notation made in patient chart as to medications received, date, and specific operating room.)

2. Maintain no stocks of controlled substances in the area. Instead, the anesthesiologist or anesthetist should take to the area the assigned stocks for each operation, delivery, or other procedure. The anesthesiologist or anesthetist would maintain the stock and all appropriate records for controlled substances, and the stock would be replenished on an as needed basis.

3. Locate a satellite pharmacy in the immediate area of the operating rooms. This annex could stock supplies that would routinely be necessary for the anesthesiologist or anesthetist. Medication could be signed out to the individual anesthesiologist or anesthetist before each operation or for all procedures scheduled for a given date.

Emergency vehicles and mobile dispensaries. If permitted by state or other applicable law, controlled substances needed for emergency vehicles may be supplied in small quantities as an extension of the hospital if the service is operated by the hospital. If it is a private ambulance service, small quantities may be supplied based on a written agreement with one hospital to supply the medications for the emergency kit. In either of these two instances, the institution is responsible for the controlled substances supplied. Local authorities should be consulted regarding basic and advanced life-support units because regulations may differ.

As an alternative, the emergency vehicle may acquire controlled substances under the registration of a consulting practitioner who must be registered at the central office location of the owner or operator of the emergency service.

The institution must develop recordkeeping and security measures that will minimize diversion potential. When the institution supplies controlled substances to a private service, no more than one kit per vehicle will be supplied; subsequent distributions will be on a replacement basis only.

The SAC may supply written approval of emergency vehicles. A written request outlining scope of operations, proposed security, and recordkeeping is required of the registrant by the SAC. If the request is adequate, written approval will be granted.

Proper state authorization for either method is required; if the operation is disapproved by the state, DEA approval will not be given.

If diversion does occur, the SAC will determine if additional safeguards are needed or if DEA approval is to be withdrawn. In either case, the registrant will be notified in writing.

Home-care setting. When injectable controlled substances are ordered in as needed doses for home-care patients, appropriate storage of large amounts of scheduled drugs in the home should be evaluated. Pharmacies providing injectable drugs to home-care patients should develop a policy on appropriate storage of injectable drugs in the home setting.

Loss or theft. Inventories of controlled substances should be performed regularly. This task is facilitated by the use of a perpetual inventory system; in that case, an audit of all purchase and issue records would identify a shortage. If the inventory shows a shortage of a particular controlled substance, it must be reported to the DEA upon discovery of such theft or loss. The federal regulations require that theft or "significant" losses of controlled substances must be reported to the DEA's Field Division Office. However, the regulations do not specifically define the term "significant." The loss or theft of controlled substances must be reported to the agency on DEA Form 106 (Report of Loss or Theft). Thefts must be reported whether or not the controlled substances are subsequently recovered or the responsible parties are identified and action is taken against them.

Pharmacies should take care not simply to file the forms and neglect procedural changes that may be indicated. Frequent filing of the forms for the same reason (e.g., consistent unexplained losses) could be a signal that actions should be taken to change departmental procedures. These reports should be analyzed and departmental procedures should be modified to attempt to avoid the problems in the future.

Placement of emergency kits containing controlled substances in (unregistered) long-term care facilities. The placement of emergency kits containing controlled substances in nonfederally registered long-term care facilities is in compliance with CSA if the appropriate state agency or regulatory authority specifically approves such placements and promulgates procedures for their use, security, recordkeeping, and accountability. The individual state authorities should be contacted to determine if such procedure is permissible in the state in which the institution is located.

Employee Screening. Registrants must screen employees who have access to controlled substances for any prior convictions or for histories of drug abuse, and employees with knowledge of illicit drug diversion by fellow employees are responsible for reporting the illicit activity to the employer. The registrant shall not employ, as an agent or employee who has access to controlled substances, any person who has been convicted of a felony offense related to controlled substances or who, at any time, had an application for registration with DEA denied, had a DEA registration revoked, or surrendered a DEA registration for cause [21 CFR 1301.76(a)].

Research, Laboratory Procedures, and Instructional Uses

Registration. General. Persons engaged in research, laboratory procedures, or instructional uses with controlled substances are required to register under the CSA and follow laws and regulations in place in their state or locality.

Use of Schedule I drugs. The conduct of research with controlled substances listed in Schedule I requires separate registration. Institutional registrations do not suffice.

Separate locations. If research or related activities are conducted with controlled substances in more than one principal place of business or professional practice at one general physical location, a separate registration is required for each principal place of business or professional practice.

Records and Reports. General requirement. Each person registered or authorized to conduct research or related activities with controlled substances is required to keep records. A registered person using a controlled substance in preclinical research or in teaching at a registered establishment does not have to maintain separate records if the establishment maintains records. The registered person must notify DEA of the name, address, and registration number of the establishment maintaining the records. Notice to DEA should be given in the form of an attachment to the application for registration or reregistration.

Inventory. The inventory requirements of a person registered to dispense or authorized to conduct research or related activities with controlled substances shall include the same information required for the inventories of dispensers (see Records and Inventory section).

Receipt and dispensing. Receipt and dispensing records must be kept by the registrant. If the registrant is a hospital, the required records should be kept by the pharmacist in the same manner as records for other controlled substances (see Records and Inventory section). It should be noted that records for substances used in chemical analysis or other laboratory work are not required. However, records must be maintained for controlled substances transferred to the laboratory and those distributed or destroyed by the laboratory.

Research. When research is conducted on human subjects, informed consent forms signed by the patients are required and must be retained in the patients' records.

Security. In a registered institution, the pharmacist should be the custodian of all controlled substances. Controlled substances may be dispensed only to or for authorized investigators, laboratory personnel, or instructors. The pharmacist should be responsible for the security of controlled substances used in research and related activities.

Methadone

Methadone for Analgesic Purposes. The allowances under DEA regulations for a registered hospital or clinic to use methadone for analgesic purposes are stated in CFR Section 1306.07, Parts (b) and (c). Section 1306.07(b) addresses physicians who are not specifically registered and allows them to administer (but not prescribe) narcotic drugs to a person for the purpose of relieving acute withdrawal symptoms when necessary while arrangements are being made for referral for treatment. Such emergency treatment may not be carried out for longer than 3 days and may not be renewed or extended.

Section 1306.07(c) notes that these regulations are not intended to impose any limitations on a physician or authorized hospital staff to administer or dispense narcotic drugs in a hospital or to maintain or detoxify a person as an adjunct to medical or surgical treatment of conditions other than addiction, or to administer or dispense narcotic drugs to persons with intractable pain in which no relief or cure is possible or none has been found after reasonable efforts.

Methadone for Narcotic Treatment Programs: Registration and Approval. General. The use of methadone in an institution for maintenance or detoxification of narcotic addicts is controlled jointly under FDA and DEA regulations. The FDA methadone regulations [21 CFR 291.501 and 291.505] provide for approved uses of methadone in institutions, medication units, and methadone treatment programs. If an institution desires to establish a methadone treatment program for detoxification and maintenance of drug-dependent persons, separate approval is required. In any case, the institution must be separately registered with DEA as a narcotic treatment program to dispense Schedule II controlled substances in addition to receiving approval under the FDA methadone regulations. Programs must submit to DEA an application for registration as a narcotic treatment program, using DEA Form 363.

Hospital use of methadone in a narcotic treatment program. The hospital shall submit to FDA and the appropriate state authority a general description of the hospital, including number of beds, specialized treatment facilities for drug dependence, and nature of patient care undertaken. The hospital shall permit FDA and the state authority to inspect supplies of these drugs at the hospital and evaluate the uses to which the drug is being put. For a hospital pharmacy lawfully to receive or dispense methadone for its approved hospital use for detoxification, the hospital must submit Form FDA-2636, Hospital Request for Methadone for Detoxification and Temporary Maintenance Treatment. The application must be approved by the responsible state authority and FDA. The form requires detailed information about the hospital, including the name of the pharmacist responsible for receiving and securing supplies of methadone.

In addition to requirements that hospitals have separate DEA registrations for narcotic treatment programs, the programs must maintain separate inventories, appropriate DEA forms, and patient records.

Program approval. Before a narcotic treatment program may be lawfully operated, the program, whether an inpatient facility, an outpatient facility, or a private practitioner, must submit the appropriate applications to FDA and the state authority and must receive the approval of both. At the time of the application for approval, the program sponsor shall indicate whether medication will be administered or dispensed at the facility.

Medication unit. A program may establish a medication unit to facilitate the needs of patients who are stabilized on an optimal dosage level. To operate a medication unit lawfully, the program shall, for each separate unit, obtain approval from FDA, DEA, and the state authority. A medication unit is limited to administering or dispensing a narcotic drug and collecting samples for drug testing or analysis for narcotic drugs.

Description of facilities. A program must have ready access to a comprehensive range of medical and rehabilitation services so that the services may be provided when necessary. The name, address, and description of each hospital, institution, clinical laboratory, or other facility available to provide the necessary services must be provided in the application submitted to FDA and the state authority. The application is also required to include the name and address of each medication unit.

Methadone treatment programs. To obtain approval to establish a methadone treatment program, the sponsor must submit Form FDA-2632, Application for Approval of Use of Methadone in a Treatment Program. The application must receive the approval of the responsible state authority and FDA with the concurrence of DEA. To ensure that each participating physician in a methadone treatment program is aware of his or her professional and administrative responsibilities, FDA requires that Form FDA-2633, Medical Responsibility Statement for Use of Methadone in a Treatment Program, be completed by each physician licensed to dispense or administer methadone in an approved program. These statements must accompany the program application. All patients in the program are required to give their consent for treatment by signing Form FDA-2635, Consent for Methadone Treatment.

Dispensing. *Authorized dispensers.* Only a licensed practitioner or an agent of the practitioner may administer or dispense methadone. The agent must be a pharmacist, registered nurse, licensed practical nurse, or other health-care professional authorized by federal and state law to administer or dispense narcotic drugs. The licensed practitioner assumes responsibility for the amounts of methadone administered or dispensed, and the licensed practitioner shall record and countersign all changes in dosage schedule.

Form. Methadone may be dispensed or administered only in an oral liquid formulation when it is used in a treatment program. Hospitalized patients under care for a medical or surgical condition are permitted to receive methadone in injectable form when the physician determines that it is needed.

Take-home medications. There are stringent requirements establishing the frequency and quantity of methadone permitted for take-home use. Take-home medication is required to be labeled with the treatment center's name, address, and telephone number. It is recommended that the liquid formulation of methadone be nonsweetened and contain a preservative so that the program staff may instruct patients not to refrigerate the product to minimize accidental ingestion by children and others or fermentation of the product.

Records and Reports. *Hospital use of methadone.* All records must be kept in compliance with the DEA requirements for Schedule I and II controlled substances. Hospitals must also maintain accurate records traceable to specific patients, and they must include dates, quantity, and batch or code marks of the drug dispensed. Methadone records must be retained for a 3-year period instead of the 2-year period required for other controlled substances. The hospital does not have to submit a detailed annual report.

Methadone treatment programs. All records must be kept in compliance with the DEA requirement for Schedule I and II controlled substances. The FDA methadone regulations require also that there be accurate records traceable to specific patients, and they must include dates, quantity, and batch or code marks of the drug dispensed. Methadone records must be retained for 3 years. The methadone treatment program is required to file an annual report with the responsible state authority and FDA. The content of the annual report is detailed in Form FDA-2634, Annual Report for Treatment Program Using Methadone.

Security. The regulations note that adequate security is required over stocks of methadone and over the manner in which it is (1) administered or dispensed, (2) distributed to medication units, and (3) stored to guard against theft and diversion of the drug. The methadone program is required to meet the security standards for the distribution and storage of controlled substances as required by DEA.

Approved by the ASHP Board of Directors, November 18, 1992. Developed by the ASHP Council on Legal and Public Affairs. Supersedes the "ASHP Technical Assistance Bulletin on Institutional Use of Controlled Substances," which was approved on November 19, 1986.

This Technical Assistance Bulletin was developed in collaboration with the staff of the Liaison and Policy Section of the Office of Diversion Control of the Drug Enforcement Administration (DEA). It is an interpretation of the Controlled Substances Act and Title 21, *Code of Federal Regulations*, for use in health-care settings and is not official DEA policy.

The bibliographic citation for this document is as follows: American Society of Hospital Pharmacists. ASHP technical assistance bulletin on use of controlled substances in organized health-care settings. *Am J Hosp Pharm.* 1993; 50:489–501.

ASHP Technical Assistance Bulletin on Repackaging Oral Solids and Liquids in Single Unit and Unit Dose Packages

To maximize the benefits of a unit dose drug distribution system, all drugs must be packaged in single unit or unit dose packages.[a] However, not all drugs are commercially available in single unit (or unit dose) packages. Therefore, the institutional pharmacist must often repackage drugs obtained in bulk containers (e.g., bottles of 500 tablets) into single unit packages so that they may be used in a unit dose system.

Certain precautions must be taken if the quality of drugs repackaged by the pharmacist is to be maintained. The guidelines presented herein will assist the pharmacist in developing procedures for repackaging drugs in a safe and acceptable manner:

1. The packaging operation should be isolated, to the extent possible, from other pharmacy activities.

2. Only one drug product at a time should be repackaged in a specific work area. No drug products other than the one being repackaged should be present in the immediate packaging area. Also, no labels other than those for the product being repackaged should be present in the area.

3. Upon completion of the packaging run, all unused stocks of drugs and all finished packages should be removed from the packaging area. The packaging machinery and related equipment should then be completely emptied, cleaned, and inspected before commencing the next packaging operation.

4. All unused labels (if separate labels are used) should be removed from the immediate packaging area. The operator should verify that none remains in the packaging machine(s). If labels are prepared as part of the packaging operation, the label plate (or analogous part of the printing apparatus) should be removed or adjusted to "blank" upon completion of the run. This will help assure that the correct label is printed during any subsequent run. There should be a procedure to reconcile the number of packages produced with the number of labels used (if any) and destroyed (if any) and the number of units or volume of drug set forth to be packaged.

5. Before beginning a packaging run, an organoleptic evaluation (color, odor, appearance, and markings) of the drug product being repackaged should be made. The bulk container should also be examined for evidence of water damage, contamination, or other deleterious effects.

6. All packaging equipment and systems should be operated and used in accordance with the manufacturer's or other established instructions. There should be valid justification and authorization by the supervisor for any deviation from those instructions on the part of the operator.

7. The pharmacist should obtain data on the characteristics of all packaging materials used. This information should include data on the chemical composition, light transmission, moisture permeability, size, thickness (alone or in laminate), recommended sealing temperature, and storage requirements.

8. Unit dose packages and labels should, to the extent possible, comply with the "ASHP Guidelines for Single Unit and Unit Dose Packages of Drugs."[1]

9. Whenever feasible, a responsible individual, other than the packaging operator, should verify that (a) the packaging system (drug, materials, and machines) is set up correctly and (b) all procedures have been performed properly. Ultimate responsibility for all packaging operations rests with the pharmacist.

10. Control records of all packaging runs must be kept. These records should include the following information: (1) complete description of the product, i.e., name, strength, dosage form, route of administration, etc.; (2) the product's manufacturer or supplier; (3) control number; (4) the pharmacy's control number if different from the manufacturer's; (5) expiration dates of the original container and the repackaged product; (6) number of units packaged and the date(s) they were packaged; (7) initials of the operator and checker (if any); (8) a sample of the label and, if feasible, a sample of the finished package, which should not be discarded until after the expiration date and which should be examined periodically for signs of deterioration; and (9) description (including lot number) of the packaging materials and equipment used.

11. It is the responsibility of the pharmacist to determine the expiration date to be placed on the package, taking into account the nature of the drug repackaged, the characteristics of the package, and the storage conditions to which the drug may be subjected. This date must not be beyond that of the original package.[b]

12. All drugs should be packaged and stored in a temperature- and humidity-controlled environment to minimize degradation caused by heat and moisture. A relative humidity of 75% at 23°C should not be exceeded. Packaging materials should be stored in accordance with the manufacturer's instructions and any applicable regulations.

13. Written procedures (both general and product specific) governing repackaging operations should be prepared and updated as required. Any deviation from these procedures should be noted and explained on the control record. Operators must understand the procedures (and operation of all packaging equipment) before commencing the run.

14. Applicable FDA and USP requirements concerning the type of package required for specific drug products must be followed.

15. Drugs and chemicals with high vapor pressures should be stored separately from other products to minimize cross contamination.

References

1. American Society of Hospital Pharmacists. ASHP

guidelines for single unit and unit dose packages of drugs. *Am J Hosp Pharm.* 1977; 34:613–4.
2. Stolar MH. Expiration dates of repackaged drug products. *Am J Hosp Pharm.* 1979; 36:170. Editorial.

---

[a]A *single unit* package is one which contains one discrete pharmaceutical dosage form, e.g., one tablet or one 5-ml volume of liquid. A *unit dose* package is one which contains the particular dose of drug ordered for the patient. A *single unit* package is a *unit dose (or single dose)* package if it contains that particular dose of drug ordered for the patient.
[b]For specific recommendations on expiration date policy, see Reference 2.

Revised by the ASHP Board of Directors, November 16–17, 1978.

Developed originally by a joint working group of the American Society of Hospital Pharmacists and the American Society of Consultant Pharmacists and representatives of the drug packaging industry. The original document subsequently was approved officially by the Boards of Directors of ASHP and ASCP. FDA reviewed the original document and commended ASHP and ASCP for developing the guidelines.

The bibliographic citation for this document is as follows: American Society of Hospital Pharmacists. ASHP technical assistance bulletin on repackaging oral solids and liquids in single unit and unit dose packages. *Am J Hosp Pharm.* 1983; 40:451–2.

ASHP Technical Assistance Bulletin on Drug Formularies

The formulary system is an ongoing process whereby an organization's pharmacy and medical staffs, working through a pharmacy and therapeutics (P&T) committee (or its equivalent), evaluate and select from among the drug products available those considered to be most useful in patient care. These products then are routinely available for use within the organization. The formulary system is a powerful tool for improving the quality and controlling the cost of drug therapy, and its use is strongly encouraged.

Formulary systems are applicable in any health-care setting including inpatient facilities, ambulatory care, and managed care organizations. Central to the operation of the formulary system is the formulary, a continually revised compilation of selected drug products plus important ancillary information about the use of the drugs and relevant organizational policies and procedures.

Since the formulary is the vehicle by which the medical staff and others make use of the formulary system, it is important that it be complete, concise, and easy to use. These guidelines are offered as an aid to pharmacists preparing a formulary or improving an existing one. They do not deal with the specific drug products that might be included in a formulary or with the selection process but, rather, with the formulary's format, organization, and content.

This document is complementary to the "ASHP Statement on the Formulary System,"[1] which should be consulted for further information on the formulary system.

Formulary Content and Organization

The primary objectives of the formulary are to provide (1) information on the drug products[a] approved for use, (2) basic therapeutic information about each item, (3) information on organizational policies and procedures governing the use of drugs, and (4) special information about drugs such as dosing guidelines and nomograms, abbreviations approved for prescribing, and sodium content of various formulary items. In accordance with these objectives, the formulary should consist of three main parts:

1. Information on organizational policies and procedures concerning drugs.
2. Drug products list.
3. Special information.

A more detailed look at each section follows.

Information on Organizational Policies and Procedures Concerning Drugs. Material to be included in this section will vary from organization to organization. Generally, the following items may be included:

1. Formulary policies and procedures, including such items as restrictions on drug use (if any) and procedures for requesting that a drug be added to the formulary.
2. Brief description of the P&T committee, including its membership, responsibilities, and operation.
3. Organizational regulations governing the prescribing, dispensing, and administration of drugs, including the

writing of drug orders and prescriptions, approved abbreviations for prescribing drugs, controlled substances considerations, generic and therapeutic equivalency policies and procedures, automatic stop orders, verbal drug orders, investigational drug policies, patients' use of their own medications, self-administration of drugs by patients, use of drug samples, policies relative to "stat" and "emergency" drug orders, use of emergency carts and kits, use of floor stock items, use of drug administration devices, prescribing by staff of medications for their own use, rules to be followed by drug manufacturers' representatives, standard drug administration times, and the reporting of adverse drug reactions and medication errors. Other topics should be included as deemed appropriate.

4. Pharmacy operating procedures such as hours of service, prescription policies, pharmacy charging policies, prescription labeling and packaging practices, drug distribution procedures, handling of drug information requests, and other services of the pharmacy (e.g., patient education programs and pharmacy bulletins).
5. Information on using the formulary, including how the formulary entries are arranged, the information contained in each entry, and the procedure for looking up a given drug product. Reference to sources of detailed information on formulary drugs [e.g., *AHFS Drug Information (AHFS-DI)* or the pharmacy's drug information service] should be included.

Drug Products List. This section is the heart of the formulary and consists of one or more descriptive entries for each drug item plus one or more indexes to facilitate use of the formulary.

Drug item entries. The entries can be arranged in several ways: (1) alphabetically by generic name, with entries for synonyms and brand names containing only a "see (generic name)" notation; (2) alphabetically within therapeutic class, usually following the *AHFS-DI* classification scheme; (3) a combination of the two systems whereby the bulk of the drugs are contained (alphabetically) in a "general" section that is supplemented by several "special" sections such as ophthalmic and otic drugs, dermatologicals, and diagnostic agents.

The type of information to be included in each entry will vary. At a minimum, each entry must include the following:

1. Generic name of the primary active drug entity or product; combination products may be listed by generic, common, or trade names.
2. Common synonym(s) and brand name(s); there should be a note in the "directions for use" section of the formulary explaining that inclusion or omission of a given brand name does not imply that it is or is not stocked by the pharmacy.
3. Dosage form(s), strength(s), packaging(s), and size(s) stocked by the pharmacy.
4. Formulation (active ingredients) of a combination product.

5. *AHFS-DI* category number.

Additional information that may be part of the drug entries includes

1. Usual adult or pediatric dosage ranges, or both.
2. Special cautions and notes such as "do not administer intravenously" or "refrigerate."
3. Controlled substances class (schedule).
4. Cost information; this information generally will be most useful where a therapeutic classification system is used or, alternatively, lists of similar drugs can be presented showing relative cost data.

Indexes to the drug products list. Two indexes will facilitate the use of the formulary:

1. Generic name–brand name/synonym cross index. The proper page number reference should be included in each entry. An example of this type of index is:

   Ophthaine: brand of proparacaine HCl, p 114
   Ophthetic: brand of proparacaine HCl, p 114
   Opium tincture, camphorated; synonym for paregoric, p 103
   Paregoric: p 103
   Proparacaine HCl: p 114

   This index can be integrated into the drug products list rather than being a separate entity. The list, in this event, must be arranged alphabetically.
2. Therapeutic/pharmacologic index. This index lists all formulary items within each therapeutic category. It is useful for ascertaining what therapeutic alternatives exist for a given situation such as patient allergy to a particular drug. An example of this type of index, beginning with the *AHFS-DI* classification code, is:

4:00	Antihistamine drugs
	Brompheniramine maleate, p 14
	Chlorpheniramine maleate, p 14
	Diphenhydramine HCl, p 14
	Promethazine HCl, p 20
8:00	Anti-infective agents
8:04	Amebicides
	Emetine HCl, p 33
	Iodoquinol, p 22

Special Information. The material to be included in this section will vary from organization to organization. However, what is included should be of general interest to the professional staff. Typically, it contains information not readily available from other sources. Examples of the type of items often found in the special information section are

1. Nutritional products list.
2. Tables of equivalent dosages of similar drugs (e.g., corticosteroids).
3. Standard parenteral nutrition formulas.
4. Guidelines for calculating pediatric dosages.
5. Table of the sodium content of drug products.
6. List of sugar-free drug products.
7. List of items (e.g., moisturizing lotion and toothpaste) typically supplied to all new inpatients.
8. Contents of emergency carts.
9. Lists of dialyzable drugs.
10. Pharmacokinetic dosing and monitoring information.
11. Metric conversion tables.
12. Examples of blank or completed organizational forms such as prescription blanks, requests for nonformulary drugs, and adverse drug reaction report forms.
13. Tables of drug interactions, drug interferences with diagnostic tests, and injectable drug incompatibilities.
14. Poison control information, including telephone numbers of poison control centers.
15. Dosages, concentrations, and standard dilutions of common emergency drugs.
16. Standard vehicles and dilutions for pediatric injections.
17. Electrolyte content of large-volume parenterals.

Format and Appearance of the Formulary

The physical appearance and structure of a printed formulary have an important influence on its use. Although elaborate and expensive artwork and materials are unnecessary, the formulary should be visually pleasing, easily readable, and professional in appearance. The need for proper grammar, correct spelling and punctuation, and neatness is obvious.

There is no single format or arrangement that all formularies must follow. A typical formulary might have the following composition:

1. Title page.
2. Table of contents.
3. Information on policies and procedures concerning drugs.
   a. Disciplines and specialties represented on the P&T committee.
   b. Objectives and operation of the formulary system.
   c. Regulations and procedures for prescribing and dispensing drugs.
   d. Pharmacy services and procedures.
   e. Instructions on use of the formulary.
4. Products accepted for use in the organization.
   a. Items added and deleted since the previous edition.
   b. Generic–brand name cross-reference list.
   c. Pharmacologic/therapeutic index with relative cost codes.
   d. Descriptions of drug products by pharmacologic/therapeutic class.
5. Appendix.
   a. Guidelines for calculating pediatric doses.
   b. Nomograms (e.g., for estimating body surface area).
   c. Schedule of standard drug administration times.

Several techniques can be used to improve the appearance and ease of use of the formulary such as

1. Using a different color paper for each section of the formulary.
2. Using an edge index.
3. Making the formulary pocket size.
4. Printing the generic name heading of each drug entry in boldface type or using some other method for making it stand out from the rest of the entry.

Distribution of the Formulary

When printed formularies are used, copies should be placed at each patient care location, including clinics, other outpatient care areas, and emergency rooms. Each pharmacist and division of the pharmacy should receive a copy. Heads of departments providing direct patient care should receive a copy, as should hospital administration. Each member of the medical staff should receive a copy. Enough copies should be printed to allow for replacement of lost or worn copies. An alternative to a printed formulary is an online formulary accessible by computer terminals.

Necessary steps should be taken to ensure that the nursing and medical staffs are familiar with the formulary and know how to use it.

Keeping the Formulary Current

Generally, the formulary will need to be revised annually. Additions and deletions to the formulary, changes in drug products, removal of drugs from the market, and changes in hospital policies and procedures all will necessitate periodic revision of the formulary.

There should be a system for including "between revision" changes in the current edition of the formulary. One method is to attach formulary supplement sheets inside the covers of the formulary books. Lists of changes can also be distributed to the medical staff. Newsletters to the medical staff may be useful as vehicles for transmitting the information. Changes to online, computer-accessible formularies can be made as they occur.

Using a different color for the cover of each printed edition of the formulary will help reduce confusion between current and past editions.

Reference

1.   American Society of Hospital Pharmacists. ASHP statement on the formulary system. *Am J Hosp Pharm.* 1983; 40:1384–5.

---

[a]"Drug product" refers to a specific drug entity/dosage form/strength/packaging/package size combination. Only certain dosage forms or strengths, for example, of a given drug entity might be included in a formulary.

Approved by the ASHP Board of Directors, November 14, 1990. Revised by the ASHP Council on Professional Affairs. Supersedes previous versions approved November 15, 1977, and November 14–15, 1984.

The bibliographic citation for this document is as follows: American Society of Hospital Pharmacists. ASHP technical assistance bulletin on drug formularies. *Am J Hosp Pharm.* 1991; 48:791–3.

ASHP Technical Assistance Bulletin on Outcome Competencies and Training Guidelines for Institutional Pharmacy Technician Training Programs

Preamble

Definitions. The term "supportive personnel" has been recommended as standard nomenclature to be used in referring collectively to all nonprofessional hospital pharmacy personnel. This document describes the training outcome competencies for those supportive personnel designated "pharmacy technicians." A technician may be defined as a person skilled in the technique of a particular art (technique being the mechanical ability required to perform an activity).

For purposes of this document, a pharmacy technician shall be defined as someone who, under the supervision of a licensed pharmacist, assists in the various activities of the pharmacy department not requiring the professional judgment of the pharmacist. Such duties include, but need not be limited to: maintaining patient records; setting up, packaging, and labeling medication doses; filling and dispensing routine orders for stock supplies of patient-care areas; maintaining inventories of drug supplies; and mixing drugs with parenteral fluids. Technicians function in strict accordance with standard, written procedures and guidelines, any deviation from which must be approved by the supervising pharmacist.

Supportive personnel primarily engaged in duties not associated with the techniques of preparing and dispensing medications (e.g., secretaries, clerks, typists, and delivery personnel) are not considered "pharmacy technicians" and their competencies are not covered in this document. Likewise, competencies of supportive personnel who administer medication ("medication technicians") are also excluded. This document addresses the training of a "generalist" technician, one who can function appropriately in most hospitals, both small and large, in the kinds of activities for which there is generally the greatest need for supportive personnel manpower.

Application of the Outcome Competencies. The competencies described in this document are representative ones, and no attempt has been made to develop an exhaustive listing. It is believed that any technician who can demonstrate attainment of these competencies should be able to perform satisfactorily in any organized health-care setting after a reasonable period of orientation. It is not expected, however, that all institutional pharmacy technicians will, in fact, possess these competencies.

The competencies are described in behavioral terms; thus, it should be possible to evaluate the trainee's attainment of each competency in the manner described in each statement. In some instances, this can be by paper and pencil tests; in other instances, it can be by oral statement; and in yet other cases, it can be by actually performing the activity or function under the observation of the evaluator. In the latter instances, it is extremely important that the evaluator judges the trainee's performance strictly on the basis of the objectives previously established for the respective training activity relating to the competency.

Omitted from most of the competency statements are references to time or error limits. Obviously, they must be taken into account in the evaluation process. It is suggested that reasonable time and error limits be imposed where indicated, based on the evaluator's experience.

The training guidelines following the list of competencies for each objective statement consist of suggested topics to be covered in the didactic portion of the training program. Again, these are not exhaustive lists; every training institution is expected to add or delete topics as it deems necessary.

The training guidelines do not include training activities necessary for the development of manipulative skills. These are clearly implied in the statements listed under the competencies for each of the 11 objectives.

The qualifications of applicants to be admitted to the training program are discussed in Appendix A. Suggestions for the training program format are given in Appendix B.

Objective I

The technician should demonstrate appropriate knowledge and understanding of the health-care institution and its pharmacy department.

Competencies. The technician should be able to

1. Interpret the institution's organizational chart in terms of the name and title of the administrative person to whom the director of pharmacy reports and the administrative and professional relationship of the pharmacy department to any other departments in the institution.
2. Describe the general responsibilities and job status of personnel in other institutional departments with whom the technician will have contact in carrying out assigned duties and activities.
3. Interpret the organizational chart for the pharmacy department in terms of names and general responsibilities of all departmental supervisory and administrative personnel.
4. Describe the location of the major hospital departments and service units, and escort another person to any department or unit.
5. State at least three reasons why information about patients must be kept confidential.
6. State at least five reasons for initiation of a disciplinary action in the institution (e.g., absenteeism, incompetency, and dishonesty).

Training Guidelines. Suggested topics include

1. Organization, functions, and responsibilities of the hospital.
2. Organization, functions, and responsibilities of the pharmacy.
3. Hospital and departmental policies and procedures.

Objective II

The technician should demonstrate a thorough knowledge and understanding of the duties and responsibilities of his/her position, including standards of ethics governing pharmacy practice.

Competencies. The technician should be able to

1. State all of the technician's primary job responsibilities, the duties falling under each, and how they differ from the primary responsibilities of the pharmacist.
2. State the institutional and departmental policies applicable to each of the primary job responsibilities, and describe the procedures for each.
3. Define what is meant by "a decision requiring a pharmacist's judgment," and cite at least 10 examples.
4. Demonstrate the use of correct telephone communication technique and protocol, both in receiving and in initiating calls.
5. Demonstrate the use of correct written communication by drafting a memorandum to the supervisor requesting a change in work assignment schedule to take care of personal business.
6. State the general requirements of any local, state, or federal laws that specifically affect any of the technician's responsibilities.

Training Guidelines. Suggested topics include

1. Orientation to technician duties (job description).
2. Relationship of technicians to pharmacists, hospital staff, and patients.
3. Communication principles and techniques.
4. Legal aspects of technician functions such as:
   a. Accountability.
   b. Pharmacy regulations.
   c. Use and storage of controlled substances.

Objective III

The technician should have a working knowledge of the pharmaceutical–medical terms, abbreviations, and symbols commonly used in the prescribing, dispensing, and charting of medications in the institution.

Competencies. The technician should be able to

1. Transcribe without error any 12 inpatient medication orders selected at random from at least four different patient units in the institution.
2. Define in lay terms the meaning of names of all clinical, diagnostic, and treatment units and services in the institution.

Training Guidelines. Suggested topics include

1. Pharmaceutical–medical terminology.
2. Pharmaceutical–medical abbreviations and symbols.
3. Drug classification systems and drug nomenclature.

Objective IV

The technician should have a working knowledge of the general chemical and physical properties of all drugs handled in manufacturing and packaging operations in the pharmacy department.

Competencies. The technician should be able to

1. Designate from a list of 50 drug names those that are light sensitive and those that must be refrigerated.
2. State what precautions and procedures must be used in handling caustic, poisonous, and flammable substances.
3. List the titles of at least four reference books where stability information on drug compounds can be found.

Training Guidelines. Suggested topics include

1. Pharmaceutical solutes, solvents, and basic solution theory.
2. Basic principles of stability (effects of heat, cold, light, and moisture on drugs and chemicals).
3. Storage requirements for drugs and chemicals.
4. Safety considerations regarding:
   a. Toxic and caustic substances.
   b. Flammable chemicals and drugs.
   c. Operating pharmacy equipment.
   d. Control of microbiological contamination.
   e. Cleaning and housekeeping.
   f. Control records.

Objective V

The technician should demonstrate an ability to carry out the calculations required for the usual dosage determinations and solutions preparation, using weight and volume equivalents in both the metric and apothecary systems.

Competencies. The technician should be able to

1. List without error the metric equivalents for the apothecary doses and for household doses written in 12 randomly selected medication orders.
2. Convert without error all metric or apothecary weights and volumes to the other system in at least four manufacturing formulas.
3. Perform the calculations necessary to prepare weight-in-volume and volume-in-volume solutions.

Training Guidelines. Suggested topics include

1. Weights and measures (apothecary and metric systems, household measures, potency units and strengths, equivalents, and conversions).
2. Review of fractions, decimals, ratios, and percentages.
3. Dosage calculations and preparation of solutions.

Objective VI

The technician should demonstrate the ability to perform the essential functions relating to drug purchasing and inventory control.

Competencies. The technician should be able to

1. Prepare a written report of a physical inventory of a representative stock of pharmacy drugs and supplies using prepared forms and records.
2. Determine from existing reorder levels which invento-

ried items should be ordered and in what quantity.

3. Demonstrate an ability to check in a drug shipment by using the packing list or invoice and purchase order, completing the receiving report, and adding the items to the inventory.

4. Demonstrate the ability to retrieve from the drug storeroom at least 10 randomly designated drug items.

5. Describe the procedure for returning outdated drugs to the manufacturer.

Training Guidelines. Suggested topics include

1. Inventory and purchasing procedures and records.
2. Maintaining controlled substances records.
3. Inspection of nursing unit drug supplies.
4. Use of computer terminals.

Objective VII

The technician should demonstrate a working knowledge of drug dosages, routes of administration, and dosage forms.

Competencies. The technician should be able to

1. List at least:
   a. Six routes of drug administration.
   b. Ten dosage forms of drugs and their respective routes.
2. State the lumen size, length, and primary use for each of five different needles.
3. Identify, by name and use, each of five different syringes.

Training Guidelines. Suggested topics include

1. Sources of drugs.
2. Rationales for drug use (preventive, curative and restorative, and limiting disease processes).
3. Dose–response relationships.
4. Absorption, biotransformation, and excretion of drugs.
5. Risk–benefit ratios.
6. Patient variables and drug therapy (age, weight, pathological conditions, and genetic factors).
7. Local administration (to skin and mucuous membranes, to ears and eyes, and irrigations).
8. Systemic administration (oral, sublingual–buccal, inhalation, rectal, and parenteral).
9. Dosage forms (tablets, capsules, solutions, suspensions, ointments, suppositories, powders, and injectables).

Objective VIII

The technician should have a working knowledge of the procedures and operations relating to the manufacturing, packaging, and labeling of drug products.

Competencies. The technician should be able to

1. Repackage and label 25 unit doses from a bulk supply of drugs and correctly complete all necessary control records.
2. Demonstrate for each of five randomly selected formulation and packaging requests:
   a. Correct selection of necessary equipment.

b. Proper assembly and use of the equipment.
c. Proper cleaning and storing of the equipment.
d. Proper selection of each ingredient.
e. Accurate calculation and measurement of each ingredient.
f. Proper completion of worksheet record of weights and volumes, manufacturers' lot numbers, and other required information.
g. Correct procedure for mixing and preparing product.
h. Proper selection and preparation of packages/containers and closures.
i. Proper packaging technique.
j. Correct selection and preparation of labels.
k. Proper quarantine procedure.

3. Identify from a list of 10 different steps in manufacturing and packaging operations those functions that must be performed by a pharmacist only.

Training Guidelines. Suggested topics include

1. Measurements of quantity (weights, volumes, and numbers).
2. Use, assembly, and maintenance of equipment and apparatus.
3. Control and recordkeeping procedures (formula mastersheets, worksheets and batch records, labeling and label control, quarantine, and product testing and monitoring).
4. Packaging considerations (drug containers and closures).
5. Storage and inventory control.
6. Lot numbers and expiration dates and times.
7. Types of drug packages and containers (multiple dose, single dose, treatment size, large-volume parenteral containers, small-volume parenteral containers, aerosols and sprays, tubes, droppers, etc.).
8. Labeling of drug containers and packages.

Objective IX

The technician should have a working knowledge of the procedures and techniques relating to aseptic compounding and parenteral admixture operations.

Competencies. The technician should be able to

1. List five different possibilities for contamination of an injectable solution during its preparation and for each possibility a precaution that would prevent the contamination.

2. Demonstrate the proper technique for using a syringe and needle for aseptic withdrawal of the contents of:
   a. A rubber-capped vial.
   b. A glass ampul.

3. Demonstrate the proper technique for aseptic reconstitution of an antibiotic injection.

4. Describe the occasions when hand washing is required, and demonstrate the proper technique.

5. Demonstrate the correct techniques and procedures for preparing at least three parenteral admixtures, including the proper preparation of the label and completion of the control records.

6. Identify the major components of a laminar-flow hood, and state their functions.

7. Define or describe:
   a. Microbial growth and transmission.
   b. Origin, pharmacologic effect, and prevention of pyrogens.
   c. Sterility.
   d. Heat sterilization.
   e. "Cold" sterilization.
8. Designate from a list of 10 different sterile preparations those that may be safely heat sterilized.
9. Demonstrate the proper technique for visual inspection of parenteral solutions.

Training Guidelines. Suggested topics include

1. Parenteral routes of administration (rationale, precautions, and problems; routes; and methods of parenteral administration).
2. Equipment and systems used in parenteral administration (needles and syringes, administration sets, fluid containers, filters, and pumps).
3. Equipment used to prepare parenteral admixtures (laminar-flow hoods, filters, pumps and vacuum sets, drug additive systems and packages, Cornwall pipetters, etc.).
4. Aseptic compounding techniques (specific to the fluid system in use and including the prefilling of syringes, preparing ophthalmic solutions, etc.).
5. Labeling and recordkeeping (bottle labels, fluid orders and profiles, and compounding records).
6. Incompatibilities (visual and chemical incompatibilities, pH and concentration effects, and reference sources).
7. Quality control (particulate matter inspection and monitoring of contamination).

Objective X

The technician should demonstrate the ability to perform the usual technician functions associated with an institutional drug distribution system.

Competencies. The technician should be able to

1. Prepare the drug profile for five newly admitted patients.
2. Pick all doses for one patient unit, and complete the necessary dispensing records.
3. Describe the special dispensing and recordkeeping procedures that apply to the dispensing of:
   a. Controlled drugs.
   b. Investigational drugs.
   c. Nonformulary drugs.
4. List for each of 30 commonly prescribed trade name drugs:
   a. The generic name.
   b. The usual dose.

Training Guidelines. Suggested topics include

1. Physicians' order sheets and patient medication profiles.
2. Setting up doses for patients.
3. Checking doses.
4. Delivery and exchange of medications.

Objective XI

The technician should demonstrate the ability to perform manipulative and recordkeeping functions associated with the dispensing of prescriptions for ambulatory patients.

Competencies. The technician should be able to

1. Carry out the following functions for any 10 randomly selected ambulatory patient prescriptions:
   a. Correctly type the label.
   b. Select the proper drug from the dispensing stock.
   c. Accurately count or measure the product, and place it in the proper container.
   d. Complete the necessary records and documents.
   e. Calculate the charge for the prescription.
2. Describe the special procedures and documentation required in dispensing ambulatory patient prescriptions for
   a. Controlled drugs.
   b. Investigational drugs.
   c. Nonprescription drugs.
3. Designate from a list of 10 steps involved in ambulatory patient prescription dispensing those functions that only a pharmacist may carry out.

Training Guidelines. Suggested topics include

1. Prescriptions and patient profiles.
2. Preparing prescription labels.
3. Counting and measuring drugs.

Appendix A: Qualifications for Training Program Applicants

Applicants to the technician training program should have certain demonstrated abilities as evidenced by successful completion of relevant high school courses or other appropriate educational programs or by acceptable grades on a written entrance examination. These abilities and knowledge include general basic chemistry, arithmetic, basic algebra, reading, and writing. Other requirements are adequate command of the English language; ability to acquire skill in the use of pharmaceutical apparatus, instruments, and equipment; ability to work with sustained attention and care on routine repetitive tasks; ability to follow oral and written instructions with accuracy, precision, and dependability; and ability to distinguish routine functions from those requiring a pharmacist's judgment. These requirements should be clearly understood by applicants to the program.

Appendix B: Training Program Format

The training course should consist of lectures, informal discussions, and practical experience sessions. The ratio of lecture material to practical experience sessions can vary, depending on the specific goals and design of the program. The course may be split into several options, with each trainee entering one of the options (e.g., parenteral admixture compounding). Alternatively, a single, more generalized course through which all trainees pass may be offered.

Each trainee should receive a course manual containing the following information:

1. General information about the hospital and hospital pharmacy (goals, organizational structures, personnel policy, etc.).
2. General information about the training program (attendance requirements, graduation requirements, and a complete schedule).
3. Detailed outline of each section of the program.
4. Detailed learning objectives in terms of behavioral outcomes for each didactic and practical training activity.
5. Other appropriate material such as pharmacy forms, lists of abbreviations, and explanatory notes.

It is suggested that topics that apply to several areas of study (e.g., safety considerations) be presented in the beginning of the course and then elaborated on as necessary for each individual section.

———————————

Approved by the ASHP Board of Directors, November 19–20, 1981.

The bibliographic citation for this document is as follows: American Society of Hospital Pharmacists. ASHP technical assistance bulletin on outcome competencies and training guidelines for institutional pharmacy technician training programs. *Am J Hosp Pharm.* 1982; 39:317–20.

ASHP Technical Assistance Bulletin on the Evaluation of Drugs for Formularies

Preamble

One of the major responsibilities of a pharmacy and thera-peutics (P&T) committee is to develop and maintain a drug formulary system. The formulary can be used as the basis for promoting optimal pharmacotherapy because it contains only those drugs judged by the P&T committee to be in the best interest of the patient's health needs in terms of efficacy and cost. The pharmacist is a key member of the drug evaluation team because of his or her knowledge of pharma-cology, pharmacokinetics, toxicology, therapeutics, and drug purchasing.

A thorough, critical review of the pharmaceutical and medical literature is necessary for evaluating drugs pro-posed for admission to a formulary. Comparative data asso-ciated with a drug's efficacy, adverse effects, and cost and the determination of its potential therapeutic advantages and deficiencies require critical evaluation by the pharmacist. Drugs may be added to or deleted from a formulary based on evaluation by the P&T committee. Alternative actions might include either conditional approval for a specific time period (with subsequent reevaluation) or temporary limitation of a drug's use to an individual medical service specialty with future reassessment.

Evaluation Report Considerations

A standardized evaluation report should be developed by the pharmacy for use in the evaluation process. It is recom-mended that each report include the following information:

1. Generic name.
   - List the officially approved name of all chemical entities in the drug product.
2. Trade name(s).
   - List the most common trade name(s) of the drug product.
3. Source(s) of supply.
   - Identify the pharmaceutical vendors from which the drug product can be procured.
   - For a generic drug product, identify the actual manufacturer; if applicable, identify the vendors distributing the product.
4. *American Hospital Formulary Service Drug Informa-tion* classification number.
   - List the number for quick access and retrieval of information.
5. Pharmacologic classification.
   - State the pharmacologic class to which the drug belongs and any similar properties it possesses compared with existing drugs.
   - State the mechanism of action; if the mechanism of action is unknown, state this. If applicable, the mechanism of action may be compared with that of another drug or class of drugs.
6. Therapeutic indications.
   - State the uses of the drug as approved by the Food and Drug Administration; indicate whether the use is prophylactic, therapeutic, palliative,

curative, adjunctive, or supportive.
   - Evaluate uses of the drug in comparison with other established forms of therapy, using, if possible, human studies for comparison. Com-parisons should emphasize therapeutics (effi-cacy, incidence of treatment success, remission, sensitivity, ease of monitoring, and treatment periods required) and include a critical analysis of clinical studies in such areas as patient popu-lation, methodology, statistics, and conclusions.
   - Identify non-FDA-labeled uses for the drug and those uses that show promise in investigational studies.
7. Dosage forms.
   - List all dosage forms available as approved by FDA; list unit cost.
8. Bioavailability and pharmacokinetics.
   - List bioavailability data for the most common route of administration and dosage of the drug. Other bioavailability data should be available on request by the P&T committee.
   - List pharmacokinetic data for absorption, distri-bution, metabolism, and excretion of the drug. For absorption, include information on the ex-tent and rate of absorption of the drug by the usual routes of administration; the factors that might affect the rate or extent of absorption; the therapeutic, toxic, and lethal blood levels; the period of time required for onset, peak, and duration of therapeutic effect; and the half-life and factors affecting it. For distribution, include information on the usual distribution of the drug in body tissues and fluids, the drug's propensity to cross the blood–brain barrier or placenta or to appear in human milk, the drug's propensity for protein binding, and the drug's volume of distri-bution. For metabolism, include information on sites of metabolism, extent of biotransforma-tion, and metabolic products and their activity. For excretion, include information on routes of elimination from the body, factors affecting elimi-nation, and the form in which the drug is elimi-nated.
9. Dosage range.
   - List the dosage range for different routes of administration of the drug.
   - List initial, maintenance, maximal, geriatric, and pediatric doses for the drug.
10. Known adverse effects and toxicities.
   - Discuss adverse effects of the drug and their frequency of occurrence from research data of human studies.
   - Discuss means or methods of preventing or treat-ing adverse effects and toxicities. Benefits of disease treatment and risks of adverse effects should be emphasized.
11. Special precautions.
   - List precautions and contraindications for cer-tain disease states or other conditions.

- Compare all of the preceding data with existing similar agents, where applicable.
- List potential drug interactions if deemed clinically important.

12. Comparisons.
- List therapeutic comparisons with other drugs or treatment regimens.
- List cost comparison data of a standard treatment regimen with the new drug versus currently used drugs.
- List unusual monitoring or drug administration requirements for the drug.

13. Recommendations.
- Formulate recommendations from analysis of all of the preceding data and consideration of other factors such as medical staff preference, distribution problems, and availability of the drug. Recommend action to be taken with regard to the drug's formulary status, as follows:

  Uncontrolled: To be available for use by all medical staff.

  Monitored: To be available for use by all medical staff, but its use is to be monitored.

  Restricted: To be available for use by the medical staff of a specific service or department.

  Conditional: To be available for use by all medical staff for a specific time period.

  Deletion: To be deleted from the current formulary.

Recommended Reference Materials

This list of recommended references includes those sources that commonly provide useful information in drug evaluation; however, review of additional specialty journals or other sources may be required.

- Texts.
  1. *American Hospital Formulary Service Drug Information.*
  2. *Drug Topics Redbook Annual Pharmacists' Reference.*
  3. *Facts and Comparisons.*
  4. *Martindale—The Extra Pharmacopoeia.*
  5. *Physicians' Desk Reference.*
  6. *The Pharmacological Basis of Therapeutics.*
- Periodicals and abstracting systems.
  1. *American Journal of Hospital Pharmacy.*
  2. *Annals of Internal Medicine.*
  3. *Archives of Internal Medicine.*

  4. *Antimicrobial Agents and Chemotherapy.*
  5. *Clinical Pharmacology and Therapeutics.*
  6. *Clinical Pharmacy.*
  7. *Drug Therapy.*
  8. Drugdex.
  9. *Drugs.*
  10. *Drug Intelligence and Clinical Pharmacy.*
  11. *Hospital Formulary.*
  12. *Hospital Therapy.*
  13. Iowa Drug Information System.
  14. *International Pharmaceutical Abstracts.*
  15. *Journal of the American Medical Association.*
  16. *The Lancet.*
  17. *Medical Letter on Drugs and Therapeutics.*
  18. *New England Journal of Medicine.*
  19. Paul de Haen Information Systems.
  20. *Pharmacotherapy.*

This technical assistance bulletin is supplementary to the "ASHP Statement on the Pharmacy and Therapeutics Committee,"[1] "ASHP Statement on the Formulary System,"[2] and "ASHP Technical Assistance Bulletin on Hospital Formularies,"[3] which should be consulted for further information on the formulary system.

References

1. American Society of Hospital Pharmacists. ASHP statement on the pharmacy and therapeutics committee. *Am J Hosp Pharm.* 1984; 41:1621.

2. American Society of Hospital Pharmacists. ASHP statement on the formulary system. *Am J Hosp Pharm.* 1983; 40:1384–5.

3. American Society of Hospital Pharmacists. ASHP technical assistance bulletin on hospital formularies. *Am J Hosp Pharm.* 1985; 42:375–7.

Developed by the ASHP Council on Professional Affairs. Approved by the ASHP Board of Directors, November 19, 1987. Supersedes an earlier version approved by the Board of Directors, April 30, 1981.

The bibliographic citation for this document is as follows: American Society of Hospital Pharmacists. ASHP technical assistance bulletin on the evaluation of drugs for formularies. *Am J Hosp Pharm.* 1988; 45:386–7.

ASHP Technical Assistance Bulletin on Handling Cytotoxic and Hazardous Drugs

In 1985, the "ASHP Technical Assistance Bulletin on Handling Cytotoxic Drugs in Hospitals"[1] summarized published information on handling hazardous drugs, referred to as cytotoxics, as of July 1984. As more information became available on the types of hazardous agents that may represent a health risk to the occupationally exposed population, and as the handling of such substances became routine in hospitals, community pharmacies, home care settings, clinics, and physicians' offices, the need to revise the Technical Assistance Bulletin became apparent.

Early concerns regarding occupational exposure to hazardous agents involved primarily drugs used in cancer therapy. Therefore, the terms "antineoplastics" (drugs used to treat neoplasms) and "chemotherapy" were used in early reports and guidelines. Although any chemical used therapeutically may be referred to as chemotherapy, this term is currently used, both in the medical and lay communities, to mean drug therapy of cancer. In an attempt to be more precise, many professionals adopted the term "cytotoxic" or "cell killer." Not all antineoplastics, however, are cytotoxic, nor are all cytotoxics used exclusively in the treatment of cancer. "Cytotoxic" is often used to refer to any agent that may be genotoxic, oncogenic, mutagenic, teratogenic, or hazardous in any way. As our knowledge of the hazardous nature of many agents grows and as new hazardous agents (e.g., genotoxic biologicals and some biotechnological agents) continue to be developed, cytotoxic is a less appropriate term. In deference to the original Technical Assistance Bulletin, cytotoxic remains in the title of this revision. The remainder of the document, however, will refer exclusively to hazardous drugs or agents, except in very specific instances.

In January 1986, the Federal Occupational Safety and Health Administration (OSHA) released recommendations on safe handling of cytotoxic drugs by health-care personnel.[2] This revised Technical Assistance Bulletin includes information from these recommendations, modified by subsequent discussions with OSHA, and from published reports by the National Institutes of Health,[3] the National Study Commission on Cytotoxic Exposure,[4] and the American Medical Association's (AMA) Council on Scientific Affairs,[5] along with other published information on this issue as of June 1988.

The safe handling of hazardous drugs is an issue that must be addressed in health-care settings and one that may even affect, in a home care environment, persons other than the patient. Inasmuch as possible, the pharmacist should take the lead in establishing policies and procedures to ensure the proper handling of all hazardous drugs in any health-care setting. The recommendations contained in this Technical Assistance Bulletin should be applied to any area where hazardous drugs are handled. Procedures specific to noninstitutional care settings have been included where available.[6-8] Because of the many questions about implementing the recommendations in the original Technical Assistance Bulletin, this revision contains detailed information in those areas of greatest concern. The recommendations contained here should be supplemented with the professional judgments of qualified staff and with newer information as it develops.

Hazardous Drug Dangers

The danger to health-care personnel from handling a hazardous drug stems from a combination of its inherent toxicity and the extent to which workers are exposed to the drug in the course of carrying out their duties. This exposure may be through inadvertent ingestion of the drug on foodstuffs (e.g., workers' lunches), inhalation of drug dusts or droplets, or direct skin contact. Drugs that may represent occupational hazards include any that exhibit the following characteristics:

1. Genotoxicity [i.e., mutagenicity and clastogenicity (see Appendix A) in short-term test systems].
2. Carcinogenicity in animal models, in the patient population, or both, as reported by the International Agency for Research on Cancer (IARC).
3. Teratogenicity or fertility impairment in animal studies or treated patients.
4. Evidence of serious organ or other toxicity at low doses in animal models or treated patients.

The oncogenic and teratogenic effects of therapeutic doses of several antineoplastic agents are well established.[9-13] The mutagenic properties of some cytotoxics, immunosuppressants, antiviral agents, and biological response modifiers have also been documented.[14] The long-term effects (e.g., cancer, impaired fertility, and organ damage) of continued exposure to small amounts of one or more of such drugs remain undetermined.

For example, it is known that long-term use of potent immunosuppressive agents may result in the development of lymphoma. It is not known, however, at what drug level or over what period of time this may occur and how this correlates with possible drug levels achieved through occupational exposure during preparation and administration of hundreds or thousands of injectable and oral doses of these agents.

Studies have attempted to assess indirectly the potential exposure of hospital pharmacists and nurses to some hazardous drugs in several health-care settings including physicians' offices.[15-21] These studies examined the urine mutagenicity or evidence of chromosome damage in subjects who prepared or administered primarily antineoplastic injections. The mutagenicity and chromosome damage that were found were thought to document exposure to and absorption of the drugs that had been handled. An association may exist between carcinogenicity and chromosome breakage or mutagenicity. Therefore, one might conclude that handling hazardous drugs entails some danger to health-care personnel. These studies, although not conclusive, support the postulated occupational risks.

However, several reports make the situation slightly more ominous. Palmer and coworkers[22] measured chromosome damage in 10 patients receiving chlorambucil. They found that the damage was cumulative and was related to both the daily dose and the duration of therapy. Another report[23] described permanent liver damage in three nurses who had worked 6, 8, and 16 years, respectively, on an oncology ward. On the basis of histories, the investigators suggested that the liver injuries may have been related to the intensity and duration of exposure to certain toxic agents. The chlorambucil study involved therapeutic doses of drug, and three cases of liver damage is a small base for drawing any final conclusions. Nevertheless, this information is disturbing in view of the fact that many health-care workers prepare or administer hundreds or even thousands of doses of hazardous drugs during their careers. If low-dose exposure to these agents is cumulative, this exposure should be minimized by strict compliance with safe handling procedures.

The value of chromosome and mutagenicity studies as indicators of the occupational risks of exposure to hazardous drugs has been questioned.[24–28] However, several researchers have employed more direct methods of determining whether or not workers have been exposed to and absorbed hazardous drugs handled in the customary manner. Demonstration that absorption has occurred would be strong support for the imposition of safety measures. (The absorption of hazardous drug is presumed to be a health risk.)

A letter[29] described a study that used the presence of thioethers in the urine as an indicator of exposure to alkylating agents (i.e., certain antineoplastic drugs). The mean urinary thioether concentration (UTC) was higher in a group of 15 oncology nurses after a 5-day rotation than it was when they returned to work after a 3-day leave ($p < 0.01$). There was no difference between the mean pre-exposure UTC and that of a group of 20 nurses who never handled antineoplastic drugs. Twelve of the 15 nurses wore gloves when handling the drugs; none wore any other form of protective apparel. Drug preparation procedures were not reported.

Using gas chromatography, Hirst's group[30] found cyclophosphamide in the urine of two nurses working in a cancer clinic who took no special precautions when handling the drug. They also demonstrated that cyclophosphamide can be absorbed through intact skin. On the other hand, another group of researchers[31] looked for (but could not detect) platinum in the urine of 10 pharmacists and nurses who frequently prepared or administered cisplatin and other platinum-containing antineoplastic agents. However, these subjects employed several protective measures when working with the drugs; this may have influenced the results (and demonstrated the effectiveness of the safety precautions employed). Also, the assay method may not have been sensitive enough.

With a different type of approach, Neal et al.[32] detected fluorouracil in the air of a drug preparation room and nearby office (where the drug was not prepared). A similar study[33] showed that routine drug manipulations in a horizontal laminar airflow hood contaminated the air in an intravenous admixture preparation room. Fluorouracil and cefazolin sodium were the test drugs employed.

Certain antineoplastic drugs have also been implicated in reproductive risks in humans. There have been reports of fetal loss or malformation occurring in pregnancies of women receiving drug therapy for cancer during the first trimester.[34] Two controlled, retrospective Finnish studies[35,36] attempted to examine the relationship between occupational exposure to antineoplastics and reproductive risks in nurses. One study of nurses reported a statistically significant correlation between the birth of children with malformations and the nurses' preparation and administration of antineoplastics more than once a week during the first trimester of pregnancy. At the time of these nurses' exposure, few protective mechanisms were used.

The second study was done in cooperation with the U.S. National Institute for Occupational Safety and Health (NIOSH); it examined only the incidence of fetal loss and did not investigate the condition of live births. The study showed a significant association between fetal loss and occupational exposure to antineoplastic drugs during the first trimester. Both studies are subject to criticism regarding recall bias and determination of exposure data. Concern about exposure of pregnant workers to hazardous drugs, at least in the first trimester, is, however, valid in light of the reproductive risk reported with therapeutic exposure to certain antineoplastics. At therapeutic doses, these drugs have also been shown to suppress testicular function and spermatogenesis.[37–39] While the relationship between occupational exposure to hazardous drugs and testicular dysfunction has not been assessed, this potential complication should be considered in light of the effects on treated patients.

To date, these reports provide the primary evidence that health-care workers exposed to hazardous drugs during the course of their work may be absorbing these drugs and may be at risk for adverse outcomes.

Additional research in this area is needed, but awareness of the problem has led to overall reduction of exposures, either by improved drug handling techniques or through the implementation of safety programs,[40,41] and thus fewer exposed health-care workers are available for study. Definitive knowledge of the occupational dangers of handling hazardous drugs may someday be available through epidemiologic studies of health-care workers.

In theory, correct and perfect preparation and handling techniques will prevent drug particles or droplets from escaping from their containers while they are being manipulated. Our opinion is that near-perfect technique is uncommon; therefore, contamination of the workplace is likely and worker exposure may increase without protective equipment and other safety measures. This is particularly true, we think, in the absence of any structured training and quality-assurance programs covering the proper handling of hazardous drugs. (Such programs are most likely to be found in health-care settings where the preparation of hazardous drugs is centralized.) Beyond problems in technique, however, contamination also will occur from inevitable spills and from the breakage of hazardous drug containers. ASHP believes that the occupational dangers of exposure to hazardous drugs can be summarized as follows:

1. If hazardous drugs are handled in the same way as other less hazardous substances (e.g., potassium chloride solutions and multivitamin tablets), contamination of the work environment is almost certain to occur.

2. The limited data available suggest that this contamination may result in exposure to and absorption of the drugs by health-care personnel and others. The amount of drug absorbed by any one individual on any given day probably is very small, except for instances of excessive exposure.

3. However, if experience with the therapeutic use of hazardous drugs indicates that the damage is cumulative, individuals whose job responsibilities require them to prepare or administer large numbers of hazardous drug doses for long periods of time (e.g., oncology or transplant nurses and pharmacy intravenous service staff) are at greater risk.

4. Considering the above, the use of procedures, equipment, and materials that demonstrably or theoretically

reduce exposure to hazardous drugs in the health-care workplace is necessary.

The question remains: What safety precautions should be employed?

Safety Precautions

Ideally, the safety precautions employed to protect health-care workers handling hazardous drugs would be those whose efficacy and cost-effectiveness have been documented. Since these drugs have many different physical and chemical properties, research studies into environmental contamination and safety-garment penetration for all questionable drugs are problematic. However, several studies have attempted to demonstrate the effectiveness of certain recommended interventions. Hoy and Stump[42] concluded that a commercial air-venting device, when used with appropriate technique, effectively reduced the release of drug aerosols during reconstitution of drugs packaged in vials. A study by Anderson et al.[16] provides support for preparing hazardous drugs in a vertical laminar airflow biological safety cabinet (BSC) (NSF Class II;[43] see Appendix B) rather than a horizontal airflow clean air work station.

A more recent air-sampling study,[44] carried out in a hospital pharmacy work area where a Class II BSC was used to prepare cytotoxic drugs, detected no fluorouracil during the study period. The study was limited to one drug and two short study periods; the results indicate that a Class II BSC, in conjunction with stringent aseptic technique and recommended procedures for handling hazardous drugs, may reduce environmental contamination by these drugs.

While common sense suggests that the airflow characteristics of containment cabinets would provide greater worker protection than open airflow workstations, it should also suggest that the front opening of the Class II BSC might present potential for environmental contamination and increased worker exposure to hazardous agents. Indeed, as demonstrated by an industrial hygiene experiment,[45] a Class II BSC may cause occasional leakage toward the operator and into the environment if it is placed in an area of strong air drafts or frequent personnel traffic. The containment characteristics of the Class II BSC are compromised whenever the intake or exhaust grilles are blocked (e.g., by placing equipment or supplies on the front grille or too near the back exhaust) or by too much movement on the part of the operator.

Gloves are a major source of protection, whether the work is performed with or without a Class II BSC. The permeability of various glove materials to selected drugs has been examined.[46-49] By using various methods to determine and quantitate penetration, researchers found that permeability of the glove material varied with the drug, contact time, and glove thickness. None of the glove materials tested was impervious to all drugs, and no material was statistically superior except as related to thickness. A thicker glove material is optimal. In addition, several glove materials showed variation in permeability within a manufacturer's lot. These studies do establish that gloves can provide protection against skin contact with the tested drugs, although the degree of protection has not been substantiated. Protection from skin contact is important since many of the problem drugs are skin irritants or even vesicants and, as Hirst et al.[30] showed, at least one (cyclophosphamide) is absorbed through the skin.

Only one study[50] looked at the permeability of gown materials to drugs. Lab coats and disposable isolation gowns were penetrated immediately and were therefore inappropriate for study. Of the four other gown materials studied, Kaycel and nonporous Tyvek had greater permeability than the coated fabrics (Saranex-laminated Tyvek and polyethylene-coated Tyvek). As with gloves, permeability was drug specific. The investigators concluded that users of garments made of Kaycel and nonporous Tyvek should be aware of the potential of these materials for permeability to certain drugs. An earlier report[51] supports the wearing of gloves and gowns. Additional research is needed in the area of protective garments and equipment. Since substantive data are still lacking, health-care professionals should choose protective measures on the basis of expert recommendations, professional judgment, and common sense as well as scientifically established facts.

Recommended Safe Handling Methods

The balance of this article presents our recommendations for policies, procedures, and safety materials for controlling, preparing, administering, containing, and disposing of hazardous drugs. The recommendations are given in a format that can be used either as a base for establishing safe handling methods or for evaluating existing procedures as part of a quality-assurance program. ASHP believes these recommendations represent a conservative but reasonable approach to the precautions that should be taken.

The recommendations are in the format of evaluation criteria organized into four groups. This format should be useful in establishing a quality-assurance system for all nontherapeutic aspects of hazardous drug use. Each group begins with a broad goal, followed by a set of specific criteria and recommendations for achieving the goal. The four goals reflect the following axioms for handling hazardous drugs:

1. Protect and secure packages of hazardous drugs.
2. Inform and educate all involved personnel about hazardous drugs and train them in the safe handling procedures relevant to their responsibilities.
3. Do not let the drugs escape from containers when they are manipulated (i.e., dissolved, transferred, administered, or discarded).
4. Eliminate the possibility of inadvertent ingestion or inhalation and direct skin or eye contact with the drugs.

The handling of hazardous drugs is a complex issue, and the advice of medical experts, occupational physicians, industrial hygienists, legal counsel, and others should be obtained when organizational policy is being established.

Goal I. Accidental contamination of the health-care environment, resulting in exposure of personnel, patients, visitors, and family members to hazardous substances, is prevented by maintaining the physical integrity and security of packages of hazardous drugs.

1. *Access to all areas where hazardous drugs are stored is limited to specified authorized staff.*
2. *A method should be present for identifying to personnel those drugs that require special precautions (e.g., cytotoxics).[52] One way to accomplish this is to apply appropriate warning labels (see Figure 1) to all hazardous drug containers, shelves, and bins*

where the drug products are stored.

3. *A method of identifying, for patients and family members, those drugs that require special precautions in the home should be in place.* This may be accomplished in the health-care setting by providing specific labeling for discharge medications, along with counseling and written instructions. Providers of home care and supplies should develop similar labeling and instructional material for the protection of patients and their families.

4. *Methods for identifying shipping cartons of hazardous drugs should be required from manufacturers and distributors of these drugs.*

5. *Written procedures for handling damaged packages of hazardous drugs should be maintained.* Personnel involved in shipping and receiving hazardous drugs should be trained in these procedures, including the proper use of protective garments and equipment. Damaged shipping cartons of hazardous drugs should be received and opened in an isolated area (e.g., in a laboratory fume hood, if available, not in a BSC used for preparing sterile products). Protective apparel—disposable closed-front gown or coveralls, disposable utility gloves over disposable latex gloves, NIOSH-approved[53] air-purifying half-mask respirator (may be disposable) equipped with a high-efficiency filter, and eye protection—should be worn. Broken containers and contaminated packaging materials should be placed in the designated receptacles as described in this article.

6. *Facilities (e.g., shelves, carts, counters, and trays) for storing hazardous drugs are designed to prevent breakage and to limit contamination in the event of leakage.* Bins, shelves with barriers at the front, or other design features that reduce the chance of drug containers falling to the floor should be used. Hazardous drugs requiring refrigeration should be stored separately from nonhazardous drugs in individual bins designed to prevent breakage and contain leakage.

7. *Methods for transporting hazardous drugs to the health-care setting should be consistent with environmental protection and national or local regulations for transporting hazardous substances.* When hazardous drugs are being transported to the home care setting, appropriate containers (e.g., lined cardboard boxes) and procedures should be used to prevent breakage and contain leakage. Hazardous drug containers should be secured to prevent handling by unauthorized persons. Transportation vehicles should be kept locked at all times.

For transporting hazardous drugs within the health-care setting, methods that do not cause breakage of or leakage from drug containers should be used. Conveyances that produce severe mechanical stress on their contents (e.g., pneumatic tubes) must not be used to transport hazardous drugs. The drugs must be securely capped or sealed and properly packaged and protected during transport to reduce further the chance of breakage and spillage in a public area such as a corridor or elevator. Adequate instruction and appropriate containers should be provided to patients for transporting discharge and home care medications that require special precautions.

Goal II. The preparation of hazardous drugs does not result in contamination of the health-care work environment or excessive exposure of personnel, patients, or family members to hazardous drug powders, dusts, liquids, or mists.

1. *Written policies and standard procedures for preparing hazardous drugs are maintained.*

   a. They should include a method for identifying for health-care personnel the particular drugs covered by these policies.

   b. Policies and procedures should be consistent with applicable government regulations, professional practice standards, and the recommendations of pharmaceutical manufacturers, hospital safety officers, and other knowledgeable parties.

   c. Since several departments, such as pharmacy, nursing, transportation, maintenance, housekeeping, and medical staff, will be involved with some aspect of the hazardous drug handling issue, preparation of safe handling policies and procedures must be a collaborative effort. Pharmacy should take the lead in this effort.

   d. All personnel who handle cytotoxic and other hazardous agents should have access to the procedures pertaining to their responsibilities. Deviations from the standard procedures must not be permitted except under defined circumstances.

2. *A method for orienting all involved personnel to the special nature of the hazardous drugs in question and the policies and procedures that govern their handling is present.*

   a. The orientation should include, as appropriate, a discussion of the known and potential hazards of the drugs and explanation of all relevant policies. Training done in association with the orientation should cover all relevant techniques and procedures and the proper use of protective equipment and materials. The contents of the orientation program and attendance should be well documented and sufficient to meet "worker right to know" statutes and regulations.

   b. While implementation of a safety program should reduce the risk of personnel exposure to hazardous drugs, the efficacy of such a program in protecting personnel during preparation or administration of these drugs has yet to be demonstrated. The limitations of such a program should be made known to hazardous drug handlers.

   c. Until the reproductive risks (or lack thereof) associated with handling hazardous drugs within

Figure 1. One example of a suitable warning label for cytotoxic and hazardous drugs. Other labels may be used.

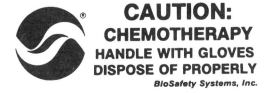

CAUTION: CHEMOTHERAPY HANDLE WITH GLOVES DISPOSE OF PROPERLY *BioSafety Systems, Inc.*

a safety program have been substantiated, staff who are pregnant or breast-feeding should be allowed to avoid contact with these drugs. Policies should be in effect that provide these individuals with alternative tasks or responsibilities if they so desire. In general, these policies should encourage personnel to solicit recommendations from their personal physicians regarding the need for restricted duties. In the case of personnel actively trying to conceive or father a child, a similar policy should be considered, and a specific time period (e.g., 3 months) should be agreed on. Legal counsel should be sought when establishing policies.

d. Prospective temporary and permanent employees who may be required to work with hazardous drugs should be so notified and should receive adequate information about the policies and procedures pertaining to their use. This notification should be documented during the interview process and retained as part of the employment record for all employees.

e. All individuals handling hazardous drugs who do not have employee status (e.g., contract workers, students, residents, medical staff, and volunteers) should be informed through proper channels of the special nature of the drugs. If they choose to handle the hazardous drugs, then they will be expected to comply with established policies and procedures for preparing, administering, and containing hazardous drugs and their associated waste.

3. *A system for verifying and documenting acceptable staff performance of and conformance with established procedures is maintained.*

a. Methods of determining adherence to departmental safety program policies and procedures should be in place. Proper technique is essential to maintain the sterility of the product being manipulated and to reduce the generation of hazardous drug contaminants. Therefore, after initial training and at regular intervals, the knowledge and competence of personnel preparing and administering these drugs should be evaluated and documented. This evaluation should include written examinations and an observed demonstration of competence in the preparation and simulated administration of practice solutions. The monitoring of staff performance and the control of hazardous drugs usually are best achieved if the storage and preparation of the drugs are centralized within one area or department.

b. All personnel involved with the transportation, preparation, administration, and disposal of cytotoxic and hazardous substances should continually be updated on new or revised information on safe handling of cytotoxic and hazardous substances. Policies and procedures should be updated accordingly.

4. *Sufficient information is maintained on safe use of the hazardous drugs in the work area.*

a. The pharmacy should provide access to information on toxicity, treatment of acute exposure (if available), chemical inactivators, solubility, and

stability of hazardous drugs (including investigational agents) used in the workplace. This information should be in addition to information required to ensure patient safety during therapy with these drugs and to be in compliance with all applicable laws and regulations. The information must be easily and readily accessible to all employees where these drugs are routinely handled.

b. Currently, a large number of investigational agents that are potentially hazardous are under clinical study. Staff members should not prepare or administer any investigational agent unless they have received adequate information and instruction about the safe and correct use of the drug. The clinical protocol should include appropriate handling and disposal techniques, if available. When information is limited, pre-clinical data should be used to assess the health risk of the agent.

5. *Appropriate engineering controls should be in place to protect the drug product from microbial contamination and to protect personnel and the environment from the potential hazards of the product.* These engineering controls should be maintained according to applicable regulations and standards.

a. Class 100 clean air work stations,[54] both horizontal and vertical airflow (with no containment characteristics), are inappropriate engineering controls for handling hazardous drugs because they provide no personnel protection and permit environmental contamination. Although there are no engineering controls designed specifically for the safe handling of hazardous chemicals as sterile products, Class II[43] contained vertical flow BSCs (biohazard cabinets) have been adopted for this use. Biohazard cabinetry is, however, designed for the handling of infectious agents, not hazardous chemicals. Therefore, the limitations of such cabinetry must be understood by purchaser and operator. Manufacturers, vendors, the National Sanitation Foundation (NSF), and some certifying agencies are appropriate sources of information regarding BSCs.

b. BSCs are available in three classes (Appendix B). Based on design, ease of use, and cost considerations, Class II contained vertical flow biohazard cabinetry is currently recommended for use in preparing sterile doses of hazardous drugs. Class II cabinetry design and performance specifications are defined in NSF Standard 49.[43] BSCs selected for use with hazardous drugs should meet NSF Standard 49 specifications to ensure the maximum protection from these engineering controls. NSF Standard 49 defines four types of Class II cabinetry, depending on the amount of contaminated air that is recirculated through high-efficiency particulate air (HEPA) filters within the cabinet (see Appendix B).

Selection criteria for Class II cabinetry should include the types and amounts of hazardous drugs prepared, the available location and amount of space, NSF Standard 49, any local requirements for handling hazardous materials and ducting contaminated air, and the cost of the cabinet and related ventilation. Minimum recommendations are a Class II, Type A cabinet (recirculating a major portion of contaminated air through a HEPA filter and back into the cabinet and exhausting a minor portion, through a HEPA filter, to the workroom). In light of the continued development of hazardous drugs having differing physical properties, selection of a Type A cabinet that can be converted to a Type B3 (greater inflow velocity, contaminated ducts and plenums under negative pressure and vented to the outside) may be a prudent investment. There are currently no data to indicate that the use of an auxiliary charcoal filter is more effective in retaining hazardous drugs than the mandatory exhaust HEPA filter of the Type A cabinet.

Type B BSCs are designed to provide more personnel protection than Type A through their greater inflow velocities and required external exhaust of contaminated air. Types B1 (exhausting approximately 70% of the contaminated air to the outside through a HEPA filter) and B2 (exhausting 100% of the contaminated air to the outside through a HEPA filter) require outside exhaust ducts with auxiliary blowers. The Type B2 cabinet is preferred, but unavailability of adequate "makeup" air may eliminate it in favor of the Type B1. All exhaust ducting of any type of BSC must meet applicable codes and ordinances. Ducting into the "dead space" in the ceiling is inappropriate and may be illegal, because it may contaminate ventilation systems and promote contamination of the environment and personnel not directly involved in hazardous drug handling.

In the selection of any BSC, ceiling height should also be considered. Several manufacturers' models have top-load HEPA filters. In workrooms with standard-height ceilings, the filters are difficult to access for certification, which may require that the entire BSC be moved when the filter must be replaced. Because of restrictions of space and cost, the 2-foot wide, Class II, Type A BSC may seem to be the only choice for smaller institutions, outpatient centers, and physician offices. There are, however, many limitations to the smaller cabinet. Because NSF testing facilities are not currently adaptable to 2-foot BSC models, no 2-foot BSC is NSF approved. Selection of a 2-foot cabinet should, therefore, include thorough investigation of cabinet design and knowledge of the reliability of the manufacturer. In all cases, the manufacturer's 2-foot cabinet should not differ extensively from designs used for its NSF-approved larger models.

c.   All Class II BSCs have an open front with inward airflow forming a "curtain" or barrier to protect the operator and the environment from contaminants released in the BSC work area. Because BSCs are subject to breaks in their containment properties if there is interference with the inward airflow through the work area access opening, placement of the BSC and operator training are critical. The placement of a BSC in an area with drafts or in close proximity to other airflow devices (e.g., horizontal flow hoods, air conditioners, air vents, fans, and doors) may interfere with the inward airflow through the opening and may release contaminants into the workroom.

The horizontal motion of an operator's arms in the opening may also result in similar workroom contamination. Because smaller BSCs are more sensitive to disruption of the inward airflow barrier, the use of a 2- to 3-foot BSC is associated with a greater risk of releasing contaminants than are larger cabinets and requires that the operator be more carefully trained and monitored. It is critical that all operators know the proper method for preparing hazardous drugs in a BSC and that they understand the limitations of BSCs.

d.   Class II BSCs should be certified according to specifications of NSF Standard 49 and Class 100 specifications of Federal Standard 209C.[54] Certification should take place on initial installation, whenever the cabinet is moved or repaired, and every 6 months thereafter. At present, there are no licensing requirements for individuals who certify Class II BSCs. It is, therefore, imperative that the pharmacist responsible for the intravenous preparation area be familiar with the certification requirements for Class II BSCs and the test procedures that should be performed.[55]

All BSCs should be tested for the integrity of the HEPA filter, velocity of the work access airflow and supply airflow, airflow smoke patterns, and integrity of external surfaces of the cabinet and filter housings. Testing of the integrity of the HEPA filter generally ensures that the particulate count in the work area is less than that required to meet Class 100 conditions of Federal Standard 209C.[54] Class II, Type B1 BSCs may be prone to exceed Class 100 particle counts and should have routine particulate testing as part of the certification process. Individuals certifying the BSC should be informed of the hazardous nature of the drugs being prepared in the BSC and should wear appropriate protective apparel (see section 5g).

e.   BSCs should be cleaned and disinfected regularly to ensure a proper environment for preparation of sterile products. For routine cleanups of surfaces between decontaminations, water should be used (for injection or irrigation) with or without a small amount of cleaner. If the contamination is soluble only in alcohol, then 70% isopropyl or ethyl alcohol may be used in addition to the cleaner. In general, alcohol is not a good cleaner, only a disinfectant, and its use in a BSC should be limited. The BSC should be disinfected with 70% alcohol before any aseptic manipulation is begun. The excessive use of alcohol should be avoided in BSCs where air is recirculated (i.e., Class II, Type A, B3, and, to a lesser extent, B1) because alcohol vapors may build up in the cabinet.

A lint-free, plastic-backed disposable liner may be used in the BSC to facilitate spill cleanup. Problems with the use of such a liner include introduction of particulates into the work area, "lumping" of a wet liner that causes unsteady placement of drug containers, poor visibility of spills, and creation of additional contaminated disposables. If used, the liner should be changed frequently and whenever it is overtly contaminated.

f. The BSC should be operated with the blower turned on continuously, 24 hours a day, 7 days a week. Hazardous drug aerosols and spills generated in the work area of the BSC routinely accumulate in the deposits of room dust and particles under the work tray. These contaminants are too heavy to be transported to the HEPA filter located at the top of the cabinet. In addition, the plenums in all of the BSCs currently available in the United States become contaminated during use; these plenums cannot be accessed for washing. Turning off the blower may allow contaminated dust to recirculate back into the workroom, especially if other sources of air turbulence, such as horizontal hoods, air intakes, air conditioners, and fans, are located near the BSC. Whether or not the BSC is vented to the outside, the downward airflow velocity is insufficient to move and "trap" room dust, spill debris, and other contaminants on the HEPA filter. If it is necessary to turn off a BSC, first the entire cabinet, including all parts that can be reached, should be thoroughly cleaned with a detergent that will remove surface contamination and then rinsed (see section 5g). Once the BSC is clean, the blower may be turned off and the work access opening of the BSC and the HEPA exhaust area may be covered with impermeable plastic and sealed with tape to prevent any contamination from inadvertently escaping from the BSC. The BSC must be sealed with plastic whenever it is moved or left inoperative for any period of time.

g. The BSC should be decontaminated on a regular basis (ideally at least weekly) and whenever there is a spill or the BSC is moved or serviced, including for certification. While NSF Standard 49 recommends decontamination with formaldehyde to remove biohazard contamination, chemical (drug) contamination is not removed by such treatment. Currently, no single reagent will deactivate all known hazardous drugs; therefore, decontamination of a BSC used for such drugs is limited to removal of contamination from a nondisposable surface (the cabinet) to a disposable surface (e.g., gauze or towels) by use of a good cleaning agent that removes chemicals from stainless steel.

The cleaning agent selected should have a pH approximating that of soap and be appropriate for stainless steel. Cleaners containing chemicals such as quaternary ammonium compounds should be used with caution, because they may be hazardous to humans and their vapors may build up in any BSC where air is recirculated (see section 5e). Similar caution should be used with any pressurized aerosol cleaner; spraying a pressurized aerosol into a BSC may disrupt the protective containment airflow, damage the HEPA filter, and cause an accumulation of the propellant within a BSC where air is recirculated, resulting in a fire and explosion hazard.

During decontamination, the operator should wear a disposable closed-front gown, disposable latex gloves covered by disposable utility gloves, safety glasses or goggles, a hair covering, and a disposable respirator, because the glass shield of the BSC occasionally must be lifted (see 5j). The blower must be left on, and only heavy toweling or gauze should be used in the BSC to prevent it from being "sucked" up the plenum and into the HEPA filter.

Decontamination should be done from top to bottom (areas of lesser contamination to greater) by applying the cleaner, scrubbing, and rinsing thoroughly with distilled or deionized water. All contaminated disposables should be contained in sealable bags for transfer to larger waste containers. The HEPA filter must not become wet during cleaning of the protective covering (e.g., grille front). This covering, therefore, should not be cleaned with spray cleaners while it is in place. Removable parts of the BSC should be cleaned within the containment area of the BSC and should not be removed from the cabinet. The work tray usually can be lifted and placed against the back wall for cleaning of the undersurface of the tray and exposure of the very bottom (or sump) of the BSC.

The drain spillage trough area collects room dust and all spills, so it is the most heavily contaminated area and must be thoroughly cleaned (at least twice with the cleaning agent). The trough provides limited access to the side and back plenums; surfaces should be cleaned as high as possible. BSCs have sharp metal edges, so disposable utility gloves are more durable and appropriate than surgical latex gloves for decontamination. Gloves should be changed immediately if torn. All plenum surfaces must be rinsed well, with frequent changes of water and gauze. If the BSC is equipped with a drainpipe and valve, it may be used to collect rinse water. The collection vessel used must fit well around the drain valve and not allow splashing. Gauze may be used around the connection to prevent aerosol from escaping. The collection vessel must have a tight-fitting cover, and all rinse water (and gauze, if used) must be disposed of as contaminated waste. The outside of the BSC should be wiped down with cleaner to remove any drip or touch contamination.

Cleaner and rinse containers are generally contaminated during the procedure and should remain in the BSC during cleaning or be placed on a plastic-backed, absorbent liner outside the BSC. All bottles must be discarded as contaminated waste after decontamination of the BSC. All protective apparel (e.g., gown, gloves, goggles, and respirator) should be discarded as contaminated waste. Work area surfaces should be disinfected with 70% alcohol before any aseptic operation is begun. With good planning, decontamination of a 4-foot BSC should take about 1 hour.

h. Because of its design and decontamination limitations, the BSC should be considered a contaminated environment and treated as such. The use of the BSC should be restricted to the preparation of sterile dosage forms of hazardous drugs. Access to the BSC should be limited to authorized personnel wearing appropriate protective clothing.

i. If a BSC previously used for biologicals will be adopted for use with hazardous drugs, the BSC should be completely decontaminated of biohazardous agents by use of NSF Standard 49 decontamination techniques. Both HEPA filters should be replaced and the cabinet tested against the *complete* requirements of NSF Standard 49 Appendix B and the particulate limitations of Class 100 conditions of Federal Standard 209C. A BSC used for hazardous drugs that will be recycled for use with hazardous drugs in another section of the institution or in another institution must be surface decontaminated (as described in section 5g), sealed (as in section 5f), and carefully transported to its new location before the filters are replaced (as in section 5j). Once in its new location, the BSC must be recertified.

j. The HEPA filters of the BSC must be replaced whenever they restrict required airflow velocity or if they are overtly contaminated (e.g., by a breach in technique that causes hazardous drug to be introduced onto the clean side of the supply HEPA filter). Personnel and environmental protection must be maintained during replacement of a contaminated HEPA filter. Because replacement of a HEPA filter generally requires breaking the integrity of the containment aspect of the cabinet, this procedure may release contamination from the filter into the pharmacy or intravenous preparation area if carried out in an inappropriate manner.

Before replacement of a HEPA filter contaminated with hazardous drugs, the BSC service agent should be consulted for a mutually acceptable procedure for replacing and subsequently disposing of a contaminated HEPA filter. One procedure would include moving the BSC to a secluded area or using plastic barriers to segregate the contaminated area. Protective clothing and equipment must be used by the servicer. The BSC should be decontaminated before filter replacement (see section 5g). The contaminated filters must be removed, bagged in thick plastic, and prepared for disposal in a hazardous waste dump site or incinerator licensed by the Environmental Protection Agency (EPA).

When arranging for disposal, precise terms should be used to describe the hazard (e.g., "toxic chemicals" or "chemical carcinogens," not "cytotoxic" or "chemotherapy") to ensure that contractors are not inadvertently misled in the classification of the hazard. Disposal of an entire contaminated BSC should be approached in the same manner. The filters should be removed, bagged, and disposed of separately from the BSC. If no available service company will

arrange for removal of the filter (or entire BSC) and its ultimate disposal, a licensed hazardous waste contractor should be used. The use of triple layers of thick plastic (e.g., 2-mil low-linear or 4-mil plastic) for initial covering of the filter or cabinet and then the construction of a plywood crate for transport to an EPA-licensed hazardous waste dump site or incinerator is suggested.

6. *Engineering controls should be supplemented with personal protective apparel and other safety materials.* Policies and procedures should be in place to ensure that these materials are used properly and consistently.

a. Workers should wear powder-free, disposable surgical latex gloves of good quality when preparing hazardous drugs. Selection criteria for gloves should include thickness (especially at the fingertips where stress is the greatest), fit, length, and tactile sensation. While no glove material has been shown to be impervious to all hazardous drugs or to be statistically superior in limiting drug penetration, thickness and time in contact with drug are crucial factors affecting permeability.[47-49]

The practice of double gloving is supported by research that indicates that many glove materials vary in drug permeability even within lots;[48,49] therefore, double gloving is recommended. This recommendation is based on currently available research findings. Evidence to show that single gloves are sufficiently protective might make this recommendation unnecessary. In general, surgical latex gloves fit better, have appropriate elasticity for double gloving and maintaining the integrity of the glove-gown interface, and have sufficient tactile sensation (even during double gloving) for stringent aseptic procedures.

b. Powdered gloves increase the particulate level in the filtered air environment of the BSC and leave a powder residue on the surfaces of supplies, final product, and the hands that may absorb contamination generated in the BSC; therefore, powdered gloves should be avoided. The use of sterile gloves is unnecessary during operations involving nonsterile surfaces. Hands must be thoroughly washed and dried before gloves are donned and when a task or batch is completed. If only powdered gloves are available, all powder must be washed off the outside of the outer glove before any operation is begun, and hands should be washed once gloves have been removed.

c. Two pairs of fresh gloves should be put on when beginning any task or batch. The outer glove should be changed immediately if contaminated. Both gloves should be changed if the outer glove is torn, punctured, or overtly contaminated with drug (as in a spill) and every hour during batch operations. During removal of gloves, care should be taken to avoid touching the inside of the glove or the skin with the contaminated glove fingers. To limit transfer of contamination from the BSC into the work area, outer gloves should be removed after each batch and should be placed in "zipper"-closure plastic bags or other sealable containers for disposal.

d. The worker should wear a protective disposable gown made of lint-free, low-permeability fabric with a solid front, long sleeves, and tight-fitting elastic or knit cuffs when preparing hazardous drugs. Washable garments are immediately penetrated by liquids and therefore provide little, if any, protection. In addition, washable garments require laundering and thus potentially expose other personnel to contamination.

e. When double gloving, one glove should be placed under the gown cuff and one over. The glove-gown interface should be such that no skin on the arm or wrist is exposed. Gloves and gowns should not be worn outside the immediate preparation area. On completion of each task or batch, the worker should, while wearing outer gloves, wipe all final products with gauze. The outer gloves should then be removed and placed, along with the gauze, in a sealable container (e.g., a zipper-closure plastic bag) within the BSC. All waste bags in the BSC should be sealed and removed for disposal. The gown should be removed and placed in a sealable container before removal of the inner gloves. The inner gloves should be removed last and placed in the container with the gown.

f. Workers who are not protected by the containment environment of a BSC should use respiratory protection when handling hazardous drugs. Respiratory protection should be an adjunct to and not a substitute for engineering controls.

g. Surgical masks of all types provide no respiratory protection against powdered or liquid aerosols of hazardous drugs.

h. In situations where workers may be exposed to potential eye contact with hazardous drugs, an appropriate plastic face shield or splash goggles should be worn. Eyewash fountains should be available in areas where hazardous drugs are routinely handled. Inexpensive alternatives include an intravenous bag of 0.9% sodium chloride solution (normal saline) or irrigation bottle of water or saline with appropriate tubing.

7. *Proper manipulative technique to maintain the sterility of injectable drugs and to prevent generation of hazardous drug contaminants is used consistently.*

a. Proper manipulative technique must be taught to all workers who will be required to prepare hazardous drugs.[56] Preparers should demonstrate competence in these techniques once training has been completed and at least annually thereafter.

b. Systems to ensure that these techniques are adhered to should exist, along with systems to ensure patient safety by providing that drugs are properly selected, calculated, measured, and delivered.

c. The work area should be designed to provide easy access to those items necessary to prepare, label, and transport final products; contain all related waste; and avoid inadvertent contamination of the work area.

d. Maintenance of proper technique requires an organized approach to the preparation of sterile

doses of hazardous drugs in a BSC. All drug and nondrug items required for completing a dose or batch and for containing the waste should be assembled and placed in the BSC; care should be taken not to overload the BSC work area. All calculations and any label preparation should be completed at this time. Appropriate gowning, hand washing and gloving (or glove changing), and glove washing should be completed before any manipulations are begun. Unnecessary moving in and out of the BSC should be avoided during aseptic manipulations.

e. Syringes and intravenous sets with Luer-lock type fittings should be used for preparing and administering hazardous drug solutions, since they are less prone to accidental separation than friction fittings. Care must be taken to ensure that all connections are secure. Syringes should be large enough so that they are not full when containing the total drug dose. This is to ensure that the plunger does not separate from the syringe barrel. Doses should be dispensed in several syringes when this problem arises.

f. The contents of an ampul should be gently tapped down from the neck and top portion of the ampul before it is opened. The ampul should be wiped with alcohol before being opened. A sterile gauze pad should be wrapped around the neck of the ampul when it is opened.

g. Substantial positive or negative deviations from atmospheric pressure within drug vials and syringes should be avoided.

h. For additional worker protection, equipment such as venting devices with 0.2-μm hydrophobic filters and 5-μm filter needles or "straws" may be used. It is critical that the worker be proficient with these devices before using them with hazardous drugs. Improper use of these devices may result in increased, rather than decreased, risk of exposure.

i. Final products should be dispensed in ready-to-administer form. If possible, intravenous administration sets should be attached to the bag or bottle in the BSC and primed with plain fluid before the hazardous drug is added. However, if total volume is a concern, intravenous sets may be primed with diluted drug solution, which is discarded into an appropriate container within the BSC. Potential disadvantages to this approach include difficulty in selecting the appropriate administration set when several methods of administering hazardous drugs exist, potential contamination of the outside of the intravenous set, and the risk of the intravenous set becoming dislodged from the bag or bottle during transport.

j. The outside of bags or bottles and intravenous sets (if used) should be wiped with moist gauze to remove any inadvertent contamination. Entry ports should be wiped with sterile, alcohol-dampened gauze pads and covered with appropriate seals or caps.

k. Final products should be placed in sealable containers (e.g., zipper-closure plastic bags) to reduce the risk of exposing ancillary personnel or contaminating the environment. Containers should be designed such that damage incurred during storage or transport is immediately visible and any leakage is fully contained. For offsite transport, appropriate storage conditions (e.g., refrigerated, padded, and locked carriers) should also be used.

l. Excess drug should be returned to the drug vial whenever possible or discarded into a closed container (empty sterile vial). Placing excess drug in any type of open container, even while working in the BSC, is inappropriate. Discarding excess drug into the drainage trough of the BSC is also inappropriate. These practices unnecessarily increase the risk of exposure to large amounts of hazardous drug.

m. All contaminated materials should be placed in leakproof, puncture-resistant containers within the contained environment of the BSC and then placed in larger containers outside the BSC for disposal. To minimize aerosolization, needles should be discarded in puncture-resistant containers without being clipped.

8. *Procedures for the preparation and dispensing of noninjectable dosage forms of hazardous drugs are established and followed.*

a. Although noninjectable dosage forms of hazardous drugs contain varying proportions of drug to nondrug (nonhazardous) components, there is potential for personnel exposure and environmental contamination with the hazardous components. Procedures should be developed to avoid the release of aerosolized powder or liquid into the environment during manipulation of these drugs.

b. Drugs designated as hazardous should be labeled or otherwise identified as such to prevent their improper handling.

c. Tablet and capsule forms of these drugs should not be placed in automated counting machines, which subject them to stress and may introduce powdered contaminants into the work area.

d. During *routine handling* of hazardous drugs and contaminated equipment, workers should wear one pair of gloves of good quality and thickness.

e. The counting and pouring of hazardous drugs should be done carefully, and clean equipment dedicated for use with these drugs should be used. Contaminated equipment should be cleaned initially with water-saturated gauze and then further cleaned with detergent and rinsed. The gauze and rinse should be disposed of as contaminated waste.

f. During *compounding* of hazardous drugs (e.g., crushing, dissolving, and preparing an ointment), workers should wear low-permeability gowns and double gloves. Compounding should take place in a protective area such as a disposable glove box. If compounding must be done in the open, an area away from drafts and traffic must be selected, and the worker should use appropriate respiratory protection.

g. When hazardous drug tablets in unit-of-use packaging are being crushed, the package should be placed in a small sealable plastic bag and crushed with a spoon or pestle; caution should be used not

to break the plastic bag.

h. Disposal of unused or unusable oral or topical dosage forms of hazardous drugs should be performed in the same manner as for hazardous injectable dosage forms and waste.

9. *Personnel know the procedures to be followed in case of accidental skin or eye contact with hazardous drugs.*

a. Each health-care setting should have an established first aid protocol for treating cases of direct contact with hazardous drugs, many of which are irritating or caustic and can cause tissue destruction. Medical care providers in each setting should be contacted for input into this protocol. The protocol should include immediate treatment measures and should specify the type and location of medical followup and work-injury reporting. Copies of the protocol, highlighting emergency measures, should be posted wherever hazardous drugs are routinely handled.

b. Hazardous drug work areas should have a sink (preferably with an eyewash fountain) and appropriate first aid equipment to treat accidental skin or eye contact according to the protocol.

c. In settings where hazardous drug handlers are offsite (e.g., home use), protocols must be part of orientation programs, and copies of the procedures should be immediately accessible to handlers, along with appropriate first aid equipment and emergency phone numbers to call for followup and reporting.

10. *All hazardous drugs are labeled with a warning label stating the need for special handling.*

a. A distinctive warning label with an appropriate CAUTION statement should be attached to all hazardous drug materials, consistent with state laws and regulations. This would include, for example, syringes, intravenous containers, containers of unit-dose tablets and liquids, prescription vials and bottles, waste containers, and patient specimens that contain hazardous drugs.

b. The hazardous drugs discussed in this Technical Assistance Bulletin are chemical hazards and *not* infectious hazards. Because the term "biohazard" refers to an infectious hazard, the use of this term or the biohazard symbol (in any variation) on the label of drugs that are chemical hazards is inappropriate and may be misleading to staff and contract workers who are familiar with the biohazard symbol. An example of a suitable label is shown in Figure 1.

c. All staff and contract workers should be informed about the meaning of the label and the special handling procedures that have been established.

d. In settings where patients or their families will be responsible for manipulating these drugs, they should be made aware of the need for special handling and the reasons behind it.

Goal III. Procedures for administering hazardous drugs prevent the accidental exposure of patients and staff and contamination of the work environment.

1. *A method for informing and training health-care professionals in these procedures is maintained.*

a. Only individuals trained to administer hazardous drugs should be allowed to perform this function. Training programs should contain information on the therapeutic and adverse effects of these drugs and the potential, long-term health risk to personnel handling them. Each individual's knowledge and technique should be evaluated before administration of these drugs. This should be done by written examination and direct observation of the individual's performance.

2. *Standard procedures for the safe administration of hazardous drugs are established and followed.* These procedures ensure the safety of both the patient and health-care personnel.

a. Intravenous administration sets (e.g., vented, nonvented, and minidrip) and infusion devices appropriate for use with the final product should be selected.

b. Syringes and intravenous sets with Luer-lock fittings should be used whenever possible.

c. Preparation of the final product for administration should take place in a clean, uncluttered area separate from other activities and excessive traffic. A plastic-backed absorbent liner should be used to cover the work area to absorb accidental spills. A single pair of disposable latex gloves and a disposable gown should be worn. The glove and gown cuffs should be worn in a manner that produces a tight fit (e.g., loose glove tucked under gown cuff; tight glove fitted over gown cuff). Hands must be thoroughly washed before gloves are donned.

Administration sets should be attached with care (if not attached during drug preparation). Administration sets and devices should be monitored for leakage.

d. Priming of intravenous sets should not allow any drug to be released into the environment. Hazardous drug solutions may be "piggybacked" into primary intravenous solutions and primed by retrograde flow of the primary solution into the secondary tubing. All Y-site connections should be taped securely. Alternatively, the intravenous set may be primed with plain solution before the hazardous drug solution bag or bottle is connected. Some intravenous sets can be primed so that the fluid enters the medication port of the intravenous bag. The priming fluid may also be discarded into a sealable plastic bag containing absorbent material if care is taken not to contaminate the sterile needle tip. Likewise, a sterile gauze pad should be placed close to the sterile needle tip when air is expelled from a syringe. The syringe plunger should first be drawn back to withdraw liquid from the needle before air is expelled. Care should be taken not to contaminate the sterile needle with gauze fibers or microorganisms.

e. Intravenous containers designed with venting tubes should not be used. If such containers must be used, gauze should be placed over the tube when the container is inverted to catch any hazardous drug solution trapped in the tube. If containers with solid stoppers are used, any vacuum present should be eliminated before the con-

tainer is attached to a primary intravenous or to a manifold. If a series of bags or bottles is used to deliver the drug, the intravenous set should be discarded with each container because removing the spike from the container is associated with a greater risk of environmental contamination than priming an intravenous set. (Use of secondary sets for administration of hazardous drugs reduces the cost of this recommendation and the risk of priming.)

f. A plastic-backed absorbent liner should be placed under the intravenous tubing during administration to absorb any leakage and prevent the solution from spilling onto the patient's skin. The use of sterile gauze around any "push" sites will reduce the likelihood of releasing drug into the environment.

g. The use of eye protection (safety glasses or goggles) during work with hazardous drugs, especially vesicants, should be considered. Work at your waist level, if possible; avoid working above the head or reaching up for connections or ports.

h. All contaminated gauze, syringes, intravenous sets, bags, bottles, etc., should be placed in sealable plastic bags and placed in a puncture-resistant container for removal from the patient-care area.

i. Gloves should be discarded after each use and immediately if contaminated. Gowns should be discarded on leaving the patient-care area and immediately if contaminated. Hands must be washed thoroughly after hazardous drugs are handled.

j. Gloves should be worn when urine and other excreta from patients receiving hazardous drugs are being handled. Skin contact and splattering should be avoided during disposal. While it may be useful to post a list of drugs that are excreted in urine and feces and the length of time after drug administration during which precautions are necessary, an alternative is to select a standard duration (e.g., 48 hours) that covers most of the drugs and is more easily remembered.

k. Disposable linen or protective pads should be used for incontinent or vomiting patients. Nondisposable linen contaminated with hazardous drug should be handled with gloves and treated similarly to that for linen contaminated with infectious material. One procedure is to place the linen in specially marked water-soluble laundry bags. These bags (with the contents) should be prewashed; then the linens should be added to other laundry for an additional wash. Items contaminated with hazardous drugs should not be autoclaved unless they are also contaminated with infectious material.

3. *Appropriate apparel and materials needed to protect staff and patients from exposure and to protect the work environment from contamination are readily available.* Supplies of disposable gloves and gowns, safety glasses, disposable plastic-backed absorbent liners, gauze pads, hazardous waste disposal bags, hazardous drug warning labels, and puncture-resistant containers for disposal of needles and ampuls should

be conveniently located for all areas where hazardous drugs are handled. Assembling a "hazardous drug preparation and administration kit" is one way to furnish nursing and medical personnel with the materials needed to reduce the risk of preparing and administering a hazardous drug.

4. *Personnel know the procedures to be followed in case of accidental skin or eye contact with hazardous drugs. (See Goal II9.)*

Goal IV. The health-care setting, its staff, patients, contract workers, visitors, and the outside environment are not exposed to or contaminated with hazardous drug waste materials produced in the course of using these drugs. (See Figure 2 for proposed flow chart for handling contaminated items.)

1. *Written policies and procedures governing the identification, containment, collection, segregation, and disposal of hazardous drug waste materials are established and maintained.* All health-care workers who handle hazardous drugs or waste must be oriented to and must follow these procedures.

2. *Throughout institutional health-care facilities and in alternative health-care settings, hazardous drug waste materials are identified, contained, and segregated from all other trash.*

   a. Hazardous drug waste should be placed in specially marked (specifically labeled CAUTION: HAZARDOUS CHEMICAL WASTE) thick plastic bags or leakproof containers. These receptacles should be kept in all areas where the drugs are commonly used. All and only hazardous drug waste should be placed in them. Receptacles used for glass fragments, needles, and syringes should be puncture resistant. Hazardous drug waste should not be mixed with any other waste. Waste containers should be handled with uncontaminated gloves.

   b. Health-care personnel providing care in a patient's home should have with them all the equipment and supplies necessary to contain properly any hazardous drug waste that is generated during the visit. Contaminated needles and syringes, intravenous containers, intravenous sets, and any broken ampuls should be placed in leakproof, puncture-resistant containers. Gloves, gowns, drug vials, etc., should be sealed in specially labeled (CAUTION: HAZARDOUS CHEMICAL WASTE) thick plastic bags or leakproof containers. All waste should be removed from the patient's home and transported to a designated area. Additional precautions should be taken during transport, including temporary storage in a spill-resistant container and ensuring that the vehicle is locked at all times. Hazardous waste should be securely stored at a designated area until it is picked up for appropriate disposal. Patients or their caregivers should be instructed on methods for the proper handling of excreta from patients receiving hazardous drugs.

   c. Unless restricted by state or local regulations, hazardous drug waste may be further divided into trace and bulk-contaminated waste, if desired, to reduce costs of disposal. As defined by the EPA, bulk-contaminated materials are solutions or containers whose contents weigh more than 3% of the capacity of the container.[57,58] For example, empty intravenous containers and intravenous administration sets usually are considered trace waste; half-empty vials of hazardous drugs and unused final doses in syringes or intravenous containers are considered bulk-contaminated waste. If trace and bulk-contaminated waste are handled separately, bulk-contaminated waste should be segregated into more secure receptacles for containment and disposal as toxic waste. While this may allow for less expensive overall disposal of hazardous waste, it also requires close monitoring of the containment and segregation process to prevent the accidental discarding of a bulk-contaminated container into a trace-waste receptacle.

   d. All hazardous waste collected from drug preparation and patient-care areas should be held in a secure place in labeled, leakproof drums or cartons (as required by state or local regulation or disposal contractor) until disposal. This waste should be disposed of as hazardous or toxic waste in an EPA-permitted, state-licensed hazardous waste incinerator. Transport to an offsite incinerator should be done by a contractor licensed to handle and transport hazardous waste. (While licenses are generally required to transport infectious waste as well as hazardous waste, these are different classes of contractors and may not be interchanged. Verification of possession and type of license should be documented before a contractor is engaged.)

   e. If access to an appropriately licensed incinerator is not available, transport to and burial in an EPA-licensed hazardous waste dump site is an acceptable alternative. While there are concerns that destruction of carcinogens by incineration may be incomplete, newer technologies and stringent licensing criteria have improved this dis-

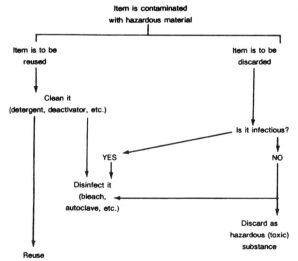

Figure 2. Proposed flow chart for handling chemical hazards versus biohazards. Disinfection of a disposable item contaminated with both infectious and hazardous material may not be necessary, depending on the degree of infectious hazard (e.g., human immunodeficiency virus versus *Escherichia coli*) and depending on the method of disposal (e.g., burial versus incineration).

posal method. (Again, the existence and type of license should be verified before use of a contract incinerator.)

    f. Chemical deactivation of hazardous drugs should be undertaken only by individuals who are thoroughly familiar with the chemicals and the procedures required to complete such a task. The IARC recently published a monograph describing methods for chemical destruction of some cytotoxic (antineoplastic) drugs in the laboratory setting.[59] The chemicals and equipment described, however, are not generally found in the clinical setting, and many of the deactivating chemicals are toxic and hazardous. Most procedures require the use of a chemical fume hood. The procedures are generally difficult, and the deactivation is not always complete. Serious consideration should be given to the negative aspects of chemical deactivation before one commits to such a course of action.

3. *Materials to clean up spills of hazardous drugs are readily available and personnel are trained in their proper use.* A standard cleanup protocol is established and followed.

    a. "Spill kits" containing all materials needed to clean up spills of hazardous drugs should be assembled or purchased. These kits should be readily available in all areas where hazardous drugs are routinely handled. If hazardous drugs are being prepared or administered in a nonroutine area (home setting or unusual patient-care area), a spill kit should be obtained by the drug handler. The kit should include two pairs of disposable gloves (one outer pair of utility gloves and one inner latex pair); low permeability, disposable protective garments (coveralls or gown and shoe covers); safety glasses or splash goggles; respirator; absorbent, plastic-backed sheets or spill pads; disposable toweling; at least two sealable thick plastic hazardous waste disposal bags (prelabeled with an appropriate warning label); a disposable scoop for collecting glass fragments; and a puncture-resistant container for glass fragments.

    b. All individuals who routinely handle hazardous drugs must be trained in proper spill management and cleanup procedures. Spills and breakages must be cleaned up immediately according to the following procedures. If the spill is not located in a confined space, the spill area should be identified and other people should be prevented from approaching and spreading the contamination. Wearing protective apparel from the spill kit, workers should remove any broken glass fragments and place them in the puncture-resistant container. Liquids should be absorbed with a spill pad; powder should be removed with damp disposable gauze pads or soft toweling. The hazardous material should be completely removed and the area rinsed with water and then cleaned with detergent. The spill cleanup should proceed progressively from areas of lesser to greater contamination. The detergent should be thoroughly rinsed and removed. All contaminated materials should be placed in the disposal bags provided and sealed and transported to a designated containment receptacle.

    c. Spills occurring in the BSC should be cleaned up immediately; a spill kit should be used if the volume exceeds 150 ml or the contents of one drug vial or ampul. If there is broken glass, utility gloves should be worn to remove it and place it in the puncture-resistant container located in the BSC. The BSC, including the drain spillage trough, should be thoroughly cleaned. If the spill is not easily and thoroughly contained, the BSC should be decontaminated after cleanup. If the spill contaminates the HEPA filter, use of the BSC should be suspended until the cabinet has been decontaminated and the HEPA filter replaced. (See Goal II 5j.)

    d. If hazardous drugs are routinely prepared or administered in carpeted areas, special equipment is necessary to remove the spill. Absorbent powder should be substituted for pads or sheets and left in place on the spill for the time recommended by the manufacturer. The powder should then be picked up with a small vacuum unit reserved for hazardous drug cleanup. The carpet should then be cleaned according to usual procedures. The vacuum bag should be removed and discarded or cleaned, and the exterior of the vacuum cleaner should be washed with detergent and rinsed before being covered and stored. The contaminated powder should be discarded into a sealable plastic bag and segregated with other contaminated waste materials. Alternatively, inexpensive wet or dry vacuum units may be purchased for this express use and used with appropriate cleaners. All such units are contaminated, once used, and must be cleaned, stored, and ultimately discarded appropriately (i.e., like BSCs).

    e. The circumstances and handling of spills should be documented. Health-care personnel exposed during spill management should also complete an incident report or exposure form.

4. *Hazardous drug waste is disposed of in accordance with all applicable state, federal, and local regulations for the handling of hazardous and toxic waste.*

    a. Regulatory agencies such as the EPA and state solid and hazardous waste agencies and local air and water quality control boards must be consulted regarding the classification and appropriate disposal of drugs that are defined as hazardous or toxic chemicals. EPA categorizes several of the antineoplastic agents (including cyclophosphamide and daunorubicin) as toxic wastes, while many states are more stringent and include as carcinogens certain cytotoxic drugs (azathioprine) and hormonal preparations (diethylstilbestrol and conjugated estrogens). EPA also allows exemptions from toxic waste regulations for "small quantity generators,"[57] whereas certain states do not. It is critical to research these regulations when disposal procedures are being established.

Other Hazardous Drug Issues

The handling of hazardous drugs, some of which are defined by the EPA as toxic chemicals, has implications that go beyond the health-care setting. Disposal of hazardous materials and toxic chemicals continues to be a controversial issue of which the disposal of hazardous drugs is but a small part. The EPA currently issues permits for both burial and incineration of hazardous waste. Some such facilities may purport to possess permits to handle these types of hazardous agents when, in fact, they do not meet the requirements or are only in the initial stages of obtaining permits. It is imperative that health-care facilities verify the license or permit status of any contractor used to remove or dispose of infectious or hazardous waste. In addition, many hazardous drugs are excreted unchanged or as equally toxic metabolites. The amount of hazardous drug transferred to the environment (primarily through the water supply) from this source may exceed that resulting from the hospital trash pathway. No good methods for reducing this source of contamination are currently known.

Definitive risks of handling these drugs may never be fully determined without epidemiologic data from a national registry of handlers of hazardous drugs (and chemicals). There is no method available for routine monitoring of personnel for evidence of hazardous drug exposure. Tests for the presence of mutagens or chromosomal damage are not drug specific and are of value only in controlled studies. Chemical analysis of urine for the presence of hazardous drugs at the sensitivity level needed to detect occupational exposure is limited to a few drugs and is not yet commercially available.

This document is designed to identify areas of risk in the handling of hazardous drugs and to provide recommendations for reducing that risk. A safety program should be coupled with a strong quality-assurance program that periodically evaluates and verifies staff adherence to and performance of the established safe handling policies and procedures. Until some type of external monitoring of exposure levels from handling hazardous drugs is commercially available, development of and compliance with a safety program remain the most logical means for minimizing occupational risk.

References

1. American Society of Hospital Pharmacists. ASHP technical assistance bulletin on handling cytotoxic drugs in hospitals. *Am J Hosp Pharm.* 1985; 42:131–7.
2. Yodaiken R. Safe handling of cytotoxic drugs by health care personnel. Washington, DC: Occupational Safety and Health Administration; 1986 Jan 29. (Instructional publication 8-1.1).
3. U.S. Public Health Service, National Institutes of Health. Recommendations for the safe handling of parenteral antineoplastic drugs. Washington, DC: U.S. Department of Health and Human Services; 1983. (NIH publication 83-2621).
4. Recommendations for handling cytotoxic agents. Providence, RI: National Study Commission on Cytotoxic Exposure; 1987 Sep.
5. AMA Council on Scientific Affairs. Guidelines for handling parenteral antineoplastics. *JAMA.* 1985; 253:1590–2.
6. Scott SA. Antineoplastic drug information and handling guidelines for office-based physicians. *Am J Hosp Pharm.* 1984; 41:2402–3.
7. Barstow J. Safe handling of cytotoxic agents in the home. *Home Healthc Nurse.* 1986; 3:46–7.
8. Barry LK, Booher RB. Promoting the responsible handling of antineoplastic agents in the community. *Oncol Nurs Forum.* 1985; 12:40–6.
9. Berk PD, Goldberg JD, Silverstein MN, et al. Increased incidence of leukemia in polycythemia vera associated with chlorambucil therapy. *N Engl J Med.* 1981; 304:441–7.
10. Penn I. Occurrence of cancer in immune deficiencies. *Cancer.* 1974; 34:858–66.
11. Schafer AI. Teratogenic effects of antileukemic therapy. *Arch Intern Med.* 1981; 141:514–5.
12. Stephens JD, Golbus MS, Miller TR, et al. Multiple congenital abnormalities in a fetus exposed to 5-fluorouracil during the first trimester. *Am J Obstet Gynecol.* 1980; 137:747–9.
13. IARC monographs on the evaluation of the carcinogenic risk of chemicals to humans. Geneva, Switzerland: World Health Organization; 1981.
14. Benedict WF, Baker MS, Haroun L, et al. Mutagenicity of cancer chemotherapeutic agents in the *Salmonella*/microsome test. *Cancer Res.* 1977; 37:2209–13.
15. Falck K, Grohn P, Sorsa M, et al. Mutagenicity in urine of nurses handling cytostatic drugs. *Lancet.* 1979; 1:1250–1.
16. Anderson RW, Puckett WH, Dana WJ, et al. Risk of handling injectable antineoplastic agents. *Am J Hosp Pharm.* 1982; 39:1881–7.
17. Norppa H, Sorsa M, Vainio H, et al. Increased sister chromatid exchange frequencies in lymphocytes of nurses handling cytostatic drugs. *Scand J Work Environ Health.* 1980; 6:299–301.
18. Waksvik H, Klepp O, Brogger A. Chromosome analyses of nurses handling cytostatic agents. *Cancer Treat Rep.* 1981; 65:607–10.
19. Nikula E, Kiviniitty K, Leisti J, et al. Chromosome aberrations in lymphocytes of nurses handling cytostatic agents. *Scand J Work Environ Health.* 1984; 10:71–4.
20. Chrysostomou A, Morley AA, Sehadri R. Mutation frequency in nurses and pharmacists working with cytotoxic drugs. *Aust N Z J Med.* 1984; 14:831–4.
21. Rogers B, Emmett EA. Handling antineoplastic agents: urine mutagenicity in nurses. *Image J Nurs Sch.* 1987; 19:108–13.
22. Palmer RG, Dore CJ, Denman AM. Chlorambucil-induced chromosome damage to human lymphocytes is dose-dependent and cumulative. *Lancet.* 1984; 1:246–9.
23. Sotaniemi EA, Sutinen S, Arranto AJ, et al. Liver damage in nurses handling cytostatic agents. *Acta Med Scand.* 1983; 214:181–9.
24. How real is the hazard? *Lancet.* 1984; 1:203.
25. Tuffnell PG, Gannon MT, Dong A, et al. Limitations of urinary mutagen assays for monitoring occupational exposure to antineoplastic drugs. *Am J Hosp Pharm.* 1986; 43:344–8.
26. Cloak MM, Connor TH, Stevens KR, et al. Occupational exposure of nursing personnel to antineoplastic agents. *Oncol Nurs Forum.* 1985; 12:33–9.
27. Connor TH, Anderson RW. Demonstrating mutagenicity testing using the Ames test. *Am J Hosp Pharm.* 1985; 42:783–4.
28. Connor TH, Theiss JC, Anderson RW, et al. Re-evaluation of urine mutagenicity of pharmacy person-

nel exposed to antineoplastic agents. *Am J Hosp Pharm.* 1986; 43:1236–9.

29. Jagun O, Ryan M, Waldrom HA. Urinary thioether excretion in nurses handling cytotoxic drugs. *Lancet.* 1982; 2:443–4.

30. Hirst M, Tse S, Mills DG, et al. Occupational exposure to cyclophosphamide. *Lancet.* 1984; 1:186–8.

31. Venitt S, Crofton-Sleigh C, Hunt J, et al. Monitoring exposure of nursing and pharmacy personnel to cytotoxic drugs: urinary mutation assays and urinary platinum as markers of absorption. *Lancet.* 1984; 1:74–6.

32. Neal A deW, Wadden RA, Chiou WL. Exposure of hospital workers to airborne antineoplastic agents. *Am J Hosp Pharm.* 1983; 40:597–601.

33. Kleinberg ML, Quinn MJ. Airborne drug levels in a laminar flow hood. *Am J Hosp Pharm.* 1981; 38:1301–3.

34. Gililland J, Weinstein L. The effects of chemotherapeutic agents on the developing fetus. *Obstet Gynecol Surv.* 1983; 38:6–13.

35. Hemminki K, Kyyronen P, Lindbohm ML. Spontaneous abortions and malformations in the offspring of nurses exposed to anesthetic gases, cytostatic drugs and other potential hazards in hospitals, based on registered information of outcome. *J Epidemiol Community Health.* 1985; 39:141–7.

36. Selevan SH, Lindbohm ML, Hornung RW, et al. A study of occupational exposure to antineoplastic drugs and fetal loss in nurses. *N Engl J Med.* 1985; 333:1173–8.

37. Richter P, Calamera JC, Morgenfeld MC, et al. Effect of chlorambucil on spermatogenesis in the human with malignant lymphoma. *Cancer.* 1970; 25:1026–30.

38. Maguire LC. Fertility and cancer therapy. *Postgrad Med.* 1979; 65:293–5.

39. Sherins JJ, DeVita VT Jr. Effect of drug treatment for lymphoma on male reproductive capacity. *Ann Intern Med.* 1973; 79:216–20.

40. Gregoire RE, Segal R, Hale KM. Handling antineoplastic-drug admixtures at cancer centers: practices and pharmacist attitudes. *Am J Hosp Pharm.* 1987; 44:1090–5.

41. Cohen IA, Newland SJ, Kirking DM. Injectable-antineoplastic-drug practices in Michigan hospitals. *Am J Hosp Pharm.* 1987; 44:1096–105.

42. Hoy RH, Stump LM. Effect of an air-venting filter device on aerosol production from vials. *Am J Hosp Pharm.* 1984; 41:324–6.

43. National Sanitation Foundation Standard: Class II (laminar flow) Biohazard Cabinetry. Standard 49. Ann Arbor, MI: National Sanitation Foundation; 1987 Jun.

44. McDiarmid MA, Egan T, Furio M, et al. Sampling for airborne fluorouracil in a hospital drug preparation area. *Am J Hosp Pharm.* 1986; 43:1942–5.

45. Clark RP, Goff MR. The potassium iodide method for determining protection factors in open-fronted microbiological safety cabinets. *J Appl Biol.* 1981; 51:461–73.

46. Connor TH, Laidlaw JL, Theiss JC, et al. Permeability of latex and polyvinyl chloride gloves to carmustine. *Am J Hosp Pharm.* 1984; 41:676–9.

47. Laidlaw JL, Connor TH, Theiss JC, et al. Permeability of latex and polyvinyl chloride gloves to 20 antineoplastic drugs. *Am J Hosp Pharm.* 1984; 41:2618–23.

48. Slevin ML, Ang LM, Johnston A, et al. The efficiency of protective gloves used in the handling of cytotoxic drugs. *Cancer Chemother Pharmacol.* 1984; 12:151–3.

49. Stoikes ME, Carlson JD, Farris FF, et al. Permeability of latex and polyvinyl chloride gloves to fluorouracil and methotrexate. *Am J Hosp Pharm.* 1987; 44:1341–6.

50. Laidlaw JL, Connor TH, Theiss JC, et al. Permeability of four disposable protective-clothing materials to seven antineoplastic drugs. *Am J Hosp Pharm.* 1985; 42:2449–54.

51. Falck K, Sorsa M, Vainio H. Use of the bacterial fluctuation test to detect mutagenicity in urine of nurses handling cytostatic drugs. *Mutat Res.* 1981; 85:236–7.

52. Myers CE. Preparing a list of cytotoxic agents. *Am J Hosp Pharm.* 1987; 44:1296, 1298. Questions and Answers.

53. National Institute of Occupational Safety and Health. Respirator decision logic. Washington, DC: U.S. Department of Health and Human Services; 1987. (DHHS, NIOSH publication 87-108).

54. Commissioner, Federal Supply Service, General Services Administration. Federal Standard 209C. Clean room and work station requirements, controlled environments. Washington, DC: U.S. Government Printing Office; 1988.

55. Bryan D, Marback MA. Laminar-airflow equipment certification: what the pharmacist needs to know. *Am J Hosp Pharm.* 1984; 41:1343–9.

56. Wilson JP, Solimando DA. Aseptic technique as a safety precaution in the preparation of antineoplastic agents. *Hosp Pharm.* 1981; 15:575–81.

57. F40 CFR 261.5.

58. Vaccari PL, Tonat K, DeChristoforo R, et al. Disposal of antineoplastic wastes at the National Institutes of Health. *Am J Hosp Pharm.* 1984; 41:87–93.

59. Castegnaro M, Adams J, Armour MA, et al., eds. Laboratory decontamination and destruction of carcinogens in laboratory wastes: some antineoplastic agents. International Agency for Research on Cancer Scientific Publication 73. Fair Lawn, NJ: Oxford University Press; 1985.

Appendix A—Glossary

Biohazard: An infectious agent presenting a real or potential risk to humans and the environment.

Carcinogen: Any cancer-producing substance.

Chemotherapy: The treatment of disease by chemical means; first applied to use of chemicals that affect the causative organism unfavorably but do not harm the patient; currently used to describe drug (chemical) therapy of neoplastic diseases (cancer).

Clastogenic: Giving rise to or inducing disruption or breakage, as of chromosomes.

Contamination: The deposition of potentially dangerous material where it is not desired, particularly where its presence may be harmful or constitute a hazard.

Cytotoxic: Possessing a specific destructive action on certain cells; used commonly in referring to antineoplastic drugs that selectively kill dividing cells.

Decontamination: Removal, neutralization, or destruction of a toxic (harmful) agent.

Exposure: The condition of being subjected to something, as to chemicals, that may have a harmful effect. Acute exposure is exposure of short duration, usually exposure of heavy intensity; chronic exposure is long-term exposure, either continuous or intermittent, usually referring to exposure of low intensity.

Genotoxic: Damaging to DNA; pertaining to agents (radiation or chemical substances) known to damage DNA, thereby causing mutations or cancer.

Hazardous: Dangerous; risky; representing a health risk.

Mutagen: Chemical or physical agent that induces or increases genetic mutations by causing changes in DNA.

Plenum: Space within a biohazard cabinet where air flows; plenums may either be under positive (greater than atmospheric pressure) or negative pressure, depending on whether the air is "blown" or "sucked" through the space.

Respirator: A National Institute of Occupational Safety and Health (NIOSH) approved, air-purifying half-mask respirator equipped with a high-efficiency filter; may be disposable (discarded after the end of its recommended period of use).

Trough: Drain spillage trough; an area below the biological safety cabinet's work surface, provided to retain spillage from the work area.

Utility gloves: Heavy, disposable gloves, similar to household latex gloves.

Appendix B—Classification of Biohazard Cabinetry (Biological Safety Cabinets)[43]

Class I: A ventilated cabinet for personnel and environmental protection, with an unrecirculated inward airflow away from the operator.
Note: The cabinet exhaust air is treated to protect the environment before it is discharged to the outside atmosphere. This cabinet is suitable for work with low- and moderate-risk biological agents when no product protection is required.

Class II: A ventilated cabinet for personnel, product, and environmental protection, having an open front with inward airflow for personnel protection, high-efficiency particulate air (HEPA) filtered laminar airflow for product protection, and HEPA-filtered exhausted air for environmental protection.
Note: When toxic chemicals or radionuclides are used as adjuncts to biological studies or pharmaceutical work, Class II cabinets designed and constructed for this purpose should be used.

- *Type A (formerly designated Type 1)*: Cabinets that (1) maintain minimum calculated average inflow velocity of 75 feet per minute (fpm) through the work area access opening; (2) have HEPA-filtered downflow air from a common plenum (i.e., plenum from which a portion of the air is exhausted from the cabinet and the remainder is supplied to the work area); (3) may exhaust HEPA-filtered air back into the laboratory; and (4) may have positive-pressure-contaminated ducts and plenums. Type A cabinets are suitable for work with low- to moderate-risk biological agents in the absence of volatile toxic chemicals and volatile radionuclides.

- *Type B1 (formerly designated Type 2)*: Cabinets that (1) maintain a minimum (calculated or measured) average inflow velocity of 100 fpm through the work area access opening; (2) have HEPA-filtered downflow air composed largely of uncontaminated recirculated inflow air; (3) exhaust most of the contaminated downflow air through a dedicated duct exhausted to the atmosphere after it passes through a HEPA filter; and (4) have all biologically contaminated ducts and plenums under negative pressure or surrounded by negative-pressure ducts and plenums. Type B1 cabinets are suitable for work with low- to moderate-risk biological agents. They may also be used with biological agents treated with minute quantities of toxic chemicals and trace amounts of radionuclides required as an adjunct to microbiological studies if work is done in the directly exhausted portion of the cabinet or if the chemicals or radionuclides will not interfere with the work when recirculated in the downflow air.

- *Type B2 (sometimes referred to as "total exhaust")*: Cabinets that (1) maintain a minimum (calculated or measured) average inflow velocity of 100 fpm through the work area access opening; (2) have HEPA-filtered downflow air drawn from the laboratory or the outside air (i.e., downflow air is not recirculated from the cabinet exhaust air); (3) exhaust all inflow and downflow air to the atmosphere after filtration through a HEPA filter without recirculation in the cabinet or return to the laboratory room air; and (4) have all contaminated ducts and plenums under negative pressure or surrounded by directly exhausted (nonrecirculated through the work area) negative-pressure ducts and plenums. Type B2 cabinets are suitable for work with low- to moderate-risk biological agents. They may also be used with biological agents treated with toxic chemicals and radionuclides required as an adjunct to microbiological studies.

- *Type B3 (sometimes referred to as "convertible cabinets")*: Cabinets that (1) maintain a minimum (calculated or measured) average inflow velocity of 100 fpm through the work access opening; (2) have HEPA-filtered downflow air that is a portion of the mixed downflow and inflow air from a common exhaust plenum; (3) discharge all exhaust air to the outdoor atmosphere after HEPA filtration; and (4) have all biologically contaminated ducts and plenums under negative pressure or surrounded by negative-pressure ducts and plenums. Type B3 cabinets are suitable for work with low- to moderate-risk biological agents treated with minute quantities of toxic chemicals and trace quantities of radionuclides that will not interfere with the work if recirculated in the downflow air.

- *Other Types*: Other cabinets may be considered Class II if they meet these requirements for performance, durability, reliability, safety, operational integrity, and cleanability.

Class III: A totally enclosed, ventilated cabinet of gas-tight construction. Operations in the cabinet are conducted through attached rubber gloves. The cabinet is maintained under negative air pressure of at least 0.5 inch (12.7 mm) water gauge (wg). Supply air is drawn into the cabinet through HEPA filters. The exhaust air is treated by double HEPA filtration or by HEPA filtration and incineration.

Revised by ASHP's Clinical Affairs Department in collaboration with Luci A. Power, M.S., Senior Consultant, Power Enterprises, San Francisco, CA. Reviewed by the officers of the ASHP Special Interest Group (SIG) on Oncology Pharmacy Practice and approved by the ASHP Council on Professional Affairs, September 20, 1989. Approved by the ASHP Board of Directors, November 15–16, 1989. Supersedes a previous version approved by the Board of Directors on November 14, 1984.

The bibliographic citation for this document is as follows: American Society of Hospital Pharmacists. ASHP technical assistance bulletin on handling cytotoxic and hazardous drugs. *Am J Hosp Pharm.* 1990; 47:1033–49.

This Technical Assistance Bulletin was reviewed in 1996 by the Council on Professional Affairs and by the Board of Directors and was found to still be appropriate.

ASHP Technical Assistance Bulletin on Assessing Cost-Containment Strategies for Pharmacies in Organized Health-Care Settings

Health-care cost-containment efforts continue to exert increased pressure on providers of care to cost justify and improve the quality of their services. As increasingly scarce resources are allocated within an organization, the administrative skills of the pharmacy manager will play a key role in determining whether the level of services offered by the department can be maintained or expanded. Pharmacists in organized health-care settings are faced with constraints on reimbursement and increasing pressure to reduce not only the cost of drug therapy but also the total cost of providing pharmaceutical services.

Pharmacy managers who are evaluating the performance and benefits of existing pharmaceutical services or the addition of new services or personnel should conduct five key analyses: environmental, internal, demand, benefit, and cost. An environmental analysis assesses the external environment of regulatory and demographic changes, payer and competitor activities, and changes in the workforce supply. Internal analyses identify the strengths and weaknesses of the pharmacy in the specific practice site.

A demand analysis uses statistics and data to assess the demand for pharmaceutical services; useful demand information includes the number and types of services, the number and intensity of patients receiving pharmaceutical care, and the use of pharmaceutical services and products per diagnosis-related group (DRG) or per member month. A benefit analysis describes and quantifies benefits that accrue to the organization because of pharmaceutical care; they could include cost savings, improvements in quality of care, reductions in length of stay, and risk management benefits. Finally, the costs of providing pharmaceutical care can be determined in a cost analysis of salaries, supplies, overhead, and other fixed and variable costs.

This document is intended as an instrument for identifying the components of the internal analysis.

In identifying areas for potential cost reductions, it is imperative that pharmacy managers evaluate the benefits and costs of the entire drug use process. Since few analytical tools are currently available for identifying and evaluating components of the drug use process, ASHP's Council on Administrative Affairs designed and recommended a checklist to assist the pharmacy manager in that task.

If the scope of pharmacy cost responsibility extends beyond the product to the entire drug use process, then it is more likely that effective cost reductions can be achieved without compromising quality. The drug use process is defined as a multistage continuum that begins with the perception of a need for a drug and ends with an evaluation of the drug's effectiveness in the patient. This continuum includes the selection of a drug regimen, the delivery of the drug product, its administration to the patient, the monitoring of its effects, and the patient's therapeutic outcome. The ultimate responsibility of the pharmacist is to ensure the safe and appropriate use of drugs at all points along this continuum.

The Council on Administrative Affairs designed the checklist as an audit to assist the pharmacy manager in assessing current cost-containment strategies and in establishing new ones. The multilevel format of the checklist allows its use by all pharmacy managers, regardless of their experience or the organization's size and level of care. This document is intended to be applicable to all organized health-care settings. Individual questions in the checklist may contain terminology that is specific to a distinct practice. For example, "per member month" and "plan pharmacies" may only be applicable to a managed care setting, and "intravenous fluid waste" may only be applicable to an acute care inpatient setting.

The purpose of the checklist is not to establish standards or to identify what services must be offered; rather, it is to assist in determining optimal services for an individual organization. It is a self-evaluation tool to be used only for internal assessment. The audit checklist examines four critical areas: drug product costs, drug therapy regimen costs, productivity, and information systems.

I. Drug Product Costs

Controlling the drug product and its cost is a primary responsibility of a pharmacy department. The definition of drug product cost includes not only the acquisition cost but the total system cost incurred in delivering the product to the patient. The questions in this section will assist in auditing nonacquisition costs.

A. *Purchasing and Inventory Control*

1. Is a single-brand purchasing policy in effect for the pharmacy department?
   a. Has the pharmacy and therapeutics (P&T) committee approved a written generic substitution policy?
   b. Has the P&T committee approved a written therapeutic interchange policy?

For questions 2–5, consider whether prime vendors or competitive bidding is used, either individually or through a group purchasing arrangement, and answer the applicable questions for your pharmacy.

2. Is competitive bidding or a pharmaceutical rebate used for
   High dollar cost items?
   High dollar volume items?
   a. Is either of these methods used:
   Guaranteed prices?
   Price ceilings for the term of the contract?
   b. Are the following considered when evaluating bids:
   Prompt payment discount?
   Terms of payment?
   Prompt payment of rebates?
   Nonperformance penalties?
   Delivery time limitations?

Returned and damaged goods policy and service?
Electronic order entry capabilities?
Value-added services?

   c.   Are contracts negotiated when appropriate?
   d.   Are contracts renegotiated on a regular basis (e.g., annually)?

3. Is group purchasing used when advantageous?

4. If group purchasing is used:
   a.   Are prices guaranteed?
   b.   Is there a mechanism for determining that group prices are not higher than those that could be obtained otherwise?

5. Are primary wholesalers or wholesale contracts used for specific drugs when appropriate?
   a.   Is the wholesaler fee equal to or less than the cost of purchasing drugs directly? (Consider all factors such as increased investment revenues, decreased number of purchase orders, reduced inventory value, and receiving costs.)
   b.   Have inventories been adequately reduced?
   c.   Have ordering and receiving costs been adequately reduced?
   d.   Do outages that require payment of premium prices occur frequently?
   e.   Are there frequent outages?

6. Are volume discounts and rebate agreements evaluated for net savings (gross savings minus increased carrying or administrative cost) before purchase?

7. Has an inventory turnover rate been calculated for your organization?
   a.   Is this rate optimal for the facility?

8. Are any of the following used in inventory control: ABC method, minimum and maximum quantities, EOQ/EOV, and just-in-time/stockless inventory arrangements?

9. Do checks occur at regular intervals to verify that appropriate purchasing and inventory control methods are being followed?
   a.   Are reorder points adjusted as needed?
   b.   Is outdated stock returned promptly?

10. Are inventories controlled in dispensing areas?
   a.   Are minimum and maximum inventories maintained?
   b.   Is the space allotted for each product restricted?
   c.   Is there a routine check for outdated drugs and excesses?
   d.   Are exchange systems used when appropriate (e.g., carts, shelf units, and boxes)?

11. Are drug inventories outside the pharmacy controlled (e.g., nursing units and emergency, operating, and recovery rooms)?
   a.   Is an approved floor stock list used for nondrug items?
   b.   Are there maximum allowable quantities for each item?
   c.   Are inventory dollar limits set for each area?
   d.   Are areas checked monthly for excesses and outdated drugs?

12. Are inventories controlled in plan pharmacies?
   a.   Are plan pharmacies audited for appropriate drug inventory and dispensing?

B. Waste and Pilferage

1. Are bid negotiating, ordering, receiving, and invoice verifying functions separated to the extent feasible?
   a.   Are packing lists and invoices matched against purchase orders for accuracy of item, quantity, and price?
   b.   Are purchase or accounts-payable ledgers verified?
   c.   Is there a periodic audit of all purchasing functions?

2. Are costs of goods sold compared with costs of goods purchased by therapeutic categories?

3. Does the distribution system account for all doses dispensed?
   a.   Are all unused medications returned to the pharmacy?
   b.   Is the number of drugs used on a p.r.n. basis reduced to a minimum?
   c.   Are multiple requests for missing doses investigated?
   d.   Is there a tracking system to monitor the frequency and number of missing doses?

4. Have diversion and pilferage of controlled substances been reduced to a minimum?
   a.   Are amounts of controlled substances purchased compared with amounts dispensed?
   b.   Are amounts of controlled substances dispensed compared with amounts administered and recorded in patient charts?
   c.   Is there accountability of controlled substances in the operating and recovery suites?

5. Are there controls to minimize waste of intravenous admixtures?
   a.   Are there written policies for use of infusion pumps, controllers, and other drug delivery devices?
   b.   Are there lists of drugs approved for use with pumps and controllers?
   c.   Have policies been established for the use of intravenous administration sets, emphasizing routine changes (with written exceptions)?
   d.   Are automatic stop orders used to reduce waste?
   e.   Are there policies restricting oral orders?
   f.   Does an intravenous therapy team exist?
   g.   Are audits conducted to determine the dollar amount of intravenous fluid waste?
   h.   Are there mechanisms for easy, efficient communication of intravenous fluid rate changes and discontinued orders?
   i.   Are standardized dosages, solutions, and volumes established for intravenous drugs?
   j.   Are total parenteral nutrition (TPN) solutions standardized?
   k.   Have manufacturers' premixed solutions been evaluated for their economic advantages?
   l.   Has the calibrated-drip-chamber method of administration of intravenous drugs been evaluated?
   m.   Have prefilled syringes been evaluated for cost-effectiveness?
   n.   Are pharmacy intravenous fluid profiles reconciled regularly with those on the nursing units?
   o.   Has the period of advance preparation been reduced to decrease waste?
   p.   Are returned intravenous solutions reused when possible?

q. Has extended use of pump cassettes or tubing been considered?

r. Have the costs and benefits of syringe pumps versus intermittent small volume containers been evaluated?

6. Is the pharmacy a secure work area?

a. Are locks in place?

b. Is the number of keys limited?

II. Drug Therapy Costs

As the pharmacy's influence over the entire drug use process expands, the opportunities for cost control are increased. Significant costs are associated with inappropriate drug choice, adverse drug reactions, and subtherapeutic treatment. Pharmacists can reduce costs and improve outcomes by adopting a patient-centered practice model referred to as pharmaceutical care. Under this model, described by Hepler and Strand (*Am J Hosp Pharm.* 1990; 47:533–43), the pharmacist is responsible for "(1) identifying potential and actual drug-related problems, (2) resolving actual drug-related problems, and (3) preventing potential drug-related problems."

By working with the patient and other professionals, the pharmacist can influence the perceived need for a drug, the selection of the product, and the patient's use of the drug throughout the duration of therapy, regardless of the setting. This integrated approach can reduce the total cost of drug therapy. The questions in this section will assist the manager in the evaluation of cost-reduction strategies.

A. Formulary Systems

1. Is there a policy for a single generic equivalent of each drug?

2. Is there a policy that combination products generally are nonformulary drugs?

3. Is there a policy that allows the pharmacy to decide which dosage sizes of a formulary drug will be stocked or reimbursed?

4. Are there procedures to discourage use of nonformulary drugs?

a. Are physicians required to complete a special form that indicates the reason for use of nonformulary drugs?

b. Is cosignature by an attending physician required before nonformulary drugs can be dispensed?

c. Do pharmacists contact prescribers of nonformulary drugs to recommend formulary equivalents?

d. Is there a policy not to stock nonformulary drugs routinely?

e. Are prescribers monitored for excessive use of nonformulary drugs?

5. Does the formulary contain cost information?

6. Is price information updated at least annually?

7. Are items in the formulary grouped by therapeutic categories?

8. Is the formulary evaluated periodically for ineffective or obsolete drugs?

B. Pharmacy and Therapeutics Committee

These questions were developed to encourage the P&T committee to establish policies for each highlighted area.

1. Are well-documented drug reviews prepared for all drugs that are being considered for formulary inclusion?

a. Does each review contain an evaluation of clinical studies?

b. Does each review contain a list of other drugs in the therapeutic category?

c. Does each review contain a cost comparison of these drugs?

d. Has the cost impact of each formulary addition been calculated?

e. Is a formal recommendation made by the pharmacy to the committee?

f. Are pertinent deletions of similar drugs suggested?

2. Are automatic stop orders in effect for selected classes of agents such as
Antibiotics?
P.R.N. analgesics?
Blood components?
Large volume injectable solutions?

3. Do automatic stop orders take effect when patients have surgery?
Are transferred to another service?
Are transferred to and from intensive care units?

4. Is there a system or P&T committee policy that limits the duration of prophylactic antibiotic therapy?

5. Are therapeutic categories containing high risk, high volume, or expensive drugs reviewed regularly to reduce therapeutic duplicates and minimize drug therapy problems? (Examples of these categories include antihistamines, broad-spectrum penicillins, cephalosporins, histamine H_2-receptor antagonists, and nonsteroidal anti-inflammatory agents.)

a. Are drugs removed from the formulary if they provide no unique benefit?

6. Is there a restricted drug category in the formulary to control expensive agents and highly toxic drugs with limited uses that cannot be removed from the formulary?

7. Has the number of controlled substances on the formulary been reduced when possible?

8. Do physicians document their experiences with newly implemented P&T committee actions?

a. Are these experiences communicated to the committee?

9. Has the P&T committee established microbial-sensitivity reporting mechanisms that reflect cost-effectiveness criteria?

10. Are there policies in place regarding P&T committee member activities and conflict of interest?

11. Are there policies in place regarding appropriate activities of pharmaceutical manufacturer representatives within the organization?

12. Are there policies in place regarding pharmaceutical industry sponsorship of presentations within the organization?

C. Clinical Pharmacy Services

Clinical pharmacy services, whose goal is improved patient outcomes, include patient and professional education, drug use evaluations and monitoring, and pharmacokinetic consulting. While documentation of discrete clinical pharmacy services is important, the underlying premise is that improved patient outcomes will result in cost reductions. ASHP's

PharmaTrend product identifies the following as measures of clinical services during a given reporting period:

1. Number of patient-care encounters.
2. Number of patient chart reviews.
3. Number of times pharmacists provided drug information to a physician or nurse.
4. Number of times pharmacists participated in patient-care rounds.
5. Number of conferences or lectures presented.
6. Number of pharmacokinetic consultations.
7. Number of literature searches with written replies.
8. Number of literature searches with oral replies.
9. Number of times pharmacists participated in cardiopulmonary resuscitation.
10. Number of drug use evaluations conducted.
11. Number of nutritional support consultations.
12. Number of inservice programs presented.
13. Number of drug information center consultations.
14. Number of pharmacy newsletter issues prepared.

Additionally, PharmaTrend provides pharmacists with six clinical service indicators: clinical service work units per pharmacy patient-day, clinical service work units per admission, clinical service hours as percentage of total personnel hours, clinical service salary cost per pharmacy patient-day, clinical service salary cost per clinical service work unit, and an estimate of clinical services productivity.

The following additional questions are provided to assist pharmacy managers in collecting data for identifying the benefits of providing clinical services.

1. Are drug use evaluations conducted to identify problem areas and determine the cost-effectiveness of drugs in general?
2. Are there criteria for evaluating the benefits of all drugs (e.g., reduction in average length of stay and reduction in cost per member month)?
3. Is there a specific plan for assessing the cost of drug therapies (e.g., a target disease program)?
4. Are physicians educated about the cost of drug therapy?
   a. Are newsletters and memos used as educational tools?
   b. Are medical rounds used?
   c. Are teaching grand rounds used?
   d. Are informal lines of communication developed with the medical staff?
   e. Do physicians hold meetings with pharmacy representatives?
   f. Do prescribers receive regular feedback on their prescribing activity and cost?
5. Is a target drug program in effect that uses pharmacists to control the use of expensive or toxic drugs that cannot be removed from the formulary?
   a. Are criteria for appropriate drug use provided?
   b. Is the target drug program preceded by an educational newsletter?
   c. Do pharmacists review patient profiles daily for use of the target drugs?
   d. Does the pharmacist recommend alternative therapy when drug use is deemed inappropriate?
   e. Is there followup communication with physicians who frequently prescribe specific drugs inappropriately?

6. Do pharmacists provide pharmacokinetic services?
7. Do pharmacists participate in the training of patients for home therapy?
8. Do pharmacists work closely with personnel responsible for intravenous drug and solution administration?
   a. Do they decrease use of intravenous solutions to keep intravenous lines open?
   b. Do they decrease duration of intravenous solution therapy?
   c. Do they decrease duration of intravenous piggyback drug therapy by changing to intramuscular or oral administration when possible?
   d. Do they decrease unnecessary intravenous drug administration?
   e. Do they target areas where waste could be decreased?
9. Are pharmacists used on the TPN team to promote cost-effective activities?
10. Do pharmacists provide any of the following services to the outpatient clinics:
    Dispensing?
    Monitoring?
    Clinical services or consultations?
    Education?
    a. Do they recommend less expensive therapy when appropriate?
    b. Do they help reduce excess medication use in this setting?
11. Do pharmacists use laboratory data to evaluate the efficacy of drug therapy and to anticipate toxicity or adverse effects?
12. Does the pharmacy actively participate in organizational cost-containment studies that address patient-care issues?
13. Do pharmacists participate in discharge planning for patients?
14. Do pharmacists participate in infection control activities within the organization?
15. Do pharmacists routinely evaluate drug therapy to prevent and identify potential adverse drug reactions?
16. Do pharmacists participate in technology assessment activities within the organization?

III. Improving Productivity

A basic definition of productivity is the ratio between goods or services produced (output) and factors that have contributed to their production (input). The PharmaTrend manual defines productivity as the ratio of the amount of time theoretically needed to produce all of the pharmacy's output to the amount of staff time actually available. However, the productivity of employees does not depend entirely on work performance; it is also influenced by technological development, skills and attitudes of supervisors, quality of materials, managerial environment, departmental job and function statements, layout and flow of work within the department, and other factors.

Monitoring departmental productivity is a key element of any cost-containment strategy. The questions in this section can be used in evaluating methods for improving departmental productivity.

A. *Effective Personnel Management Skills*

1. Have job analyses been conducted?

2. Are job descriptions rewritten periodically (e.g., annually)?
3. Have alternative staffing methods been considered such as job sharing, part-time hours, flextime, 10-hour shifts, and use of on-call personnel?
4. Is there an effective performance appraisal system in the department?
5. Are work methods and redistribution of staffing regularly reviewed?
6. Do supportive personnel perform all functions that do not require a pharmacist?
7. Has departmental personnel turnover been evaluated?
8. Are evaluations of performance appraisal, work methods, supportive personnel, and turnover used regularly in designing the department's staffing?
9. Has overtime been analyzed?
10. Have behavioral and motivational factors affecting productivity been assessed?
11. Is there a cost-effective orientation and training program?
12. Is a participative problem-solving program (e.g., quality improvement) used to build productive attitudes?
13. Is improved productivity a pharmacy objective and commitment?
14. Is the organization managed in a way that positively develops productive employee attitudes?

B. Development of Systems to Improve Productivity

1. Have new technologies been evaluated for increasing efficiency or decreasing required personnel hours (e.g., premixed intravenous admixtures, new drug delivery systems, and automation)?
2. Have all systems in the drug use process been evaluated for maximum efficiency (e.g., delivery and transportation, unit dose system, intravenous admixture system, billing, and claims processing system)?
3. Have productivity measurements been established?
4. Have management systems (e.g., total quality management) that support improved productivity been implemented?
5. Is computerization used effectively?
   a. Is the charging system computerized or automated?
   b. Is the drug distribution system computerized?
   c. Is adequate computer support available for clinical services?
6. Does the facility design promote efficient work?
   a. Have optimal workflow patterns been examined for each area of the pharmacy?
7. Are communication devices properly used?
   a. Is the telephone system used efficiently?
   b. Are state-of-the-art communication devices and systems used?
   c. Is communication effective between departmental sections, between shifts, among personnel, and among multiple providers?

IV. Information Management

Providers cannot function under the prospective pricing system without accurate and timely access to internal information. There is a need for identifying and capturing the necessary data in a form that pharmacy managers can use. Changes in health care will create new information needs

that can be best met by combining clinical and financial data into a common system.

The success of the information system in addressing managers' needs will depend strongly on the development of an indepth strategy by those who will use this system. In general terms, the strategy for developing clinical and financial reporting systems should include the following steps:

1. Evaluate the pharmacy's information needs.
2. Determine the availability of data within the organization.
3. Obtain and use the data currently available in the department and organization.
4. Plan methods for obtaining needed data that are not currently available.

The pharmacy manager must rapidly collect, evaluate, and act on complex information. Adequate information systems support is needed to collect and evaluate data pertinent to pharmacy operations, clinical services, and management functions. The questions in this section will assist the pharmacy manager in evaluating the usefulness and relevance of specific information systems.

1. Does the pharmacy receive adequate and appropriate reports, in a timely manner, from the organization's data processing or management information systems (MIS) department for cost-containment planning?
   a. Are detailed expense, revenue, and cost-of-goods reports received for each accounting period?
   b. Are reports adequate in explanation of detail?
   c. Are variance reports available that show actual versus budgeted use?
   d. Are reports matched with statistics maintained within the pharmacy?
   e. Do the reports detail expenses by drug or by drug category, especially for high cost items?
   f. Does the pharmacy receive regular full-time equivalent (FTE) use reports (e.g., how many FTEs are used and the variance between budget and actual)?
   g. Does the department receive adequately detailed expense reports that itemize products purchased from central warehousing, from wholesalers, and directly from manufacturers?
2. Are appropriate and comprehensive reports regularly prepared by pharmacy management for the organization's administration?
   a. Does the pharmacy prepare evaluative reports of activities and expenditures to include:
      1) A report of drug purchases, detailing actual dollar purchases for the given time period?
      2) A report per drug or drug category?
   b. Are computers used effectively for supporting the following departmental functions:
      1) Purchasing and inventory control?
      2) Drug information service?
      3) Drug preparation and distribution systems?
      4) Clinical pharmacy services?
      5) Drug use evaluation?
      6) Pharmacokinetic services?
      7) Drug therapy monitoring systems?
      8) Outpatient or ambulatory care systems?
      9) Claims processing and benefits design?
   c. Is the pharmacy computer system appropriately

connected with the organization's mainframe system?

    d.   Are microcomputers available for support of services that the hospital mainframe cannot support?

3.   Have applicable federal and state regulations been reviewed?

4.   Is information on national or regional departmental performance data (e.g., Monitrend and PharmaTrend) used for comparison?

Approved by the ASHP Board of Directors, September 27, 1991. Supersedes an April 25, 1985 version which was developed by the ASHP Council on Administrative Affairs. The questions in the checklist sections on drug product costs and drug therapy costs were adapted from the following article: Abramowitz PW. Controlling financial variables—changing prescribing patterns. *Am J Hosp Pharm.* 1984; 41:503–15.

The bibliographic citation for this document is as follows: American Society of Hospital Pharmacists. ASHP technical assistance bulletin on assessing cost-containment strategies for pharmacies in organized health-care settings. *Am J Hosp Pharm.* 1992; 49:155–60.

ASHP Technical Assistance Bulletin on Surgery and Anesthesiology Pharmaceutical Services

Surgical suites and anesthesiology areas have traditionally been areas of the hospital without direct pharmacist involvement. Drugs for these areas have often been available through a stock distribution system maintained by operating room personnel, and documentation of controlled substances use has often been handled by personnel other than those actually administering the drugs. As an alternative, drug use control in these areas can be assumed by pharmacists, often through a direct presence in the areas. In many hospitals, this is accomplished through an onsite pharmacy satellite.[1-5] This Technical Assistance Bulletin is intended to assist pharmacists in implementing and managing such a pharmacy satellite.

Each organization has its own specific needs, and the pharmaceutical services described should be tailored to patients' needs and the individual practice environment. The practices described are relatively new and still evolving. Thus, this document discusses issues and procedures that may change as this practice area matures. In general, pharmacy practice in this area should have goals consistent with those in other areas of hospital pharmacy practice.

The term "surgery and anesthesiology pharmaceutical services" should not be interpreted too literally. Many satellite pharmacies serving surgery and anesthesiology areas also serve other areas. They may include cystoscopy and endoscopy suites, cardiac catheterization laboratories or suites, postanesthesia care units, recovery rooms, labor and delivery rooms, freestanding surgical centers, and critical care areas. It is common for such satellites to be termed "operating room (OR) pharmacy satellites" and for the pharmacist to be termed an "OR pharmacist." This bulletin does not attempt to make a distinction among these terms, as they may be applied differently in various settings. Throughout the bulletin, the terms "satellite" and "pharmacist" are used in the broadest senses.

Justification

Justification of a satellite is a critical step in the overall process of establishing pharmaceutical services in surgery and anesthesiology areas.[5,6]

Familiarization with Surgery and Anesthesiology Pharmaceutical Services Concepts. As an initial step, the individual in charge of the project should become familiar with typical surgery and anesthesiology satellite pharmacy services. Review of pertinent literature, discussions with pharmacists in other organizations, and site visits to established satellites are methods of accomplishing this step. The site visit is especially useful, as it can reinforce and further define information gained by other means. At the conclusion of this step, the pharmacist should have a realistic view of the type and scope of services typically provided.

Obtaining Support for the Concept. If justification is to be successful, the support of key individuals from the major departments affected by the service should be obtained.[5] In most institutions the major parties affected are hospital administration, anesthesiology, surgery, operating room nurs-

ing, and certified registered nurse anesthetists.

The support of the anesthesiology department is crucial. A request for satellite services from the director of the anesthesiology department can eliminate a substantial amount of time that may otherwise be spent in "selling" the concept. If the request for satellite services does not originate with the anesthesiology department, the process can be more time consuming. Data gathered in the preliminary review of the site and information obtained from the literature can be used in discussing the concept with the director of anesthesiology. If some anesthesiologists have been especially receptive to pharmacy involvement, it may be valuable to solicit their support. The proposal for a satellite might then be presented jointly by pharmacy personnel and anesthesiologists.

Hospital administration should also be approached at this time. The administration's reaction will provide some guidance on how difficult the approval process for the satellite will be.

If conceptual support from the aforementioned groups is present, development of a formal proposal can begin. If certain departments or key individuals have doubts about the need for a satellite, it may be wise to propose a compromise to keep the process moving forward. One possible compromise would be to conduct a pilot project, with the establishment of a permanent satellite pending favorable results in the pilot experience.

Initial Assessment of Setting. A general review of the surgery and anesthesiology areas should be performed after familiarity with the overall concept is gained. At this time, it is not essential that detailed information be obtained. Useful information to collect includes

1. Location and quantity of drugs stored in the setting.
2. Location and storage of controlled substances.
3. Controlled substances accountability systems used.
4. Drug preparation and distribution procedures used in the setting.
5. Billing systems used for all drugs.
6. Stock replenishment and rotation systems used.

Nurses, anesthesiologists, anesthetists, supply technicians, and surgeons may be able to assist in the collection of this information.

Formal Proposal. The development of a formal proposal is an important part of the justification process. It is essential that the proposal be well organized and factual. The writers should expect the proposal to be examined in great detail by hospital administration and others during the decisionmaking process. The proposal should expand on the information obtained in the initial review of the surgical suite. Information that should be in the proposal includes

1. Dollar value of current drug inventory in the setting.
2. Dollar value of drugs used per time period (e.g., per year).
3. Dollar value of patient charges currently generated.
4. Average cost of drugs used per surgical case.

5. Estimated cost of drug waste per time period.
6. General quality and completeness of controlled substances records.
7. Number of controlled substances discrepancies reported per month.
8. Number of drug-related incident reports received per month.
9. Time currently spent by personnel in the setting performing pharmacy-related activities.
10. Time currently spent by pharmacy personnel performing functions for the setting.

Collection of the above information can be facilitated through the formation of a multidisciplinary team. Representatives from the departments of anesthesiology, nursing, and surgery can be included. This approach has several benefits. Data collection can be expedited, because the expertise of each individual can be used. The concept of a satellite will be continuously reinforced to these individuals, and all affected groups will have input in the decisionmaking process.

A formal proposal can be prepared once the required information has been collected. Minimally, the proposal should contain the following sections: introduction, statement of problems and anticipated benefits, summary of the proposed services, and cost–benefit analysis.[5] In preparing these sections, it is important to be as specific as possible and to assign dollar values whenever they are available.

The proposal should be endorsed by the members of the multidisciplinary team and should be submitted to the administration by the director of pharmacy. Careful planning, data collection, analysis, and presentation of the information gathered will make approval more likely.

Implementation

Implementation should begin as soon as possible after administrative approval.[5] Implementation steps should be planned and executed in a clear, concise manner. In the plan, an implementation time line can be developed that lists the steps to be taken and the expected amount of time required for each activity. The amount of time required for each activity may vary from institution to institution, but the order in which the steps should be performed will be reasonably standard.

The major implementation steps and an approximate order in which they should be performed are as follows:[5]

1. Obtain formal commitment of space in the setting.
2. Assign a project leader. (This person should be responsible for the project's development. This person need not be the pharmacist that will be assigned to staff the satellite. Often, it is valuable for the project leader to be a supervisor or assistant director.)
3. Identify construction and equipment needs.
4. Do construction work.
5. Obtain and install equipment.
6. Draft policies and procedures.
7. Develop job descriptions.
8. Select staff (pharmacists and supportive personnel).
9. Design and print forms.
10. Formalize policies and procedures.
11. Determine satellite drug stock levels.
12. Train staff.
13. Train backup and relief staff.
14. Educate nursing staff.
15. Educate anesthesiology department staff.
16. Educate surgeons.
17. Open satellite for operation.

Many of these steps can be expedited by working closely with members of the anesthesiology and nursing departments.

The satellite's services should be monitored and evaluated on an ongoing basis through the use of workload statistics, financial data, and patient outcomes. In addition, the satisfaction levels of the nursing and anesthesiology staffs should be periodically assessed.

Pharmaceutical Services

Numerous activities and services may be improved in surgery and anesthesiology areas through the presence of a pharmacy satellite and pharmacy staff. Often these include

- Drug preparation and distribution.
- Drug inventory control.
- Waste reduction.
- Drug cost reduction.
- Improved revenue generation through accurate patient billing.
- Improved documentation of drugs administered to patients.[7]
- Drug accountability and control.
- Quality assurance.
- Clinical activities.
- Educational and research activities.
- Involvement with the use of drug administration devices.
- Enhanced interdisciplinary decisionmaking.

Drug Preparation and Distribution. Drug preparation and distribution can be accomplished in various ways. For nonanesthesiology drugs and drugs that are not case specific, a general supply (e.g., in cart or cassette format) can be provided with the understanding that these drugs may be used for any patient. Anesthesiology medications can be supplied on a case-specific basis or through a daily restocking of a drug supply (e.g., an "anesthesia" cart).

The methods chosen may depend on the wishes and needs of the anesthesiologists and the surgery staff and, fundamentally, should be based on the provision of accurate and timely supplies to meet the needs of patients. Secondarily, the methods chosen may be influenced by staffing levels in the setting and charge capture mechanisms. Common to all of the methods, however, is the objective of eliminating nursing and anesthesiology staff time spent in gathering and preparing drugs.

Drug Accountability and Control. The pharmacist should be responsible for all general drugs and controlled substances dispensed and distributed in the setting. To the extent possible, all drug inventories should be centralized in the satellite. Minimal, if any, drug stock should be maintained in each surgical suite. As a generalization, the satellite should be staffed during all hours and days when the surgery and anesthesiology areas are normally staffed.

If the satellite is not open 24 hours per day, it may be necessary to establish an after-hours drug supply (e.g., a cart) for use in the setting. The pharmacist should determine the drug levels required for the supply, and the supply levels should be checked and replenished daily. Trends in drug usage or disappearance should be noted and reconciled.

Clinical Activities. The pharmacist should be familiar with all drugs used in the setting, including drugs used for general and regional anesthesia, neuromuscular blockade, analgesia, preoperative management, hemodynamic control, diagnosis and manipulation during surgery, prevention of infection, and treatment of intraoperative emergencies. Knowledge may be gained by observation of surgery and anesthesia procedures, attendance at anesthesia and surgery conferences, reading the literature, and direct clinical involvement in patient care.

Clinical pharmacy services and activities provided in surgery and anesthesiology settings should coincide with those provided to all other patient areas as outlined in the "ASHP Statement on the Pharmacist's Clinical Role in Organized Health-Care Settings"[8] and the "ASHP Technical Assistance Bulletin on Assessment of Departmental Directions for Clinical Practice in Pharmacy."[9] Clinical services and activities may include the following.

Drug information. The pharmacist should provide timely and accurate drug information in response to needs noted and inquiries. Inquiries may originate from any staff, including surgery and recovery room staff, anesthesia staff, residents, nurse anesthetists, nurses, perfusionists, residents, and students. Drug information may be provided in oral or written form, as appropriate, and may necessitate detailed literature searches with accompanying interpretation.

The satellite should maintain a body of pharmaceutical literature containing current primary, secondary, and tertiary literature sources. Scientific and professional practice journals in pharmacy and medicine should be directly available or readily accessible in a timely enough manner to enable clinical decisionmaking on behalf of immediate patients. Reference texts should be current and provide detailed information in at least the following areas: drug action, drug side effects, adverse drug effects, doses, drugs of choice, efficacy, formulations, incompatibilities, indications, interactions, laws and regulations, pharmacology, nonprescription drugs, pathophysiology, pharmacokinetics, toxicology, surgery, and anesthesia. The pharmacist may also wish to develop and distribute a newsletter and make available specific literature articles of interest to others in the setting. The pharmacist should have access to a formal drug information center.

Formulary system. The pharmacist should continually evaluate the organization's formulary and advise the medical staff and pharmacy and therapeutics committee with respect to drug efficacy, adverse effect experiences, and cost.

Drug regimen review. Whenever possible, drug requests from surgery or anesthesiology staff should be evaluated before dispensing the drug with respect to appropriateness, dose, route of administration, timing of administration, and cost. The choice of drug should be based on its appropriateness for a specific patient and cost. Doses, timing, and choices of prophylactic antibiotics should be monitored.

The pharmacist should review the surgery schedule, routinely screen patient profiles or charts prior to surgery for allergies (commonly antibiotics and narcotics), and notify appropriate personnel of pertinent findings. Profiles or charts should also be reviewed whenever possible for potential intraoperative drug–drug or drug–disease interactions and

for proper continuation of maintenance medications and discontinuation of unnecessary medications postoperatively.

Rounds. When possible, the pharmacist should participate actively in patient care rounds with anesthesia, surgery, and recovery room staff. The pharmacist may wish to limit rounds to specific types of patients (such as cardiothoracic surgery or transplant patients) for whom the pharmacist's preoperative or postoperative involvement may be most beneficial. The pharmacist should participate in anesthesia "grand rounds," morbidity and mortality reviews, and other scheduled educational sessions as appropriate.

Drug use evaluation. The pharmacist should participate in the drug use evaluation of selected drugs, assisting in the establishment of criteria, data collection, analysis, recommendations, and followup.[10] Data collection is often more easily accomplished prospectively or concurrently in the setting by coordination with surgery and anesthesiology staff.

Drug research. The pharmacist should strive to initiate and participate in drug research related to use in surgery, both as a principal investigator and one who supports the studies of others (e.g., providing randomization, preparing drugs, and assisting in study design and data collection).

Education. Educational presentations on drug-related topics should be made regularly by the pharmacist to surgery and anesthesiology residents and staff, nursing staff, and other personnel. The pharmacist should provide education about drugs added to the organization's formulary, drug precautions, and drugs used during cardiac and respiratory arrest. The pharmacist should educate other pharmacy staff members about drugs used in the setting, with special attention to neuromuscular blocking agents, anesthetic gases, and the management of malignant hyperthermia.

Formal educational rotations in the satellite and its functions may be conducted for undergraduate and graduate pharmacy students, pharmacy residents, or pharmacy fellows. Specific learning and experiential goals and objectives should be developed, and the "student" should learn about satellite services and preoperative, intraoperative, and postoperative drug therapy through didactic instruction, observation, project participation, and selected reading. Rotations should be coordinated with the anesthesiology department.

Adverse drug reaction monitoring and reporting. The pharmacist should monitor, detect, document, report, and recommend appropriate management of adverse drug reactions that occur in the setting.[11]

Participation in emergency life support. The pharmacist should participate in the drug treatment of cardiac or respiratory arrests that occur in the setting. This participation should be based on a formal policy endorsement of the pharmacist's role in such events. At the minimum, the pharmacist should possess a current certification in basic cardiac life support (BCLS) procedures and preferably in advanced cardiac life support (ACLS).

The pharmacist should also participate in the treatment of malignant hyperthermia by preparing and maintaining malignant hyperthermia emergency kits and in the preparation and administration of medications used to treat malignant hyperthermia.

Pharmacokinetic management and consultation. The pharmacist should participate in the pharmacokinetic management of patients and should serve as a consultant to surgery and anesthesiology staff on pharmacokinetic drug dosing.

Pain management. The pharmacist should participate

actively in patient-controlled analgesia or other pain management programs. Participation may include the development of such a program, identification of appropriate patients, patient education, drug preparation, and educational presentations to other staff.

Documentation of clinical activities. The pharmacist should document clinical activities and identify those leading to improved patient outcomes and cost reductions.

Controlled Substances

All controlled substances procedures should comply with applicable federal and state statutes and regulations and organizational policies and procedures.[12] Procedures for the satellite and the setting it serves should address the following:

1. Controlled substances (and other drugs) to be monitored.
2. Methods of distribution.
3. Records.
4. Ordering.
5. Storage, access, and inventorying.
6. Reconciliation and disposal.

Controlled Substances (and Other Drugs) to Be Monitored. The pharmacist should be responsible for monitoring the use of all controlled substances used in the setting. As required (e.g., because of abuse or diversion potential), drugs other than controlled substances may be handled via accountability procedures similar (or identical) to those used for controlled substances.

Methods of Distribution. A per case distribution system is recommended. This approach should ensure that the exact drugs required per case are available and should enable accurate recordkeeping and monitoring. It should minimize the potential for diversion. If a per case approach is not possible, the distribution of a daily supply of controlled substances to each anesthesiologist is an alternative. A per case approach is more labor intensive for satellite staff, and it requires more "transaction" documentations. As necessary in individual settings, those considerations should be balanced against the need for closer control.

To the extent possible, controlled substances should be distributed only in response to signed orders or requests from prescribers. Given the urgency of need often present during surgical procedures and the necessity for prescribers to devote undivided attention to anesthesia procedures and sterility safeguard procedures during surgery, it may not always be possible to comply with such a requirement. When it *is* possible, the organization's standard physician order sheet or a special controlled substances request form developed specifically for the surgical suite may be used.

In the per case approach, the order sheet can be designed with multiple copies to allow the original to be placed in the patient's chart and a duplicate to be retained by the satellite. Regardless of the methods used, clear documentation, signed by the responsible prescribers, that all controlled substances used were administered to the patient should exist at the end of each surgical procedure.

Records. Records should be kept of the following:

1. Controlled substances dispensed.

2. Controlled substances inventories.
3. Controlled substances returned and records reconciled.
4. Controlled substances disposed.
5. Controlled substances use, categorized by prescriber.

If the satellite does not provide 24-hour services, it is desirable for the documentation procedures for after-hours use to be as similar as possible to those used when the satellite is staffed. This will help ensure staff efficiency and familiarity with the recordkeeping requirements in after-hours occasions. Forms specific to the setting and to the after-hours circumstance may have to be developed.

Ordering. The pharmacist should be responsible for ordering all controlled substances for the satellite. Once received, the controlled substances should be added to the satellite's stock and recorded in inventory records. If the satellite does not provide 24-hour services, the pharmacist is responsible for ensuring that adequate supplies are available in designated after-hours locations.

The pharmacist should maintain controlled substances inventory amounts sufficient only to meet the needs of the setting for a reasonable time period. This time period should be dependent on the frequency and timeliness with which controlled substances are available from the central pharmacy. Less inventory is required, for example, if supplies are ordered on a daily basis than if ordering occurs less often.

Shortly after the initial opening of a satellite and after use has stabilized, stock levels should be reassessed and adjusted as needed. During ordering, the pharmacist should note developing trends with respect to use.

Storage, Access, and Inventorying. Controlled substances should be stored in a locked space (e.g., cabinet, drawer, or cart) within the satellite. These storage spaces should remain locked when controlled substances are not being dispensed. Access to the spaces should be limited to satellite personnel.

If 24-hour satellite services are not provided, a separate, locked, after-hours storage space within the setting will be required. "Kits" of after-hours controlled substances may be useful, as may carts of controlled substances that can be moved from one surgical suite to another as required. Regardless of how they are configured or located, all after-hours supplies should be checked and all records reconciled by satellite staff on the first working day after the after-hours supplies are entered.

If possible, one individual per shift should be identified as responsible for controlled substances (and related procedures) when the satellite is not staffed. That person should have access (key or code) to locked after-hours supplies. This approach will enable more consistent recordkeeping, limit the number of people with access to after-hours supplies, and enable more reliable monitoring of controlled substances usage. In each setting, the most logical person for this assignment must be determined. Individuals often assigned this responsibility include an "in charge" nurse or the "first-call" anesthesiology resident.

Controlled substances inventories should be verified by physical count at least once daily. Occasional documented, unscheduled audits of controlled substances in the satellite setting should be performed by staff not normally assigned to the satellite.

Reconciliation and Disposal. Reconciliation of controlled substances use can be accomplished via various methods[13–15] such as

- *Comparison of quantities dispensed with quantities documented as administered.* Controlled substances returned to the satellite should be compared with the quantity dispensed. The amount dispensed should equal the amount returned (unopened and partially filled containers and partially used syringes) plus the amount documented as administered.
- *Verification of use through review of anesthesia record.* The anesthesia record should be reviewed to ensure that the amount documented as administered (in records returned to the satellite) is identical to that documented in the patient's anesthesia record. This verification is ideally performed on all cases but may be performed by periodic audits of randomly selected cases if anesthesia records are not readily available from every case.
- *Qualitative testing of returned controlled substances.* To verify that unadulterated drug is contained in partially used containers returned to the satellite, a refractometer or other device can be used.

The pharmacist should account for all controlled substances dispensed and should report all discrepancies to internal and external authorities as required.

Disposal of controlled substances (e.g., partially used syringes) should be performed in the satellite by the pharmacist in the presence of a witness. This action should be documented in the satellite's controlled substances records.

Quality Assurance

The pursuit of continuous improvement in the quality of services provided should be a philosophy of practice of the pharmacist and the satellite staff. In that light, many of the pharmacist's (and the satellite's) activities may be seen as pertinent to quality-assurance efforts. Some of these activities are

- Adverse drug reaction (ADR) monitoring and reporting.
- Medication error monitoring and reporting.
- Periodic inspections of all drug storage sites.
- Drug therapy monitoring.
- Drug use evaluations.
- Drug interaction monitoring.
- Controlled substances monitoring.
- Quality control of compounded parenterals (e.g., cardioplegic solutions).

Some of these activities should not be difficult to implement in a satellite setting, since ongoing procedures developed for the organization overall should already exist. In some cases, it may be necessary to develop new programs or variations of existing ones tailored to the surgery and anesthesiology setting.

The Pharmacist's Role

The pharmacist should be responsible for the development, implementation, management, and evaluation of all satellite activities and services. The pharmacist should be responsible for providing appropriate storage, distribution, and accountability for all drugs; provision of clinical pharmacy services; and supervision of satellite staff. The pharmacist should perform or supervise all drug preparation, labeling, and distribution, including the preparation of injectable drugs used in the setting. The pharmacist should be responsible for all production activities (including preparation of per case or per prescriber kits, if applicable), drug charging, controlled substances accounting, and recordkeeping associated with these activities.

The pharmacist should be responsible for maintaining adequate stocks of drugs, proper storage of drugs, and removal of expired drug products from the setting. The pharmacist should provide drug information and perform other clinical functions as required. The pharmacist should develop and maintain quality-assurance programs for the satellite and its services.

Policies and Procedures. The pharmacist should develop and maintain policies and procedures for the satellite and its services. Policies and procedures should exist for the production of drug kits (if applicable), distribution systems, controlled substances handling, hours of operation, preparation of parenteral drugs, expiration dating, recycling of products, drug inventory levels, staff training, and after-hours drug distribution.

Interdisciplinary Interfaces. The pharmacist should function as a liaison between the pharmacy department and all staff in the setting served, including anesthesiology, nursing, and surgery staff; perfusionists; and management staff. The pharmacist should represent the pharmacy department on appropriate interdisciplinary committees designed to evaluate or make recommendations about services in the setting. A committee specifically designed to focus on pharmacy matters may be appropriate.

Financial Analysis. The pharmacist should document drug costs, service costs, revenues, and savings attributable to the satellite and the activities of its staff. Financial reports should be prepared periodically and provided to the organization's administration.

The Pharmacy Technician's Role

Pharmacy technicians assigned to the satellite should be trained to perform their assigned functions and tasks. Within the overall work force of pharmacy technicians in the organization, it is desirable to have some technicians trained as available backup staff for the satellite. Technicians should be trained in general technical activities as outlined in the "ASHP Technical Assistance Bulletin on Outcome Competencies and Training Guidelines for Institutional Pharmacy Technician Training Programs."[16]

Technicians should receive training and experience in injectable drug preparation, drug distribution procedures, physician order interpretation, and controlled substances recordkeeping specific to the satellite. The training should include a review of

1. Procedures unique to surgical suites, including special apparel (e.g., caps, masks, and foot covers) and restricted movements within surgical suites.
2. Surgical suite terminology, including abbreviations and acronyms used to name surgical procedures.
3. Drug classes, indications, and proper handling of drugs

routinely used in surgical suites (e.g., special packaging and preservative requirements for spinal and epidural drugs).

4. Controlled substances procedures.
5. Emergency drugs that are typically used in surgical suites.

Typical pharmacy technician activities performed in the satellite under the supervision of the pharmacist include drug distribution, controlled substances handling, injectable drug preparation, ordering drugs and restocking the satellite, orientation and training of new staff, and quality-assurance activities. Each of these activities is discussed in greater detail below.

Drug Distribution. The technician typically distributes general drugs to storage sites in the setting and prepares per case or per prescriber kits of drugs and distributes them. Given the nature of surgical procedures and the urgency of need for the requested drugs, these distributions often will have to occur on the basis of oral requests. The pharmacist should screen such requests to ensure proper choices of drugs for specific patients.

The technician typically returns unused drugs to stock and charges patients or departments for drugs used.

The technician typically checks and replenishes after-hours drug supplies and charges drugs used to appropriate patients or departments.

Controlled Substances Handling. The technician typically distributes controlled substances and creates appropriate records according to the distribution procedures of the satellite and in accordance with federal and state statutes and regulations. Typical activities include assisting with inventory counts, maintaining perpetual inventory records, disposal of controlled substances with the pharmacist, and participation in audits, assays, and preparation of reports.

Injectable Drug Preparation. The technician typically aseptically compounds, packages, and labels injectable drugs and documents all products made.

Ordering Drugs and Restocking the Satellite. The technician typically routinely orders replenishment supplies of drugs for the satellite, checks the supplies delivered in response to the orders, and then places the stock in appropriate places.

Orientation and Training of New Staff. The technician typically assists in the orientation and training of new staff (including other technicians).

Quality Assurance. The technician should be involved in quality-assurance activities of the satellite. Such activities may include regular controlled substances audits or assays, microbiological monitoring of injectable drugs prepared, and inspections of drug supplies.

References

1. Powell PJ, Maland L, Bair JN, et al. Implementing an operating room pharmacy satellite. *Am J Hosp Pharm.* 1983; 40:1192–8.

2. Opoien D. Establishment of surgery satellite pharmacy services in a large community hospital. *Hosp Pharm.* 1984; 19:485–90.

3. Keicher PA, McAllister JC III. Comprehensive pharmaceutical services in the surgical suite and recovery room. *Am J Hosp Pharm.* 1985; 42:2454–62.

4. Buchanan EC, Gaither MW. Development of an operating room pharmacy substation on a restricted budget. *Am J Hosp Pharm.* 1986; 43:1719–22.

5. Vogel DP, Barone J, Penn F, et al. Ideas for action: the operating room pharmacy satellite. *Top Hosp Pharm Manage.* 1986; 6:63–80.

6. Ziter CA, Dennis BW, Shoup LK. Justification of an operating-room satellite pharmacy. *Am J Hosp Pharm.* 1989; 46:1353–61.

7. Donnelly AJ. Multidisciplinary approach to improving documentation of medications used during surgical procedures. *Am J Hosp Pharm.* 1989; 46:724–8.

8. American Society of Hospital Pharmacists. ASHP statement on the pharmacist's clinical role in organized health-care settings. *Am J Hosp Pharm.* 1989; 46:805–6.

9. American Society of Hospital Pharmacists. ASHP technical assistance bulletin on assessment of departmental directions for clinical practice in pharmacy. *Am J Hosp Pharm.* 1989; 46:339–41.

10. American Society of Hospital Pharmacists. ASHP guidelines on the pharmacist's role in drug-use evaluation. *Am J Hosp Pharm.* 1988; 45:385–6.

11. American Society of Hospital Pharmacists. ASHP guidelines on adverse drug reaction monitoring and reporting. *Am J Hosp Pharm.* 1989; 46:336–7.

12. American Society of Hospital Pharmacists. ASHP technical assistance bulletin on institutional use of controlled substances. *Am J Hosp Pharm.* 1987; 44:580–9.

13. Satterlee GB. System for verifying use of controlled substances in anesthesia. *Am J Hosp Pharm.* 1989; 46:2506–8.

14. Shovick VA, Mattei TJ, Karnack CM. Audit to verify use of controlled substances in anesthesia. *Am J Hosp Pharm.* 1988; 45:1111–3.

15. Gill DL, Goodwin SR, Knudsen AK, et al. Refractometer screening of controlled substances in an operating room satellite pharmacy. *Am J Hosp Pharm.* 1990; 47:817–8.

16. American Society of Hospital Pharmacists. ASHP technical assistance bulletin on outcome competencies and training guidelines for institutional pharmacy technician training programs. *Am J Hosp Pharm.* 1982; 39:317–20.

Approved by the ASHP Board of Directors, November 14, 1990. Developed by the ASHP Council on Professional Affairs.

The bibliographic citation for this document is as follows: American Society of Hospital Pharmacists. ASHP technical assistance bulletin on surgery and anesthesiology pharmaceutical services. *Am J Hosp Pharm.* 1991; 48:319–25.

ASHP Technical Assistance Bulletin on the Pharmacist's Role in Immunization

Pharmacists can play active roles in the prevention of disease through the advocacy of immunizations. This activity is consistent with the preventive aspects of pharmaceutical care.[1] These guidelines address the pharmacist's role in promoting proper immunization of patients in all organized health-care settings. The pharmacist's role in promoting disease prevention through participation in community efforts is also discussed.

Each year, 60,000 Americans die of vaccine-preventable infections such as influenza, pneumococcal disease, and diphtheria. Most of these people visited health-care providers as either inpatients or outpatients in the year preceding their deaths but were not vaccinated.[2-6] Tens of millions of Americans are susceptible to these infections despite the availability of effective vaccines. In the United States, vaccination rates of individual antigens required for children at the time they enter school are greater than 95%. However, in 1991, a retrospective assessment of vaccination levels among school-aged children in nine major cities found that fewer than half had completed their primary series by the age of 2 years.[7] Most American adults are inadequately vaccinated, particularly against influenza, pneumococcal disease, hepatitis B, tetanus, and diphtheria.[2]

Five ways in which pharmacists can promote immunization are (1) formulary management, (2) administrative measures, (3) history and screening, (4) counseling and documentation, and (5) public education.

Formulary Management

Formulary systems in organized health-care settings should include vaccines, toxoids, and immune globulins available for use in preventing diseases in patients and staff. Appropriate decisions by the pharmacy and therapeutics committee (or its equivalent) on immunologic drug choices require consideration of relevant immunologic pharmaceutics, immunopharmacology, and disease epidemiology. Because of their expertise and training, pharmacists are well equipped to provide information and recommendations on which these decisions may be based.

It is the pharmacist's responsibility to develop and maintain product specifications to aid in the purchase of drugs under the formulary system.[8] The pharmacist should also establish and maintain standards to ensure the quality, proper storage, and proper use of all pharmaceuticals dispensed. Pharmacists must choose between single dose or multidose containers of vaccines on the basis of efficiency, safety, and economic considerations. Pharmacists in institutions should also develop guidelines on the routine stocking of immunologic drugs in certain high use patient-care areas.

Proper storage is an important consideration for immunologic drugs, since many require storage at refrigerated or frozen temperatures. Detailed references on this topic have been published.[9-15] Pharmacists must also ensure that immunologic drugs received by the pharmacy have been transported under suitable storage conditions.

It is important that methods be established for detecting and properly disposing of outdated and partially administered immunologic agents. Live viral (e.g., yellow fever) or bacterial (e.g., bacillus Calmette-Guérin) vaccines should be disposed of in the same manner as other infectious waste.

Administrative Measures

Pharmacists on key committees (e.g., infection control and risk management) in organized health-care settings can promote adequate immunization delivery among staff and patients by encouraging the development of sound organizational policies on immunization. Health-care organizations should develop policies and protocols that address the following:

1. Hepatitis B preexposure prophylaxis for health-care workers at risk for exposure to blood products and other contaminated items.[16]
2. Hepatitis B postexposure (e.g., needle-stick) prophylaxis for previously unvaccinated patients and health-care personnel.[16]
3. Rabies preexposure and postexposure prophylaxis.[17]
4. Wound management guidelines designed to prevent tetanus and diphtheria.[18,19]
5. Valid contraindications to vaccination to ensure patient safety and minimize inappropriate exclusions from vaccination.[18,20,21]
6. Requirements for employee immunization against measles, rubella, influenza, and other diseases.[22]
7. Tuberculosis screening of patients and staff.[23-25]
8. Immunization of persons with certain underlying health conditions (e.g., pregnant or immunocompromised patients). Current authoritative guidelines on this subject should be consulted.[22,26-29]
9. Emergency measures necessary in the event of vaccine-related adverse reactions. Such measures should address the availability of epinephrine and other emergency drugs, as well as advanced cardiac life support.

History and Screening

Pharmacists can promote proper immunization of their patients through identification of patients in need of immunization. Tasks that support this objective include gathering immunization histories, encouraging use of vaccine profiles, issuing vaccination records to patients,[30-37] preventing immunologic drug interactions,[38,39] and screening patients for immunization needs.[31-36,40-42]

Immunization screening should be a component of all clinical routines, regardless of the practice setting. Quality indicators and monitoring systems should be implemented to ensure that all patients are assessed for immunization adequacy before they leave the facility. In clinics where a large number of patients at high risk for contracting vaccine-preventable diseases are seen (e.g., in diabetic, asthmatic, heart disease, and geriatric clinics), special emphasis should be placed on immunization screening and appropriate vaccine use.

Screening for immunization needs may be organized in several ways; a prototype screening form has previously been published.[42] Pharmacists can be involved in some or all of the following forms of immunization screening.

Occurrence Screening. This screening involves identification of vaccine needs at the time of particular events, such as hospital or nursing home admission or discharge, ambulatory or emergency room visits, mid-decade birthdays (years 25, 35, 45, etc.),[22,43] and any contact with a health-care delivery system for patients under 8 years or over 64 years of age.

Diagnosis Screening. This screening involves review of vaccine needs among patients with conditions that place them at increased risk of preventable infections. Diagnoses such as hemophilia, thalassemia, most types of cancer, sickle-cell anemia, chronic alcoholism, cirrhosis, human immunodeficiency virus infection, and certain other disorders should prompt specific attention to the patient's vaccine needs.[22,36]

Procedure Screening. This screening identifies immunization needs on the basis of medical or surgical procedures. These procedures include splenectomy, heart or lung surgery, organ transplantation, antineoplastic therapy, radiation therapy, immunosuppression of other types, dialysis, and prescription of certain medications used to treat conditions that place patients at risk of preventable infections.[22,36] When designing and implementing automated prescription databases, pharmacy managers may wish to consider specifications that allow retrieval of lists of patients receiving drugs that suggest the need for immunization.[36,40]

Periodic Mass Screening. This screening involves the comprehensive assessment of immunization adequacy in selected populations at a given time. This type of screening may be conducted, for example, during autumn influenza programs or outbreaks of certain vaccine-preventable illnesses (e.g., measles).[32,35,36] Schools and other institutions can perform mass screening when registering new students or residents. Mass screening may also be appropriate in areas where no comprehensive immunization program has been conducted recently. This type of screening helps improve vaccine coverage rates at a given time, but long-term benefits are much greater when such intermittent programs are combined with ongoing comprehensive screening efforts.

Occupational Screening. This screening focuses on the immunization needs of health-care personnel whose responsibilities place them at risk of exposure to certain vaccine-preventable diseases. Health-care employers frequently provide immunization screening and vaccination of employees as part of employee health programs. The Occupational Safety and Health Administration requires that health-care employers provide hepatitis B vaccination at no cost, on a voluntary basis, to all employees at risk for occupational exposure to bloodborne pathogens.[44] Depending on their risk of exposure, members of the pharmacy staff may need to receive hepatitis B vaccine.

Patient Counseling

Once patients in need of immunization have been identified, they should be advised of their infection risk and encouraged to accept the immunizations they need. Counseling and documentation issues related to immunizations have been discussed elsewhere.[37,45] The patient's physician(s) should

also be informed of the patient's need for vaccination. Patients who need immunizations should be vaccinated during the current health-care contact unless valid contraindications exist. Delaying the vaccination until a future appointment increases the risk that the patient will not be vaccinated.

Advising patients of their need for immunization can take several forms. In the ambulatory care setting, individualized or form letters or postcards can be mailed to patients, patients can be called by telephone, or an insert can be included with prescriptions informing patients of their infection risk and the availability and efficacy of vaccines.[33,36,46] Adhesive warning labels can also be affixed to prescription containers for drugs used to treat conditions that may indicate the need for vaccination against influenza and pneumococcal disease (e.g., digoxin, warfarin, theophylline, and insulin[36]); these labels would be analogous to labels currently in widespread use (e.g., "Shake well" and "Take with food or milk"). Such labels might read, "You may need flu or pneumonia vaccine: Ask your doctor or pharmacist." For inpatients and institutional residents, chart notes, consultations, messages to patients, and similar means can be used.[31,34,47]

The Centers for Disease Control and Prevention now requires that health-care providers who administer certain vaccines provide relevant printed information to any adult to whom the vaccine is to be administered or to the legal representative of any child to whom the vaccine is to be administered.[48] These vaccines include those that immunize against diphtheria, tetanus, and pertussis; measles, mumps, and rubella; and polio.

Documentation

The National Childhood Vaccine Injury Act of 1986 (NCVIA) requires all health-care providers who administer vaccines to maintain permanent vaccination records and to report occurrences of certain adverse events specified in the Act.[26] The recipient's permanent medical record (or the equivalent) must state the date the vaccine was administered, the vaccine's manufacturer and lot number, and the name, address, and title of the person administering the vaccine. Pharmacists in organized health-care settings may encourage compliance with this requirement by providing reminder notices each time doses of vaccines are dispensed.[49] Automated databases that allow for long-term storage of patient immunization information may provide an efficient method for maintaining and retrieving immunization records.[42]

NCVIA also mandates that selected adverse effects noted after any inoculation be reported to the Vaccine Adverse Event Reporting System.[26,50] Because pharmacists have experience with adverse drug reaction reporting, they can take the lead in developing and implementing a program to meet this requirement.

Patients should maintain personal immunization records that include both inpatient and outpatient immunization experiences and function as a backup in the event of loss of clinicians' immunization records. Several personal immunization record forms are available, including Public Health Service Form 731 (International Certificate of Vaccination), colloquially called the "yellow shot record." Form 731 is used to document vaccines indicated for international travel but can also serve as a convenient common document for a patient's personal record of vaccinations. Additionally, each state as well as the District of Columbia prints its own uniform immunization record form, often designed for both pediatric and adult immunizations, which also is a suitable personal patient record. It has been recommended that adults carry personal immunization records in their wallets.[27]

Reimbursement Issues

Immunization has repeatedly been shown to be cost effective[51-53] and is likely the most cost-effective practice in medicine. However, third-party reimbursement programs often do not provide coverage for recommended vaccines. Pharmacists should closely monitor immunization reimbursement policies and advocate third-party coverage for immunizations as a cost-effective preventive measure.

Public Education

Pharmacists have ample opportunities to advance the public health through immunization advocacy. Pharmacists can facilitate disease prevention strategies, since many potential victims of influenza and pneumococcal disease visit pharmacies and are seen by pharmacists daily.

Pharmacists can lead local activities in observance of National Adult Immunization Week each October.[40] Working through various patient support groups (e.g., local diabetes, heart, lung, and retired persons' associations), pharmacists may help to increase vaccination rates among high risk populations. Newsletters, posters, brochures, and seminars may be used to explain the risk of preventable infections to pharmacy staff, other health-care personnel, and patients.

Summary

Pharmacists can play an important role in health promotion and disease prevention by advocating proper immunization. To do so, pharmacists must actively practice and promote preventive medicine. As primary contact persons in the health-care system, pharmacists have the opportunity to screen and counsel their patients to help protect them from preventable infections.

References

1. Hepler CD, Strand LM. Opportunities and responsibilities in pharmaceutical care. *Am J Hosp Pharm.* 1990; 47:533–43.
2. Williams WW, Hickson MA, Kane MA, et al. Immunization policies and vaccine coverage among adults: the risk for missed opportunities. *Ann Intern Med.* 1988; 108:616–25.
3. Fedson DS, Harward MP, Reid RA, et al. Hospital-based pneumococcal immunization—epidemiologic rationale from the Shenandoah study. *JAMA.* 1990; 264:117–22.
4. Fedson DS. Influenza and pneumococcal immunization strategies for physicians. *Chest.* 1987; 91:436–43.
5. Fedson DS. Improving the use of pneumococcal vaccine through a strategy of hospital-based immunization: a review of its rationale and implications. *J Am Geriatr Soc.* 1985; 33:142–50.
6. Magnussen CR, Valenti WM, Mushlin AI. Pneumococcal vaccine strategy: feasibility of a vaccination program directed at hospitalized and ambulatory patients. *Arch Intern Med.* 1984; 144:1755–7.
7. Retrospective assessment of vaccination coverage among school-aged children—selected U.S. cities, 1991. *MMWR.* 1992; 41:103–7.
8. American Society of Hospital Pharmacists. ASHP technical assistance bulletin on hospital drug distribution and control. *Am J Hosp Pharm.* 1980; 37:1097–103.
9. Vaccine management: recommendations for handling and storage of selected biologicals. Atlanta, GA: Division of Immunization, Centers for Disease Control; 1991.
10. Casto DT, Brunell PA. Safe handling of vaccines. *Pediatrics.* 1990; 87:108–12.
11. Ross MB. Additional stability guidelines for routinely refrigerated drug products. *Am J Hosp Pharm.* 1988; 45:1498–9. Letter.
12. Sterchele JA. Update on stability guidelines for routinely refrigerated drug products. *Am J Hosp Pharm.* 1987; 44:2698, 2701. Letter.
13. Miller LG, Loomis JH. Advice of manufacturers about effects of temperature on biologicals. *Am J Hosp Pharm.* 1985; 42:843–8.
14. Vogenberg FR, Souney PF. Stability guidelines for routinely refrigerated drug products. *Am J Hosp Pharm.* 1983; 40:101–2.
15. Wolfert RR, Cox RM. Room temperature stability of drug products labeled for refrigerated storage. *Am J Hosp Pharm.* 1975; 32:585–7.
16. Immunization Practices Advisory Committee, Centers for Disease Control. Protection against viral hepatitis. *MMWR.* 1990; 39(RR-2):1–26.
17. Immunization Practices Advisory Committee, Centers for Disease Control. Rabies prevention—United States, 1991: Recommendations of the Immunization Practices Advisory Committee. *MMWR.* 1991; 40(RR-3):1–19.
18. Immunization Practices Advisory Committee, Centers for Disease Control. Diphtheria, tetanus, and pertussis: guidelines for vaccine prophylaxis and other preventive measures. *MMWR.* 1985; 34:405–26.
19. Grabenstein JD. Stop buying tetanus toxoid (with one exception). *Hosp Pharm.* 1990; 25:361–2.
20. Immunization Practices Advisory Committee, Centers for Disease Control. Pertussis immunization: family history of convulsions and use of antipyretics, supplementary ACIP statement. *MMWR.* 1987; 36:281–2.
21. American Academy of Pediatrics. The relationship between pertussis vaccine and brain damage: reassessment. *Pediatrics.* 1991; 88:397–400.
22. American College of Physicians. Guide for adult immunization, 2nd ed. Philadelphia, PA: American College of Physicians; 1990.
23. Centers for Disease Control. Prevention and control of tuberculosis in facilities providing long-term care to the elderly. *MMWR.* 1990; 39(RR-10):7–15.
24. Centers for Disease Control. Screening for tuberculosis and tuberculous infection in high-risk populations. *MMWR.* 1990; 39(RR-8):1–8.
25. Centers for Disease Control. Purified protein derivative (PPD)-tuberculin anergy and HIV infection: guidelines for anergy testing and management of anergic persons at risk of tuberculosis. *MMWR.* 1991; 40(RR-5):27–33.
26. Centers for Disease Control. Update on adult immunization: recommendations of the Immunization Practices Advisory Committee. *MMWR.* 1991; 4 (RR-12):1–94.

27. Canadian National Advisory Committee on Immunization. Canadian immunization guide, 3rd ed. Ottawa: Ministry of National Health and Welfare; 1989.

28. Centers for Disease Control. Health information for international travel, 1991. Washington, DC: U.S. Government Printing Office; 1991.

29. Immunization during pregnancy. Washington, DC: American College of Obstetricians and Gynecologists; 1991 Oct.

30. Huff PS, Hak SH, Caiola SM. Immunizations for international travel as a pharmaceutical service. *Am J Hosp Pharm*. 1982; 39:30–3.

31. Spruill WJ, Cooper JW, Taylor WJR. Pharmacist-coordinated pneumonia and influenza vaccination program. *Am J Hosp Pharm*. 1982; 39:1904–6.

32. Grabenstein JD, Smith LJ, Carter DW, et al. Comprehensive immunization delivery in conjunction with influenza vaccination. *Arch Intern Med*. 1986; 146:1189–92.

33. Williams DM, Daugherty LJ, Aycock DG, et al. Effectiveness of improved targeting efforts for influenza immunization in an ambulatory-care setting. *Hosp Pharm*. 1987; 22:462–4.

34. Morton MR, Spruill WJR, Cooper JW. Pharmacist impact on pneumococcal vaccination rates in long-term-care facilities. *Am J Hosp Pharm*. 1988; 45:73. Letter.

35. Grabenstein JD, Smith LJ, Watson RR, et al. Immunization outreach using individual need assessments of adults at an Army hospital. *Public Health Rep*. 1990; 105:311–6.

36. Grabenstein JD, Hayton BD. Pharmacoepidemiologic program for identifying patients in need of vaccination. *Am J Hosp Pharm*. 1990; 47:1774–81.

37. Grabenstein JD. Get it in writing: documenting immunizations. *Hosp Pharm*. 1991; 26:901–4.

38. Grabenstein JD. Drug interactions involving immunologic agents, I. Vaccine–vaccine, vaccine–immunoglobulin, and vaccine–drug interactions. *DICP Ann Pharmacother*. 1990; 24:67–81.

39. Grabenstein JD. Drug interactions involving immunologic agents, II. Immunodiagnostic and other immunologic drug interactions. *DICP Ann Pharmacother*. 1990; 24:186–93.

40. Grabenstein JD. Pneumococcal pneumonia: don't wait, vaccinate. *Hosp Pharm*. 1990; 25:866–9.

41. Grabenstein JD, Casto DT. Recommending vaccines for your patients' individual needs. *Am Pharm*. 1991; 31(9):58–67.

42. Grabenstein JD. Screening patients for need of vaccines and immunologic tests: using a standardized form. *Consult Pharm*. 1990; 5:735–9.

43. Polis MA, Davey VJ, Collins ED, et al. The emergency department as part of a successful strategy for increasing adult immunization. *Ann Emerg Med*. 1988; 17:1016–8.

44. 29 CFR 1910.1030. Occupational exposure to bloodborne pathogens. 1991 Dec.

45. Kirk JK, Grabenstein JD. Interviewing and counseling patients about immunisations. *Hosp Pharm*. 1991; 26:1006–10.

46. Grabenstein JD, Hartzema AG, Guess HA, et al. Community pharmacists as immunization advocates: a pharmacoepidemiologic experiment. *Int J Pharm Pract*. 1993; 2:5–10.

47. Casto DT. Prevention, management, and control of influenza: roles for the pharmacist. *Am J Med*. 1987; 82(Suppl 6A):64–7.

48. 42 CFR 110. Vaccine information materials. 1991 Oct.

49. Perkins LD. Complying with the national childhood vaccine injury act. *Am J Hosp Pharm*. 1990; 47:1260–6.

50. Food and Drug Administration. New vaccine adverse event reporting system. *FDA Drug Bull*. 1990; 20:7–8, 13–4.

51. Gable CB, Holzer SS, Engelhart L, et al. Pneumococcal vaccine: efficacy and associated cost savings. *JAMA*. 1990; 264:2910–5.

52. Koplan JP. The benefits and costs of immunizations revisited. *Drug Info J*. 1988; 22:379–83.

53. Riddiough MA, Sisk JE, Bell JC. Influenza vaccination: cost-effectiveness and public policy. *JAMA*. 1983; 249:3189–95.

Approved by the ASHP Board of Directors, November 18, 1992. Developed by the ASHP Council on Professional Affairs.

The bibliographic citation for this document is as follows: American Society of Hospital Pharmacists. ASHP technical assistance bulletin on the pharmacist's role in immunization. *Am J Hosp Pharm*. 1993; 50:501–5.

ASHP Technical Assistance Bulletin on Pharmacy-Prepared Ophthalmic Products

Pharmacists are frequently called on to prepare sterile products intended for ophthalmic administration when a suitable sterile ophthalmic product is not available from a licensed manufacturer. These products may be administered topically or by subconjunctival or intraocular (e.g., intravitreal and intracameral) injection and may be in the form of solutions, suspensions, or ointments.

The sterility of these products, as well as accuracy in the calculation and preparation of doses, is of great importance. Ocular infections and loss of vision caused by contamination of extemporaneously prepared ophthalmic products have been reported.[1,2] Drugs administered by subconjunctival or intraocular injection often have narrow therapeutic indices. In practice, serious errors in technique have occurred in the preparation of intravitreal solutions, which resulted in concentrations up to double the intended amounts.[3] To ensure adequate stability, uniformity, and sterility, ophthalmic products from licensed manufacturers should be used whenever possible.

The following guidelines are intended to assist pharmacists when extemporaneous preparation of ophthalmic products is necessary. These guidelines do not apply to the manufacturing of sterile pharmaceuticals as defined in state and federal laws and regulations. Other guidelines on extemporaneous compounding of ophthalmic products also have been published.[4,5]

1. Before compounding any product for ophthalmic use, the pharmacist should review documentation that substantiates the safety and benefit of the product when administered into the eye. If no such documentation is available, the pharmacist must employ professional judgment in determining suitability of the product for ophthalmic administration.

2. Important factors to be considered in preparing an ophthalmic medication include the following:[6]
   a. Sterility.
   b. Tonicity.
   c. pH, buffering.
   d. Inherent toxicity of the drug.
   e. Need for a preservative.
   f. Solubility.
   g. Stability in an appropriate vehicle.
   h. Viscosity.
   i. Packaging and storage of the finished product.

3. A written procedure for each ophthalmic product compounded should be established and kept on file and should be easily retrievable. The procedure should specify appropriate steps in compounding, including aseptic methods, and whether microbiologic filtration or terminal sterilization (e.g., autoclaving) of the finished product is appropriate.

4. Before preparation of the product is begun, mathematical calculations should be reviewed by another person or by an alternative method of calculation in order to minimize error. This approach is especially important for products, such as intraocular injections, for which extremely small doses are frequently ordered,

necessitating multiple dilutions. Decimal errors in the preparation of these products may have serious consequences.

5. Accuracy in compounding ophthalmic products is further enhanced by the use of larger volumes, which tends to diminish the effect of errors in measurement caused by the inherent inaccuracy of measuring devices. Larger volumes, however, also necessitate special attention to adequate mixing procedures, especially for ointments.

6. Strict adherence to aseptic technique and proper sterilization procedures are crucial in the preparation of ophthalmic products. All extemporaneous compounding of ophthalmic products should be performed in a certified laminar airflow hood (or, for preparing cytotoxic or hazardous agents, a biological safety cabinet).[5] Only personnel trained and proficient in the techniques and procedures should prepare ophthalmic products. Quality-assurance principles for compounding sterile products should be followed, and methods should be established to validate all procedures and processes related to sterile product preparation. In addition, the following should be considered:
   a. Ingredients should be mixed in sterile empty containers. Individual ingredients often can first be drawn into separate syringes and then injected into a larger syringe by insertion of the needles into the needle-free tip of the larger syringe. The larger syringe should be of sufficient size to allow for proper mixing of ingredients.
   b. To maximize measurement accuracy, the smallest syringe appropriate for measuring the required volume should be used. When the use of a single syringe would require estimation of the volume (e.g., measuring 4.5 ml in a 5-ml syringe with no mark at the 4.5-ml level), the use of two syringes of appropriate capacities (or two separate syringe "loads") should be considered in order to provide a more accurate measurement.
   c. A fresh disposable needle and syringe should be used at each step to avoid contamination and prevent error due to residual contents.
   d. When multiple dilutions are required, the containers of interim concentrations should be labeled to avoid confusion.
   e. In the preparation of an ophthalmic product from either (1) a sterile powder that has been reconstituted or (2) a liquid from a glass ampul, the ingredients should be filtered through a 5-μm filter to remove any particulate matter.

7. For ophthalmic preparations that must be sterilized, an appropriate and validated method of sterilization should be determined on the basis of the characteristics of the particular product and container. Filtration of the preparation through a 0.22-μm filter into a sterile final container is a commonly used method; however, this method is not suitable for sterilizing ophthalmic sus-

pensions and ointments.[7] When an ophthalmic preparation is compounded from a nonsterile ingredient, the final product must be sterilized before it is dispensed. Sterilization by autoclaving in the final container may be possible, provided that product stability is not adversely affected and appropriate quality control procedures are followed.[6]

8. Preservative-free ingredients should be used in the preparation of intraocular injections, since some preservatives are known to be toxic to many of the internal structures of the eye.[6]

9. In the preparation of ophthalmic products from cytotoxic or other hazardous agents, the pharmacist should adhere to established safety guidelines for handling such agents.[8,9]

10. The final container should be appropriate for the ophthalmic product and its intended use and should not interfere with the stability and efficacy of the preparation.[10] Many ophthalmic liquids can be packaged in sterile plastic bottles with self-contained dropper tips or in glass bottles with separate droppers. Ophthalmic ointments should be packaged in sterilized ophthalmic tubes. Injectables that are not for immediate use should be packaged in sterile vials rather than in syringes, and appropriate overfill should be included. All containers should be adequately sealed to prevent contamination.

11. The pharmacist should assign appropriate expiration dates to extemporaneously prepared ophthalmic products; these dates should be based on documented stability data as well as the potential for microbial contamination of the product.[11] The chemical stability of the active ingredient, the preservative, and packaging material should be considered in determining the overall stability of the final ophthalmic product.[12]

12. Ophthalmic products should be clearly and accurately labeled. In some cases, it may be appropriate to label the products with both the weight and concentration of active ingredients and preservatives. Labels should also specify storage and handling requirements and expiration dates. Extemporaneously prepared ophthalmic products dispensed for outpatient use should be labeled in accordance with applicable state regulations for prescription labeling.

References

1. Associated Press. Pittsburgh woman loses eye to tainted drugs; 12 hurt. *Baltimore Sun*. 1990; Nov 9:3A.
2. Associated Press. Eye drop injuries prompt an FDA warning. *N Y Times*. 1990; 140(Dec 9):39I.
3. Jeglum EL, Rosenberg SB, Benson WE. Preparation of intravitreal drug doses. *Ophthalmic Surg*. 1981; 12:355–9.
4. Reynolds LA. Guidelines for preparation of sterile ophthalmic products. *Am J Hosp Pharm*. 1991; 48:2438–9.
5. Reynolds LA, Closson R. Ophthalmic drug formulations. A handbook of extemporaneous products. Vancouver, WA: Applied Therapeutics; (in press).
6. The United States Pharmacopeia, 22nd rev., and The National Formulary, 17th ed. Rockville, MD: The United States Pharmacopeial Convention; 1989:1692–3.
7. Allen LV. Indomethacin 1% ophthalmic suspension. *US Pharm*. 1991; 16(May):82–3.
8. American Society of Hospital Pharmacists. ASHP technical assistance bulletin on handling cytotoxic and hazardous drugs. *Am J Hosp Pharm*. 1990; 47:1033–49.
9. OSHA work-practice guidelines for personnel dealing with cytotoxic (antineoplastic) drugs. *Am J Hosp Pharm*. 1986; 43:1193–204.
10. Ansel HC, Popovich NG. Pharmaceutical dosage forms and drug delivery systems. 5th ed. Philadelphia: Lea & Febiger; 1990:354–7.
11. Stolar MH. Expiration dates of repackaged drug products. *Am J Hosp Pharm*. 1979; 36:170. Editorial.
12. Remington's pharmaceutical sciences. 19th ed. Gennaro AR, ed. Easton, PA: Mack Publishing; 1990:1581–959.

Approved by the ASHP Board of Directors, April 21, 1993. Developed by the ASHP Council on Professional Affairs.

The bibliographic citation for this document is as follows: American Society of Hospital Pharmacists. ASHP technical assistance bulletin on pharmacy-prepared ophthalmic products. *Am J Hosp Pharm*. 1993; 50:1462–3.

ASHP Technical Assistance Bulletin on Quality Assurance for Pharmacy-Prepared Sterile Products

Pharmacists are responsible for the correct preparation of sterile products.[a] Patient morbidity and mortality have resulted from incorrectly prepared or contaminated pharmacy-prepared products.[1–5] These ASHP recommendations are intended to help pharmacists ensure that pharmacy-prepared sterile products are of high quality.

The National Coordinating Committee on Large Volume Parenterals (NCCLVP), which ceased to exist in the 1980s, published a series of recommendations in the 1970s and early 1980s,[6–12] including an article on quality assurance (QA) for centralized intravenous admixture services in hospitals.[7] The NCCLVP recommendations, however, are somewhat dated and do not cover the variety of settings in which pharmacists practice today nor the many types of sterile preparations pharmacists compound in current practice settings.

The Joint Commission on Accreditation of Healthcare Organizations (JCAHO) publishes only general standards relating to space, equipment and supplies, and record keeping for the preparation of sterile products in hospitals.[13] The 1993 JCAHO home care standards provide somewhat more detailed, nationally recognized pharmaceutical standards for home care organizations.[14] These standards, however, also lack sufficient detail to provide pharmacists with adequate information on quality assurance activities.

The Food and Drug Administration (FDA) publishes regulations on Current Good Manufacturing Practices[15,16] that apply to sterile products made by pharmaceutical manufacturers for shipment in interstate commerce. The FDA has also published a draft guideline on the manufacture of sterile drug products by aseptic processing.[17] Both of these documents apply to the manufacture of sterile products by licensed pharmaceutical manufacturers. The Centers for Disease Control and Prevention (CDC) has published guidelines for hand washing, prevention of intravascular infections,[18] and hospital environmental control.[19] The United States Pharmacopeial Convention, Inc. (USPC) establishes drug standards for packaging and storage, labeling, identification, pH, particulate matter, heavy metals, assay, and other requirements[16]; as of this writing, there is an effort under way at USPC to develop an informational chapter on compounding sterile products intended for home use.[20]

Although the aforementioned guidelines provide assistance to pharmacists, each has certain limitations (e.g., outdated, limited scope). None of these guidelines addresses sterile product storage and administration with newer types of equipment (e.g., portable infusion devices,[21,22] indwelling medication reservoirs) or the use of automated sterile-product compounding devices.[23]

This document was developed to help pharmacists establish quality assurance procedures for the preparation of sterile products. The recommendations in this Technical Assistance Bulletin are applicable to pharmacy services in various practice settings including but not limited to hospitals, community pharmacies, nursing homes, and home health care organizations. ASHP has published a practice standard on handling cytotoxic and hazardous drugs[24]; when preparing sterile preparations involving cytotoxic or hazardous drugs, pharmacists should consider the advice in that document.

The ASHP Technical Assistance Bulletin on Quality Assurance for Pharmacy-Prepared Sterile Products *does not* apply to the *manufacture* of sterile pharmaceuticals, as defined in state and federal laws and regulations, *nor* does it apply to the preparation of medications by pharmacists, nurses, or physicians in emergency situations for immediate administration to patients. Not all recommendations may be applicable to the preparation of pharmaceuticals.

These recommendations are referenced with supporting scientific data when such data exist. In the absence of published supporting data, recommendations are based on expert opinion or generally accepted pharmacy procedures. Pharmacists are urged to use professional judgment in interpreting these recommendations and applying them in practice. It is recognized that, in certain emergency situations, a pharmacist may be requested to compound products under conditions that do not meet the recommendations. In such situations, it is incumbent upon the pharmacist to employ professional judgment in weighing the potential patient risks and benefits associated with the compounding procedure in question.

Objectives. The objectives of these recommendations are to provide

1. Information to pharmacists on quality assurance and quality control activities that may be applied to the preparation of sterile products in pharmacies; and
2. A scheme to match quality assurance and quality control activities with the potential risks to patients posed by various types of products.

Multidisciplinary Input. Pharmacists are urged to participate in the quality improvement, risk management, and infection control programs of their organizations. In so doing, pharmacists should report findings about quality assurance in sterile preparations to the appropriate staff members or committees (e.g., risk management, infection control practitioners) when procedures that may lead to patient harm are known or suspected to be in use. Pharmacists should also cooperate with managers of quality improvement, risk management, and infection control to develop optimal sterile product procedures.

Definitions. Definitions of selected terms, as used for the purposes of this document, are located in the appendix. For brevity in this document, the term *quality assurance* will be used to refer to both quality assurance and quality control (as defined in the appendix), as befits the circumstances.

Risk Level Classification

In this document, sterile products are grouped into three levels of risk to the patient, increasing from least (level 1) to greatest (level 3) potential risk and having different associated quality assurance recommendations for product integrity and patient safety. This classification system should assist pharmacists in selecting which sterile product preparation procedures to use. Compounded sterile products in risk levels 2 and 3 should meet or exceed all of the quality assurance recommendations for risk level 1. When circumstances make risk level assignment unclear, recommendations for the higher risk level should prevail. Pharmacists must exercise their own professional judgment in deciding which risk level applies to a specific compounded sterile product or situation. Consideration should be given to factors that increase potential risk to the patient, such as multiple system breaks, compounding complexities, high-risk administration sites, immunocompromised status of the patient, use of nonsterile components, microbial growth potential of the finished sterile drug product, storage conditions, and circumstances such as time between compounding and initiation of administration. The following risk assignments, based on the expertise of knowledgeable practitioners, represent one logical arrangement in which pharmacists may evaluate risk. Pharmacists may construct alternative arrangements that could be supported on the basis of scientific information and professional judgment.

Risk Level 1. Risk level 1 applies to compounded sterile products that exhibit characteristics 1, 2, *and* 3 stated below. All risk level 1 products should be prepared with sterile equipment (e.g., syringes, vials), sterile ingredients and solutions, and sterile contact surfaces for the final product. Of the three risk levels, risk level 1 necessitates the least amount of quality assurance. Risk level 1 includes the following:

1. Products
   a. Stored at room temperature (see the appendix for temperature definitions) and completely administered within 28 hours from preparation; or
   b. Stored under refrigeration for 7 days or less before complete administration to a patient over a period not to exceed 24 hours (Table 1); or
   c. Frozen for 30 days or less before complete administration to a patient over a period not to exceed 24 hours.
2. Unpreserved sterile products prepared for administration to one patient, or batch-prepared products containing suitable preservatives prepared for administration to more than one patient.
3. Products prepared by closed-system aseptic transfer of sterile, nonpyrogenic, finished pharmaceuticals obtained from licensed manufacturers into sterile final containers (e.g., syringe, minibag, portable infusion-device cassette) obtained from licensed manufacturers.

Risk Level 2. Risk level 2 sterile products exhibit characteristic 1, 2, *or* 3 stated below. All risk level 2 products should be prepared with sterile equipment, sterile ingredients and solutions, and sterile contact surfaces for the final product and by using closed-system transfer methods. Risk level 2 includes the following:

1. Products stored beyond 7 days under refrigeration, or stored beyond 30 days frozen, or administered beyond 28 hours after preparation and storage at room temperature (Table 1).
2. Batch-prepared products without preservatives that are intended for use by more than one patient. (Note: Batch-prepared products without preservatives that

Table 1.

Assignment of Products to Risk Level 1 or 2 According to Time and Temperature Before Completion of Administration

Risk Level	Room Temperature (15 to 30 °C)	Days of Storage Refrigerator (2 to 8 °C)	Freezer (−20 to −10 °C)
1	Completely administered within 28 hr	≤ 7	≤ 30
2	Storage and administration exceeds 28 hr	> 7	> 30

will be administered to multiple patients carry a greater risk to the patients than products prepared for a single patient because of the potential effect of product contamination on the health and well-being of a larger patient group.)

3. Products compounded by combining multiple sterile ingredients, obtained from licensed manufacturers, in a sterile reservoir, obtained from a licensed manufacturer, by using closed-system aseptic transfer before subdivision into multiple units to be dispensed to patients.

Risk Level 3. Risk level 3 products exhibit either characteristic 1 *or* 2:

1. Products compounded from nonsterile ingredients or compounded with nonsterile components, containers, or equipment.
2. Products prepared by combining multiple ingredients—sterile or nonsterile—by using an open-system transfer or open reservoir before terminal sterilization or subdivision into multiple units to be dispensed.

Quality Assurance for Risk Level 1

RL 1.1: Policies and Procedures. Up-to-date policies and procedures for compounding sterile products should be written and available to all personnel involved in these activities. Policies and procedures should be reviewed at least annually by the designated pharmacist and department head and updated, as necessary, to reflect current standards of practice and quality. Additions, revisions, and deletions should be communicated to all personnel involved in sterile compounding and related activities. These policies and procedures should address personnel education and training requirements, competency evaluation, product acquisition, storage and handling of products and supplies, storage and delivery of final products, use and maintenance of facilities and equipment, appropriate garb and conduct for personnel working in the controlled area, process validation, preparation technique, labeling, documentation, and quality control.[9] Further, written policies and procedures should address personnel access and movement of materials into and near the controlled area. Policies and procedures for monitoring environmental conditions in the controlled area should take into consideration the amount of exposure of the product to the environment during compounding. Before compounding sterile products, all personnel involved should read the policies and procedures and sign to verify their understanding.

RL 1.2: Personnel Education, Training, and Evaluation.
Pharmacy personnel preparing or dispensing sterile products should receive suitable didactic and experiential training and competency evaluation through demonstration, testing (written or practical), or both. Some aspects that should be included in training programs include aseptic technique; critical-area contamination factors; environmental monitoring; facilities, equipment, and supplies; sterile product calculations and terminology; sterile product compounding documentation; quality assurance procedures; aseptic preparation procedures; proper gowning and gloving technique; and general conduct in the controlled area. In addition to knowledge of chemical, pharmaceutical, and clinical properties of drugs, pharmacists should also be knowledgeable about the principles of Current Good Manufacturing Practices.[15,16] Videotapes[25] and additional information on the essential components of a training, orientation, and evaluation program are described elsewhere.[7,12,26,27] All pharmacy personnel involved in cleaning and maintenance of the controlled area should be knowledgeable about cleanroom design (if applicable), the basic concepts of aseptic compounding, and critical-area contamination factors. Non-pharmacy personnel (e.g., housekeeping staff) involved in the cleaning or maintenance of the controlled area should receive adequate training on applicable procedures.

The aseptic technique of each person preparing sterile products should be observed and evaluated as satisfactory during orientation and training and at least on an annual basis thereafter. In addition to observation, methods of evaluating the knowledge of personnel include written or practical tests and process validation.

RL 1.3: Storage and Handling. Solutions, drugs, supplies, and equipment used to prepare or administer sterile products should be stored in accordance with manufacturer or USP requirements. Temperatures in refrigerators and freezers used to store ingredients and finished sterile preparations should be monitored and documented daily to ensure that compendial storage requirements are met. Warehouse and other pharmacy storage areas where ingredients are stored should be monitored to ensure that temperature, light, moisture, and ventilation remain within manufacturer and compendial requirements. To permit adequate floor cleaning, drugs and supplies should be stored on shelving areas above the floor. Products that have exceeded their expiration dates should be removed from active storage areas. Before use, each drug, ingredient, and container should be visually inspected for damage, defects, and expiration date.

Unnecessary personnel traffic in the controlled area should be minimized. Particle-generating activities, such as removal of intravenous solutions, drugs, and supplies from cardboard boxes, should not be performed in the controlled area. Products and supplies used in preparing sterile products should be removed from shipping containers outside the controlled area before aseptic processing is begun. Packaging materials and items generating unacceptable amounts of particles (e.g., cardboard boxes, paper towels, reference books) should not be permitted in the controlled area or critical area. The removal of immediate packaging designed to retain the sterility or stability of a product (e.g., syringe packaging, light-resistant pouches) is an exception; obviously, this type of packaging should not be removed outside the controlled area. Disposal of packaging materials, used syringes, containers, and needles should be performed at least daily, and more often if needed, to enhance sanitation and avoid accumulation in the controlled area.

In the event of a product recall, there should be a mechanism for tracking and retrieving affected products from specific patients to whom the products were dispensed.

RL 1.4: Facilities and Equipment. The controlled area should be a limited-access area sufficiently separated from other pharmacy operations to minimize the potential for contamination that could result from the unnecessary flow of materials and personnel into and out of the area. Computer entry, order processing, label generation, and record keeping should be performed outside the critical area. The controlled area should be clean, well lighted, and of sufficient size to support sterile compounding activities. For hand washing, a sink with hot and cold running water should be in close proximity. Refrigeration, freezing, ventilation, and room temperature control capabilities appropriate for storage of ingredients, supplies, and pharmacy-prepared sterile products in accordance with manufacturer, USP, and state or federal requirements should exist. The controlled area should be cleaned and disinfected at regular intervals with appropriate agents, according to written policies and procedures. Disinfectants should be alternated periodically to prevent the development of resistant microorganisms. The floors of the controlled area should be nonporous and washable to enable regular disinfection. Active work surfaces in the controlled area (e.g., carts, compounding devices, counter surfaces) should be disinfected, in accordance with written procedures. Refrigerators, freezers, shelves, and other areas where pharmacy-prepared sterile products are stored should be kept clean.

Sterile products should be prepared in a Class 100 environment.[28] Such an environment exists inside a certified horizontal- or vertical-laminar-airflow hood. Facilities that meet the recommendations for risk level 3 preparation would be suitable for risk level 1 and 2 compounding. Cytotoxic and other hazardous products should be prepared in a Class II biological-safety cabinet.[24] Laminar-airflow hoods are designed to be operated continuously. If a laminar-airflow hood is turned off between aseptic processing, it should be operated long enough to allow complete purging of room air from the critical area (e.g., 15–30 minutes), then disinfected before use. The critical-area work surface and all accessible interior surfaces of the hood should be disinfected with an appropriate agent before work begins and periodically thereafter, in accordance with written policies and procedures. The exterior surfaces of the laminar-airflow hood should be cleaned periodically with a mild detergent or suitable disinfectant; 70% isopropyl alcohol may damage the hood's clear plastic surfaces. The laminar-airflow hood should be certified by a qualified contractor at least every six months or when it is relocated to ensure operational efficiency and integrity.[29] Prefilters in the laminar-airflow hood should be changed periodically, in accordance with written policies and procedures.

A method should be established to calibrate and verify the accuracy of automated compounding devices used in aseptic processing.

RL 1.5: Garb. Procedures should generally require that personnel wear clean clothing covers that generate low amounts of particles in the controlled area. Clean gowns or closed coats with sleeves that have elastic binding at the cuff are recommended. Hand, finger, and wrist jewelry should be minimized or eliminated. Head and facial hair should be covered. Masks are recommended during aseptic preparation procedures.

Personnel preparing sterile products should scrub their hands and arms (to the elbow) with an appropriate antimicrobial skin cleanser.

RL 1.6: Aseptic Technique and Product Preparation. Sterile products should be prepared with aseptic technique in a Class 100 environment. Personnel should scrub their hands and forearms for an appropriate length of time with a suitable antimicrobial skin cleanser at the beginning of each aseptic compounding process and when re-entering the controlled area. Personnel should wear appropriate attire (see RL 1.5: Garb). Eating, drinking, and smoking should be prohibited in the controlled area. Talking should be minimized in the critical area during aseptic preparation.

Ingredients used to compound sterile products should be determined to be stable, compatible, and appropriate for the product to be prepared, according to manufacturer or USP guidelines or appropriate scientific references. The ingredients of the preparation should be predetermined to be suitable to result in a final product that meets physiological norms for solution osmolality and pH, as appropriate for the intended route of administration. Each ingredient and container should be inspected for defects, expiration date, and product integrity before use. Expired, inappropriately stored, or defective products should not be used in preparing sterile products. Defective products should be promptly reported to the FDA.[30]

Only materials essential for preparing the sterile product should be placed in the laminar-airflow hood. The surfaces of ampuls, vials, and container closures (e.g., vial stoppers) should be disinfected by swabbing or spraying with an appropriate disinfectant solution (e.g., 70% isopropyl alcohol) before placement in the hood. Materials used in aseptic preparation should be arranged in the critical area of the hood in a manner that prevents interruption of the unidirectional airflow between the high-efficiency particulate air (HEPA) filter and critical sites of needles, vials, ampuls, containers, and transfer sets. All aseptic procedures should be performed at least 6 inches inside the front edge of the laminar-airflow hood, in a clear path of unidirectional airflow between the HEPA filter and work materials (e.g., needles, stoppers). The number of personnel preparing sterile products in the hood at one time should be minimized. Overcrowding of the critical work area may interfere with unidirectional airflow and increase the potential for compounding errors. Likewise, the number of units being prepared in the hood at one time should be consistent with the amount of work space in the critical area. Automated compounding devices and other equipment placed in or adjacent to the critical area should be cleaned, disinfected, and placed to avoid contamination or disruption of the unidirectional airflow between the HEPA filter and sterile surfaces.

Aseptic technique should be used to avoid touch contamination of sterile needles, syringe parts (e.g., plunger, syringe tip), and other critical sites. Solutions from ampuls should be properly filtered to remove particles. Solutions of reconstituted powders should be mixed carefully, ensuring complete dissolution of the drug with the appropriate diluent. Needle entry into vials with rubber stoppers should be done cautiously to avoid the creation of rubber core particles. Before, during, and after the preparation of sterile products, the pharmacist should carefully check the identity and verify the amounts of the ingredients in sterile preparations against the original prescription, medication order, or other appropriate documentation (e.g., computerized patient profile, label generated from a pharmacist-verified order) before the product is released or dispensed. Additional information on aseptic technique is available elsewhere.[6,25,31]

For preparation involving automated compounding devices, data entered into the compounding device should be verified by a pharmacist before compounding begins and end-product checks should be performed to verify accuracy of ingredient delivery. These checks may include weighing and visually verifying the final product. For example, the expected weight (in grams) of the final product, based on the specific gravities of the ingredients and their respective volumes, can be documented on the compounding formula sheet, dated, and initialed by the responsible pharmacist. Once compounding is completed, each final product can be weighed and its weight compared with the expected weight. The product's actual weight should fall within a pre-established threshold for variance.[32] Visual verification may be aided by marking the beginning level of each bulk container before starting the automated mixing process and checking each container after completing the mixing process to determine whether the final levels appear reasonable in comparison with expected volumes. The operator should also periodically observe the device during the mixing process to ensure that the device is operating properly (e.g., check to see that all stations are operating).[33] If there are doubts whether a product or component has been properly prepared or stored, then the product should not be used. Refractive index measurements may also be used to verify the addition of certain ingredients.[34]

RL 1.7: Process Validation. Validation of aseptic processing procedures provides a mechanism for ensuring that processes consistently result in sterile products of acceptable quality. For most aseptic preparation procedures, process validation is actually a method of assessing the adequacy of a person's aseptic technique. It is recommended that each individual involved in the preparation of sterile products successfully complete a validation process on technique before being allowed to prepare sterile products. The validation process should follow a written procedure that includes evaluation of technique through process simulation.[35–37]

Process simulation testing is valuable for assessing the compounding process, especially aseptic fill operations.[17] It allows for the evaluation of opportunities for microbial contamination during all steps of sterile product preparation. The sterility of the final product is a cumulative function of all processes involved in its preparation and is ultimately determined by the processing step providing the lowest probability of sterility.[38] Process simulation testing is carried out in the same manner as normal production except that an appropriate microbiological growth medium is used in place of the actual products used during sterile preparation. The growth medium is processed as if it were a product being compounded for patient use; the same personnel, procedures, equipment, and materials are involved. The medium samples are then incubated and evaluated. If no microbial growth is detected, this provides evidence that adequate aseptic technique was used. If growth is detected, the entire sterile preparation process must be evaluated, corrective action taken, and the process simulation test performed again.[17,38] No products intended for patient use should be prepared by an individual until the process simulation test indicates that the individual can competently perform aseptic procedures. It is recommended that personnel competency be revalidated at least annually, whenever the quality assurance program yields an unacceptable result, and whenever unacceptable techniques are observed; this revalidation should be documented.

RL 1.8: Expiration Dating. All pharmacy-prepared sterile products should bear an appropriate expiration date. The expiration date assigned should be based on currently available drug stability information and sterility considerations. Sources of drug stability information include references (e.g., *Remington's Pharmaceutical Sciences, Handbook on Injectable Drugs*), manufacturer recommendations, and reliable, published research. When interpreting published drug stability information, the pharmacist should consider all aspects of the final sterile product being prepared (e.g., drug reservoir, drug concentration, storage conditions).[15,16] Methods used for establishing expiration dates should be documented. Appropriate inhouse (or contract service) stability testing may be used to determine expiration dates.

RL 1.9: Labeling. Sterile products should be labeled with at least the following information:

1. For patient-specific products: the patient's name and any other appropriate patient identification (e.g., location, identification number); for batch-prepared products: control or lot number;
2. All solution and ingredient names, amounts, strengths, and concentrations (when applicable);
3. Expiration date (and time, when applicable);
4. Prescribed administration regimen, when appropriate (including rate and route of administration);
5. Appropriate auxiliary labeling (including precautions);
6. Storage requirements;
7. Identification (e.g., initials) of the responsible pharmacist;
8. Device-specific instructions (when appropriate); and
9. Any additional information, in accordance with state or federal requirements.

It may also be useful to include a reference number for the prescription or medication order in the labeling; this information is usually required for products dispensed to outpatients. The label should be legible and affixed to the final container in a manner enabling it to be read while the sterile product is being administered (when possible).

RL 1.10: End-Product Evaluation. The final product should be inspected and evaluated for container leaks, container integrity, solution cloudiness, particulates in the solution, appropriate solution color, and solution volume when preparation is completed and again when the product is dispensed. The responsible pharmacist should verify that the product was compounded accurately with respect to the use of correct ingredients, quantities, containers, and reservoirs; different methods may be used for end-product verification (e.g., observation, calculation checks, documented records).

RL 1.11: Documentation. The following should be documented and maintained on file for an adequate period of time, according to organizational policies and procedures and state regulatory requirements: (1) the training and competency evaluation of employees in sterile product procedures, (2) refrigerator and freezer temperatures, and (3)

certification of laminar-airflow hoods. Pharmacists should also maintain appropriate dispensing records for sterile products, in accordance with state regulatory requirements.

Quality Assurance for Risk Level 2

Because the risks associated with contamination of a sterile product are increased with long-term storage and administration, more stringent requirements are appropriate for risk level 2 preparation.

RL 2.1: Policies and Procedures. In addition to all recommendations for risk level 1, the written quality assurance program should define and identify necessary environmental monitoring devices and techniques to be used to ensure an adequate environment for risk level 2 sterile product preparation. Examples include the use of airborne particle counters, air velocity and temperature meters, viable particle samplers (e.g., slit samplers), agar plates, and swab sampling of surfaces and potential contamination sites. All aspects of risk level 2 sterile product preparation, storage, and distribution, including details such as the choice of cleaning materials and disinfectants and the monitoring of equipment accuracy, should be addressed in written policies and procedures. Limits of acceptability (threshold or action levels) for environmental monitoring and process simulation and actions to be implemented when thresholds are exceeded should be defined in written policies. For sterile batch compounding, written policies and procedures should be established for the use of master formulas and work sheets and for appropriate documentation. Policies and procedures should also address personnel attire in the controlled area, lot number determination and documentation, and any other quality assurance procedures unique to compounding risk level 2 sterile products.

RL 2.2: Personnel Education, Training, and Evaluation. All recommendations for risk level 1 should be met. In addition to recommendations for risk level 1, assessment of the competency of personnel preparing risk level 2 sterile products should include an appropriate process simulation procedure (as described in RL 1.7: Process validation). However, process simulation procedures for assessing the preparation of risk level 2 sterile products should be representative of all types of manipulations, products, and batch sizes personnel preparing risk level 2 products are likely to encounter.

RL 2.3: Storage and Handling. All storage and handling recommendations for risk level 1 should be met.

RL 2.4: Facilities and Equipment. In addition to all recommendations for risk level 1, the following are recommended for risk level 2 sterile product preparation:

1. Risk level 2 products should be prepared in a Class 100 horizontal- or vertical-laminar-airflow hood that is properly situated in a controlled area that meets Class 100,000 conditions (or better) for acceptable airborne particle levels. Class 100,000 conditions mean that no more than 100,000 particles 0.5 μm and larger may exist per cubic foot of air.[28] A positive pressure relative to adjacent pharmacy areas is recommended.
2. Cleaning materials (e.g., mops, sponges, germicidal disinfectants) for use in the controlled area or cleanroom

should be carefully selected. They should be made of materials that generate a low amount of particles. If reused, cleaning materials should be cleaned and disinfected between uses.

3. The critical-area work surfaces (e.g., interior of the laminar-airflow hood) should be disinfected frequently and before and after each batch preparation process with an appropriate agent, according to written policies and procedures. Floors should be disinfected at least daily. Carpet or porous floors, porous walls, and porous ceiling tiles are not desirable in the controlled area because these surfaces cannot be properly disinfected. Exterior hood surfaces and other hard surfaces in the controlled area, such as shelves, carts, tables, and stools, should be disinfected weekly and after any unanticipated event that could increase the risk of contamination. Walls should be cleaned at least monthly.

4. To ensure that an appropriate environment is maintained for risk level 2 sterile product preparation, an effective written environmental monitoring program is recommended.[26] Sampling of air and surfaces according to a written plan and schedule is recommended.[17,26] The plan and frequency should be adequate to document that the controlled area is suitable and that the laminar-airflow hood(s) or biological-safety cabinet(s) meet the Class 100 requirements. Limits of acceptability (thresholds or action levels) and appropriate actions to be taken in the event thresholds are exceeded should be specified.

5. To help reduce the number of particles in the controlled area, an adjacent support area (e.g., anteroom) of high cleanliness, separated from the controlled area by a barrier (e.g., plastic curtain, partition, wall), is desirable. Appropriate activities for the support area include, but are not limited to, hand washing, gowning and gloving, removal of packaging and cardboard items, and cleaning and disinfecting hard-surface containers and supplies before placing these items in the controlled area.

RL 2.5: Garb. All recommendations for risk level 1 should be met. Gloves, gowns, and masks are recommended for the preparation of all risk level 2 sterile products. It must be emphasized that, even if sterile gloves are used, gloves do not remain sterile during aseptic compounding; however, they do assist in containing bacteria, skin, and other particles that may be shed, even from scrubbed hands. Clean gowns, coveralls, or closed jackets with sleeves having elastic binding at the cuff are recommended; these garments should be made of low-shedding materials. Shoe covers may be helpful in maintaining the cleanliness of the controlled area. During sterile product preparation, gloves should be rinsed frequently with a suitable agent (e.g., 70% isopropyl alcohol) and changed when their integrity is compromised (i.e., when they are punctured or torn).

RL 2.6: Aseptic Technique and Product Preparation. All recommendations for risk level 1 sterile production preparation should be met.

A master work sheet should be developed for each batch of sterile products to be prepared. Once approved by the designated pharmacist, a verified duplicate (e.g., photocopy) of the master work sheet should be used as the preparation work sheet from which each batch is prepared

and on which all documentation for that batch occurs. A separate preparation work sheet should be used for each batch prepared. The master work sheet should consist of the formula, components, compounding directions or procedures, a sample label, and evaluation and testing requirements.[39] The preparation work sheet should be used to document the following:

1. Identity of all solutions and ingredients and their corresponding amounts, concentrations, or volumes;
2. Manufacturer lot number for each component;
3. Component manufacturer or suitable identifying number;
4. Container specifications (e.g., syringe, pump cassette);
5. Lot or control number assigned to batch;
6. Expiration date of batch-prepared products;
7. Date of preparation;
8. Identity (e.g., initials, codes, signatures) of personnel involved in preparation;
9. End-product evaluation and testing specifications;
10. Storage requirements;
11. Specific equipment used during aseptic preparation (e.g., a specific automated compounding device); and
12. Comparison of actual yield to anticipated yield, when appropriate.

A policy and procedure could be developed that allows separate documentation of batch formulas, compounding instructions, and records. However documentation is done, a procedure should exist for easy retrieval of all records pertaining to a particular batch. Each group of sterile batch-prepared products should bear a unique lot number. Under no circumstances should identical lot numbers be assigned to different products or different batches of the same product. Lot numbers may be alphabetic, numeric, or alphanumeric.

The process of combining multiple sterile ingredients into a single, sterile reservoir for subdivision into multiple units for dispensing may necessitate additional quality control procedures. It is recommended that calculations associated with this process be verified by a second pharmacist, when possible; this verification should be documented. Because this process often involves making multiple entries into the intermediate sterile reservoir, the likelihood of contamination may be greater than that associated with the preparation of other risk level 2 sterile products.

RL 2.7: Process Validation. Each individual involved in the preparation of risk level 2 sterile products should successfully complete a validation process, as recommended for risk level 1. Process simulation procedures for compounding risk level 2 sterile products should be representative of all types of manipulations, products, and batch sizes that personnel preparing risk level 2 sterile products are likely to encounter.

RL 2.8: Expiration Dating. All recommendations for risk level 1 should be met.

RL 2.9: Labeling. All recommendations for risk level 1 should be met.

RL 2.10: End-Product Evaluation. All recommendations for risk level 1 should be met. Additionally, the growth media fill procedure should be supplemented with a program of end-product sterility testing, according to a formal sampling plan.[40–42] Written policies and procedures should specify measurements and methods of testing. Policies and procedures should include a statistically valid sampling plan and acceptance criteria for the sampling and testing. The criteria should be statistically adequate to reasonably ensure that the entire batch meets all specifications. Products not meeting all specifications should be rejected and discarded. There should be a mechanism for recalling all products of a specific batch if end-product testing procedures yield unacceptable results. On completion of final testing, products should be stored in a manner that ensures their identity, strength, quality, and purity. Detailed information on end-product sterility testing is published elsewhere.[7,16]

RL 2.11: Documentation. All recommendations for risk level 1 should be met. Additionally, documentation of end-product sampling and batch-preparation records should be maintained for an adequate period of time, according to organizational policies and procedures and state regulatory requirements. Documentation for sterile batch-prepared products should include the

1. Master work sheet;
2. Preparation work sheet; and
3. End-product evaluation and testing results.

Quality Assurance for Risk Level 3

General Comment on Risk Level 3. Risk level 3 addresses the preparation of products that pose the greatest potential risk to patients. The quality assurance activities described in this section are clearly more demanding—in terms of processes, facilities, and final product assessment—than for risk levels 1 and 2. Ideally, the activities described for risk level 3 would be used for all high-risk products. The activities may be viewed as most important in circumstances in which the medical need for such high-risk products is *routine*. In circumstances where the medical need for such a product is immediate (and there is not a suitable alternative) or when the preparation of such a product is rare, professional judgment must be applied as to the extent to which some activities (e.g., strict facility design, quarantine and final product testing before product dispensing) should be applied.

RL 3.1: Policies and Procedures. There should be written policies and procedures related to every aspect of preparation of risk level 3 sterile products. These policies and procedures should be detailed enough to ensure that all products have the identity, strength, quality, and purity purported for the product.[13,16] All policies and procedures should be reviewed and approved by the designated pharmacist. There should be a mechanism designed to ensure that policies and procedures are communicated, understood, and adhered to by personnel cleaning or working in the controlled area or support area. Policies and procedures should be reviewed at least annually by the designated pharmacist and department head. Written policies and procedures should define and identify the environmental monitoring activities necessary to ensure an adequate environment for risk level 3 sterile product preparation.

In addition to the policies and procedures required for risk levels 1 and 2, there should be written policies and procedures for the following:

1. Component handling and storage;
2. Any additional personnel qualifications commensurate with the preparation of risk level 3 sterile products;
3. Personnel responsibilities in the controlled area (e.g., cleaning, maintenance, access to controlled area);
4. Equipment use, maintenance, calibration, and testing;
5. Sterilization;
6. Master formula and master work sheet development and use;
7. End-product evaluation and testing;
8. Appropriate documentation for preparation of risk level 3 sterile products;
9. Use, control, and monitoring of environmentally controlled areas and calibration of monitoring equipment;
10. Validation of processes for preparing risk level 3 sterile products;
11. Quarantine of products and release from quarantine, if applicable;
12. A mechanism for recall of products from patients in the event that end-product testing procedures yield unacceptable results; and
13. Any other quality control procedures unique to the preparation of risk level 3 sterile products.

RL 3.2: Personnel Education, Training, and Evaluation. Persons preparing sterile products at risk level 3 must have specific education, training, and experience to perform all functions required for the preparation of risk level 3 sterile products. However, final responsibility should lie with the pharmacist, who should be knowledgeable in the principles of good manufacturing practices and proficient in quality assurance requirements, equipment used in the preparation of risk level 3 sterile products, and other aspects of sterile product preparation. The pharmacist should have sufficient education, training, experience, and demonstrated competency to ensure that all sterile products prepared from sterile or nonsterile components have the identity, strength, quality, and purity purported for the products.[7,13] In addition to the body of knowledge required for risk levels 1 and 2, the pharmacist should possess sufficient knowledge in the following areas:

1. Aseptic processing[17,38,43];
2. Quality control and quality assurance as related to environmental, component, and end-product testing;
3. Sterilization techniques[16]; and
4. Container, equipment, and closure system selection.

All pharmacy personnel involved in the cleaning and maintenance of the controlled area should be specially trained and thoroughly knowledgeable in the special requirements of Class 100 critical-area technology and design. There should be documented, ongoing training for all employees to enable retention of expertise.

RL 3.3: Storage and Handling. In addition to recommendations for risk levels 1 and 2, risk level 3 policies and procedures for storage and handling should include the procurement, identification, storage, handling, testing, and recall of components and finished products.

Components and finished products ready to undergo end-product testing should be stored in a manner that prevents their use before release by a pharmacist, minimizes the risk of contamination, and enables identification. There should be identifiable storage areas that can be used to quarantine products, if necessary, before they are released.[15]

RL 3.4: Facilities and Equipment. Preparation of risk level

3 sterile products should occur in a Class 100 horizontal- or vertical-laminar-airflow hood that is properly situated in a controlled area that meets Class 10,000 conditions for acceptable airborne particle levels *or* in a properly maintained and monitored Class 100 cleanroom (without the hood).[28] The controlled area should have a positive pressure differential relative to adjacent, less clean areas of at least 0.05 inch of water.[17] Solutions that are to be terminally sterilized may be prepared in a Class 100 laminar-airflow hood located inside a controlled area that meets Class 100,000 conditions.

To allow proper cleaning and disinfection, walls, floors, and ceilings in the controlled area should be nonporous. To help reduce the number of particles in the controlled area, an adjacent support area (e.g., anteroom) should be provided.

During the preparation of risk level 3 sterile products, access to the controlled area or cleanroom should be limited to those individuals who are required to be in the area and are properly attired. The environment of the main access areas directly adjacent to the controlled area (e.g., anteroom) should meet at least Federal Standard 209E Class 100,000 requirements.[28] To help maintain a Class 100 critical-area environment during compounding, the adjacent support area (e.g., anteroom) should be separated from the controlled area by a barrier (e.g., plastic curtain, partition, wall). Written policies and procedures for monitoring the environment of the controlled area and adjacent areas should be developed.[17,26]

No sterile products should be prepared in the controlled area if it fails to meet established criteria specified in the policies and procedures. A calibrated particle counter capable of measuring air particles 0.5 μm and larger should be used to monitor airborne particulate matter. Before product preparation begins, the positive-pressure air status should meet or exceed the requirements. Air samples should be taken at several places in the controlled area with the appropriate environmental monitoring devices (e.g., nutrient agar plates). Surfaces on which work actually occurs, including laminar-airflow hood surfaces and tabletops, should be monitored using surface contact plates, the swab-rinse technique, or other appropriate methods.[37,42]

Test results should be reviewed and criteria should be pre-established to determine the point at which the preparation of risk level 3 sterile products will be disallowed until corrective measures are taken. When the environment does not meet the criteria specified in the policies and procedures, sterile product processing should immediately cease and corrective action should be taken. In the event that this occurs, written policies and procedures should delineate alternative methods of sterile product preparation to enable timely fulfillment of prescription orders.

Equipment should be adequate to prevent microbiological contamination. Methods should be established for the cleaning, preparation, sterilization, calibration, and documented use of all equipment.

Critical-area work surfaces should be disinfected with an appropriate agent before the preparation of each product. Floors in the controlled area should be disinfected at least daily. Exterior hood surfaces and other hard surfaces in the controlled area, such as shelves, tables, and stools, should be disinfected weekly and after any unanticipated event that could increase the risk of contamination. Walls and ceilings in the controlled area or cleanroom should be disinfected at least weekly.

Large pieces of equipment, such as tanks, carts, and tables, used in the controlled area or cleanroom should be made of a material that can be easily cleaned and disinfected; stainless steel is recommended. Equipment that does not come in direct contact with the finished product should be properly cleaned, rinsed, and disinfected before being placed in the controlled area. All nonsterile equipment that will come in contact with the sterilized final product should be properly sterilized before introduction into the controlled area; this precaution includes such items as tubing, filters, containers, and other processing equipment. The sterilization process should be monitored and documented.[17]

RL 3.5: Garb. All recommendations for risk levels 1 and 2 should be met. Additionally, cleanroom garb should be worn inside the controlled area at all times during the preparation of risk level 3 sterile products. Attire should consist of a low-shedding coverall, head cover, face mask, and shoe covers. These garments may be either disposable or reusable. Head and facial hair should be covered. Before donning these garments over street clothes, personnel should thoroughly wash their hands and arms up to the elbows with a suitable antimicrobial skin cleanser.[19] Sterile disposable gloves should be worn and rinsed frequently with an appropriate agent (e.g., 70% isopropyl alcohol) during processing. The gloves should be changed if the integrity is compromised. If persons leave the controlled area or *support area* during processing, they should regown with clean garments before re-entering.

RL 3.6: Aseptic Technique and Product Preparation. All recommendations for risk levels 1 and 2 should be met. Methods should ensure that components and containers remain free from contamination and are easily identified as to the product, lot number, and expiration date. If components are not finished sterile pharmaceuticals obtained from licensed manufacturers, pharmacists should ensure that these components meet USP standards. Products prepared from nonsterile ingredients should be tested to ensure that they do not exceed specified endotoxin limits.[16] As each new lot of components and containers is received, the components should be quarantined until properly identified, tested, or verified by a pharmacist.

The methods for preparing sterile products and using process controls should be designed to ensure that finished products have the identity, strength, quality, and purity they are intended to have. Any deviations from established methods should be documented and appropriately justified.

A master work sheet should be developed for the preparation of each risk level 3 sterile product. Once approved by the pharmacist, a verified duplicate of the master work sheet should be used as the controlling document from which each sterile end product or batch of prepared products is compounded and on which all documentation for that product or batch occurs. The master work sheet should document all the requirements for risk level 2 plus the following:

1. Comparison of actual with anticipated yield;
2. Sterilization method(s); and
3. Quarantine specifications.

The preparation work sheet should serve as the batch record for each time a risk level 3 sterile product is prepared. Each batch of pharmacy-prepared sterile products should bear a unique lot number, as described in risk level 2.

There should be documentation on the preparation work sheet of all additions of individual components plus the signatures or initials of those individuals involved with the measuring or weighing and addition of these components.

The selection of the final packaging system (including container and closure) for the sterile product is crucial to maintaining product integrity. To the extent possible, pre-sterilized containers obtained from licensed manufacturers should be used. If an aseptic filling operation is used, the container should be sterile at the time of the filling operation. If nonsterile containers are used, methods for sterilizing these containers should be established. Final containers selected should be capable of maintaining product integrity (i.e., identity, strength, quality, and purity) throughout the shelf life of the product.[44]

For products requiring sterilization, selection of an appropriate method of sterilization is of prime importance. Methods of product sterilization include sterile filtration, autoclaving, dry heat sterilization, chemical sterilization, and irradiation.[16,45] Selection of the sterilization technique should be based on the properties of the product being processed. The pharmacist must ensure that the sterilization method used is appropriate for the product components and does not alter the pharmaceutical properties of the final product. A method of sterilization often used by pharmacists is sterile filtration.[46] In sterile filtration, the product should be filtered into presterilized containers under aseptic conditions. Sterilizing filters of 0.22 μm or smaller porosity should be used in this process. Colloidal or viscous products may require use of a 0.45-μm filter; however, extreme caution should be exercised in these circumstances, and more stringent end-product sterility testing is essential.[26,47,48]

To ensure that a bacteria-retentive filter did not rupture during filtration of a product, an integrity test should be performed on all filters immediately after filtration. This test may be accomplished by performing a bubble point test, in which pressurized gas is applied to the upstream side of the filter with the downstream outlet immersed in water and the pressure at which a steady stream of bubbles begins to appear is noted.[46,48] The observed pressure is then compared with the manufacturer's specification for the filter. To compare the used filter with the manufacturer's specifications, which would be based on the filtration of water through the filter, it is necessary to first rinse the filter with sterile water for injection. An observed value lower than the manufacturer's specification indicates that the filter was defective or ruptured during the sterilization process. Methods should be established for handling, testing, and resterilizing any product processed with a filter that fails the integrity test.

RL 3.7: Process Validation. In addition to risk level 1 and 2 recommendations, written policies and procedures should be established to validate all processes involved in the preparation of risk level 3 sterile products (including all procedures, equipment, and techniques) from sterile or nonsterile components. In addition to evaluating personnel technique, process validation provides a mechanism for determining whether a particular process will, when performed by qualified personnel, consistently produce the intended results.

RL 3.8: Expiration Dating. In addition to risk level 2 recommendations, there should be reliable methods for establishing all expiration dates including laboratory testing of products for sterility, pyrogenicity, and chemical content, when necessary. These tests should be conducted in a manner based on appropriate statistical criteria, and the results documented.

RL 3.9: Labeling. All recommendations for risk levels 1 and 2 should be met.

RL 3.10: End-Product Evaluation. For each preparation of a sterile product or a batch of sterile products, there should be appropriate laboratory determination of conformity with established written specifications and policies. Any reprocessed material should undergo complete final product testing. It is advisable to quarantine sterile products compounded from nonsterile components, pending the results of end-product testing. If products prepared from nonsterile components must be dispensed before satisfactory completion of end-product testing, there must be a procedure to allow for immediate recall of the products from patients to whom they were dispensed.

RL 3.11: Documentation. In addition to the recommendations for risk levels 1 and 2, documentation for risk level 3 sterile products should include

1. Preparation work sheet;
2. Sterilization records of final products (if applicable);
3. Quarantine records (if applicable); and
4. End-product evaluation and testing results.

Appendix A—Glossary

Aseptic Preparation: The technique involving procedures designed to preclude contamination (of drugs, packaging, equipment, or supplies) by microorganisms during processing.

Batch Preparation: Compounding of multiple sterile-product units, in a single discrete process, by the same individual(s), carried out during one limited time period.

Cleanroom: A room in which the concentration of airborne particles is controlled and there are one or more clean zones. (A clean zone is a defined space in which the concentration of airborne particles is controlled to meet a specified airborne-particulate cleanliness class.) Cleanrooms are classified based on the maximum number of allowable particles 0.5 μm and larger per cubic foot of air. For example, the air particle count in a Class 100 cleanroom may not exceed a total of 100 particles of 0.5 μm and larger per cubic foot of air.[28]

Closed-System Transfer: The movement of sterile products from one container to another in which the container-closure system and transfer devices remain intact throughout the entire transfer process, compromised only by the penetration of a sterile, pyrogen-free needle or cannula through a designated stopper or port to effect transfer, withdrawal, or delivery. Withdrawal of a sterile solution from an ampul in a Class 100 environment would generally be considered acceptable; however, the use of a rubber-stoppered vial, when available, would be preferable.

Compounding: For purposes of this document, compounding simply means the mixing of substances to prepare a medication for patient use. This activity would include dilution, admixture, repackaging, reconstitution, and other manipulations of sterile products.

Controlled Area: For purposes of this document, a controlled area is the area designated for preparing sterile products.

Critical Areas: Any area in the controlled area where

products or containers are exposed to the environment.[37]

Critical Site: An opening providing a direct pathway between a sterile product and the environment or any surface coming in contact with the product or environment.

Critical Surface: Any surface that comes into contact with previously sterilized products or containers.[37]

Expiration Date: The date (and time, when applicable) beyond which a product should not be used (i.e., the product should be discarded beyond this date and time). NOTE: Circumstances may occur in which the expiration date and time arrive while an infusion is in progress. When this occurs, judgment should be applied in determining whether it is appropriate to discontinue that infusion and replace the product. Organizational policies on this should be clear.

HEPA Filter: A high-efficiency particulate air (HEPA) filter composed of pleats of filter medium separated by rigid sheets of corrugated paper or aluminum foil that direct the flow of air forced through the filter in a uniform parallel flow. HEPA filters remove 99.97% of all air particles 0.3 µm or larger. When HEPA filters are used as a component of a horizontal- or vertical-laminar-airflow hood, an environment can be created consistent with standards for a Class 100 cleanroom.[49]

Quality Assurance: For purposes of this document, quality assurance is the set of activities used to ensure that the processes used in the preparation of sterile drug products lead to products that meet predetermined standards of quality.

Quality Control: For purposes of this document, quality control is the set of testing activities used to determine that the ingredients, components (e.g., containers), and final sterile products prepared meet predetermined requirements with respect to identity, purity, nonpyrogenicity, and sterility.

Repackaging: The subdivision or transfer from a container or device to a different container or device, such as a syringe or ophthalmic container.

Sterilizing Filter: A filter that, when challenged with a solution containing the microorganism *Pseudomonas diminuta,* at a minimum concentration of 10^7 organisms per square centimeter of filter surface, will produce a sterile effluent.[16,17]

Temperatures (USP): Frozen means temperatures between –20 and –10 °C (–4 and 14 °F). Refrigerated means temperatures between 2 and 8 °C (36 and 46 °F). Room temperature means temperatures between 15 and 30 °C (59 and 86 °F).[16]

Validation: Documented evidence providing a high degree of assurance that a specific process will consistently produce a product meeting its predetermined specifications and quality attributes.[17]

References

1. Hughes CF, Grant AF, Leckie BD, et al. Cardioplegic solution: a contamination crisis. *J Thorac Cardiovasc Surg.* 1986; 91:296–302.

2. Associated Press. Pittsburgh woman loses eye to tainted drugs; 12 hurt. *Baltimore Sun.* 1990; Nov 9:3A.

3. Anon. ASHP gears up multistep action plan regarding sterile drug products. *Am J Hosp Pharm.* 1991; 48:386, 389–90. News.

4. Dugleaux G, Coutour XL, Hecquard C, et al. Septicemia caused by contaminated parenteral nutrition pouches: the refrigerator as an unusual cause. *J Parenter Enter Nutr.* 1991; 15:474–5.

5. Solomon SL, Khabbaz RF, Parker RH, et al. An outbreak of *Candida parapsilosis* bloodstream infections in patients receiving parenteral nutrition. *J Infect Dis.* 1984; 149:98–102.

6. National Coordinating Committee on Large Volume Parenterals. Recommended methods for compounding intravenous admixtures in hospitals. *Am J Hosp Pharm.* 1975; 32:261–70.

7. National Coordinating Committee on Large Volume Parenterals. Recommended guidelines for quality assurance in hospital centralized intravenous admixture services. *Am J Hosp Pharm.* 1980; 37:645–55.

8. National Coordinating Committee on Large Volume Parenterals. Recommendations for the labeling of large volume parenterals. *Am J Hosp Pharm.* 1978; 35:49–51.

9. National Coordinating Committee on Large Volume Parenterals. Recommended standard of practice, policies, and procedures for intravenous therapy. *Am J Hosp Pharm.* 1980; 37:660–3.

10. National Coordinating Committee on Large Volume Parenterals. Recommended procedures for in-use testing of large volume parenterals suspected of contamination or of producing a reaction in a patient. *Am J Hosp Pharm.* 1978; 35:678–82.

11. National Coordinating Committee on Large Volume Parenterals. Recommended system for surveillance and reporting of problems with large volume parenterals in hospitals. *Am J Hosp Pharm.* 1975; 34:1251–3.

12. Barker KN, ed. Recommendations of the NCCLVP for the compounding and administration of intravenous solutions. Bethesda, MD: American Society of Hospital Pharmacists; 1981.

13. Joint Commission on Accreditation of Healthcare Organizations. 1993 Accreditation manual for hospitals. Oakbrook Terrace, IL: Joint Commission on Accreditation of Healthcare Organizations; 1992.

14. Joint Commission on Accreditation of Healthcare Organizations. 1993 Accreditation manual for home care. Vol. 1. Standards. Oakbrook Terrace, IL: Joint Commission on Accreditation of Healthcare Organizations; 1993.

15. Food and Drug Administration. Title 21 Code of Federal Regulations. Part 21—current good manufacturing practice for finished pharmaceuticals, United States.

16. The United States Pharmacopeia, 22nd rev., and The National Formulary, 17th ed. Rockville, MD: The United States Pharmacopeial Convention; 1989.

17. Division of Manufacturing and Product Quality, Office of Compliance, Food and Drug Administration. Guideline on sterile drug products produced by aseptic processing. Rockville, MD: Food and Drug Administration; 1987.

18. Centers for Disease Control. Guideline for prevention of intravascular infections. *Am J Infect Control.* 1983; 11(5):183–93.

19. Centers for Disease Control. Guideline for handwashing and hospital environmental control. *Am J Infect Control.* 1986; 4(8):110–29.

20. Anon. Sterile drug products for home use. *Pharmacopeial Forum.* 1993; 19:5380–409.

21. Stiles ML, Tu Y-H, Allen LV Jr. Stability of morphine sulfate in portable pump reservoirs during storage and simulated administration. *Am J Hosp Pharm.* 1989; 46:1404–7.

22. Duafala ME, Kleinberg ML, Nacov C, et al. Stability of morphine sulfate in infusion devices and containers for intravenous administration. *Am J Hosp Pharm.* 1990; 47:143–6.

23. Seidel AM. Quality control for parenteral nutrition compounding. Paper presented at 48th ASHP Annual Meeting; San Diego, CA: 1991 Jun 6.

24. American Society of Hospital Pharmacists. ASHP technical assistance bulletin on handling cytotoxic and hazardous drugs. *Am J Hosp Pharm.* 1990; 47:1033–49.

25. American Society of Hospital Pharmacists. Aseptic preparation of parenteral products. (Videotape and study guide.) Bethesda, MD: American Society of Hospital Pharmacists; 1985.

26. Avis KE, Lachman L, Lieberman HA, eds. Pharmaceutical dosage forms: parenteral medications. Vol 2. New York: Marcel Dekker; 1992.

27. American Society of Hospital Pharmacists. ASHP technical assistance bulletin on outcome competencies and training guidelines for institutional pharmacy technician training programs. *Am J Hosp Pharm.* 1982; 39:317–20.

28. Federal Standard No. 209E. Airborne particulate cleanliness classes in cleanrooms and clean zones. Washington, DC: General Services Administration; 1992.

29. Bryan D, Marback RC. Laminar-airflow equipment certification: what the pharmacist needs to know. *Am J Hosp Pharm.* 1984; 41:1343–9.

30. Kessler DA. MedWatch: the new FDA medical products reporting program. *Am J Hosp Pharm.* 1993; 50:1921–36.

31. Hunt ML. Training manual for intravenous admixture personnel, 4th ed. Chicago: Baxter Healthcare Corporation and Pluribus Press, Inc.; 1989.

32. Murphy C. Ensuring accuracy in the use of automatic compounders. *Am J Hosp Pharm.* 1993; 50:60. Letter.

33. Brushwood DB. Hospital liable for defect in cardioplegia solution. *Am J Hosp Pharm.* 1992; 49:1174–6.

34. Meyer GE, Novielli KA, Smith JE. Use of refractive index measurement for quality assurance of pediatric parenteral nutrition solutions. *Am J Hosp Pharm.* 1987; 44:1617–20.

35. Morris BG, Avis KN, Bowles GC. Quality-control plan for intravenous admixture programs. II: validation of operator technique. *Am J Hosp Pharm.* 1980; 37:668–72.

36. Dirks I, Smith FM, Furtado D, et al. Method for testing aseptic technique of intravenous admixture personnel. *Am J Hosp Pharm.* 1982; 39:457–9.

37. Brier KL. Evaluating aseptic technique of pharmacy personnel. *Am J Hosp Pharm.* 1983; 40:400–3.

38. Validation of aseptic filling for solution drug products. Technical monograph no. 2. Philadelphia: Parenteral Drug Association, Inc.; 1980.

39. Boylan JC. Essential elements of quality control. *Am J Hosp Pharm.* 1983; 40:1936–9.

40. Choy FN, Lamy PP, Burkhart VD, et al. Sterility-testing program for antibiotics and other intravenous admixtures. *Am J Hosp Pharm.* 1982; 39:452–6.

41. Doss HL, James JD, Killough DM, et al. Microbiologic quality assurance for intravenous admixtures in a small hospital. *Am J Hosp Pharm.* 1982; 39:832–5.

42. Posey LM, Nutt RE, Thompson PD. Comparison of two methods for detecting microbial contamination in intravenous fluids. *Am J Hosp Pharm.* 1982; 28:659–62.

43. Frieben WR. Control of aseptic processing environment. *Am J Hosp Pharm.* 1983; 40:1928–35.

44. Neidich RL. Selection of containers and closure systems for injectable products. *Am J Hosp Pharm.* 1983; 40:1924–7.

45. Phillips GB, O'Neill M. Sterilization. In: Gennaro AR, ed. Remington's pharmaceutical sciences. 18th ed. Easton, PA: Mack Publishing; 1990:1470–80.

46. McKinnon BT, Avis KE. Membrane filtration of pharmaceutical solutions. *Am J Hosp Pharm.* 1993; 50:1921–36.

47. Olson W. Sterilization of small-volume parenteral and therapeutic proteins by filtration. In: Olson W, Groves MJ, eds. Aseptic pharmaceutical manufacturing: technology for the 1990s. Prairie View, IL: Interpharm; 1987:101–49.

48. Eudailey WA. Membrane filters and membrane filtration processes for health care. *Am J Hosp Pharm.* 1983; 40:1921–3.

49. Turco S, King RE. Extemporaneous preparation. In: Turco S, King RE, eds. Sterile dosage forms. Philadelphia: Lea & Febiger; 1987:55–61.

---

^aUnless otherwise stated in this document, the term "sterile products" refers to sterile drug or nutritional substances that are prepared (e.g., compounded or repackaged) by pharmacy personnel.

Approved by the ASHP Board of Directors, September 24, 1993. Developed by the ASHP Council on Professional Affairs.

The bibliographic citation for this document is as follows: American Society of Hospital Pharmacists. ASHP technical assistance bulletin on quality assurance for pharmacy-prepared sterile products. *Am J Hosp Pharm.* 1993; 50:2386–98.

ASHP Technical Assistance Bulletin on Compounding Nonsterile Products in Pharmacies

Introduction

Pharmacists are the only health care providers formally trained in the art and science of compounding medications.[1,2] Therefore, pharmacists are expected, by the medical community and the public, to possess the knowledge and skills necessary to compound extemporaneous preparations. Pharmacists have a responsibility to provide compounding services for patients with unique drug product needs.

This Technical Assistance Bulletin is intended to assist pharmacists in the extemporaneous compounding of nonsterile drug products for individual patients. Included in this document is information on facilities and equipment, ingredient selection, training, documentation and record keeping, stability and beyond-use dating, packaging and labeling, and limited batch compounding. This document is not intended for manufacturers or licensed repackagers.

Facilities and Equipment

Facilities. It is not necessary that compounding activities be located in a separate facility; however, the compounding area should be located sufficiently away from routine dispensing and counseling functions and high traffic areas. The area should be isolated from potential interruptions, chemical contaminants, and sources of dust and particulate matter. To minimize chemical contaminants, the immediate area and work counter should be free of previously used drugs and chemicals. To minimize dust and particulate matter, cartons and boxes should not be stored or opened in the compounding area. The compounding area should not contain dust-collecting overhangs (e.g., ceiling utility pipes, hanging light fixtures) and ledges (e.g., windowsills). Additionally, at least one sink should be located in or near the compounding area for hand washing before compounding operations. Proper temperature and humidity control within the compounding area or facility is desirable.

Work areas should be well lighted, and work surfaces should be level and clean. The work surface should be smooth, impervious, free of cracks and crevices (preferably seamless), and nonshedding. Surfaces should be cleaned at both the beginning and the end of each distinct compounding operation with an appropriate cleaner or solvent. The entire compounding facility should be cleaned daily or weekly (as needed) but not during the actual process of compounding.

Equipment. The equipment needed to compound a drug product depends upon the particular dosage form requested. Although boards of pharmacy publish lists of required equipment and accessories, these lists are not intended to limit the equipment available to pharmacists for compounding.[2] Equipment should be maintained in good working order. Pharmacists are responsible for obtaining the required equipment and accessories and ensuring that equipment is properly maintained and maintenance is documented.

Weighing Equipment. In addition to a torsion balance, pharmacists who routinely compound may need to use a top-loading electronic balance that has a capacity of at least 300 g, a sensitivity of ±1 mg (or 0.1 mg), and 1-mg, 100-mg, 1-g, and 100-g weights for checking. Balances should be maintained in areas of low humidity and should be stored on flat, nonvibrating surfaces away from drafts. At least annually, the performance of balances should be checked according to the guidelines found in *Remington's Pharmaceutical Sciences,*[3] *USP XXII NF XVII: The United States Pharmacopeia–The National Formulary (USP–NF),*[4] or *USP DI Volume III: Approved Drug Products and Legal Requirements*[5] or the instructions of the balance manufacturer. Performance should be documented.

Weights should be stored in rigid, compartmentalized boxes and handled with metal, plastic, or plastic-tipped forceps—not fingers—to avoid scratching or soiling. Since most Class III prescription balances are only accurate to ±5 or 10 mg, Class P weights may be used for compounding purposes.[4] The *USP–NF* recommends that the class of weights used be chosen to limit the error to 0.1%. In practical terms this means that Class P weights can be used for weighing quantities greater than 100 mg.

The minimum weighable quantity must be determined for any balance being used for compounding. To avoid errors of 5% or more on a Class III balance with a sensitivity requirement of 6 mg, quantities of less than 120 mg of any substance should not be weighed. Smaller quantities may be weighed on more sensitive balances. If an amount is needed that is less than the minimum weighable quantity determined for a balance, an aliquot method of measurement should be used.

Measuring Equipment. The pharmacist should use judgment in selecting measuring equipment. The recommendations given in the *USP–NF* General Information section on volumetric apparatus should be followed. For maximum accuracy in measuring liquids, a pharmacist should select a graduate with a capacity equal to or slightly larger than the volume to be measured. The general rule is to measure no less than 20% of the capacity of a graduate. Calibrated syringes of the appropriate size may be preferred over graduated cylinders for measuring viscous liquids such as glycerin or mineral oil, since these liquids drain slowly and incompletely from graduated cylinders. Viscous liquids may also be weighed if this is more convenient, provided that the appropriate conversions from volume to weight are made by using the specific gravity of the liquid. Thick, opaque liquids should be weighed. For example, if a formulation specifies 1.5 mL of a liquid, it is better to use a 3-mL syringe with appropriate graduations to measure 1.5 mL than to use a 10-mL graduated cylinder, since quantities of less than 2.0 mL cannot be accurately measured in a 10-mL graduate. Also, if an opaque, viscous chemical, such as Coal Tar, USP, must be measured, it is more accurate to weigh the substance than to try to read a meniscus on a graduated cylinder or a fill line on a syringe.

For volumes smaller than 1 mL, micropipettes are recommended, in sizes to cover the range of volumes measured. Two or three variable pipettes can usually cover the range from about 50 µL to 1 mL.

Although conical graduates are convenient for mixing

solutions, the error in reading the bottom of the meniscus increases as the sides flare toward the top of the graduate. Therefore, for accurate measurements, cylindrical graduates are preferred. Conical graduates having a capacity of less than 25 mL should not be used in prescription compounding.[4]

Compounding Equipment. Pharmacists need at least two types of mortars and pestles—one glass and one Wedgwood or porcelain. The sizes of each will depend on the drug products being compounded. Glass mortars should be used for liquid preparations (solutions and suspensions) and for mixing chemicals that stain or are oily. Generally, glass mortars should be used for antineoplastic agents. Because of their rough surface, Wedgwood mortars are preferred for reducing the size of dry crystals and hard powder particles and for preparing emulsions. Porcelain mortars have a smoother surface than Wedgwood mortars and are ideal for blending powders and pulverizing soft aggregates or crystals. When Wedgwood mortars are used for small amounts of crystals or powders, the inside surface may first be lightly dusted with lactose to fill any crevices in which the crystals or powders might lodge. If the contact surfaces of the mortar and pestle become smooth with use, rubbing them with a small amount of sand or emery powder may adequately roughen them. Over extended use, a pestle and a mortar become shaped to each other's curvature. Thus, to ensure maximum contact between the surface of the head of each pestle and the interior of its corresponding mortar, pestles and mortars should not be interchanged.[3]

The compounding area should be stocked with appropriate supplies. Although supply selection depends on the types of products compounded, all areas should have weighing papers, weighing cups, or both to protect balance pans and spatulas. Glassine weighing papers (as opposed to bond weighing paper) should be used for products such as ointments, creams, and some dry chemicals. Disposable weighing dishes should also be stocked for substances like Coal Tar, USP.

Each compounding area should have stainless steel and plastic spatulas for mixing ointments and creams and handling dry chemicals. The pharmacist should exercise judgment in selecting the size and type of spatula. Small spatula blades (6 inches long or less) are preferred for handling dry chemicals, but larger spatula blades (>6 inches) are preferred for large amounts of ointments or creams and for preparing compactible powder blends for capsules. Plastic spatulas should be used for chemicals that may react with stainless steel blades. A variety of spatulas should be stocked in the compounding area, including 4-, 6-, and 8-inch stainless steel spatulas (one each) and 4- and 6-inch plastic spatulas (one each). Imprinted spatulas should not be used in compounding, since the imprinted ink on the spatula blade may contaminate the product.

The compounding area should contain an ointment slab, pill tile, or parchment ointment pad. Although parchment ointment pads are convenient and reduce cleanup time, parchment paper cannot be used for the preparation of creams because it will absorb water. Therefore, an ointment slab or pill tile is necessary. If suppositories are compounded, appropriate suppository molds, either reusable or disposable, should be available.

Other useful equipment and supplies may include funnels, filter paper, beakers, glass stirring rods, a source of heat (hot plate or microwave oven), a refrigerator, and a freezer—in some cases, an ultrafreezer capable of maintaining temperatures as low as –80 °C.

Ingredients

Ideally, only USP or NF chemicals manufactured by FDA-inspected manufacturers should be used for compounding. Although chemicals labeled USP or NF meet *USP–NF* standards for strength, quality, and purity for human drug products, the facilities in which the chemicals were manufactured may not meet FDA Good Manufacturing Practice (GMP) standards. In the event that a needed chemical is not available from an FDA-inspected facility, the pharmacist should, by next best preference, obtain a USP or NF product. If that is not available, the pharmacist should use professional judgment and may have to obtain the highest-grade chemical possible. Chemical grades that may be considered in this situation are ACS grade (meeting or exceeding specifications listed for reagent chemicals by the American Chemical Society) and FCC grade (meeting or exceeding requirements defined by the Food Chemicals Codex). Additional professional judgment is especially necessary in cases of chemical substances that have not been approved for *any* medical use. Particularly in these cases, but also in others as needed, the pharmacist, prescriber, and patient should be well informed of the risks involved.

Selection of ingredients may also depend on the dosage form to be compounded. In most cases, the prescriber specifies a particular dosage form, such as a topical ointment, oral solution or rectal suppository. Sometimes, however, the prescriber relies on the pharmacist to decide on an appropriate form. Irrespective of how the drug order is written, the pharmacist should evaluate the appropriateness of ingredients and the drug delivery system recommended. Factors to consider in selecting the dosage form include (1) physical and chemical characteristics of the active ingredient, (2) possible routes of administration that will produce the desired therapeutic effect (e.g., oral or topical), (3) patient characteristics (e.g., age, level of consciousness, ability to swallow a solid dosage form), (4) specific characteristics of the disease being treated, (5) comfort for the patient, and (6) ease or convenience of administration.

In checking the physical form of each ingredient, the pharmacist should not confuse drug substances that are available in more than one form. For example, coal tar is available as Coal Tar, USP, or Coal Tar Topical Solution, USP; phenol is available as Liquified Phenol, USP, or Phenol, USP; sulfur is available as Precipitated Sulfur, USP, or Sublimed Sulfur, USP. If ingredients are liquids, the pharmacist should consider compounding liquid dosage forms such as solutions, syrups, or elixirs for the final product. If ingredients are crystals or powders and the final dosage form is intended to be a dry dosage form, options such as divided powders (powder papers) or capsules should be considered. If ingredients are both liquids and dry forms, liquid formulations such as solutions, suspensions, elixirs, syrups, and emulsions should be considered.

Care must be exercised when using commercial drug products as a source of active ingredients. For example, extended-release or delayed-release products should not be crushed. Also, since chemicals such as preservatives and excipients in commercial products may affect the overall stability and bioavailability of the compounded product, their presence should not be ignored. Information on preservatives and excipients in specific commercial products can be found in package inserts and also in the dosage form section of selected product monographs in *USP DI Volume I*.[6]

If an injectable drug product is a possible source of active ingredient, the pharmacist should check the salt form of the injectable product to make sure it is the same salt form ordered. If it is necessary to use a different salt because of physical or chemical compatibility considerations or product availability, the pharmacist should consult with the prescriber. Some injectable products contain active constituents in the form of prodrugs that may not be active when administered by other routes. For example, if an injectable solution is a possible source of active ingredient for an oral product, the pharmacist must consider the stability of the drug in gastric fluids, the first-pass effect, and palatability. Also, if injectable powders for reconstitution are used, expiration dating may have to be quite short.

Storage

All chemicals and drug products must be stored according to *USP–NF* and manufacturer specifications. Most chemicals and drug products marketed for compounding use are packaged by the manufacturer in tight, light-resistant containers. Chemicals intended for compounding should be purchased in small quantities and stored in the manufacturer's original container, which is labeled with product and storage information. This practice fosters the use of fresh chemicals and ensures that the manufacturer's label remains with the lot of chemical on hand. Certificates of purity for chemical ingredients should be filed for a period of time no less than the state's time requirement for retention of dispensing records.

The manufacturer's label instructions for storage should be followed explicitly to ensure the integrity of chemicals and drug products and to protect employees. Most chemicals and commercial drug products may be stored at controlled room temperature, between 15 and 30 °C (59 and 86 °F); however, the pharmacist should always check the manufacturer's label for any special storage requirements. Storage information provided for specific commercial drug products in *USP DI Volume I* and on product labels follows the definitions for storage temperatures found in the General Notices and Requirements section of *USP–NF*. An acceptable refrigerator maintains temperatures between 2 and 8 °C (36 and 46 °F); an acceptable freezer maintains temperatures between –20 and –10 °C (– 4 and –14 °F).

To protect pharmacy employees and property, hazardous products such as acetone and flexible collodion must be stored appropriately. Safety storage cabinets in various sizes are available from laboratory suppliers.

Personnel

Compounding personnel include pharmacists and supportive personnel engaged in any aspect of the compounding procedures.

Training. The pharmacist—who is responsible for ensuring that the best technical knowledge and skill, most careful and accurate procedures, and prudent professional judgment are consistently applied in the compounding of pharmaceuticals—must supervise all compounding activities and ensure that supportive personnel are adequately trained to perform assigned functions. Both pharmacists and the compounding personnel they supervise should participate in programs de-

signed to enhance and maintain competence in compounding. Training programs should include instruction in the following areas:

- Proper use of compounding equipment such as balances and measuring devices—including guidelines for selecting proper measuring devices, limitations of weighing equipment and measuring apparatus, and the importance of accuracy in measuring.
- Pharmaceutical techniques needed for preparing compounded dosage forms (e.g., levigation, trituration, methods to increase dissolution, geometric dilution).
- Properties of dosage forms (see Pharmaceutical Dosage Forms in *USP–NF*) to be compounded and related factors such as stability, storage considerations, and handling procedures.
- Literature in which information on stability, solubility, and related material can be found (see suggested references at the end of this document).
- Handling of nonhazardous and hazardous materials in the work area, including protective measures for avoiding exposure, emergency procedures to follow in the event of exposure, and the location of Material Safety Data Sheets (MSDSs) in the facility.[7–10]
- Use and interpretation of chemical and pharmaceutical symbols and abbreviations in medication orders and in product formulation directions.
- Pharmaceutical calculations.

Procedures should be established to verify the ability of staff to meet established competencies. These procedures may include observation, written tests, or quality control testing of finished products.

Attire. Personnel engaged in compounding should wear clean clothing appropriate for the duties they perform. Protective apparel, such as head, face, hand, and arm coverings, should be worn as necessary to preclude contamination of products and to protect workers.

Generally, a clean laboratory jacket is considered appropriate attire for most personnel performing nonsterile compounding activities. Personnel involved in compounding hazardous materials should wear safety goggles, gloves, a mask or respirator, double gowns, and foot covers as required, depending on the substance being handled. To avoid microbial contamination of compounded drug products, written policies should be established that address appropriate precautions to be observed if an employee has an open lesion or an illness. Depending on the situation, an affected employee may be required to wear special protective apparel, such as a mask or gloves, or may be directed to avoid all contact with compounding procedures.

Reference Materials

Pharmacists and supportive personnel must have ready access to reference materials on all aspects of compounding (see suggested references at the end of this document). Earlier editions of some references, such as *Remington's Pharmaceutical Sciences,* provide more comprehensive compounding information than do the later editions. Information on compounding extemporaneous dosage forms from commercially available products can sometimes be obtained from the product's FDA-approved labeling (package insert), the manufacturer, a local pharmacy college, or a drug information center. It is essential that the stability and proper storage conditions for extemporaneous products be thoroughly researched. Therefore, the availability of adequate references and appropriate training in the use of the references is important.

Documentation and Record Keeping

Each step of the compounding process should be documented. Pharmacists should maintain at least four sets of records in the compounding area: (1) compounding formulas and procedures, (2) a log of all compounded items, including batch records and sample batch labels (see section on packaging and labeling), (3) equipment-maintenance records, including documentation of checks of balances, refrigerators, and freezers, and (4) a record of ingredients purchased, including certificates of purity for chemicals (see section on ingredient selection) and MSDSs.

Compounding procedures should be documented in enough detail that preparations can be replicated and the history of each ingredient can be traced. Documentation should include a record of who prepared the product (if the compounder is not a pharmacist, the supervising pharmacist should also sign the compounding record); all names, lot numbers, and quantities of ingredients used; the order of mixing, including any interim procedures used (such as preparing a solution and using an aliquot); the assigned beyond-use date; and any special storage requirements (see section on stability and expiration dating). Compounding formulas and procedures should be written in a typeface that can be read easily. If formulas originate from published articles, copies of the articles should be attached to or filed with the written procedures.

Equipment maintenance and calibrations should be documented and the record maintained in an equipment-maintenance record file. Refrigerator and freezer thermometers should be checked and documented routinely, as should alarm systems indicating that temperatures are outside of acceptable limits.

Follow-up contact with patients who have received extemporaneously compounded products is recommended to ascertain that the product is physically stable and that no adverse effects have occurred from use of the product. Documentation of the contact and the findings is recommended.

Stability, Expiration, and Beyond-Use Dating

The USP–NF[4] defines stability as the extent to which a dosage form retains, within specified limits and throughout its period of storage and use, the same properties and characteristics that it possessed at the time of its preparation. The USP–NF lists the following five types of stability:

- Chemical
- Physical
- Microbiological
- Therapeutic
- Toxicological

Factors affecting stability include the properties of each ingredient, whether therapeutically active or inactive. Environmental factors such as temperature, radiation, light, humidity, and air can also affect stability. Similarly, such factors as particle size, pH, the properties of water and other solvents employed, the nature of the container, and the presence of other substances resulting from contamination or from the intentional mixing of products can influence stability.[4]

Since compounded drug products are intended for consumption immediately or storage for a very limited time, stability evaluation and expiration dating are different for these products than for manufactured drug products. According to criteria for assigning dating in the USP–NF[4] General Notices and Requirements section and the Code of Federal Regulations,[11] the pharmacist labeling extemporaneously compounded drug products should be concerned with the beyond-use date as used by USP–NF or the expiration date as used by the Code of Federal Regulations. For uniformity, the term beyond-use date will be used in the remainder of this bulletin. The beyond-use date is defined as that date after which a dispensed product should no longer be used by a patient.

Determination of the period during which a compounded product may be usable after dispensing should be based on available stability information and reasonable patient needs with respect to the intended drug therapy. When a commercial drug product is used as a source of active ingredient, its expiration date can often be used as a factor in determining a beyond-use date. For stability or expiration information on commercial drug products, the pharmacist can refer to USP DI Volume I.[6] If no information is available, the manufacturer should be contacted. When the active ingredient is a USP or NF product, the pharmacist may be able to use the expiration dating of similar commercial products for guidance in assigning a beyond-use date. In addition, the pharmacist can often refer to published literature to obtain stability data on the same active ingredient under varying conditions and in different formulations.[12]

The pharmacist must assess the potential for instability that may result from the new environment for the active ingredients—from the combination of ingredients and the packaging materials. According to USP–NF,[4] hydrolysis, oxidation-reduction, and photolysis are the most common chemical reactions that cause instability. When the possibility of such reactions exists, the pharmacist should seek additional stability data or consider other approaches. These could, in extreme cases, include the preparation and dispensing of more than one compounded drug product or the use of alternative methods of dosing. For some drugs, the latter methods might include, for example, crushing a tablet or emptying the contents of a hard gelatin capsule into an appropriate food substance at each dosing time.

In assigning a beyond-use date for compounded drug products, the pharmacist should use all available stability information, plus education and experience in deciding how factors affecting product stability should be weighted. In the absence of stability data to the contrary or any indication of a stability problem, the following general criteria for assigning maximum beyond-use dates are recommended. It must be emphasized that these are general criteria. Professional judgment as discussed elsewhere in this section must be used in deciding when these general criteria may not be appropriate.

- When a manufactured final-dosage-form product is used as a source of active ingredient, use no more than 25% of the manufacturer's remaining expiration dating or six months, whichever is less;

- When a USP or NF chemical not from a manufactured final-dosage-form product is used, use no more than six months;
- In other cases, use the intended period of therapy or no more than 30 days, whichever is less.

All compounded products should be observed for signs of instability. Observations should be performed during preparation of the drug product and any storage period that may occur before the compounded drug product is dispensed. A list of observable indications of instability for solid, liquid, and semisolid dosage forms appears in *USP–NF*.

Packaging and Labeling

The packaging of extemporaneously compounded products for ambulatory patients should comply with regulations pertaining to the Poison Prevention Packaging Act of 1970. These regulations can be found in *USP–NF*.[4]

Containers for compounded products should be appropriate for the dosage form compounded. For example, to minimize administration errors, oral liquids should never be packaged in syringes intended to be used for injection.

The drug product container should not interact physically or chemically with the product so as to alter the strength, quality, or purity of the compounded product. Glass and plastic are commonly used in containers for compounded products. To ensure container inertness, visibility, strength, rigidity, moisture protection, ease of reclosure, and economy of packaging, glass containers have been the most widely used for compounded products.[3] Amber glass and some plastic containers may be used to protect light-sensitive products from degradation; however, glass that transmits ultraviolet or violet light rays (this includes green, blue, and clear ["flint"] glass) should not be used to protect light-sensitive products.

The use of plastic containers for compounded products has increased because plastic is less expensive and lighter in weight than glass. Since compounded products are intended for immediate use, most capsules, ointments, and creams should be stable in high-density plastic vials or ointment jars. Only plastic containers meeting *USP–NF* standards should be used.[4] Reclosable plastic bags may be acceptable for selected divided powders that are intended to be used within a short period of time.

Each compounded product should be appropriately labeled according to state and federal regulations. Labels should include the generic or chemical name of active ingredients, strength or quantity, pharmacy lot number, beyond-use date, and any special storage requirements. If a commercial product has been used as a source of drug, the generic name of the product should be used on the label. The trade name should not be used because, once the commercial drug product has been altered, it no longer exists as the approved commercial product. Listing the names and quantities of inactive ingredients on labels is also encouraged. The coining of short names for convenience (e.g., "Johnson's solution") is strongly discouraged; these names provide no assistance to others who may need to identify ingredients (e.g., in emergency circumstances).

Capsules should be labeled with the quantity (micrograms or milligrams) of active ingredient(s) per capsule. Oral liquids should be labeled with the strength or concentration per dose (e.g., 125 mg/5 mL or 10 meq/15 mL). If the quantity of an active ingredient is a whole number, the number should not be typed with a decimal point followed by a zero. For example, the strength of a capsule containing 25 mg of active ingredient should be labeled as 25 mg and not 25.0 mg. In cases where the dosage strength is less than a whole number, a zero should precede the decimal point (e.g., 0.25 µg).[13]

In expressing salt forms of chemicals on a label, it is permissible to use atomic abbreviations. For example, HCl may be used for hydrochloride, HBr for hydrobromide, Na for sodium, and K for potassium.

Vehicles should also be stated on labels, especially if similar products are prepared with different vehicles. For example, if a pharmacist prepares two potassium syrups, one using Syrup, USP, as the vehicle and one using a sugar-free syrup as the vehicle, the name of the vehicle should be included on the labels.

Liquids and semisolid concentrations may be expressed in terms of percentages. When the term "percent" or the symbol "%" is used without qualification for solids and semisolids, percent refers to weight in weight; for solutions or suspensions, percent refers to weight in volume; for solutions of liquids in liquids, percent refers to volume in volume.[4]

Labels for compounded products that are prepared in batches should include a pharmacy-assigned lot number. Assignment of a pharmacy lot number must enable the history of the compounded product to be traced, including the person compounding the product and the product's formula, ingredients, and procedures. Being able to trace the history of a batch is essential in cases of a drug product recall or withdrawal.

In the preparation of labels for batches of compounded products, all extra labels should be destroyed, since pharmacy lot numbers change with each batch. If computers, memory typewriters, or label machines are used to print batch labels, care must be taken to ensure that the memory and printing mechanism have been cleared and the correct information is programmed before any additional labels are made. It is a good practice to run a blank label between each batch of labels to ensure that the memory has been erased or cleared. To document the information printed on each set of labels, a sample label printed for the batch should be attached to the compounded-product log. If labels are sequentially prepared for different drug products, procedures should exist to minimize the risk of mislabeling the compounded products. These procedures should ensure, for example, that labels for one drug product are physically well separated from labels for any other drug product.

Auxiliary labels are convenient for conveying special storage or use information. Auxiliary labels should be attached conspicuously to containers, if possible. If the container is too small for both a general label and an auxiliary label, special storage and use instructions should appear on the label in a format that will emphasize the instructions.

Limited Batch Compounding

The purpose of extemporaneously compounding products is to provide individualized drug therapy for a particular patient. When a pharmacist is repeatedly asked to prepare identical compounded products, it may be reasonable and more efficient for the pharmacist to prepare small batches of the compounded product.

Batch sizes should be consistent with the volume of drug orders or prescriptions the pharmacist receives for the compounded product and the stability of the compounded product. The pharmacist should use judgment in deciding reasonable batch sizes. Product assays should be performed by a chemical analysis laboratory on a regular basis to ensure product consistency among various lots, product uniformity, and stability. Analyses should be repeated every time an ingredient (active or inert) or procedure is changed. Documentation of assay findings should be filed for a period no less than the state's time requirement for the retention of dispensing records.

General Compounding Considerations

To provide the patient with the most stable drug product, the pharmacist should take the following steps upon receiving a prescription order that requires compounding.

First, the pharmacist should determine if a similar commercial product is available. A pharmacist can refer to various reference texts to check the availability of identical or similar products. Package Inserts from commercially available products also contain information on inactive ingredients that can be compared with the requested formulation. If there is a commercially manufactured identical product, the local availability of the product should be determined.

When a similar product is commercially available, the pharmacist should determine which ingredients are different from the requested formulation to decide whether or not the commercial product can be used. At this stage, the pharmacist should seek answers to the following questions:

- Are all of the ingredients appropriate for the condition being treated?
- Are the concentrations of the ingredients in the drug order reasonable?
- Are the physical, chemical, and therapeutic properties of the individual ingredients consistent with the expected properties of the ordered drug product?

If the answers to these questions are positive, the pharmacist should consult the prescriber about the possibility of dispensing the commercial product. (In some states, pharmacists may not be required to obtain permission from the prescriber to dispense a commercial product if the formulation is identical to the drug order.) Dispensing a commercial product is preferable to extemporaneously compounding a drug product because commercial products carry the manufacturer's guarantee of labeled potency and stability.

If there is not a commercial product available with the same or similar formulation, the pharmacist should consider asking the prescriber the following questions:

- What is the purpose of the order? There may be another way to achieve the purpose without compounding a product.
- Where did the formula originate (article, meeting, colleague)?
- How will the drug product be used?
- Does the patient have other conditions that must be considered?
- For how long will the drug product be used?

If possible, the pharmacist should obtain a copy of the original formula to determine the extent to which the formulation has been tested for stability. When documentation is not available, the pharmacist should review the ingredients for appropriateness and reasonable concentrations.

For drug products that must be compounded, the pharmacist should closely observe the compounded drug product for any signs of instability. Such observations should be performed during preparation of the drug product and during any storage period that may occur before the compounded drug product is dispensed.

If specific packaging information is not available, a light-resistant, tight container, such as an amber vial or bottle, should be used to maximize stability (see section on packaging and labeling).

The pharmacist should label the compounded drug product, including an appropriate beyond-use date and storage instructions for the patient.

Specific Compounding Considerations

Accepted, proven compounding procedures for products including solutions, suspensions, creams, ointments, capsules, suppositories, troches, emulsions, and powders may be found in reference sources or the pharmacy literature. For additional information, pharmacists should check references cited in this document or consult colleagues or colleges of pharmacy with known expertise in compounding.

Glossary

For the purposes of this document, the following terms are used with the meanings shown.

Active Ingredient: Any chemical that is intended to furnish pharmacologic activity in the diagnosis, cure, mitigation, treatment, or prevention of disease or to affect the structure or function of the body of man or other animals.[4]

Batch: Multiple containers of a drug product or other material with uniform character and quality, within specified limits, that are prepared in anticipation of prescription drug orders based on routine, regularly observed prescribing patterns.

Cold: Any temperature not exceeding 8 °C (46 °F).[4]

Commercially Available Product: Any drug product manufactured by a producer registered with the Department of Health and Human Services as a pharmaceutical manufacturer.

Compounding: The mixing of substances to prepare a drug product.

Container: A device that holds a drug product and is or may be in direct contact with the product.[3]

Cool: Any temperature between 8 and 15 °C (46 and 59 °F).[4]

Drug Product: A finished dosage form that contains an active drug ingredient usually, but not necessarily (in the case of a placebo), in combination with inactive ingredients.[4]

Extemporaneous: Impromptu; prepared without a standard formula from an official compendium; prepared as required for a specific patient.

Inactive Ingredient: Any chemical other than the active ingredients in a drug product.[4]

Manufacturer: Anyone registered with the Department of Health and Human Services as a producer of drug products.[14]

Sensitivity Requirements: The maximal load that will

cause one subdivision of change on the index plate in the position of rest of the indicator of the balance.[4]

Stability: The chemical and physical integrity of a drug product over time.[4]

Trituration: The reducing of substances to fine particles by rubbing them in a mortar with a pestle.[3]

Warm: Any temperature between 30 and 40 °C (86 and 104 °F).[4]

Suggested References

Product Availability
American Drug Index
Drug Facts & Comparisons
Physicians' Desk Reference
The Extra Pharmacopoeia (Martindale)
CHEMSOURCES
AHFS Drug Information

Compounding Techniques
Compounding Companion PC-Based Software
King's *Dispensing of Medications*
Remington's Pharmaceutical Sciences
Contemporary Compounding column in *U.S. Pharmacist*

Pharmaceutical Calculations
Stoklosa and Ansel's *Pharmaceutical Calculations*
Math—Use It or Lose It column in *Hospital Pharmacy*
Calculations in Pharmacy column in *U.S. Pharmacist*

Drug Stability and Compatibility
American Journal of Hospital Pharmacy
ASHP's *Handbook on Extemporaneous Formulations*
ASHP's *Handbook on Injectable Drugs*
International Pharmaceutical Abstracts
Journal of the Parenteral Drug Association (now *Journal of Pharmaceutical Science and Technology*)
Canadian Society of Hospital Pharmacists *Extemporaneous Oral Liquid Dosage Preparations*
Pediatric Drug Formulations
Physicians' Desk Reference
Contemporary Compounding column in *U.S. Pharmacist*
AHFS Drug Information
The Merck Index

References

1. Pancorbo SA, Campagna KD, Devenport JK, et al. Task force report of competency statements for pharmacy practice. *Am J Pharm Educ.* 1987; 51:196–206.

2. Allen LV Jr. Establishing and marketing your extemporaneous compounding service. *US Pharm.* 1990; 15(Dec):74–7.

3. Remington's pharmaceutical sciences. 18th ed. Gennaro AR, ed. Easton, PA: Mack Publishing; 1990; 1630–1, 1658, 1660.

4. The United States Pharmacopeia, 22nd rev., and The National Formulary, 17th ed. Rockville, MD: The United States Pharmacopeial Convention; 1989.

5. USP DI Volume III: Approved drug products and legal requirements. 14th ed. Rockville, MD: The United States Pharmacopeial Convention; 1994.

6. USP DI Volume I: Drug information for the health care professional. 14th ed. Rockville, MD: The United States Pharmacopeial Convention; 1994.

7. 29 §C.F.R. 1910. 1200(1990).

8. ASHP technical assistance bulletin on handling cytotoxic and hazardous drugs. *Am J Hosp Pharm.* 1990; 47:1033–49.

9. Feinberg JL. Complying with OSHA's Hazard Communication Standard. *Consult Pharm.* 1991; 6:444, 446, 448.

10. Myers CE. Applicability of OSHA Hazard Communication Standard to drug products. *Am J Hosp Pharm.* 1990; 47:1960–1.

11. 21 C.F.R. §211.137.

12. Connors KA, Amidon GL, Stella VJ. Chemical stability of pharmaceuticals: a handbook for pharmacists. 2nd ed. New York: Wiley; 1986.

13. American Society of Hospital Pharmacists. ASHP guidelines on preventing medication errors in hospitals. *Am J Hosp Pharm.* 1993; 50:305–14.

14. Fitzgerald WL Jr. The legal authority to compound in pharmacy practice. *Tenn Pharm.* 1990; 26(Mar): 21–2.

Approved by the ASHP Board of Directors, April 27, 1994. Developed by the Council on Professional Affairs.

The bibliographic citation for this document is as follows: American Society of Hospital Pharmacists. ASHP technical assistance bulletin on compounding nonsterile products in pharmacies. *Am J Hosp Pharm.* 1994; 51:1441–8.

ASHP Technical Assistance Bulletin on the Recruitment, Selection, and Retention of Pharmacy Personnel

This Technical Assistance Bulletin is intended to assist the pharmacy manager in the recruitment, selection, and retention of qualified employees. The pharmacy manager working in an organized health care system must work with a centralized human resources department and within the framework of the specific recruitment, hiring, and selection policies of the organization.

Position Description

A well-developed position description is critical to the success of any recruitment effort. The position description should contain detailed information on the knowledge, skills, experience, and abilities that an acceptable candidate should possess. The following information may be included in a position description:

- Position title and position number, if applicable.
- Duties, essential job functions, and responsibilities of the position.
- Education, training, experience, and licensure required.
- Knowledge, skills, and abilities required based on assigned duties.
- Reporting relationships.
- Pay grade and salary range (optional).
- Education required to maintain competence.
- Other specifications of the position that may be required to meet legal requirements (e.g., the Americans with Disabilities Act).

A revised position description should be reviewed with staff currently in that position, as well as the supervisor of that position. In many workplaces, human resources departments maintain files and may require approval of all position descriptions in the organization. Procedures specific to the workplace should be followed. Review by staff with legal expertise is advisable in order to determine compliance with organizational and legal requirements.

Recruitment Sources

Recruitment of individuals from within the organization (e.g., from another department) may be less expensive than recruitment from other sources and may result in greater employee retention and loyalty among staff through internal growth opportunities. To facilitate internal recruitment, notice of a vacant position can be posted within the organization before the information is made available to potential candidates outside the organization. Posting can be accomplished by various means, including memorandums, electronic mail, voice mail, newsletters, and bulletin boards.

Recruitment of outside candidates expands the number of potential candidates and the talent available to the organization. It brings new skills and viewpoints into the organization and discourages a reliance on seniority alone as the basis for promotion. Budgetary constraints and the urgency to fill a position may affect the recruitment method(s) selected for external candidates. These methods may include the following:

- Advertisements in professional journals, newspapers, state professional society newsletters, and electronic bulletin boards.
- Personnel placement services provided by national or state professional societies.
- Oral and written recommendations from colleagues.
- Personal discussion or correspondence with potential candidates.
- Recruitment visits to colleges of pharmacy for pharmacists or, for technicians, to facilities conducting technician-training programs.
- Tuition assistance programs for students in exchange for future work commitments.
- Professional recruiting firms.
- Familiarizing students with the organization by offering summer jobs or participating in college of pharmacy experiential rotations.
- Initial screening interviews conducted by the human resources department.
- A "prospect list" of individuals applying for previous job openings.
- Contacts established through networking.

The ability to recruit qualified candidates may depend on the financial stability and location of the organization; the organization's compensation program, which includes salary, fringe benefits, and raise structure; and the reputation and scope of pharmaceutical services offered.

Pre-Interview Information

The applicant's correspondence, résumé or curriculum vitae, letters of recommendation, academic records, and completed application form (if any) should be carefully evaluated on the basis of the position description to determine the suitability of the candidate for an interview. The position description should be provided in advance to all interviewers.

There are certain legal restrictions on the type of information that may be requested from candidates on an application form. As a generalization, an application form may request only information that has been shown to be related to the job for which the candidate is applying. If an application form different from that of the organization is used, it is advisable to forward it to the human resources department for review before distributing it to potential candidates.

Initial Screening Interview

An initial screening interview may be necessary if several qualified candidates have been identified. The screening interview is generally a brief interview conducted by human resources department staff or the direct supervisor for the position; it offers a quick assessment of the suitability of the candidate for the position. This interview is often conducted by telephone, especially if the candidate lives far away.

The Interview Process

A successful interview is one that matches the best available candidate with a specific position. The process should allow the interviewer to predict the future performance of candidates as accurately as possible. One style of interview is the individual interview—one interviewer and one interviewee. Individual interviews offer the advantages of simplicity, ease of scheduling, and consistency of perspective. Team interviewing involves a group of interviewers. Members of the team may interview the candidate individually and then pool their results, or they may interview the candidate as a group. The well-prepared team approach offers multiple perspectives within a standardized evaluation scheme. Its disadvantage is extra time consumed to train the team and to conduct interviews. Its advantage is that it incorporates more individuals into the process of analyzing a candidate to determine whether that person will succeed in the position and to discern the best applicant.[1] It also provides an opportunity to observe the candidate's ability to interact with groups, which may be important if the position will require that type of activity.

The composition of the team will depend on the position being filled. The team should include people with a common interest in the outcome of the selection process and people who have been in the organization long enough to share with the applicant some history of the organization and the department.[1]

Characteristics of an effective interview process include the following:

- The interviewer provides the candidate with travel directions to the organization in advance and clarifies what interview expenses, if any, will be covered by the organization.
- The interview is carefully planned. An itinerary is developed in advance, taking into consideration the availability of those who need to participate in the process and allowing adequate time for each event, including a tour of the facility as needed. The candidate should receive a copy of the itinerary prior to the interview.
- Interviewers are well prepared. Pre-interview information submitted by the candidate is distributed to and reviewed by participants in advance.
- Carefully planned, open-ended questions are developed in advance. Literature can be consulted to obtain sample questions for interviewers to ask candidates, as well as questions that are inadvisable or prohibited by law.[1-4] Human resources departments can usually assist in the development of questions. (Refer to the appendix for sample questions.)
- To the extent possible, a core group of questions are asked of all candidates as a means of comparing them. This does not negate the need to investigate different areas for each candidate and to pursue specific questions that surface during the conversation.
- Questions focus on predetermined criteria for the position and the qualifications of the candidates. The goal is to match the best candidate available with the vacant position. Questions should also focus on past performance, which often is a good indicator of future performance.
- The interviewer gives the candidate a realistic view of the position. Candidates should be given favorable and unfavorable information about the position. If the candidate is "oversold" on the position, dissatisfaction will set in once the truth is known.
- Performance standards and methods used for evaluation are fully explained.
- A follow-up letter is sent to the candidate after the interview to express thanks for interest in the position and the organization and advising the candidate of the next steps.

Each interview should be documented to help keep track of each candidate's responses and avoid confusion later. Documentation could include interview questions and the candidate's responses or could simply be a rating of impressions of the candidate's responses to specific questions. Documentation should take place immediately after the interview.[1] The interviewer should look for punctuality, completeness and accuracy of the résumé or curriculum vitae, communication skills, compensation expectations, and skills and knowledge pertinent to the position when considering a potential employee.

Background Verification

The accuracy of information provided by the candidate should be verified by the human resources department. Information may be obtained from the following sources:

- Personal reference letters provided by the applicant.
- Reference letters provided by previous employers, with the applicant's permission.
- State board of pharmacy records.
- Academic records.

Job Offer

The job offer should be made as quickly as possible. The information about candidate selection should be kept confidential until after the offer has been accepted. The organization may have specific policies and procedures regarding job offers.[1]

The salary offered to a candidate generally will be competitive with salaries for similar jobs in other organizations in the same market and compatible with the organization's existing salary structure. The market may vary, depending on the position. For example, the market for a pharmacy technician may be local, whereas the market for a pharmacist or pharmacy manager may be regional or national. The salary offered to a candidate generally should be consistent with salaries of current staff in that position in order to preserve equity within the organization. When or if exceptions must be made, it may become necessary to reassess the compensation of existing staff.

In addition to salary, other commitments made to a candidate should be expressed in writing as part of the formal job offer. These may include the following:

- Date on which employment will begin.
- Supervisor's name and position.
- Position description.
- Performance standards and evaluation system.
- Next performance review date.
- Next compensation increase date.
- Expected work schedule, and whether it is subject to change depending on future needs of the department.
- Employee benefits, such as insurance, vacation, tuition assistance, sick leave, holidays, and retirement and pension benefits.

- Miscellaneous commitments (if any), including an employment bonus, relocation expenses, licensure reimbursement, payment for professional association memberships, and payment for attendance at professional education programs.
- Potential drug screening as applicable and in keeping with the law or employee physical examination.

Retention

Staff turnover is costly in terms of the time required to recruit and retrain and the temporary loss of productivity in the workplace.[5] Because individuals have varied needs and wants that may change over time, there is no consistent formula for managers to apply to ensure employee retention.[6-8] Reasons why people remain in the job can be as varied as the number of employees in an organization. Each organization will be different based on such factors as the age of employees, their stage in life, their stage in career, the organizational structure, the work environment, and the work itself.

Often, factors affecting retention compete with those affecting recruitment. For example, creating staff positions with exclusively morning shifts may help in the retention of existing staff but may decrease the ability to recruit new staff. (Candidates interested in evening and night shifts may not be available.) When issues such as these arise, they must be balanced with the short-term and long-term departmental goals and the current economic demand for employment.

Each organization should identify and assess retention factors by examining the unique aspects of the respective department. On the basis of this assessment, a retention plan should be developed. A committee should be established to determine the major retention factors important to that organization. The plan should be reviewed periodically as the needs of employees change. Surveys of existing employees may help in determining primary factors for retention. The following factors may be considered in analyzing staff retention:

- *Intent to Stay.* Existing employees can simply be asked whether they intend to stay. This refers to the perceptions of an individual rather than a behavior; a person's internal orientation. This factor is part of a person's values or attitudes, and, while an important consideration, it may be influenced by a manager. In several studies, this factor was the best predictor of staff retention.[9]
- *Job Satisfaction.* Existing employees can be asked how satisfied they are with their jobs. This refers to the degree to which individuals like their jobs. Studies have linked job satisfaction with retention to various degrees. Job satisfaction is often considered an important part of the retention "equation," although the relationship with retention may be direct or indirect. It is important to remember that dissatisfaction does not necessarily lead to staff turnover, if other factors are more important to the individual.[9,10]
- *Pay and Benefits.* These refer to the remuneration for work performed and the organization's overall benefit plan. Pay may be hourly (a wage) or salaried and may include overtime premiums or bonuses and incentive plans. A benefit plan may include life, medical, dental, disability, and liability insurance; tuition payments; retirement packages; paid organizational membership

dues; sick leave; paid vacation; and prescription benefits. The value of specific benefits to an employee will most likely change over time. Many organizations offer a benefits plan that gives the employee the option of choosing benefits individually suited to stages in his or her life, employment, and career.
- *Recognition and Awards.* These include both formal and informal feedback mechanisms. Recognition is often identified as lacking in the workplace.[6,9]
- *Promotion Opportunities.* These may be in the form of formal promotions, career advancement programs, or special project or committee appointments. Flat organizational structures provide fewer formal opportunities for staff promotion. Employees who have made personal investments in the organization—through expanded responsibilities associated with promotion—may have stronger feelings of loyalty that translate into increased retention.
- *Job Design.* This refers to the general tasks an employee performs—the content of the work. Factors included are autonomy and the complexity of tasks. Some motivational theories suggest that the job itself can motivate intrinsically and lead to increased employee satisfaction. Some studies have found that job content is more highly correlated with retention as the degree of an employee's education increases.[9]
- *Peer Relations.* This refers to working relationships with peers, nursing and physician staff, and technical support staff. This factor is often rated highly as a reason to stay with an organization. While this element is important, it is difficult to screen for it during an interview process.
- *Kinship Responsibilities.* This refers to family considerations, such as child care needs and spouse-employment transfers. Child care needs are important for working parents.
- *Opportunity.* This refers to other options in the job market. Obviously, tight job markets (a relative lack of alternative positions) increase retention, whereas open job markets (those with many other open positions) may lead to increased turnover. Managers in open job markets should be attentive to retaining good employees.
- *Staff-Development Opportunities.* This refers to job training, educational opportunities, and tuition reimbursement or other educational and personal growth opportunities for staff within an organization.
- *Management Style/Availability.* This refers to the organizational structure and prevalent management style in the organization (e.g., on the spectrum from autocratic to participative). The accessibility of management staff may be a factor. The extent to which staff input is encouraged may be a factor. Each employee will be comfortable with different styles of management. Managers, when concerned about retention, must be sensitive to the management styles that are effective for their staff. No one style works equally well for every employee.
- *Physical Working Conditions.* This refers to the physical characteristics of the workplace, such as space, equipment, noise levels, parking accommodations, and cleanliness.
- *Scheduling.* This refers to opportunities for varied scheduling, vacation time, shift rotation, job sharing, and part-time work.

- *Motivational Factors.* Motivational theories, such as Maslow's hierarchy of needs theory and Herzberg's motivation–hygiene theory, are often cited as being related to retention.[11,12]

References

1. Nimmo CM, ed. Human resources management. ACCRUE level II. Bethesda, MD: American Society of Hospital Pharmacists; 1991.
2. Yate M. Hiring the best. 3rd ed. Holbrook, MA: Adams; 1990.
3. Wilson R. Conducting better job interviews. Hauppauge, NY: Barrons; 1991.
4. Smart B. The smart interviewer. New York: Wiley; 1989.
5. Donovan L. The shortage. *RN.* 1980; 8:21–7.
6. Smith SN, Stewart JE, Grussing PG. Factors influencing the rate of job turnover among hospital pharmacists. *Am J Hosp Pharm.* 1986; 43:1936–41.
7. Porter LW, Stears RM. Organizational work and personal factors in employee turnover and absenteeism. *Psychol Bull.* 1973; 80:151–76.
8. Loveridge CE. Contingency theory: explaining staff nurse retention. *J Nurs Adm.* 1988; 18(6):22–5.
9. Cavanagh SJ. Predictions of nursing staff turnover. *J Adv Nurs.* 1990; 15:373–80.
10. Johns G. Organizational behavior: understanding life at work. Glenview, IL: Scott, Foresman; 1983.
11. Maslow AH. Motivation and personality. 2nd ed. New York: Harper & Row; 1970.
12. Herzberg F, Mausner B, Snyderman BB. The motivation to work. 2nd ed. New York: Wiley; 1959.

Appendix—Sample Questions to Ask of Job Candidates[1]

Suggested questions to ask of experienced pharmacists and technicians

- How did you become interested in pharmacy?
- What skills or traits do you think a pharmacist needs in order to be successful?
- What is the single greatest contribution you have made in your present (or most recent) position?
- What is something you have recommended or tried in your present (or most recent) position that did not work? Why didn't it?
- How are you evaluated in your present (most recent) job?
- What would your present (most recent) employer say are your strong points? How about your weak points?
- Why did you (do you want to) leave your last (present) job?

- Do you prefer working on a team or alone? Why?
- What part of the job did you like the best and least?

Suggested questions to ask of recent pharmacy school graduates

- What was your most rewarding college experience?
- Why did you want to study pharmacy?
- What would you change about your college experience if you could?
- Do you think your grades accurately reflect your academic achievements?
- What subjects did you like most and least? Why?

General questions

- What qualities are you looking for in your next supervisor?
- What supervisory style do you think you have?
- What are your long-term career goals?
- How does this position fit in with your long-term career goals?
- What are you looking for in your next position that has been lacking in previous positions?

Subjects you may not ask about

- Race
- National origin
- Religion
- Age
- Marital or family status
- Child care arrangements or childbearing plans
- Arrest records (although convictions related to drug use would be appropriate)
- Credit rating and other financial information (unless the position involves financial responsibilities)
- Military discharge status, unless resulting from a military conviction
- General information that would point out handicaps or health problems unrelated to job performance

Approved by the ASHP Board of Directors, April 27, 1994. Developed by the ASHP Council on Administrative Affairs.

The bibliographic citation for this document is as follows: American Society of Hospital Pharmacists. ASHP technical assistance bulletin on the recruitment, selection, and retention of pharmacy personnel. *Am J Hosp Pharm.* 1994; 51:1811–5.

ASHP
Therapeutic Position Statements

ASHP Therapeutic Position Statement on the Use of the International Normalized Ratio System to Monitor Oral Anticoagulant Therapy

Statement of Position

ASHP supports the use of the International Normalized Ratio (INR) as a standardized method for reporting prothrombin time in patients receiving oral anticoagulant therapy. ASHP encourages the use of the INR system in all organized health care settings and clinical laboratories that measure prothrombin times, because the INR system reduces the differences in prothrombin time test results that are caused by using thromboplastins with varying sensitivities. ASHP encourages the education of all health care providers on the importance and appropriate use of the INR system.

Background

Oral anticoagulant therapy (primarily warfarin) must be closely monitored, because the anticoagulant response to fixed dosages varies among individuals and the safety and efficacy of the drugs are dependent on maintaining the anticoagulant effect within a defined therapeutic range.[1-3] Prothrombin time (PT) or "pro time" has been used for laboratory monitoring since its introduction by Quick et al. in 1935.[4] The PT is used because it measures the depression of three of the clotting factors of the extrinsic coagulation pathway (II, VII, and X). Warfarin inhibits the production of these vitamin K-dependent clotting factors. The PT test is performed by adding calcium and tissue thromboplastin to citrated plasma to activate the coagulation cascade. The time required for clotting to occur is expressed in seconds. To monitor warfarin therapy, the PT ratio had been traditionally calculated as the patient's PT divided by a mean normal PT.

The source of thromboplastin reagents used in North America has changed from human brain (1950) to rabbit brain (1970s and 1980s).[5] The change occurred primarily because rabbit brain thromboplastins, which are less responsive to the anticoagulant effects of warfarin than human brain thromboplastins are, were more readily available from commercial sources and less expensive than human brain thromboplastins. Although this was thought to be an inconsequential substitution, the change to less responsive rabbit brain thromboplastins resulted in a substantial decrease in the sensitivity of the PT test and, hence, lower measurements of PT values. Because this substitution was largely unrecognized by many clinicians, the average dose of warfarin used to treat thromboembolic disorders unnecessarily *increased* during the 1970s and 1980s in an attempt to maintain PT ratios at therapeutic goals.[5]

In response to this problem, the World Health Organization (WHO) developed an international reference standard, the International Sensitivity Index (ISI), to determine the responsiveness of the PT to the reduction in coagulation factors, as measured with a given thromboplastin.[6-11] Each lot of thromboplastin can be characterized by an ISI that calibrates the reagent with the first WHO reference human brain thromboplastin, which was assigned an ISI of 1.0.[11] In 1985, the International Committee on Thrombosis and Hemostasis/International Committee for Standardization in Haematology recommended adoption of a uniform calibration system in which the PT ratio is expressed in terms of the International Normalized Ratio (INR).[12] The INR is the PT ratio that would have been obtained if the WHO standard for thromboplastin reagent had been used.

Calculation Method

Any PT system (i.e., a combination of the thromboplastin reagent and the clotting instrument) can be related to the INR scale by calibration. The calibration is performed by measuring, with both the local thromboplastin and the WHO standard reagent, the PT of 20 healthy individuals and a number of patients receiving oral anticoagulants (60 patients are recommended). The PTs are plotted on double logarithmic scales, and the ISI is calculated by orthogonal regression analysis.[12] The commercial manufacturer of the thromboplastin reagent calculates the ISI and includes it in the product package insert. The ISI is specific for each lot. The lower the ISI, the more "sensitive" the reagent, and the closer the derived INR will be to the observed PT ratio. The INR, an exponential function, is calculated as follows:

$$\text{INR} = (\text{PT}/\bar{\chi})^{\text{ISI}} \text{ or } \text{INR} = (\text{PT ratio})^{\text{ISI}}$$

where PT = patient prothrombin time expressed in seconds and $\bar{\chi}$ = mean of the range of the normal prothrombin time expressed in seconds.[a] Current literature indicates that thromboplastin reagents available in the United States have an ISI between 1.0 and 2.88.[13]

Calculation of the INR is relatively simple and can be performed with a hand-held calculator. For example, if the PT ratio is 1.7 and the ISI of thromboplastin is 2.6, the calculated INR = $1.7^{2.6} = 3.97$. The relationship between the INR and PT ratio over a range of ISI values is shown in Figure 1.[14] Calculation should not be necessary for the practicing clinician if clinical laboratories routinely report INRs instead of PT ratios.

Failure to rely on the INR system may have resulted in significant errors in anticoagulant therapy due to the variability in thromboplastin reagent sensitivity.[15] Because of the large range of sensitivities of available commercial thromboplastins, it is no longer possible to establish standardized therapeutic ranges of anticoagulation by using the PT ratio or the uncorrected PT in seconds.[15] This variability in thromboplastin sensitivity is of particular concern if a patient's PT is measured at a variety of laboratories with different thromboplastin reagents. Although the INR system has not eliminated interlaboratory differences in PT, it does reduce the differences.[16,17] The INR system provides the best method of standardizing PT monitoring for the variable sensitivities of different thromboplastin reagents. Recommended therapeutic ranges of INRs are beyond the scope of this document, but readers are encouraged to review the October 1992 supplement to *Chest* for this information.

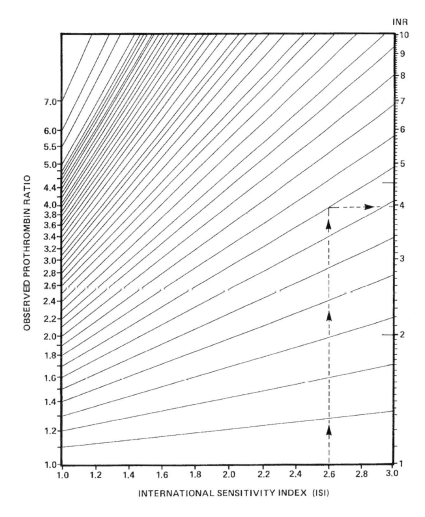

Figure 1. Nomogram showing relationship between INR and PT ratio over a range of ISI values. In the example shown, the INR is 3.97 when the observed PT ratio is 1.7 and the thromboplastin ISI is 2.6. Reprinted from reference 14, with permission.

Limitations of the INR System

As the use of the INR system to monitor warfarin therapy has increased, concerns have been raised about the reliability of this system. The specific problems, as identified by Hirsh and Poller,[18] include (1) lack of reliability of the INR system when used at the onset of warfarin therapy, (2) loss of INR system accuracy and precision when thromboplastins with high ISI values are used, (3) loss of accuracy of the INR with automated clot detectors, (4) lack of reliability of the ISI result provided by the manufacturer, (5) incorrect calculation of the INR resulting from the use of inappropriate control plasma, and (6) high INR values in overanticoagulated patients, producing unnecessary alarm. Hirsh and Poller offer potential solutions to these problems: (1) using INRs during the induction phase of warfarin treatment, on the basis of evidence that the PT ratio is less reliable than the INR and lack of evidence that the INR is not as reliable; (2) using sensitive thromboplastins with ISI values close to 1.0; (3) calibrating each new batch of thromboplastin with lyophilized plasmas with certified INR values; (4) calibrating with certified lyophilized plasma samples with known INR values to determine instrument-specific ISI; (5) educating laboratory personnel about the differences between mean normal PT and control PT; and (6) following a standard approach to treating patients with high INR values.

Summary

The INR system of standardizing PT measurements can minimize variability between laboratories, PT reagents, and instruments. The INR system can also facilitate international agreement on therapeutic ranges and allow direct comparison of clinical trials. This should provide greater uniformity in the management of oral anticoagulant therapy and ultimately may improve patient outcomes.[11] ASHP supports the use of the INR system on the basis of studies demonstrating that this system permits warfarin dosing that is less dependent on the variability of thromboplastin reagent sensitivity.

References

1. Hirsh J, Dalen JE, Deykin D, et al. Oral anticoagulants: mechanism of action, clinical effectiveness, and optimal therapeutic range. *Chest.* 1992; 102(Suppl):312S–326S.

2. Hull R, Hirsh J, Carter C, et al. Different intensities of oral anticoagulant therapy in the treatment of proximal vein thrombosis. *N Engl J Med.* 1982; 307:1676–81.

3. Turpie AGG, Gunstensen J, Hirsh J, et al. Randomized comparison of two intensities of oral anticoagu-

lant therapy after tissue valve replacement. *Lancet.* 1988; 1:1242–5.

4. Quick AJ, Stanley-Brown M, Bancroft FW. A study of the coagulation defect in hemophilia and in jaundice. *Am J Med Sci.* 1935; 190:501–11.

5. Hirsh J, Poller L, Deykin D, et al. Optimal therapeutic range for oral anticoagulants. *Chest.* 1989; 95(suppl 25):5S–11S.

6. Bailey EL, Harper TA, Pinkerton PG. The "therapeutic range" of one-stage prothrombin time in control of anticoagulant therapy: the effect of different thromboplastin preparations. *Can Med Assoc J.* 1971; 105:1041–3.

7. Zucker S, Cathey MG, Sox PJ, et al. Standardization of laboratory tests for controlling anticoagulant therapy. *Am J Clin Pathol.* 1970; 53:348–54.

8. Latatto ZA, Thomson JM, Poller L. An evaluation of chromogenic substrates in the control of oral anticoagulant therapy. *Br J Haematol.* 1981; 47:301–18.

9. Poller L. Laboratory control of anticoagulant therapy. *Semin Thromb Haemost.* 1986; 12:13–9.

10. Poller L. Progress in standardisation in anticoagulant control. *Hematol Rev.* 1987; 1:225–41.

11. Eckman MH, Levine HJ, Pauker SG. Effect of laboratory variation in the prothrombin time ratio results of oral anticoagulant therapy. *N Engl J Med.* 1993; 329:696–702.

12. Loelinger EA. ICSH/ICTH recommendations for reporting prothrombin time in oral anticoagulant control. *J Clin Pathol.* 1985; 38:133–4.

13. DuPont Pharma. ADOPT-INR. Accurate determination of prothrombin times; International Normalized Ratio. Wilmington, DE; 1993.

14. Poller L. A simple nomogram for the derivation of international normalised ratios for the standardisation of prothrombin times. *Thromb Haemost.* 1988; 60:18–20.

15. Bussey HI, Force RW, Bianco TM, et al. Reliance on prothrombin time ratio causes significant errors in anticoagulant therapy. *Arch Intern Med.* 1992; 152:278–82.

16. Ng VL, Levin J, Corash L, et al. Failure of the international normalized ratio to generate consistent results within a local medical community. *Am J Clin Pathol.* 1993; 99:689–94.

17. Le DT, Weibert RT, Sevilla BK, et al. The International Normalized Ratio (INR) for monitoring warfarin therapy: reliability and relation to other monitoring methods. *Ann Intern Med.* 1994; 120:552–8.

18. Hirsh J, Poller L. The international normalized ratio: a guide to understanding and correcting its problems. *Arch Intern Med.* 1994; 154:282–9.

---

[a]A well-defined mean normal PT must be used. The mean normal PT is determined by measuring the PT for fresh plasma samples obtained from at least 20 healthy individuals from both sexes over a range of age groups. The mean normal PT should be determined with the same thromboplastin reagent and on the same instrument as the patient's PT. The mean normal PT is reestablished for each new lot of reagent.

Approved by the ASHP Board of Directors November 16, 1994. Developed by the ASHP Commission on Therapeutics.

The bibliographic citation for this document is as follows: American Society of Health-System Pharmacists. ASHP therapeutic position statement on the use of the International Normalized Ratio system to monitor oral anticoagulant therapy. *Am J Health-Syst Pharm.* 1995; 52:529–31.

ASHP Therapeutic Position Statement on the Institutional Use of 0.9% Sodium Chloride Injection to Maintain Patency of Peripheral Indwelling Intermittent Infusion Devices

Statement of Position

0.9% Sodium chloride injection is a safe and effective means for maintaining catheter patency of peripheral indwelling intermittent infusion devices (PIIIDs) in adults. ASHP supports the use of 0.9% sodium chloride injection in preference to heparin-containing flush solutions (heparin flush) in the institutional setting, on the basis of clinical evidence indicating that 0.9% sodium chloride injection (1) is as effective as heparin flush in maintaining the patency of PIIIDs when blood is not aspirated into the device, (2) is safer to use than heparin flush because of less potential for adverse effects, (3) avoids drug incompatibilities associated with heparin flush, and (4) is a cost-effective alternative to heparin flush. Because of limited available scientific evidence to date, this recommendation is not applicable to children under the age of 12 years, patients in the home or other outpatient settings, catheters used for central venous or arterial access (including peripherally inserted central catheters and midline catheters), or the maintenance of patency in indwelling venipuncture devices used to obtain blood samples. Further research on PIIID patency in the aforementioned patient populations and settings is warranted.

Background

PIIIDs, commonly referred to as "heparin locks," are used to provide convenient intravenous (i.v.) access in patients who require intermittent i.v. administration of medications without a continuous infusion of i.v. fluids. The advantages of PIIIDs include patient mobility and comfort and reduced fluid load.[1–4] PIIIDs most commonly consist of an intravenously inserted catheter attached to a short external cannula with a resealable injection port that is designed to facilitate multiple needle entries; thus, these devices eliminate the unnecessary trauma of multiple venipunctures.[4]

A problem frequently encountered with a PIIID is the loss of patency because of clot formation within the catheter. To prevent clot formation, catheters are commonly flushed after each administration of i.v. medication and every 8 to 12 hours when the device is not in use.[5] Because of heparin's anticoagulant effects, dilute solutions of heparin in 0.9% sodium chloride injection (e.g., 10–100 units/mL) have traditionally been used to periodically flush and fill these devices and hence to prevent the formation of clots. Dilute heparin solutions are used to maintain patency while avoiding the systemic effects associated with therapeutic doses of heparin.[6] The optimum concentration of heparin and whether the drug is needed at all have not been established.[4,7–11]

Efficacy. Studies indicate that 0.9% sodium chloride injection alone is as effective as heparin-containing solutions in maintaining PIIID patency.[5,9,10,12–19] In several randomized, double-blind studies in which PIIIDs composed principally of fluoroethylene propylene (FEP-Teflon®) were used, 0.9% sodium chloride injection for flushing was associated with patency rates similar to those achieved with flush solutions containing 10 or 100 units of heparin sodium per milliliter.[13–15] The frequency of phlebitis associated with the use of these solutions was also similar.[7–11,13–15] The type of solution used to maintain PIIID patency may not be as important as the positive pressure maintained in the i.v. line by the capped (sealed) injection device, which appears to prevent blood reflux and clot formation in the device.[10,11] Several studies provide a scientific basis for using heparin,[6,20,21] but most published research supports 0.9% sodium chloride injection as an effective alternative to heparin flush in maintaining the patency of PIIIDs. Limited data from children four weeks to 18 years of age suggest no difference between 0.9% sodium chloride injection alone and 0.9% sodium chloride injection with heparin 10 units/mL in maintaining device patency.[22] Until further controlled studies are conducted in this patient population, heparin, if it is used, should be administered in the smallest amount necessary to maintain patency of the device. One survey showed that it is common practice to flush catheter devices in neonates with heparin 1–2 units/mL.[23]

Adverse Effects of Heparin Flush Therapy. Heparin, even when used in small doses, may elicit adverse reactions in some patients. The potential for bleeding complications increases when patients receive multiple, unmonitored heparin flushes.[24] Repeated injections of heparin even in small doses can alter activated partial thromboplastin time results.[25] Allergic reactions are an inherent risk of using heparin. Although rare, heparin flush-associated thrombocytopenia and hemorrhage have been reported.[24,26–28] The risks of these adverse effects may be avoided by using 0.9% sodium chloride injection instead of heparin flush.

Drug Incompatibility. Heparin has been shown to be incompatible with many commonly used i.v. drugs.[29] If heparin flush has been used to maintain the patency of a PIIID and a drug must be administered that is incompatible with heparin, it is necessary to flush the catheter with 0.9% sodium chloride injection before and after administering the incompatible drug and then to refill the PIIID with heparin. This procedure is commonly referred to as "SASH" (sodium chloride—administration [of drug]—sodium chloride—heparin).[30] The use of 0.9% sodium chloride injection as a flushing agent avoids the numerous drug incompatibilities associated with heparin and obviates the need for SASH.

Cost Implications. Enhanced quality of patient care should be the primary reason for deciding to use 0.9% sodium chloride injection for flushing. Secondarily, the choice of 0.9% sodium chloride injection may avoid substantial costs associated with drugs, related supplies, and staff time.[11]

Summary

Because of current therapeutic evidence supporting the efficacy of 0.9% sodium chloride and the inherent risks associated with heparin, ASHP believes the use of 0.9% sodium chloride injection is appropriate for maintaining the patency of PIIIDs in adults in institutional settings.

References

1. Millam DA. Intermittent devices. *NITA*. 1981; 4(Mar–Apr):142–5.

2. Larkin M. Heparin locks. *NITA*. 1979; 2(May–Jun):18–9.

3. Thomas RB, Salter FJ. Heparin locks: their advantages and disadvantages. *Hosp Formul.* 1975; 10:536–8.

4. Deeb EN, Di Mattia PE. How much heparin in the lock? *Am J IV Ther.* 1976; 3(Dec–Jan):22–6.

5. Tuten SH, Gueldner SH. Efficacy of sodium chloride versus dilute heparin for maintenance of peripheral intermittent intravenous devices. *Appl Nurs Res.* 1991; 2:63–71.

6. Hanson RL, Grant AM, Majors KR. Heparin-lock maintenance with ten units of sodium heparin in one milliliter of normal saline solution. *Surg Gynecol Obstet.* 1976; 142:373–6.

7. Garrelts JC. White clot syndrome and thrombocytopenia: reasons to abandon heparin i.v. lockflush solution. *Clin Pharm.* 1992; 11:797–9.

8. Weber DR. Is heparin really necessary in the lock and, if so, how much? *DICP Ann Pharmacother.* 1991; 25:399–407.

9. Barrett PJ, Lester RL. Heparin versus saline flushing solutions in a small community hospital. *Hosp Pharm.* 1990; 25:115–8.

10. Dunn DL, Lenihan SF. The case for the saline flush. *Am J Nurs.* 1987; 87:798–9.

11. Goode CJ, Titler M, Rakel B, et al. *Nurs Res.* 1991; 40:324–30.

12. Fry B. Intermittent heparin flushing protocols. A standardization issue. *J Intraven Nurs.* 1992; 15 (May–Jun):160–3.

13. Epperson EL. Efficacy of 0.9% sodium chloride injection with and without heparin for maintaining indwelling intermittent injection sites. *Clin Pharm.* 1984; 3:626–9.

14. Garrelts JC, LaRocca J, Ast D, et al. Comparison of heparin and 0.9% sodium chloride injection in the maintenance of indwelling intermittent IV devices. *Clin Pharm.* 1989; 8:34–9.

15. Hamilton RA, Plis JM, Clay C, et al. Heparin sodium versus 0.9% sodium chloride injection for maintaining patency of indwelling intermittent infusion devices. *Clin Pharm.* 1988; 7:439–43.

16. Shearer J. Normal saline versus dilute heparin flush: a study of peripheral intermittent IV devices. *NITA.* 1987; 10:425–7.

17. Miracle V, Fangman B, Kayrouz P, et al. Normal saline vs. heparin lock flush solution: one institution's findings. *Ky Nurse.* 1989; 37(Jul–Aug):1, 6–7.

18. Ashton J, Gibson V, Summers S. Effects of heparin versus saline solution on intermittent infusion device irrigation. *Heart Lung.* 1990; 19:608–12.

19. Hook ML, Ose P. Heparin vs. normal saline. *J Intraven Nurs.* 1990; 13:150.

20. Cyganski JM, Donahue JM, Heaton JS. The case for the heparin flush. *Am J Nurs.* 1987; 87:796–7.

21. Holford NH, Vozeh S, Coates P, et al. More on heparin lock. *N Engl J Med.* 1977; 296:1300–1. Letter.

22. Lombardi TP, Gundersen B, Zammett LO, et al. Efficacy of 0.9% sodium chloride injection with or without heparin sodium for maintaining patency of intravenous catheters in children. *Clin Pharm.* 1988; 7:8332–6.

23. Romanowski GL, Zenk KE. Intravenous flush solutions for neonates. Paper presented at 26th Annual ASHP Midyear Clinical Meeting. New Orleans, LA: 1991 Dec 10.

24. Passannante A, Macik BG. Case report: the heparin flush syndrome: a cause of iatrogenic hemorrhage. *Am J Med Sci.* 1988; 296(Jul):71–3.

25. AHFS Drug Information 93. McEvoy GK, ed. Heparin sodium. Bethesda, MD: American Society of Hospital Pharmacists; 1993: 833.

26. Heeger PS, Backstrom JT. Heparin flushes and thrombocytopenia. *Ann Intern Med.* 1986; 105:143.

27. Doty JR, Alving BM, McDonnell DE, et al. Heparin-associated thrombocytopenia in the neurosurgical patient. *Neurosurgery.* 1986; 19:69–72.

28. Cines DB, Tomaski A, Tannenbaum S. Immune endothelial-cell injury in heparin-associated thrombocytopenia. *N Engl J Med.* 1987; 316:581–9.

29. Trissel LA. Handbook on injectable drugs. 7th ed. Bethesda, MD: American Society of Hospital Pharmacists; 1992.

30. Intravenous Nurses Society. Intravenous Nursing Standards of Practice. *J Intraven Nurs.* 1990; 13:S77–8.

Approved by the ASHP Board of Directors April 27, 1994. Developed by the Commission on Therapeutics.

The bibliographic citation for this document is as follows: American Society of Hospital Pharmacists. ASHP therapeutic position statement on the institutional use of 0.9% sodium chloride injection to maintain patency of peripheral indwelling intermittent infusion devices. *Am J Hosp Pharm.* 1994; 51:1572–4.

ASHP Therapeutic Position Statement on Strategies for Identifying and Preventing Pneumococcal Resistance

Statement of Position

The emergence of penicillin-resistant strains of *Streptococcus pneumoniae* heightens the importance of implementing strategies for limiting the spread of this pathogen and preventing the serious health consequences of pneumococcal infection. The pneumococcal vaccine can prevent invasive pneumococcal infection and thereby decrease the associated morbidity and mortality. Vaccination may also reduce the potential for further development of penicillin-resistant strains. Thus, ASHP encourages vaccination of all patients at high risk for acquiring pneumococcal disease. ASHP also encourages the establishment of local, state, and national surveillance programs to track the prevalence of antimicrobial-resistant organisms so that appropriate empirical antimicrobial regimens can be used. ASHP supports continued educational efforts to promote the rational use of antimicrobials.

Background

Epidemiology. Infections due to *S. pneumoniae* are among the leading causes of illness and death worldwide. *S. pneumoniae* (pneumococcus) is the most common cause of community-acquired pneumonia and the leading cause of meningitis and sepsis. Infants, children, and the elderly are the most susceptible to invasive pneumococcal infection. Acute otitis media is the second leading cause of physician office visits and the leading cause of emergency room visits. Approximately 30–50% of episodes of acute otitis media are caused by *S. pneumoniae*.[1] *S. pneumoniae* is the most prominent pathogen in community-acquired infections.

Penicillin has historically been considered the drug of choice for the treatment of infections caused by *S. pneumoniae*. However, in recent years the prevalence of penicillin-resistant strains has increased, rendering this inexpensive first-line agent ineffective in some parts of the world. Newer, more expensive agents are now being used against this common community-acquired pathogen. The clinical impact of penicillin-resistant *S. pneumoniae* on morbidity and mortality is unknown. However, the increase in infections due to resistant organisms presents a challenge for clinicians treating pneumococcal disease.

Until the late 1980s, penicillin-resistant strains of *S. pneumoniae* were thought to be uncommon in the United States. However, the prevalence is rapidly increasing. The Centers for Disease Control and Prevention (CDC) has reported that 14.1% of *S. pneumoniae* isolates are intermediately resistant to penicillin and 3.2% are highly resistant.[2] These data were collected from 12 sentinel hospitals in 11 states and provide only a snapshot of pneumococcal resistance at selected hospitals. One of the first reports of penicillin-resistant *S. pneumoniae* came from Tennessee and Kentucky in 1993.[3] These two states reported that approximately 30% of *S. pneumoniae* isolates from ambulatory children were resistant to penicillin. A more recent outpatient study conducted in 30 medical centers across the United States found an overall rate of pneumococcal resistance to penicillin of 23.6% (14.1% intermediate and 9.5% high-level resistance).[4] This study showed distinct geographic variations in the prevalence of pneumococcal resistance. In the eight-county metropolitan Atlanta area, 25% of the pneumococcal strains causing invasive disease in hospitalized patients were penicillin resistant.[5]

The true prevalence of pneumococcal resistance in the United States is unknown because drug-resistant pneumococcal infection is not generally considered reportable to local, state, or federal health agencies. However, concern over increasing antimicrobial resistance has led several state health departments to require clinical laboratories to report all cases of invasive drug-resistant pneumococcal infection.[6] In addition, the CDC has fostered the initiation of several multicenter surveillance projects, such as the Intensive Care Antibiotic Resistance Epidemiology (ICARE) project, a program that is tracking resistant organisms and antimicrobial-use patterns in intensive care units. However, until a comprehensive national surveillance plan is in effect, the burden of tracking drug-resistant *S. pneumoniae* will be on individual hospitals and communities.

Several factors are postulated to contribute to the emergence and spread of resistant bacteria. Major contributors are the abuse and misuse of antimicrobials for empirical therapy and the widespread use of broad-spectrum antimicrobials for questionable indications in the community setting. Patients and their caregivers also contribute to the misuse of antimicrobials by pressuring physicians to provide treatment. Another postulated cause is the widespread use of antimicrobial agents in agriculture; however, the actual impact of this practice is unknown.[1]

Definitions and Mechanism of Resistance. *S. pneumoniae* resistant to penicillin is defined in terms of the minimum inhibitory concentration (MIC) of penicillin. Strains may be distinguished as being susceptible (MIC ≤ 0.06 µg/mL), intermediately resistant (MIC 0.1–1.0 µg/mL), or highly resistant (MIC ≥ 2.0 µg/mL). Highly resistant strains of *S. pneumoniae* are less likely to respond to β-lactam agents and are often resistant to other classes of antimicrobials as well, while intermediately resistant strains may respond to high-dose penicillin therapy or to other β-lactam agents such as the cephalosporins.[7] Multidrug-resistant *S. pneumoniae* is defined as a strain resistant to three or more classes of antimicrobials, such as the penicillins, cephalosporins, macrolides, tetracyclines, and trimethoprim–sulfamethoxazole.[5]

Strains of *S. pneumoniae* tolerant to penicillin have also been described. Tolerant strains require a much higher concentration of penicillin for bactericidal activity than the concentration required to inhibit growth.[5] The clinical significance of this phenomenon is not clear, but tolerance has been implicated as the cause of therapeutic failures of penicillin.

Resistance of *S. pneumoniae* to penicillin is due to alterations in the penicillin-binding proteins (PBPs). These proteins are involved in the synthesis of bacterial cell walls and are the sites of action for the β-lactam agents. Alterations in the PBPs may result in structural modifications of the cell wall that allow the organism to avoid the inhibitory effects of penicillin.[8] Resistance may also be conferred onto all agents in the penicillin class of antimicrobials, including extended-spectrum agents such as mezlocillin and piperacillin. It is important to note that plasmid-mediated β-lactamase enzymes have not been identified in penicillin-resistant strains of pneumococci. Therefore, the addition of a β-lactamase inhibitor should have no effect on the susceptibility of these strains to the penicillin antimicrobials.

Detection of Resistance. The National Committee on Clinical Laboratory Standards (NCCLS) has established criteria for testing pneumococcal susceptibilities with the disk diffusion method. The E test method has been shown to be as accurate as the disk diffusion method in determining pneumococcal susceptibilities. Commercial automated microdilution systems, such as MicroScan and Vitek, may inaccurately indicate sensitivity to penicillin for strains of *S. pneumoniae* that are actually intermediately or highly resistant to penicillin.[9] Therefore, the automated systems should be used with caution or not at all.

In the disk diffusion method, either a methicillin or an oxacillin disk may be used to determine pneumococcus susceptibility to penicillin. An oxacillin disk is preferred because of its greater worldwide availability. A 1-μg oxacillin disk is used with a zone cutoff of 20 mm. If the zone of inhibition is >20 mm, the pneumococcal strain is considered susceptible to penicillin. Even though zones of <19 mm indicate resistance, the penicillin MIC should still be determined for the purpose of differentiating between intermediate and high-level resistance.[9]

The E test is a new and simpler method of determining MICs. It uses a calibrated, antimicrobial-impregnated plastic strip. The antimicrobial gradient produces an elliptical zone of inhibition. The area where the ellipse meets the plastic strip determines the MIC for the organism. This method has been shown to give MIC results equivalent to those obtained with other standard methods.[9,10] The E test is becoming a widely accepted method for determining pneumococcal MICs because of its reproducibility and the ease of performing the test.

The NCCLS suggests that all isolates of *S. pneumoniae* cultured from usually sterile sites be tested for penicillin resistance. If resistance to penicillin is detected, then quantitative tests for penicillin, extended-spectrum cephalosporin, chloramphenicol, and vancomycin MICs should be performed; quantitative MIC determinations for other antimicrobials that may be clinically indicated for the treatment of the patient may also be performed.[6]

Establishment of Surveillance Systems

Surveillance systems should be established at the local level to determine the prevalence of penicillin-resistant *S. pneumoniae* within an individual community. Health systems within a community or region should work together to identify the prevalence of the resistant strains, which may vary widely among institutions within the same community. Collaboration among medical, pharmacy, clinical microbiology laboratory, and nursing personnel is imperative so that appropriate empirical antimicrobial therapy can be selected for patients.

Vaccination of High-Risk Patients

Several national organizations and the CDC Advisory Committee on Immunization Practices (ACIP) have recommended that adults at age 50 years have a complete review of their vaccination status and determination of risk factors that may indicate the need for the pneumococcal vaccine.[11] The ACIP recommends use of the pneumococcal vaccine in adults considered to be at high risk for acquiring pneumococcal infection and in children ≥2 years old with certain chronic illnesses (Table 1).[11,12] Individuals should be revaccinated every six years.

There are currently two 23-valent pneumococcal vaccines on the U.S. market: Pneumovax 23 by Merck and Pnu-Imune 23 by Wyeth-Ayerst. These vaccines include 23 pneumococcal capsular types that cause 88% of bacteremic pneumococcal infections in the United States. Also, there is cross-reactivity with other capsular types for an additional 8% of bacteremic illnesses. These vaccines are approximately 60% effective in preventing invasive pneumococcal disease.[12] A conjugated pneumococcal vaccine is being developed for use in children <2 years of age.

The pneumococcal vaccine is underused in that it is estimated to be administered to less than 30% of individuals >65 years old. Although studies testing the effectiveness of the pneumococcal vaccine have been criticized, its use in the elderly is thought to be a cost-effective prevention measure.[13,14] Use of the pneumococcal vaccine has not been shown to decrease the prevalence of penicillin-resistant *S. pneumoniae*; however, 89% of the intermediately resistant organisms isolated by the CDC Pneumococcal Sentinel Surveillance System are serotypes in the 23-valent pneumococcal vaccine.[3] In addition, prevention of invasive pneumococcal infection may decrease the potential for further development of resistant organisms. Therefore, comprehensive vaccination programs should be instituted with the intent of decreasing the morbidity and mortality associated with invasive pneumococcal infection.

Promotion of Rational Antimicrobial Use

Overuse of antimicrobial agents promotes the development and spread of resistant organisms. Factors contributing to antimicrobial overuse include inappropriate use of antimicrobials for viral infections, inadequate diagnostic criteria for some respiratory tract infections, unnecessary use of broad-spectrum agents covering all possible infecting organisms in order to avoid legal liability, and pressure from patients or caregivers on physi-

Table 1.
Candidates for Pneumococcal Vaccine[11,12]

Immunocompetent Adults
  Persons ≥65 years of age
  Persons with cardiovascular disease, pulmonary disease, diabetes mellitus, alcoholism, cirrhosis, or cerebrospinal fluid (CSF) leaks
Immunosuppressed Adults
  All, including those with HIV infection
Children
  Those ≥2 years with anatomic or functional asplenia, nephrotic syndrome, CSF leaks, immunosuppression, or previous invasive pneumococcal disease

cians to provide treatment.[6] Educational efforts to promote the rational use of antimicrobials will need to be directed at health care providers, third-party payers, and the public.

Summary

The increasing prevalence of antibiotic-resistant *S. pneumoniae* in the United States underscores the need for adequate treatment, monitoring, and prevention of pneumococcal infections. Clinicians need to be informed of the prevalence and patterns of drug resistance within their communities in order to optimize empirical antimicrobial regimens. Use of the pneumococcal vaccine in high-risk populations should be promoted. Educational efforts to encourage the rational use of antimicrobials must be instituted or continued.

References

1. Public and Scientific Affairs Board. Report of the ASM task force on antibiotic resistance. Washington, DC: American Society for Microbiology; 1995.

2. Butler JC, Hofmann JC, Cetron MS, et al. The emergence of drug-resistant *Streptococcus pneumoniae* in the United States: an update from the Centers for Disease Control and Prevention's pneumococcal sentinel surveillance system. *J Infect Dis.* 1996; 174:986–93.

3. Centers for Disease Control and Prevention. Drug resistant *Streptococcus pneumoniae*—Kentucky and Tennessee, 1993. *MMWR.* 1994; 43:23–5.

4. Doern GV, Brueggemann A, Holley HP et al. Antimicrobial resistance of *Streptococcus pneumoniae* recovered from outpatients in the United States during the winter months of 1994 to 1995: results of a 30-center national surveillance study. *Antimicrob Agents Chemother.* 1996; 40:1208–13.

5. Hofman J, Cetron MS, Farley MM, et al. The prevalence of drug-resistant *Streptococcus pneumoniae* in Atlanta. *N Engl J Med.* 1995; 333:481–6.

6. Centers for Disease Control and Prevention. Defining the public health impact of drug-resistant *Streptococcus pneumoniae*: report of a working group. *MMWR.*
1996; 45(RR-1):1–14.

7. Friedland IR, McCracken GH. Management of infections caused by antibiotic-resistant *Streptococcus pneumoniae*. *N Engl J Med.* 1994; 331:377–82.

8. Caputo GM, Appelbaum PC, Liu HH. Infections due to penicillin-resistant pneumococci: clinical, epidemiologic, and microbiologic features. *Arch Intern Med.* 1993; 153:1301–10.

9. Jacobs MR. Treatment and diagnosis of infections caused by drug-resistant *Streptococcus pneumoniae*. *Clin Infect Dis.* 1992; 15:119–27.

10. Jorgensen JH. Detection of antimicrobial resistance in *Streptococcus pneumoniae* by use of standardized susceptibility testing methods and recently developed interpretive criteria. *Clin Microbiol News.* 1994; 16 (Jul 1):97–101.

11. Centers for Disease Control and Prevention. Assessing adult vaccination status at age 50 years. *MMWR.* 1995; 44:561–3.

12. Centers for Disease Control. Update on adult immunization—pneumococcal disease. *MMWR.* 1991; 40(RR-12):42–5.

13. Hirschmann JV, Lipsky BA. The pneumococcal vaccine after 15 years of use. *Arch Intern Med.* 1994; 154:373–7.

14. Fedson DS, Shapiro ED, LaForce FM, et al. Pneumococcal vaccine after 15 years of use, another view. *Arch Intern Med.* 1994; 154:2531–5.

This official ASHP practice standard was developed through the ASHP Commission on Therapeutics and approved by the ASHP Board of Directors on November 16, 1996.

The bibliographic citation for this document is as follows: American Society of Health-System Pharmacists. ASHP therapeutic position statement on strategies for identifying and preventing pneumococcal resistance. *Am J Health-Syst Pharm.* 1997; 54:575–8.

ASHP Therapeutic Position Statement on Strategies for Preventing and Treating Multidrug-Resistant Tuberculosis

Statement of Position

ASHP encourages the implementation of strategies for preventing and treating multidrug-resistant tuberculosis (MDR-TB). To reduce the occurrence of MDR-TB resulting from nonadherence to medication regimens, ASHP supports the use of directly observed therapy and other efforts to promote medication adherence in all patients with tuberculosis. In addition, ASHP encourages the establishment of patient screening programs for early detection of tuberculosis and the use of methods to ensure appropriate drug selection and monitoring of patients with tuberculosis.

Background

Tuberculosis remains a significant cause of morbidity and mortality worldwide. It is estimated that more than one third of the world's population, or 1.7 billion persons, are infected with *Mycobacterium tuberculosis*,[1] with approximately 3 million deaths occurring per year. In the United States, attempts to eradicate tuberculosis have failed. Along with other factors, the increase in MDR-TB has limited the success of antimicrobial chemotherapy. MDR-TB is a result of inadequate therapy and a cause of poor treatment outcomes.

MDR-TB is defined as infection due to a strain of *M. tuberculosis* that is resistant to both isoniazid and rifampin, with or without concurrent resistance to other antituberculosis agents.[2] Isoniazid and rifampin are the most important antituberculosis agents used today. Effective use of these agents enables high (>95%) success rates with a short duration of therapy (six to nine months) and minimal adverse effects.[3] When these drugs cannot be used because of resistance, clinicians are forced to use more toxic, less efficacious drugs for longer periods of time. It is estimated that treatment of MDR-TB has a failure rate 80 times greater than for treatment of drug-susceptible TB.[4] In patients infected with the human immunodeficiency virus (HIV), the prognosis may be even worse.[5] Efforts to treat MDR-TB strain health care budgets. The average cost for treating a case of MDR-TB has been estimated at $180,000,[6] compared with $12,000 for a case caused by a drug-susceptible strain.[7]

Most cases of MDR-TB result from the evolution in a particular patient of drug-susceptible tuberculosis to a drug-resistant form (primary resistance). This occurs when small subpopulations of resistant bacteria survive and ultimately become the predominant population. This emergence of resistant bacterial mutants occurs for one or more of the following reasons: therapy is discontinued before all bacteria have been eradicated, the patient does not take all of the prescribed medications appropriately, an inadequate number of drugs are prescribed for active tuberculosis, or drug concentrations in vivo are too low to effectively eradicate bacteria. These examples of medication mismanagement are common,[6] but they can often be corrected through the use of appropriate protocols for treatment and follow-up.

MDR-TB can also develop through transmission of resistant organisms from one person to another (secondary resistance). Traditionally, secondary resistance has been considered a less common cause of MDR-TB than primary resistance, but recent studies suggest that acquisition through secondary resistance is increasing in the United States.[8,9] Secondary acquisition of MDR-TB is particularly common in HIV-infected persons, immigrants, persons residing in certain institutions (e.g., homeless shelters, prisons, HIV wards), and close contacts of index cases of MDR-TB. Health professionals must be aware of epidemiologic causes of MDR-TB and should manage high-risk patients accordingly.[10]

Since 1985, the proportion of *M. tuberculosis* strains resistant to isoniazid and rifampin has more than doubled. In the United States, approximately 1 strain in 7 is resistant to at least one antituberculosis agent, and 1 in 30 can be classified as multidrug resistant.[11] The increase in drug-resistant isolates is particularly dramatic in New York City; residents are 50 times more likely to be infected with a strain of MDR-TB than those living outside New York City.[12] A history of previous antituberculosis drug therapy is associated with a marked increase in the likelihood of drug resistance, particularly to rifampin or multiple drugs. One study noted that the frequency of MDR-TB was twice as high in previously treated patients as in those without prior treatment.[11]

Much of the association between prior antituberculosis therapy and MDR-TB can be attributed to nonadherence. Medication nonadherence is a particularly important risk factor for MDR-TB and is common in settings where supervised therapy is not used. It is estimated that, on average, one in three patients will be nonadherent with antituberculosis therapy. However, nonadherence rates as high as 80% may be observed in some populations.[13]

Directly Observed Therapy

Pharmacists and other health care professionals should develop and implement measures to reduce the adverse effects of MDR-TB and thereby improve outcomes in patients with tuberculosis. First and foremost, the risk for drug resistance resulting from patient nonadherence should be eliminated. This can be accomplished through the establishment of treatment protocols using directly observed therapy (DOT).[14] DOT is defined as the administration of drugs or other therapies under the supervision of one or more health care workers or other responsible caregivers for the purpose of ensuring adherence. DOT regimens can involve twice- or thrice-weekly administration of antituberculosis agents, which has been shown to be as effective as daily administration.[4,15] In fact, because of the improvement in adherence, DOT programs often result in higher efficacy rates and lower primary and secondary resistance rates than daily unsupervised therapy.[16,17] Furthermore, DOT provides a regular opportunity for patient education and may also result in earlier detection of adverse effects, thereby preventing serious complications of therapy.

Homeless persons and other underprivileged individuals have generally been characterized as unreliable in completing their therapy and thus as candidates for DOT, whereas "responsible" patients of private physicians may be treated with daily unsupervised therapy. A presumption of adherence in the privately treated patient may be erroneous. A study conducted in Baltimore, Maryland, compared the outcomes (sputum culture conversion to negative for *M. tuberculosis* at three months) in patients with pulmonary tuberculosis who were treated by private physicians with those in patients receiving DOT in a city-run clinic. The three-month culture conversion rate was only 40% in the private patients, compared with 90% in the public clinic patients.[18] The need for DOT should be considered in all patients with tuberculosis.

Other Methods of Promoting Adherence

In patients for whom DOT may not be practical, other methods should be used to ensure adherence to the antituberculosis regimen. Patients should be educated about their disease and its therapy. They should be asked routinely about adherence during follow-up visits or in telephone calls. Adherence can also be checked by performing pill counts or periodic urine tests to identify the presence of drug metabolites. Adherence in adult patients can be enhanced through the use of fixed-dose combination capsules or tablets. The patient's sputum cultures should also be monitored for bacteriologic conversion to negative. DOT should be considered for patients whose sputum remains positive for *M. tuberculosis* after two months of therapy.[19]

Patient Screening for MDR-TB

In addition to their efforts to improve adherence to drug treatment regimens, pharmacists and other health professionals should identify patients who may already be infected with drug-resistant strains. All isolates of *M. tuberculosis* from infected patients should be tested for drug susceptibility with rapid assay techniques,[20] and therapy should be modified appropriately when resistance is detected.

All health care institutions should establish procedures for effective screening of patients with suspected pulmonary tuberculosis and for respiratory isolation of patients at risk until an alternate diagnosis is established. In the case of suspected pulmonary MDR-TB, isolation should be continued until susceptibility results are known or a microbiologic response is observed. All cases of tuberculosis (including MDR-TB) should be reported to the appropriate state health department as well as to the Centers for Disease Control and Prevention.

Drug Selection

Most patients should initially receive a regimen of four drugs (isoniazid, rifampin, pyrazinamide, and ethambutol). The regimen can be tailored when susceptibility results are known. Initiating therapy with three drugs is adequate only in areas where the rate of isoniazid resistance is documented to be less than 4%.[21] For patients in whom MDR-TB is suspected (previously treated patients, immigrants, homeless persons, HIV-infected patients, documented contacts of persons with MDR-TB), initial empirical drug therapy should include five or more drugs until susceptibility results are known.[21] Health professionals should be aware of rates of resistance to isoniazid and rifampin in their community and modify empirical

therapy in all patients accordingly if resistance rates exceed 4%.[2]

Patient Monitoring

Finally, all patients with tuberculosis should be monitored closely throughout therapy to ensure success. Although DOT will ensure adherence to drug therapy, follow-up roentgenographic and microbiologic testing is still important for documenting successful treatment. If drug therapy appears to be failing (i.e., sputum smear remains positive for acid-fast bacilli after two months of therapy; sputum culture remains positive after three months of therapy; elevated temperature, cough, or other symptoms persist after one month of therapy), MDR-TB should be suspected and at least two previously unused antituberculosis agents added to the regimen until susceptibility can be documented.[2,3] If treatment fails despite appropriate drug therapy and documented adherence, pharmacokinetic studies may be indicated to determine whether inadequate drug bioavailability or altered drug disposition may be contributing to failure.[22]

Summary

MDR-TB is usually the result of mismanagement of tuberculosis and requires intensive and costly therapeutic strategies. Prevention is the most effective means of managing MDR-TB. Pharmacists and other health professionals should work together to plan and implement programs for effective screening and therapy of tuberculosis. DOT is an important therapeutic tool that should be considered in all patients. Interdisciplinary management programs can be effective in reducing the rate of drug resistance and maximizing efficacy.

References

1. Raviglione MC, Snider DE Jr, Kochi A. Global epidemiology of tuberculosis: morbidity and mortality of a worldwide epidemic. *JAMA.* 1995; 273:220–6.
2. Centers for Disease Control and Prevention. Initial therapy for tuberculosis in the era of multidrug resistance: recommendations of the advisory council for the elimination of tuberculosis. *MMWR.* 1993; 42(RR-7):1–8.
3. American Thoracic Society. Treatment of tuberculosis and tuberculosis infection in adults and children. *Am J Respir Crit Care Med.* 1994; 149:1359–74.
4. Goble M, Iseman MD, Madsen LA, et al. Treatment of 171 patients with pulmonary tuberculosis resistant to isoniazid and rifampin. *N Engl J Med.* 1993; 328:527–32.
5. Busillo CP, Lessmau KD, Sanjana V, et al. Multidrug-resistant *Mycobacterium tuberculosis* in patients with human immunodeficiency virus infection. *Chest.* 1992; 102:797–801.
6. Mahmoudi A, Iseman MD. Pitfalls in the care of patients with tuberculosis: common errors and their association with the acquisition of drug resistance. *JAMA.* 1993; 270:65–8.
7. Cohen ML. Epidemiology of drug resistance: implications for a post-antibiotic era. *Science.* 1992; 257:1050–5.
8. Beck-Sague C, Dooley SW, Hutton MD, et al. Hospital outbreak of multidrug-resistant *Mycobacterium tu-*

berculosis infections: factors in transmission to staff and HIV-infected patients. *JAMA.* 1992; 268:1280–6.

9. Small PM, Shafer RW, Hopewell PC, et al. Exogenous reinfection with multidrug-resistant *Mycobacterium tuberculosis* in patients with advanced HIV infection. *N Engl J Med.* 1993; 328:1137–44.

10. Centers for Disease Control and Prevention. Screening for tuberculosis and tuberculosis infection in high-risk patients. *MMWR.* 1995; 44(RR-11):19–32.

11. Bloch AB, Cauthen GM, Onorato IM, et al. Nationwide survey of drug-resistant tuberculosis in the United States. *JAMA.* 1994; 271:665–71.

12. Frieden TR, Sterling T, Pablos-Mendez A, et al. The emergence of drug-resistant tuberculosis in New York City. *N Engl J Med.* 1993; 328:521–6.

13. Brudney K, Dobkin J. Resurgent tuberculosis in New York City: human immunodeficiency virus, homelessness, and the decline of tuberculosis control programs. *Am Rev Respir Dis.* 1991; 144:745–9.

14. Schluger N, Ciotoli C, Cohen D, et al. Comprehensive tuberculosis control for patients at high risk for noncompliance. *Am J Respir Crit Care Med.* 1995; 151:1486–90.

15. Hong Kong Chest Service/British Medical Research Council. Controlled trial of 2, 4, and 6 months of pyrazinamide in 6-month, three-times-weekly regimens for smear-positive pulmonary tuberculosis, including an assessment of a combined preparation of isoniazid, rifampin, and pyrazinamide. *Am Rev Respir Dis.* 1991; 143:700–6.

16. Weis SE, Slocum PC, Blais FX, et al. The effect of directly observed therapy on the rates of drug resistance and relapse in tuberculosis. *N Engl J Med.* 1994; 330:1179–84.

17. Lowe C, ed. New York City Department of Health. Summary of reportable diseases and conditions, 1994. *City Health Inf.* 1995; 14(4):1–24.

18. Chaulk CP, Moore-Rice K, Rizzo R, et al. 11 years of community-based directly observed therapy for tuberculosis. *JAMA.* 1995; 274:945–51.

19. Core curriculum on tuberculosis. 3rd ed. Atlanta: Centers for Disease Control and Prevention; 1994.

20. Centers for Disease Control and Prevention. Laboratory practices for diagnosis of tuberculosis—United States, 1994. *MMWR.* 1995; 44:587–90.

21. Centers for Disease Control and Prevention. Meeting the challenge of multidrug-resistant tuberculosis: summary of a conference. *MMWR.* 1992; 41(RR-11):51–7.

22. Peloquin CA, Berning SE. Infection caused by *Mycobacterium tuberculosis. Ann Pharmacother.* 1994; 28:72–84.

This official ASHP practice standard was developed through the ASHP Commission on Therapeutics and approved by the ASHP Board of Directors on November 16, 1996.

The bibliographic citation for this document is as follows: American Society of Health-System Pharmacists. ASHP Therapeutic Position Statement on Strategies for Preventing and Treating Multidrug-Resistant Tuberculosis. *Am J Health-Syst Pharm.* 1997; 54:428–31.

ASHP Therapeutic Position Statement on Strict Glycemic Control in Selected Patients with Insulin-Dependent Diabetes Mellitus

Statement of Position

ASHP supports the maintenance of strict glycemic control in selected patients with insulin-dependent diabetes mellitus (IDDM). Strict glycemic control has been shown to reduce the appearance and progression of the chronic diabetic complications nephropathy, retinopathy, and neuropathy in patients with IDDM.[1] Biochemical mechanisms by which hyperglycemia causes tissue damage have been demonstrated[2]; this evidence may help to further support the benefits of strict glycemic control. For the purposes of this document, strict glycemic control is defined as the use of intensive insulin treatment regimens to maintain optimal blood glucose concentrations. Intensive insulin administration methods consist of multiple daily injections of insulin or the use of subcutaneous insulin-infusion pumps combined with frequent blood glucose monitoring (at least three times per day).

Strict glycemic control is probably beneficial for the majority of patients; however, it may be inappropriate for some patients because of the risks associated with severe hypoglycemia. Therefore, intensive treatment regimens should be initiated with caution, and they may not be appropriate in patients with poor perception of the symptoms of hypoglycemia and those with a history of frequent, severe hypoglycemic episodes. Additionally, the risk–benefit ratio of strict glycemic control may be unfavorable in patients less than 13 years of age, obese patients, and patients with advanced complications such as end-stage renal disease or cardiovascular or cerebrovascular disease.

The effects of strict glycemic control in patients with non-insulin-dependent diabetes mellitus (NIDDM) are undetermined but are being evaluated in two major prospective, controlled trials.[3,4] Studies have suggested that poor glycemic control is associated with the development of chronic diabetic complications in both IDDM and NIDDM patients.[5] Further research on the benefits of strict glycemic control in patients with NIDDM is warranted.

Background

Several studies have demonstrated a correlation between glycemic control and development of diabetic complications.[6-11] The most conclusive evidence of this correlation was found in the 1993 Diabetes Control and Complications Trial (DCCT), a multicenter, randomized clinical trial evaluating 1441 patients with IDDM.[1] The study addressed two questions: (1) Does the institution of strict glycemic control reduce the rate of progression of chronic complications that are present at the initiation of intensive treatment? (secondary intervention cohort) and (2) Does strict glycemic control prevent the appearance of chronic complications? (primary prevention cohort). The primary prevention cohort included 726 patients and the secondary intervention cohort, 715. Patients from both cohorts were randomized into one of two groups, the intensive therapy group or the conventional therapy group. Conventional therapy consisted of one or two daily injections of insulin, including mixed intermediate and rapid-acting insulins; daily self-monitoring of urine or blood glucose; diet; and exercise. Intensive therapy included the administration of insulin three or more times daily by injection or the use of an external pump. The dosage was adjusted according to the results of self-monitoring of blood glucose performed at least four times per day, dietary intake, and anticipated exercise. Patients were followed in the study for a mean of 6.5 years. The study data overwhelmingly demonstrated that intensive therapy delays the onset and slows the progression of retinopathy, nephropathy, and neuropathy in patients with IDDM.

The main adverse effect related to intensive treatment was severe hypoglycemia. The DCCT also demonstrated that early and transient worsening of retinopathy could occur with intensive insulin therapy. Other studies have suggested that rapid improvement of glycemic control could cause transient retinal deterioration,[12-14] and subsequent studies have confirmed that these untoward changes were in fact transient.[15,16]

Levels of Glycemic Control

Desired blood glucose levels and methods of glucose control for patients with IDDM depend upon a number of factors including the patient's age, risk of hypoglycemia, capacity and motivation to follow complex treatment regimens, the presence or absence of advanced complications, concurrent life-shortening disease, and the duration and age of onset of disease.

Patients should be fully informed of the treatment options for achieving strict glycemic control. While the practitioner has some latitude in establishing a glycemic target range, it appears that blood glucose concentrations in all patients with diabetes should be maintained as close to normal as possible, given the constraints of hypoglycemic episodes and reasonable treatment regimens as determined by patient-specific characteristics. Guidelines for glycemic control published by the American Diabetes Association (ADA) should be followed (Table 1).[17]

The ADA has also established guidelines for the use of self-monitoring of blood glucose in patients with diabetes. An expert panel concluded that self-monitoring of blood glucose should be used for achieving and maintaining a

Table 1.
Glycemic Control for People with Diabetes[a,b]

Biochemical Index	Nondiabetic	Goal	Action Suggested
Preprandial glucose (mg/dL)	<115	80–120	<80 or >140
Bedtime glucose (mg/dL)	<120	100–140	<100 or >160
Hemoglobin A$_{1c}$	<6	<7	>8

[a]These values are for nonpregnant individuals. "Action suggested" depends on individual patient circumstances. Hemoglobin A$_{1c}$ is referenced to a nondiabetic range of 4.0–6.0% (mean ± S.D., 5.0 ± 0.5%)
[b]Reprinted with permission of the American Diabetes Association.

specific level of glycemic control, preventing and detecting hypoglycemia, avoiding severe hypoglycemia, adjusting dosages in patients undergoing lifestyle changes, and determining the need for initiating insulin therapy in gestational diabetes mellitus.[18] These recommendations apply to virtually every patient with diabetes.

Treatment Plan

Strict glycemic control in patients with IDDM is best achieved by intensive insulin administration methods as described in the DCCT (multiple daily injections or subcutaneous insulin infusion pump). Risk factor reduction, diet, and exercise should be incorporated into the treatment plan of all patients with diabetes.

Pharmacist's Role

An informed patient is critical to the success or failure of any treatment plan. Knowledgeable patients adhere more closely to prescribed drug regimens and thus have improved therapeutic outcomes. Therefore, pharmacists, by virtue of their training and expertise, have a responsibility to inform patients about their medication therapy.[19] The pharmacist, in collaboration with other members of the health care team, should actively participate in educating, counseling, and monitoring patients with diabetes. Pharmacists should provide other health care professionals and patients with information about the effects of strict glycemic control, discuss treatment options, and promote adherence to treatment regimens. Pharmacists should work with other health care professionals in designing treatment regimens for patients with diabetes that incorporate considerations such as age, weight, diabetes type, renal function, level of motivation, and cognitive function. Pharmacists should ensure that patients are able to self-monitor blood glucose. They should advocate monitoring of fasting blood glucose and glycosylated hemoglobin levels at regular intervals. Pharmacists should also encourage screening for accompanying risk factors (e.g., hyperlipidemia, hypertension).

Summary

ASHP supports strict glycemic control in selected patients with IDDM on the basis of studies demonstrating that strict glycemic control delays the onset and slows the progression of diabetic retinopathy, nephropathy, and neuropathy. Because of the increased risk of hypoglycemia, intensive treatment regimens may not be appropriate in patients with poor perception of hypoglycemic symptoms and those with a history of frequent, severe hypoglycemic episodes. The pharmacist can play a key role in implementing and monitoring this therapy by collaborating with other members of the health care team and by counseling patients.

References

1. Diabetes Control and Complication Trial Research Group. The effect of intensive treatment of diabetes on the development and progression of long-term complications in insulin-dependent diabetes mellitus. *N Engl J Med*. 1993; 329(14):977–86.

2. Brownlee M, Cerami A, Vlassara H. Advanced glycosylation end products in tissue and the biochemical basis of diabetic complications. *N Engl J Med*. 1988; 318:1315–21.

3. UK Prospective Diabetes Study: VIII. Study design, progress, performance. *Diabetologia*. 1991; 34:877–90.

4. Abraira C, Johnson N, Colwell J. The VACSDM Group: VA cooperative study on glycemic control and complications in type II diabetes. *Diabetes*. 1994; 43:59A. Abstract.

5. Colwell JA. DCCT findings, applicability and implications for NIDDM. *Diabetes Rev*. 1994; 2(3):277–90.

6. Keiding NR, Root HF, Marble A. Importance of control of diabetes in prevention of vascular complications. *JAMA*. 1952; 150:964–9.

7. Johnsson S. Retinopathy and nephropathy in diabetes mellitus: comparison of the effects of two forms of treatment. *Diabetes*. 1960; 9:1–8.

8. Job D, Eschwege E, Guyot-Argenton C et al. Effect of multiple daily insulin injections on the course of diabetic retinopathy. *Diabetes*. 1976; 25:463–9.

9. Pirart J. Diabetes mellitus and its degenerative complications: a prospective study of 4,400 patients observed between 1947 and 1973. *Diabetes Care*. 1978; 1(3):168–88, 253–63.

10. Feldt-Rasmussen B, Mathiesen ER, Deckert T. Effect of two years of strict metabolic control on progression of incipient nephropathy in insulin-dependent diabetes. *Lancet*. 1986; 2:1300–4.

11. Rosenstock J, Friberg T, Raskin P. Effect of glycemic control on microvascular complications in patients with type I diabetes mellitus. *Am J Med*. 1986; 81:1012–7.

12. Kroc Collaborative Study Group. Blood glucose control and the evolution of diabetic retinopathy and albuminuria: a preliminary multicenter trial. *N Engl J Med*. 1984; 311:365–72.

13. Dahl-Jorgensen K, Brinchmann-Hansen O, Hanssen KF, et al. for the Aker Diabetes Group. Rapid tightening of blood glucose control leads to transient deterioration of retinopathy in insulin dependent diabetes mellitus: the Oslo study. *Br Med J*. 1985; 290:811–5.

14. Lauritzen T, Frost-Larsen K, Larsen HW, et al. for the Steno Study Group. Effect of 1 year of near-normal blood glucose levels on retinopathy in insulin-dependent diabetics. *Lancet*. 1983; 1:200–4.

15. Lauritzen T, Frost-Larsen IK, Larsen HW, et al. for the Steno Study Group. Two-year experience with continuous subcutaneous insulin infusion in relation to retinopathy and neuropathy. *Diabetes*. 1985; 34:74–9.

16. Dahl-Jorgensen K, Brinchmann-Hansen O, Hanssen KF, et al. Effect of near normoglycemia for two years on the progression of early diabetic retinopathy, nephropathy, and neuropathy: the Oslo study. *Br Med J*. 1986; 293:1195–9.

17. American Diabetes Association. Standards of medical care for patients with diabetes mellitus. *Diabetes Care*. 1995; 18(suppl 1):8–15.

18. American Diabetes Association. Self monitoring of blood glucose. *Diabetes Care*. 1994; 17(1):81–6.

19. American Society of Hospital Pharmacists. ASHP guidelines on pharmacist-conducted patient counseling. *Am J Hosp Pharm*. 1993; 50:505–6.

Approved by the ASHP Board of Directors on September 22, 1995. Developed by the ASHP Commission on Therapeutics.

ASHP
Therapeutic Guidelines

ASHP Therapeutic Guidelines on Angiotensin-Converting-Enzyme Inhibitors in Patients with Left Ventricular Dysfunction

Heart failure (HF) is one of the most important cardiovascular diseases treated with drug therapy. It affects approximately 1.5% of the U.S. adult population, causing a dramatic decline in quality of life and a shortened life expectancy. HF is a syndrome characterized by fatigue, exercise intolerance, shortness of breath, peripheral edema, and pulmonary congestion. These symptoms result from the heart's inability to pump effectively enough to meet the body's metabolic demands.

Approximately 3 million people in the United States have HF. The incidence is approximately 3 per 1000 per year at the ages of 35–64 years and increases with advancing age to about 10 per 1000 per year at ages 65–94.[1] Accordingly, the prevalence of HF approximately doubles for each decade of life.[2]

HF is the most common hospital discharge diagnosis in patients over the age of 65 and the fourth most common discharge diagnosis overall.[3] In the United States, more than 400,000 new cases are diagnosed annually, and HF is the only major cardiovascular disease for which the incidence is increasing.[4] The prognosis for patients with HF is poor; data from control groups in large clinical trials indicate that patients with HF have a five-year mortality rate of approximately 50% and that patients with the most severe symptoms have approximately a 50% one-year mortality.

The economic impact of HF is also significant. In the United States, annual expenditures for the diagnosis and treatment of HF exceed $10 billion.[5] Of this, approximately $230 million is spent on drug therapy and $7.5 billion on hospitalizations. The remainder is spent on nursing home days ($1.9 billion) and physician office visits ($690 million). The average length of hospitalization for HF is approximately nine days, at an average cost of more than $12,000.[6]

Because of the high morbidity, mortality, and cost associated with the disease, HF is likely to remain a significant public health concern. Innovations in the medical management of HF should be evaluated for their ability to ameliorate symptoms, prevent hospitalizations, reduce medical costs, and increase life span. Recent trials with various angiotensin-converting-enzyme inhibitors (ACEIs) have documented progress toward these goals. This document contains scientific and clinical information intended to guide health care professionals in the optimal use of ACEIs in patients with HF.

Scope

HF is a clinical syndrome with a variety of signs and symptoms and numerous underlying causes. A majority (60–80%) of patients with symptoms of HF have poor myocardial contractile performance (systolic dysfunction), but in a small subset of patients HF is due solely to improper relaxation during diastole (diastolic dysfunction).[7] The largest proportion of patients with HF have both systolic and diastolic dysfunction. These guidelines address the outcome of patients receiving ACEIs for systolic dysfunction, which is well characterized. The use of ACEIs in patients with diastolic dysfunction may be warranted, but outcome data

supported by large clinical trials are not available. Furthermore, mortality from primary diastolic dysfunction is low, particularly compared with systolic dysfunction.[8] The recommendations provided in these guidelines are for adult patients with systolic dysfunction, generally defined as those with a left ventricular ejection fraction of less than 40%. Heart failure in pediatric patients is not addressed, since little is known about the use of ACEIs and outcomes in that population.

The most common underlying disorder predisposing patients to HF is myocardial ischemia due to coronary artery disease.[9] Idiopathic dilated cardiomyopathy and hypertension (previously the most common cause of HF) are other common disorders of patients enrolled in the clinical trials documenting the benefits of ACEI therapy in HF. Less common underlying diagnoses include valvular disease or dysfunction (rheumatic heart disease, valvular regurgitation, or stenosis), effects of myocardial toxins (alcohol, cocaine), thyrotoxicosis, atrial fibrillation, viral infection, and postpartum cardiomyopathy. The benefits of ACEIs in improving long-term outcomes have been studied primarily in patients with coronary artery disease and idiopathic cardiomyopathy.

Agency for Health Care Policy and Research Clinical Guidelines

In 1994 the federal Agency for Health Care Policy and Research (AHCPR) released a clinical practice guideline for the diagnosis and management of patients with left ventricular systolic dysfunction.[5] The AHCPR guideline covers the use of ACEIs, diuretics, digitalis, and other drug therapies for HF. It also provides recommendations on diagnostic tests, including echocardiograms and cardiac catheterization, cardiac transplantation, and revascularization procedures. This ASHP document is intended to expand upon the section of the AHCPR guideline that covers ACEIs and to provide more detailed information for pharmacists and other health care professionals on the selection, implementation, and monitoring of ACEI therapy in patients with HF.

Pharmacist's Role in ACEI Therapy for HF

Pharmacists, through direct contacts with both the patient and the patient's prescribing physician, can promote the rational use of drugs to achieve optimal patient outcomes. ACEI therapy is underused in patients with HF, despite the growing body of clinical evidence supporting this therapy. The AHCPR Expert Panel estimated that 20–40% of eligible patients are receiving an ACEI.[5] Many patients are not treated with ACEIs because of concerns about adverse effects on blood pressure or renal function, and many others are given ACEIs at dosages below those shown to be beneficial. Moreover, mortality rates for HF are increasing, despite numerous clinical trials showing reduced mortality from HF in patients receiving optimal therapy with ACEIs.[3] For these reasons, it is imperative that the pharmacist be intimately familiar with the indications, contraindications, and dosing guidelines for ACEIs in patients with HF.

Despite the documented benefits of ACEI therapy in HF, some patients will remain intolerant even when every effort is made to safely introduce these agents. This document covers adverse effects of ACEIs, definitions of ACEI intolerance, and the clinical utility of therapeutic alternatives.

Guideline Development and Use

The ASHP Therapeutic Guidelines on Angiotensin-Converting-Enzyme Inhibitors in Patients with Left Ventricular Dysfunction were prepared by the University of Cincinnati under contract to ASHP. The project was coordinated by a pharmacy specialist with expertise in cardiology and critical care, who consulted with a pharmacy specialist in drug information and two board-certified cardiologists on staff at the University of Cincinnati. The project coordinator worked in conjunction with an independent panel of six pharmacy clinical specialists with expertise in cardiology who were appointed by ASHP. Panel members and contractors were required to disclose any possible conflicts of interest prior to their appointment. The guidelines underwent multidisciplinary field review to evaluate their validity, reliability, and utility in clinical practice. The final document was approved by the ASHP Commission on Therapeutics and the ASHP Board of Directors.

The recommendations in this document may not be appropriate for use in all clinical situations. Decisions to follow these recommendations must be based on the professional judgment of the clinician and take into account individual patient circumstances and available resources.

These guidelines reflect current knowledge (at the time of publication) on the effective and appropriate use of ACEIs in HF. Given the dynamic nature of scientific information and technology, periodic review, updating, and revision are to be expected. Contact the ASHP Professional Practice and Scientific Affairs division at 301-657-3000, ext. 1283 to determine the status of this document.

Level of Evidence for Recommendations

To prepare this report, the panel members reviewed clinical trials of ACEIs in HF. A MEDLINE search of the medical literature for the years 1975–1995 identified more than 450 articles on the use of ACEIs in HF. These studies were placed in categories based on the information provided, such as effects on mortality, comparisons with other treatments for HF, drug interactions, and pharmacokinetics. Studies supporting the recommendations in this report were classified according to the following criteria[10,11]:

Level I: Supportive evidence from large, well-conducted randomized, controlled clinical trials

Level II: Supportive evidence from small, well-conducted randomized, controlled clinical trials

Level III: Supportive evidence from well-conducted cohort studies

Level IV: Supportive evidence from well-conducted case–control studies

Level V: Supportive evidence from uncontrolled studies that were not well conducted

Level VI: Conflicting evidence, but tending to favor the recommendation

Level VII: Expert opinion

The same system was used by the AHCPR expert panel to classify the strength of evidence for a variety of therapeutic or diagnostic recommendations. Each recommendation in the ASHP therapeutic guidelines is assigned a category corresponding to the strength of evidence:

Category A: Levels I–III
Category B: Levels IV–VI
Category C: Level VII

A category C recommendation represents a consensus of the panel based on the clinical experience of the individual panel members and a paucity of quality supporting literature. Where opinions were markedly divided, recommendations will indicate that a substantial number of panel members supported an alternative approach.

Effect of ACEI Therapy on Mortality

ACEI therapy has been shown to reduce mortality from either symptomatic or asymptomatic left ventricular dysfunction. The defining criterion for left ventricular dysfunction is an ejection fraction of less than 40% (a normal ejection fraction is at least 50–55%). Although 10 ACEIs have received FDA approval for use in hypertension, only 6 agents bear FDA-approved labeling for HF: captopril, enalapril, fosinopril, lisinopril, quinapril, and ramipril. Captopril, enalapril, lisinopril, and ramipril have been studied for their effects on mortality in heart failure.

The trials documenting a reduction in mortality generally stratify study patients according to their severity of symptoms as outlined by the following classification developed by the New York Heart Association (NYHA):

Class I: Asymptomatic left ventricular dysfunction (no limitations in physical activity)

Class II: Mild left ventricular dysfunction (some limitations in physical activity)

Class III: Moderate left ventricular dysfunction (marked limitation in physical activity)

Class IV: Severe left ventricular dysfunction (HF symptoms at rest)

Mortality trials with ACEIs have enrolled patients with class IV HF (severe symptoms), classes II and III HF (mild to moderate symptoms), and class I HF (asymptomatic). The effect of ACEIs on mortality can be summarized according to the severity of symptoms.

Class IV HF. Only enalapril has been evaluated for effects on mortality in patients with class IV HF. The Cooperative North Scandinavian Enalapril Survival Study (CONSENSUS) evaluated clinical outcomes in 253 patients randomly assigned to enalapril maleate (2.5–40 mg per day) or placebo added to conventional therapy that could include other vasodilators.[12] At an average dosage of 18 mg per day, enalapril therapy resulted in significant reductions in mortality (40% reduction at six months and 31% reduction at one year). Mortality was reduced primarily through slowing the progression of heart failure. Two-year follow-up showed that enalapril had a marked carryover effect on mortality, lasting for an additional 15 months.[13] Thus, this trial supports the use of ACEIs in severe heart failure at dosages documented to achieve significant reductions in mortality. It supports the following recommendation:

Recommendation 1. Patients with severe, symptomatic HF due to systolic dysfunction, and without documented contraindications, should receive targeted dosages of recommended ACEIs to reduce mortality over the ensuing 6–12 months. (Strength of evidence = A) (*See recommendation 9 for recommended ACEIs and the "patient monitoring" section for a discussion of the targeted dosing concept.*)

Class II–III HF. There have been two well-conducted prospective trials evaluating the effects of ACEIs on mortality in patients with NYHA class II or III (mild to moderate) HF. The second Veterans Administration Heart Failure Trial (V-HeFT II) randomly assigned 804 men with NYHA class II–III HF stabilized on digoxin and diuretics to receive either enalapril or the combination of hydralazine and isosorbide dinitrate to compare the relative efficacies of two differing vasodilator strategies.[14] After two years of follow-up, enalapril maleate, at an average daily dosage of 15 mg, resulted in a significantly (28%) greater reduction in mortality than the hydralazine–isosorbide dinitrate combination. Mortality at two years was 18% with enalapril compared with 25% with hydralazine–isosorbide dinitrate. This compares to a two-year mortality of 34% in the placebo group of the first Veterans Administration Heart Failure Trial (V-HeFT I), which recruited patients similar to those in V-HeFT II.[15] Thus, enalapril reduced two-year mortality by approximately 47% compared with placebo.

The other major mortality trial in mild to moderate HF was the Studies of Left Ventricular Dysfunction (SOLVD) treatment trial.[16] Patients with HF symptoms and an ejection fraction of 35% or less were randomly assigned to receive placebo or enalapril maleate at dosages of 2.5 to 10 mg twice daily. Enalapril maleate, given at an average daily dosage of 16.6 mg, resulted in a significant (16%) reduction in mortality at 41 months of follow-up.

The effects of captopril on mortality have been studied in four small trials in patients with mild to severe HF. The captopril dosages ranged from 25 to 300 mg per day. Significant reductions in mortality were observed in three of the four studies, including one retrospective analysis.[17–20] However, the small number of patients and the few events recorded make it difficult to determine the effect of captopril on mortality in patients with symptomatic HF.

In summary, large, well-conducted clinical trials support the use of enalapril to reduce mortality in patients with NYHA class II and III HF. Trials with reduced mortality as an outcome have not been conducted with other agents in this subset of HF patients. The dosage associated with a reduction in mortality is approximately 15–17 mg/day, with a majority of patients receiving 10 mg twice daily. In patients without contraindications to ACEI therapy, enalapril maleate should be tried and, if tolerated, increased to a dosage of 10 mg twice daily.

Recommendation 2. Patients with mild to moderate HF due to left ventricular systolic dysfunction, and in the absence of documented contraindications, should receive a recommended ACEI to reduce mortality over the next three to four years. (Strength of evidence = A)

Class I (Asymptomatic) HF. ACEIs have most recently been evaluated for their ability to delay the onset of HF symptoms in patients at high risk for developing symptomatic left ventricular dysfunction. These patients are usually identified as having a recent myocardial infarction. In this setting, an ACEI is not being used to control symptoms but may be useful in slowing progressive ventricular dilatation, a process called remodeling.[21] During the early phases of a myocardial infarction, prompt medical intervention with an ACEI delays the onset of symptomatic HF, possibly through reduced intramyocardial pressures, improved myocardial perfusion, and neuroendocrine mechanisms, specifically the renin–angiotensin–aldosterone system and the sympathetic nervous system. These effects are translated into clinical benefits of reduced mortality and morbidity from HF.

The Survival and Ventricular Enlargement (SAVE) trial randomized patients with an ejection fraction of 40% or less to captopril or placebo between 3 and 16 days after myocardial infarction.[22] After 3.5 years of follow-up, mortality was 19% lower in the captopril group (targeted dosage of 50 mg three times a day). This translates into one life saved for every 85 patients treated per year. The reduction in mortality was due primarily to a reduction in cardiovascular death, particularly from progressive HF. The size of the effect was not influenced by use of aspirin, a thrombolytic agent, or a β-blocker, suggesting that the reduction in mortality from captopril was additive to traditional medical therapies for myocardial infarction.

In a similar group of patients enrolled in Gruppo Italiano per lo Studio della Sopravvivenza nell'Infarto Miocardico III (GISSI-3), early (within 24 hours) use of oral lisinopril 5–10 mg/day reduced six-week mortality by 11%.[23] Although ejection fraction was not determined at randomization, fewer patients receiving lisinopril than receiving placebo had an ejection fraction of 35% or less at the end of the study.

Enalapril has been evaluated in asymptomatic patients with reduced ejection fractions. The SOLVD prevention trial compared enalapril maleate (mean daily dosage 17 mg) with placebo in patients in NYHA classes I (67%) and II (33%) who had ejection fractions of 35% or less, but not necessarily related to a recent myocardial infarction.[24] The mortality rate for the enalapril group was 8%, not significantly different from the placebo rate. Enalapril was associated with a 29% reduction in the combined endpoints of mortality and the development of HF.

Taken together, these three major trials support the early use of ACEIs to slow the progression of HF in asymptomatic patients at high risk for the development of the disease.

Recommendation 3. Patients with asymptomatic left ventricular systolic dysfunction (ejection fractions of 35–40%), and in the absence of documented contraindications, should receive an ACEI to reduce mortality and slow the rate of progression to symptomatic HF. (Strength of evidence = A)

Effect of ACEI Therapy on Hospitalizations for Heart Failure

The ability of ACEI therapy to reduce the frequency of hospitalizations due to HF has only recently been evaluated. Approximately 35% of all patients diagnosed with HF require at least one hospitalization for exacerbation of symptoms over the ensuing 12 months.[5] Hospitalizations for HF exacerbations are frequently due to progression of the disease, but noncompliance with diet or medications is a major factor as well.

Data from the SOLVD treatment trial indicate that ACEI therapy reduces the number of hospitalizations for exacerbations of HF in patients with mild to moderate HF by approximately 30%.[16,25] Therefore, treating 1000 patients for three years with an ACEI prevents approximately 350 hospitalizations, with a corresponding savings of approximately $4 million to the health care system. This figure does not include potential additional savings in physician's office and emergency room visits. The reduction in hospitalization frequency is greatest after one year of therapy (approximately 40%) and gradually declines to 27% after four years of therapy. The relative risk for first hospitalization for HF was reduced by 36% in the SOLVD prevention trial with enalapril and by 22% in the SAVE trial with captopril. The rate of hospitalizations for HF does not appear to differ between ACEIs and the alternative vasodilator combination of hydralazine and isosorbide dinitrate (see "alternatives and concomitant therapies").[14]

Recommendation 4. Patients with either symptomatic or asymptomatic left ventricular systolic dysfunction, and in the absence of documented contraindications, should receive an ACEI to reduce the number of hospitalizations for HF. (Strength of evidence = A)

Effect of ACEI Therapy on Quality of Life

Patients with HF suffer from a reduced capacity to perform even the simplest daily activities. Physical limitations become more debilitating as the disease progresses, to the point that NYHA class IV patients have symptoms of HF at rest. Improvement in a patient's quality of life is a major benefit of appropriate medical therapy for HF. Improvements in quality of life can be measured as increases in exercise capacity, daily activity, social interactions, or cognitive function; improvement in NYHA functional class; or, more subjectively, a positive change in quality of life as assessed by the patient.

Increased Exercise Capacity. Almost all ACEIs have been evaluated for their ability to increase exercise duration in patients with mild, moderate, and severe HF.[26-31] Exercise capacity has usually been determined by performance on a standardized protocol with a treadmill or a bicycle. Improvements in exercise performance have been observed in 50–100% of patients, with greater improvements seen as therapy continues.[26,27,29] Improvements in exercise capacity appear to be dose related, with the greatest increases seen at higher ACEI dosages. Although increases in life span have been greater with enalapril than with the combination of hydralazine and isosorbide dinitrate, improvements in exercise capacity with the two regimens have been similar.[14]

Reduction in Severity of Symptoms. In trials of ACEIs, reduction in the severity of HF symptoms is indicated by an improvement in NYHA functional class. The symptoms assessed include dyspnea on exertion, orthopnea, peripheral edema, fatigue, and paroxysmal nocturnal dyspnea. When added to a drug regimen of diuretics plus digoxin, ACEI therapy usually improves symptoms enough that the NYHA functional class is reduced by 0.5–1.0. Approximately half of patients with severe HF (Class IV) have shown improvement as reflected by NYHA functional class, while 30–85% of patients with mild to moderate HF have improvements in NYHA functional class.[12,26,27,32–36] Similar results are seen when ACEI therapy is added to monotherapy with a diuretic.[37] However, the reduction in symptoms gained when an ACEI is added to long-term diuretic therapy is no greater than that achieved by the addition of digoxin.[38–40]

Improvements in Quality-of-Life Questionnaires. Quality-of-life questionnaires completed by patients provide subjective information on the severity of their disease and its impact on daily living.[41–46] The questionnaires usually have patients rate their ability to walk, complete errands, work around the house, and participate in recreational activities. Other measurements may include their ability to concentrate, drug side effects, medical costs, need for rest during the day, and feelings of depression. ACEI therapy results in significant improvements in overall quality-of-life scores.[46] However, despite ACEIs having a greater impact on mortality, improvements in these measures of quality of life are similar for enalapril and the combination of hydralazine–isosorbide dinitrate.[45] Differences in quality of life between individual ACEIs are poorly documented, although longer-acting ACEIs may have a better effect on quality of life than ACEIs requiring multiple daily doses, even with similar improvements in NYHA functional class.[47]

Recommendation 5. Patients with symptomatic left ventricular systolic dysfunction, and in the absence of documented contraindications, should receive ACEI therapy to reduce symptoms, improve exercise performance, and enhance overall quality of life. (Strength of evidence = A)

Contraindications to ACEI Therapy

Despite the well-documented benefits of ACEI therapy for patients with HF, certain clinical situations represent either absolute or relative contraindications to ACEI therapy. The clinician should make every effort to include an ACEI in the therapy of every HF patient, because positive patient outcomes (reduced morbidity and mortality) are seen most consistently when the drug regimen includes an ACEI.

Absolute contraindications to ACEI therapy include pregnancy, history of angioedema or other documented hypersensitivity to an ACEI, bilateral renal artery stenosis, and history of well-documented intolerance due to hypotension, decline in renal function, hyperkalemia, or cough. Relative contraindications include hypotension (systolic blood pressure <90 mm Hg), renal dysfunction, hyperkalemia (serum potassium >5.5 meq/L), and cough documented as due to an ACEI.

To ensure appropriate dosing and monitoring so that patients can achieve maximum benefits, the clinician must be intimately familiar with the clinical pharmacology of ACEIs. Only 20–50% of patients with a diagnosis of HF receive an ACEI, primarily because of concerns about hypotension, renal dysfunction, hyperkalemia, and cough.[5,48] Therefore, clinician awareness of the frequency and management of these conditions will allow patients to achieve optimal therapeutic outcomes with ACEIs. Other adverse effects of ACEIs must be considered but are beyond the scope of this document.

Hypotension. Blood pressure should be determined in all patients before the initiation of ACEI therapy for HF. Blood pressure should then be re-evaluated for up to six hours after the first dose of ACEI to monitor for hypotension, which may be symptomatic or asymptomatic. The time during

Table 1.
Dosing of Angiotensin-Converting-Enzyme Inhibitors (ACEIs) in Heart Failure

Drug	Initial Dose[a] (mg)	Targeted Dosage[b,c] (mg)	Maximum Dosage (mg)	Time (hr) to Peak Effect on Blood Pressure
Captopril[d]	6.25–12.5	50 t.i.d.[e]	100 t.i.d.	1–2
Enalapril maleate[d]	2.5–5	10 b.i.d.[e]	20 b.i.d.	4–6
Fosinopril sodium[f]	5–10	20 daily	40 daily	2–6
Lisinopril[f]	2.5–5	10–20 daily[g]	40 daily	4–6
Quinapril hydrochloride[f]	5–10	20 b.i.d.	20 b.i.d.	2–4
Ramipril[d]	1.25–2.5	5 b.i.d.[e]	10 b.i.d.	4–6

[a]Lower initial dose recommended for patients with low serum sodium or elevated serum creatinine concentration, systolic blood pressure below 100 mm Hg, recent aggressive diuretic therapy (hypovolemia), or concurrent therapy with a potassium-sparing diuretic.

[b]When switching from one ACEI to another, the percentage of the targeted dosage achieved may be used (e.g., enalapril maleate 5 mg b.i.d. is 50% of the targeted dosage, and the equivalent fosinopril sodium dosage would be 10 mg daily).

[c]t.i.d. = three times a day; b.i.d. = twice a day.

[d]Has FDA approved-labeling for symptomatic improvement and mortality reduction in heart failure.

[e]Targeted dosage established by clinical trials with reduced mortality as an outcome.

[f]Has FDA approved-labeling for symptomatic improvement in heart failure.

[g]Targeted dosage of 10 mg daily was effective in GISSI-3; however, most clinical data support 20 mg daily.

which to monitor for maximum hypotensive response varies with the individual ACEI. This critical monitoring interval is indicated in Table 1. Blood pressure should be checked at the expected maximum response time; it should also be checked before that time if symptoms occur.

In large-scale, placebo-controlled trials, symptomatic hypotension occurred in as many as 28% of patients but was severe enough for discontinuation of therapy in only 0–10% of patients.[12,13,23,32,34,38,40] In CONSENSUS, patients at risk for hypotension were identified as those with a low serum sodium concentration (<130 meq/L), a recent (within one week) increase in diuretic dosage, concurrent therapy with a potassium-sparing diuretic, or serum creatinine concentration >1.7 mg/dL.[12] Patients with any of these conditions should receive an initial dose of enalapril maleate 2.5 mg or captopril 6.25 mg and be observed during the appropriate time interval (Table 1) for hypotension. Higher initial doses may lead to symptomatic hypotension in a substantial number of patients.[12] Patients at high risk for hypotension may be admitted to the hospital for 24 hours to receive their initial doses of ACEI; however, this strategy was necessary in only 1.2% of patients in the SOLVD treatment trial.[16] Some patients may require a reduction in diuretic dosage or brief discontinuation to better tolerate the initial dose of ACEI.[38,49] In the absence of risk factors for hypotension, an ACEI may be safely initiated at one half the targeted dosage (e.g., for captopril or its equivalent, 25 mg three times a day), although some clinicians prefer to always use small initial dosages even in the absence of risk factors for hypotension.[50] If the initial ACEI dosage is tolerated, the dosage should be increased, at three- to seven-day intervals, toward the targeted dosage. Longer intervals may be indicated if the clinician believes the patient is at increased risk for hypotension or renal dysfunction, or if the clinical situation

requires (for example, coordination with clinic visits). Once the maintenance dosage is reached, the average fall in blood pressure from baseline can be expected to range from 5 to 10 mm Hg systolic and 3 to 6 mm Hg diastolic.[13,16,24,26,34,38]

Reports in the literature do not specify a blood pressure below which an ACEI should not be initiated. Some clinicians recommend that maintenance dosages be reduced by 50% in patients whose systolic blood pressure is below 100 mm Hg and further reduced or discontinued if the systolic blood pressure is below 90 mm Hg.[23] Most clinicians would not administer an ACEI to a patient with HF whose systolic blood pressure was below 90 mm Hg. Conversely, some clinicians would not withhold ACEI therapy if the systolic blood pressure was below 90 mm Hg unless there were signs and symptoms of hypotension or reductions in renal function.

Renal Dysfunction. Another major barrier to the use of an ACEI in a patient with HF is a concern about deterioration of renal function. The adaptive response to reduced cardiac output in HF leads to activation of the renin–angiotensin–aldosterone axis, with significant increases in intrarenal and plasma angiotensin II levels that preserve glomerular filtration rate.[51] Decreases in arterial and intraglomerular pressure as a result of ACEI treatment may reduce renal perfusion. Increases in blood urea nitrogen (BUN) and serum creatinine concentrations are reported to occur in 6–38% of patients and are more likely in those with advanced HF and a baseline serum creatinine >2.0 mg/dL.[12,16,26,52,53] The increase in serum creatinine and BUN is generally small (less than 0.4 mg/dL and 4.0 mg/dL, respectively).[14,16,54]

In most major clinical trials, patients with HF who received placebo had further deterioration in renal function, with increases in BUN and serum creatinine similar to those observed with long-term ACEI therapy.[12,23,24] Most of the increase in serum creatinine due to ACEI therapy is observed in the first six weeks of therapy; concentrations then stabilize with continued treatment.[55,56] As many as 25% of patients may have improvements in renal function with continued therapy.[23,56,57]

In some trials, patients with elevated baseline serum creatinine concentrations were at greater risk for increases in serum creatinine, but this was not observed in other trials.[23,52] Increases in serum creatinine of 30–100% are seen in approximately one fourth of patients, with an additional 11% having increases of 100% or greater.[57] In a vast majority of cases, an increase in sodium intake, with or without a reduction in diuretic dosage, normalizes renal function in less than two weeks with no reduction in ACEI dosage.[47,57] The evidence from most studies indicates that renal function changes are not predicted by baseline renal function; therefore, ACEI therapy should not be ruled out in patients with mild renal insufficiency because of concerns about further decline in renal function.[58] Fewer than 2% of patients require discontinuation of ACEIs because of renal dysfunction.[23,38,56]

Some investigators have reported that the risks of hypotension and renal dysfunction are greater with longer-acting ACEIs. In one randomized, nonblinded clinical trial, treatment with enalapril was associated with greater reductions in creatinine clearance and larger increases in BUN than was captopril treatment, possibly because of prolonged reductions in blood pressure between enalapril doses.[59] However, the dosages of the two ACEIs—enalapril maleate 20 mg twice daily and captopril 50 mg three times daily—may not have been comparable, since the enalapril dosage was larger than those now known to provide improvements in patient outcomes. Notably, other investigators using midrange doses of ACEIs found no major clinical differences in renal function between captopril, enalapril, and lisinopril.[60-63]

Hyperkalemia. The use of ACEIs partially reverses the effects of aldosterone on the distal tubule in the nephron, thereby reducing urinary potassium excretion. The resultant increase in serum potassium concentration is often beneficial and offsets potassium wasting from commonly prescribed loop diuretics, such as furosemide.

Hyperkalemia (serum potassium concentration >5.5 meq/L) developed in approximately 6% of patients in the SOLVD treatment trial receiving recommended dosages of enalapril.[16] However, in large-scale clinical trials, recommended dosages of enalapril maleate (20 mg per day) usually resulted in only mild increases in serum potassium of between 0.1 and 0.2 meq/L.[16,24] In CONSENSUS, all patients who had hyperkalemia were receiving potassium sparing diuretics or potassium supplements.[12] Renal impairment does not appear to increase the risk of ACEI-associated hyperkalemia, but diabetes may.[12,47,52] Comparative clinical trials with various ACEIs have usually shown no difference between agents in the frequency of hyperkalemia; in the one trial that showed a difference in potassium response, the observed difference could be explained by the use of potassium-sparing diuretics.[47]

Clinicians should consider stopping all potassium supplements and potassium-sparing diuretics before initiating therapy with an ACEI. This may not be necessary in some patients whose baseline serum potassium concentration remains low despite treatment with a potassium-sparing diuretic or a potassium supplement. Serum potassium concentration should be determined approximately one week after ACEI therapy is initiated, and the ACEI dosage reduced for those with hyperkalemia. In patients who remain hypokalemic on recommended dosages of an ACEI, small doses of potassium supplements or a potassium-sparing diuretic can be instituted and serum potassium further monitored.

Cough. Cough is the most frequent adverse effect of ACEI therapy and is a major reason for discontinuation of these drugs. Clinicians should understand the occurrence of cough and its management in order to give patients the full benefits of ACEI therapy. Cough due to ACEIs is believed to stem from accumulation of bradykinins, mediated by ACEI blockade of kininase II, which is responsible for breakdown of kinins.[64] Kinins are known to mediate bronchoconstriction, which produces hyperreactive airways and a dry, nonproductive cough.[65] However, cough can be due to pulmonary edema, and discontinuation of ACEIs because of cough is often unnecessary.

The frequency of ACEI-induced cough in patients with HF is difficult to establish because of differences in reporting (e.g., whether cough is reported as a reason for discontinuation of therapy). In three of the largest clinical trials, cough was reported to occur in 34–37% of patients receiving ACEIs, compared with 27–31% of patients receiving placebo.[14,16,24] The high frequency of cough in the placebo groups underscores the fact that in patients with HF, cough can be a manifestation of the disease.

Although it is often described as a nuisance rather than a hazard, cough can affect quality of life by producing sleeplessness or vomiting. However, cough is rarely severe enough to require discontinuation of therapy; only 1% of patients in V-HeFT II, 0.5% in GISSI-3, and 2.4% in the SAVE trial required ACEI discontinuation.[14,22,23] Patients who experience cough should be questioned to determine whether this symptom is due to the ACEI or to pulmonary edema. If cough is likely due to the ACEI, dosage reduction or switching to an alternative ACEI is sometimes helpful. A recent report suggests that cough severity may be lessened with the use of inhaled cromolyn.[66] In most cases the patient (and patient's family) can be advised that if the cough is bothersome but not intolerable the benefits of ACEI therapy outweigh this adverse effect.

Recommendation 6. Absolute contraindications to ACEIs include pregnancy, bilateral renal artery stenosis, angioedema or other allergic responses, and documented persistent intolerance because of hypotension, severe renal dysfunction, hyperkalemia, or cough. (Strength of evidence = B)

Initial Dosage

Patients not at risk for an acute hypotensive response to an ACEI can receive initial dosages of enalapril maleate 5 mg twice a day, captopril 12.5 mg three times a day, lisinopril 5 mg daily, or equivalent dosages of other ACEIs. These dosages were proved to be safe in large clinical trials.[12,14,16,22-24] ACEIs should be initiated at one half the usual initial dosage (2.5 mg for enalapril maleate, 6.25 mg for captopril, and 2.5 mg for lisinopril) in patients with the following risk factors for hypotension, identified in CONSENSUS and other trials[12,67]: serum sodium concentration <130 meq/L, recent increase (within one week) in diuretic therapy (with evidence of volume depletion), serum creatinine concentration >1.7 mg/dL, or concurrent therapy with a potassium-sparing diuretic.

Recommendation 7. Patients who have a serum sodium concentration of <130 meq/L, recent increase in diuretic therapy, or serum creatinine concentration >1.7 mg/dL or are receiving concurrent therapy with a potassium-sparing diuretic should receive initial ACEI therapy at one half the normal starting dosage to minimize the risk for clinically important hypotension. (Strength of evidence = A)

Patient Monitoring

All patients being considered for ACEI therapy should have baseline determinations of serum electrolytes (sodium and potassium), renal function (serum creatinine and BUN), and blood pressure. Their recent use of diuretics should be determined. Once ACEI therapy is selected and initiated, blood pressure should be monitored for peak effect at one to two hours for captopril and four to six hours for enalapril and lisinopril.[47] If hypotension occurs, the patient should be monitored until blood pressure stabilizes and signs and symptoms of hypotension resolve. Once patient tolerance is established, the dosage should be increased at three- to seven-day intervals until targeted dosages are reached. Longer intervals between increases may be indicated either for patient convenience or if the patient is still at risk for hypotension or renal dysfunction. In most clinical trials, ACEIs have been withheld from patients with systolic blood pressures below 90 mm Hg; however, there are few clinical data documenting a specific blood pressure below which an ACEI should absolutely not be given.

Within one week of the start of therapy, determinations of serum potassium and creatinine and BUN should be repeated. If these values are stable, they should be monitored at three-month intervals or within one week of a change in the ACEI or diuretic dosage.

Patients with clinically important declines in renal function (as indicated by elevated BUN or serum creatinine) resulting from ACEI therapy should initially have the dosage of their diuretic reduced by 25%, which often results in normalization of renal function.[47] In some cases, diuretic therapy may need to be discontinued altogether for one or two days before the initiation of ACEI therapy.[68] Once ACEI therapy is stabilized, the need for and dosage of diuretic can be reassessed.

The targeted dosage concept for ACEIs should be used to achieve reductions in hospitalizations and improvements in quality of life (e.g., symptoms), as well as the ultimate goal of prolonged survival. Because ACEI dosages in the major clinical trials were adjusted to achieve a targeted dosage, not to achieve a reduction in symptoms, it is not known whether dosages that result in symptom reduction would also result in prolonged survival. Targeted dosages associated with prolonged survival are 10 mg twice a day for enalapril maleate, 50 mg three times a day for captopril, and 10 mg daily for lisinopril.[12,14,16,22,23] Even if patients do not receive the targeted dosage, their survival may still be prolonged by ACEI therapy; only about 50% of patients in the SOLVD treatment trial received enalapril maleate at 10 mg twice daily, while 10% received 10 mg daily.[16] Similarly, in GISSI-3 less than half the patients (47.5%) received the targeted dosage of lisinopril (10 mg daily).[23] Although prospective, controlled clinical trials showed prolonged survival even without achievement of targeted dosages, a retrospective review showed a greater increase in survival with enalapril maleate at a mean dosage of 17 mg/day than with captopril at a comparatively lower mean daily dosage of 54 mg.[69] The results of other trials indicate that higher ACEI dosages may be necessary to adequately interrupt the neurohormonal systems associated with morbidity and mortality in HF.[70] Therefore, every attempt should be made to increase individual patients' dosages to the recommended (targeted) dosage (Table 1), even though many patients will require dosage reductions to avoid undesirable adverse effects.

Recommendation 8. BUN, serum creatinine and potassium concentrations, and blood pressure should be determined before the initiation of ACEI therapy. These values should be monitored as the ACEI dosage is increased to the level associated with reductions in morbidity and mortality. (Strength of evidence = B)

Recommended ACEIs

The panel strongly believes that an ACEI that has been shown to prolong survival should be recommended over an ACEI that is labeled for symptom reduction in HF but lacks evidence of effect on mortality. The ACEIs that are labeled for use in patients with left ventricular dysfunction and have been shown to prolong survival are enalapril, captopril, and lisinopril.[12,14,16–18,20,22,23] Quinapril and fosinopril are labeled for symptom reduction in HF but lack data on mortality.[71–77] In 2.5 years of follow-up, post-myocardial-infarction patients with heart failure symptoms who received ramipril had a 27% reduction in mortality.[78] The panel thinks that positive patient outcomes can be achieved with certainty and in a cost-beneficial fashion by using an ACEI that has been shown to reduce morbidity and prolong survival at recom-

mended dosages. This is reflected in Table 1.

Recommendation 9. Captopril, enalapril, lisinopril, and ramipril are preferred ACEIs for patients with HF at dosages shown to reduce hospitalizations, reduce symptoms, and prolong survival. (Strength of evidence = A)

Special Populations: The Elderly

As noted previously, the incidence of HF increases with advancing age. As the fastest-growing segment of the U.S. population, the elderly deserve special attention in relation to the risks and benefits of ACEI therapy for HF. No mortality trial has been conducted specifically in an elderly population; however, the average age of patients in CONSENSUS was 71 years.[12] The average age of patients in clinical trials of ACEIs was 60–65 years; however, 27% of patients in GISSI-3 and 15% in the SAVE trial were older than 70.[22,23] Thus, the available data indicate prolonged survival of elderly patients receiving ACEIs.

In up to 40% of cases, the elderly patient with HF symptoms has a normal (>50%) ejection fraction.[79] The prognosis in elderly patients with HF and a normal ejection fraction is much better than for elderly patients with impaired left ventricular function. In one small prospective trial, the four-year survival in elderly patients (mean age >80 years) was 44% in those with normal left ventricular function compared with 15% in those with reduced left ventricular function.[79] Therefore, confirming that the diagnosis of HF is due to systolic dysfunction is an important step in directing therapy to achieve desired clinical benefits.

The elderly have reduced elimination of most ACEIs. Elimination half-life and area under the serum concentration–time curve (AUC) are 15–40% higher in patients 60–80 years old than in younger patients with similar renal function.[80–82] The exception is fosinopril; age is not a factor in reducing elimination of this drug, possibly because of compensatory hepatic elimination.[83]

Despite these modest changes in pharmacokinetics, the use of ACEIs in elderly patients with normal renal function is not associated with an increased frequency of adverse effects.[82,84,85] However, the use of ACEIs in elderly patients with compromised renal function (serum creatinine >1.9 mg/dL) may result in marked deterioration in renal function, which may limit the ability to increase ACEI dosages to effective levels.[51,86] Acute deterioration in renal function may indicate severe renal artery stenosis, which may exist unrecognized in up to 45% of patients with peripheral and coronary artery atherosclerosis.[87,88] Because atherosclerosis increases with advancing age, the elderly may need to have their ACEI dosages stabilized in an institutional setting, with careful monitoring of blood pressure and renal function prior to discharge.

The elderly require special pharmaceutical care to improve compliance and reduce hospital admissions for worsening HF symptoms. The primary reason for hospitalizations in the SOLVD treatment trial was noncompliance with diet and medications.[16] Up to 40% of hospital readmissions for heart failure in elderly patients are potentially preventable through encouragement of dietary and medication compliance, appropriate discharge planning, patient follow-up, assurance of adequate social support, and patient education about the need to seek medical attention.[88]

Recommendation 10. ACEI therapy should be instituted

cautiously in the elderly patient with HF. Because of age-related reductions in renal function, the elderly may be particularly susceptible to ACEI-induced reductions in blood pressure and renal function. The elderly require more careful and prolonged monitoring when ACEI therapy is instituted. (Strength of evidence = B)

Drug Interactions

The ACEIs are relatively free of clinically important drug interactions. Patients may experience postural hypotension when ACEIs are used in combination with other peripheral vasodilators, such as calcium-channel blockers, hydralazine, phenothiazines, and tricyclic antidepressants. In addition, the risk of hyperkalemia with ACEIs is higher when the drugs are used in combination with potassium-sparing diuretics or potassium supplements.

The best-documented drug interaction with ACEIs is their interaction with lithium, which can result in threefold to fourfold increases in serum lithium concentration.[89,91] The mechanism of this interaction is not clear. The increase in lithium concentration may be observed after two to four days of concomitant therapy, and frequent monitoring is recommended so that lithium dosages can be adjusted downward to maintain therapeutic serum levels.

Aspirin and other nonsteroidal anti-inflammatory drugs (NSAIDs) may result in fluid accumulation, decline in renal function, or loss of ACEI-associated improvements in hemodynamics. These counterproductive effects may be due to NSAID inhibition of the prostaglandin component of ACEIs' mechanism of action. Aspirin at a dose of 350 mg has been shown to reduce the hemodynamic response to enalapril; however, the clinical benefit of ACEIs in reducing mortality was maintained in the SAVE trial even in patients receiving aspirin.[22,92] Conversely, a retrospective analysis of SOLVD showed no reduction in mortality in HF patients receiving enalapril and aspirin.[93] The concomitant use of aspirin and an ACEI may also lead to additive declines in renal function; however, only 10% of an elderly population had a decline in creatinine clearance when aspirin was used along with an ACEI at dosages intended for antiplatelet effects.[94] There are no prospective data documenting the clinical importance of an aspirin–ACEI interaction, nor is there information on its likely mechanism. Since most patients with HF have evidence of coronary artery disease, the benefits of aspirin warrant its use in conjunction with an ACEI. An ongoing trial will prospectively examine the relative effects on mortality of aspirin compared with warfarin and placebo.[95]

Recommendation 11. In patients receiving the combination of lithium and an ACEI, serum lithium concentration must be monitored and the lithium dosage decreased if serum lithium concentrations increase. Potassium-sparing diuretics and potassium supplements should be used in combination with ACEIs only in patients with documented hypokalemia during ACEI therapy. In patients with severe HF, the concurrent use of aspirin or other NSAIDs may lead to sodium retention, declines in renal function, and increased signs and symptoms of HF. Caution is advised when using NSAIDs in patients with HF. (Strength of evidence = B)

Concomitant and Alternative Therapies

The initiation of ACEI therapy in relation to other pharmacologic therapy of left ventricular dysfunction is depicted in Figure 1. In patients already receiving diuretic therapy, ACEIs should be considered the next treatment step. Digoxin should clearly be added to the therapeutic regimen of HF patients when there is a second indication for digoxin therapy (e.g., a supraventricular arrhythmia for which digoxin is specifically indicated). In other patients, the point at which digoxin should be added to the therapeutic regimen remains controversial. Compared with digoxin, patients on ACEI therapy show greater improvements in exercise performance and NYHA functional class with fewer adverse clinical events.[38,40,96–98] However, approximately one third of patients experience worsening of HF symptoms when digoxin is withdrawn from existing therapy with diuretics and ACEIs.[99] Recently, the results of a large NIH-sponsored clinical trial of digoxin (Digitalis Investigation Group [DIG] study) were presented and revealed that digoxin had no adverse or beneficial effect on mortality in HF (unpublished data). However, there were significant reductions in hospitalizations for HF. Therefore, most panel members consider it appropriate to use digoxin in the patient still symptomatic after therapy with a diuretic and an ACEI has been optimized. A minority of panel members believe the addition of digoxin to ACEI and diuretic therapy (when volume overload is present) should be considered early in therapy. This contrasts with current recommendations from AHCPR and American Heart Association/American College of Cardiology guidelines (published before the DIG trial) that suggest adding digoxin after optimal or maximal doses of an ACEI are tried.

The only alternative therapy that has been compared with ACEIs for patients with left ventricular dysfunction is the combination of hydralazine and isosorbide dinitrate. V-HeFT I documented that this combination reduces three-year mortality from 47% to 36% in patients primarily with NYHA functional class II–III heart failure.[15] However, enalapril was superior to the combination of hydralazine and isosorbide dinitrate in V-HeFT II, with enalapril reducing mortality by 28% relative to the combination.[14] Several factors favor the use of ACEIs over the combination of hydralazine and isosorbide dinitrate. In addition to the direct effect on mortality, most of the benefit of the combination has been seen in the first 12 months of therapy and thus the benefits of the combination beyond one year are unknown.[100] Second, despite similarities between the combination and an ACEI in improvements in quality of life and reductions in hospitalizations, fewer patients tolerate the combination vasodilator therapy.[14,45,100,101] Greater improvements in dyspnea, tiredness, exercise tolerance, and ejection fraction are seen with ACEIs.[102] Finally, more patients receiving hydralazine plus isosorbide dinitrate than receiving ACEIs die of sudden cardiac death (presumably from ventricular arrhythmias).[14,103] Every attempt should be made to institute ACEI therapy in patients with HF, but hydralazine plus isosorbide dinitrate is a viable alternative for patients with documented intolerance to ACEIs.

In the future, more therapies may become available. Ongoing clinical trials are being conducted with spironolactone, calcium-channel blockers (amlodipine, felodipine), losartan, and β-blockers.[104–109] These studies will undoubtedly lead to specific indications for the use of these drugs in patients with HF. The documented benefits of ACEIs in HF will influence the design of trials of new agents. For ethical reasons, ACEI therapy will likely be included as concomitant therapy for both the placebo and treatment groups. As these new alterna-

Figure 1. Drug therapy for heart failure (HF) due to systolic dysfunction. ACEI = angiotensin-converting-enzyme inhibitor. ISDN = isosorbide dinitrate. A-II = angiotensin II.

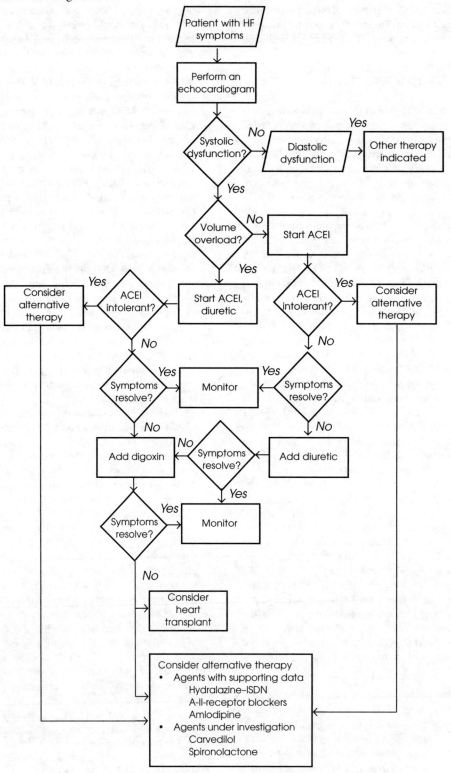

tives become available, they will probably be indicated for use in addition to ACEIs, rather than as replacements.

Recommendation 12. The greatest improvements in patient outcome are achieved with ACEIs. Digoxin may be added to the regimen to further reduce symptoms and hospitalizations. Therapy with alternative vasodilator regimens should be reserved for patients who are still symptomatic after optimal triple-drug therapy (diuretic, ACEI, digoxin) or documented intolerance to ACEIs. (Strength of evidence = A)

Conclusion

ACEIs have become the cornerstone of therapy for HF, but they are often not used or used in insufficient dosages. The clinician caring for patients with documented HF due to systolic dysfunction should be familiar with the recommendations in these guidelines and make every attempt to institute ACEI therapy in patients with HF to alleviate symptoms, reduce hospitalizations, and prolong the patient's life. The role of ACEIs in HF will continue to evolve as newer therapies are fully investigated; however, current practice is to rely on ACEIs for optimizing outcomes in the patient with HF.

References

1. Kannel WB, Cupples A. Epidemiology and risk profile of cardiac failure. *Cardiovasc Drugs Ther.* 1988; 2:387–95.

2. Smith WM. Epidemiology of congestive heart failure. *Am J Cardiol.* 1985; 55:3A–8A.

3. Gillum RF. Epidemiology of heart failure in the United States. *Am Heart J.* 1993; 126:1042–7.

4. Kannel WB, Belanger AJ. Epidemiology of heart failure. *Am Heart J.* 1991; 121:951–7.

5. Konstam MA, Dracup K, Bottorff MD, et al. Evaluation and care of patients with left-ventricular systolic dysfunction. Clinical practice guideline 11. Washington, DC: Agency for Health Care Policy and Research, U.S. Department of Health and Human Services, June 1994. AHCPR Publication No. 94-0612.

6. Detailed diagnoses and procedures national hospital discharge survey, 1989. Hyattsville, MD: National Center for Health Statistics; 1991 Sep:32. DHHS publication no. 91-1769. (Vital and health statistics, series 13, no. 108.)

7. Bonow RO, Udelson JE. Left ventricular dysfunction as a cause of congestive heart failure. *Ann Intern Med.* 1992; 117:502–10.

8. Brutsaert DL, Sys SU, Gillebert TC. Diastolic failure: pathophysiology and therapeutic implications. *J Am Coll Cardiol.* 1993; 22:318–25.

9. Teerlink JR, Goldhaber SZ, Pfeffer MA. An overview of contemporary etiologies of congestive heart failure. *Am Heart J.* 1991; 121:1852–3. Editorial.

10. Chalmers TC, Smith H Jr, Blackburn B, et al. A method for assessing the quality of a randomized control trial. *Controlled Clin Trials.* 1981; 2:31–49.

11. Liberati A, Himel HN, Chalmers TC. A quality assessment of randomized control trials of primary treatment of breast cancer. *J Clin Oncol.* 1986; 4:942–51.

12. CONSENSUS Trial Study Group. Effects of enalapril on mortality in severe congestive heart failure. Results of the Cooperative North Scandinavian Enalapril Survival Study (CONSENSUS). *N Engl J Med.* 1987; 316:1429–35.

13. Kjekshus J, Swedberg K, Snapinn S. Effects of enalapril on long-term mortality in severe congestive heart failure. *Am J Cardiol.* 1992; 69:103–7.

14. Cohn JN, Johnson G, Ziesche S, et al. A comparison of enalapril with hydralazine–isosorbide dinitrate in the treatment of chronic congestive heart failure. *N Engl J Med.* 1991; 325:303–10.

15. Cohn JN, Archibald DG, Ziesche S, et al. Effect of vasodilator therapy on mortality in chronic congestive heart failure: results of a Veterans Administration Cooperative Study. *N Engl J Med.* 1986; 314:1547–52.

16. SOLVD Investigators. Effect of enalapril on survival in patients with reduced left ventricular ejection fractions and congestive heart failure. *N Engl J Med.* 1991; 325:293–302.

17. Newman TJ, Maskin CS, Dennick LG, et al. Effects of captopril on survival in patients with heart failure. *Am J Cardiol.* 1988; 84(suppl 3A):140–4.

18. Kleber FX, Niemoller L, Doering W. Impact of converting enzyme inhibition on progression of chronic heart failure: results of the Munich Mild Heart Failure Trial. *Br Heart J.* 1992; 67:289–96.

19. Fonarow GC, Chelimsky-Fallick C, Stevenson LW, et al. Effect of direct vasodilation with hydralazine versus angiotensin-converting enzyme inhibition with captopril on mortality in advanced heart failure: the HY-C Trial. *J Am Coll Cardiol.* 1992; 19:842–50.

20. Ajayi AA, Osodi OO, Akintomide AO. The influence of captopril on intra-hospital mortality and duration of hospitalization in Nigerians with congestive heart failure. *Int J Cardiol.* 1992; 36:341–3.

21. Rumberger JA. Ventricular dilatation and remodeling after myocardial infarction. *Mayo Clin Proc.* 1994; 69:664–74.

22. Pfeffer MA, Braunwald E, Moye LA, et al. Effect of captopril on mortality and morbidity in patients with left ventricular dysfunction after myocardial infarction: results of the Survival and Ventricular Enlargement Trial. *N Engl J Med.* 1992; 327:669–77.

23. Gruppo Italiano per lo Studio della Sopravvivenza nell'Infarto Miocardico. GISSI-3: effects of lisinopril and transdermal glyceryl trinitrate singly and together on 6-week mortality and ventricular function after acute myocardial infarction. *Lancet.* 1994; 343:1115–22.

24. SOLVD Investigators. Effect of enalapril on mortality and the development of heart failure in asymptomatic patients with reduced left ventricular ejection fractions. *N Engl J Med.* 1992; 327:685–91.

25. Coats AJS. Therapeutic interventions to reduce rates of hospitalization and death in patients with heart failure: new clinical evidence. *Cardiology.* 1992; 81:1–7.

26. Colfer HT, Ribner HS, Gradman A, et al. Effects of once-daily benazepril therapy on exercise tolerance and manifestations of chronic congestive heart failure. *Am J Cardiol.* 1992; 70:354–8.

27. Riegger GAJ. The effects of ACEI inhibitors on exercise capacity in the treatment of congestive heart failure. *J Cardiovasc Pharmacol.* 1990(suppl 2):S41–6.

28. Lewis GR. Comparison of lisinopril versus placebo for congestive heart failure. *Am J Cardiol.* 1989; 63:12D–16D.

29. Boschetti E, Tantucci CL, Cocchieri M, et al. Sympathetic activation on effort in patients with chronic heart failure: long term effects of captopril. *Acta Cardiol.* 1988; 43:569–82.

30. Sharpe DN, Murphy J, Coxon R, et al. Enalapril in patients with chronic heart failure: a placebo-controlled, randomized, double-blind study. *Circulation.* 1984; 70:271–8.

31. Franciesco P, Borghi A, Ruggieri A, et al. Changes in pulmonary hemodynamics predict benefits in exercise capacity after ACE inhibition in patients with mild to moderate congestive heart failure. *Clin Cardiol.* 1993; 16:607–12.

32. Barabino A, Galbariggi G, Pizzorni C, et al. Comparative effects of long-term therapy with captopril and ibopamine in chronic congestive heart failure in old patients. *Cardiology.* 1991; 78:243–56.

33. Kiowski W, Drexler H, Meinertz T, et al. Cilazapril

in congestive heart failure. *Drugs.* 1991; 41(suppl 1):54–61.

34. DiBianco R. A large-scale trial of captopril for mild to moderate heart failure in the primary care setting. *Clin Cardiol.* 1991; 14:676–82.

35. Bach R, Zardini P. Long-acting angiotensin-converting enzyme inhibition: once-daily lisinopril versus twice-daily captopril in mild-to-moderate heart failure. *Am J Cardiol.* 1992; 70:70C–77C.

36. Zannad F, van den Broek SAJ, Bory M. Comparison of treatment with lisinopril versus enalapril for congestive heart failure. *Am J Cardiol.* 1992; 70:78C–83C.

37. Yodfat Y. Functional status in the treatment of heart failure by captopril: a multicentre, controlled, double-blind study in family practice. *Fam Pract.* 1991; 8:409–11.

38. The Captopril-Digoxin Multicenter Research Group. Comparative effects of therapy with captopril and digoxin in patients with mild to moderate heart failure. *JAMA.* 1988; 259:539–44.

39. Kholeif MA, Pringle S, Kesson E, et al. A comparison of the efficacy and safety of ramipril and digoxin added to maintenance diuretic treatment in patients with chronic heart failure. *J Cardiovasc Pharmacol.* 1991; 18(suppl 2):S180–3.

40. Herlitz J and the Lisinopril–Digoxin Study Group. Comparison of lisinopril versus digoxin for congestive heart failure during maintenance diuretic therapy. *Am J Cardiol.* 1992; 70:84C–90C.

41. Bergner M, Bobbitt RA, Carter WB, et al. The Sickness Impact Profile: development and final revision of a health status measure. *Med Care.* 1981; 19:787–805.

42. Hunt SM, McKenna SP, McEwen J. A quantitative approach to perceived health. *J Epidemiol Community Health.* 1980; 34:281–5.

43. Kaplan RM, Bush JW. Health related quality of life measurement for research evaluation and policy analysis. *Health Psychol.* 1982; 1:61–80.

44. Spitzer WO, Dobson AJ, Hall J, et al. Measuring quality of life of cancer patients. *J Chron Dis.* 1981; 34:585–97.

45. Rector TS, Johnson G, Dunkman B, et al. Evaluation by patients with heart failure of the effects of enalapril compared with hydralazine plus isosorbide dinitrate on quality of life: VHeFT II. *Circulation.* 1993; 87(suppl 6):71–7.

46. Rector TS, Cab SH, Cohn JN. Validity of the Minnesota Living with Heart Failure Questionnaire as a measure of therapeutic response to enalapril or placebo. *Am J Cardiol.* 1993; 71:1106–7.

47. Giles T, Katz R, Sullivan JM, et al. Short and long acting angiotensin converting enzyme inhibitors: a randomized trial of lisinopril versus captopril in the treatment of congestive heart failure. *J Am Coll Cardiol.* 1989; 13:1240–7.

48. Ackman ML and the CQI Network Investigators. Practice patterns and outcome in congestive heart failure. Paper presented at Canadian Society of Hospital Pharmacists 26th Annual Professional Practice Conference. Toronto, Ontario; 1995 Feb 5–9.

49. Flapan AD, Davies E, Williams BC, et al. The relationship between diuretic dose, and the haemodynamic response to captopril in patients with cardiac failure. *Eur Heart J.* 1992; 13:971–5.

50. McLay JS, McMurray J, Bridges A, et al. Practical issues when initiating captopril therapy in chronic heart failure: what is the appropriate dose and how long should patients be observed? *Eur Heart J.* 1992; 13:1521–7.

51. Packer M, Lee WH, Kessler PD. Preservation of glomerular filtration rate in human heart failure by activation of the renin-angiotensin system. *Circulation.* 1986; 74:766–74.

52. Schwartz D, Averbuch M, Pines A, et al. Renal toxicity of enalapril in very elderly patients with progressive, severe congestive heart failure. *Chest.* 1991; 100:1558–61.

53. Moyses C, Higgins TJC. Safety of long-term use of lisinopril for congestive heart failure. *Am J Cardiol.* 1992; 70:91C–97C.

54. Desche P, Antony I, Lerebours G, et al. Acceptability of perindopril in mild-to-moderate chronic congestive heart failure. *Am J Cardiol.* 1993; 71:61E–68E.

55. Ljungman S, Kjekshus J, Swedberg K, for the CONSENSUS Trial Group. Renal function in severe congestive heart failure during treatment with enalapril (the Cooperative North Scandinavian Enalapril Survival Study [CONSENSUS] Trial). *Am J Cardiol.* 1992; 70:479–87.

56. Mirvis DM, Insel J, Boland MJ, et al. Chronic therapy for congestive heart failure with benazepril HCl, a new angiotensin converting enzyme inhibitor. *Am J Med Sci.* 1990; 300:354–60.

57. Packer M, Lee WH, Medina N, et al. Functional renal insufficiency during long-term therapy with captopril and enalapril in severe chronic heart failure. *Ann Intern Med.* 1987; 106:346–54.

58. Levine TB. Effect of angiotensin converting enzyme inhibition on renal function in the treatment of heart failure. *Clin Ther.* 1989; 11:495–502.

59. Packer M, Lee WH, Yushak M, et al. Comparison of captopril and enalapril in patients with severe heart failure. *N Engl J Med.* 1986; 315:847–53.

60. Osterziel KJ, Dietz R, Harder K, et al. Comparison of captopril with enalapril in the treatment of heart failure: influence on hemodynamics and measures of renal function. *Cardiovasc Drugs Ther.* 1992; 6:173–80.

61. Osterziel KJ, Karr M, Lemmer B, et al. Effect of captopril and lisinopril on circadian blood pressure rhythm and renal function in mild-to-moderate heart failure. *Am J Cardiol.* 1992; 70:147C–150C.

62. Bach R, Zardini P. Long-acting angiotensin-converting enzyme inhibition: once-daily lisinopril versus twice-daily captopril in mild-to-moderate heart failure. *Am J Cardiol.* 1992; 70:70C–77C.

63. Zannad F, van den Broek SAJ, Bory M. Comparison of treatment with lisinopril versus enalapril for congestive heart failure. *Am J Cardiol.* 1992; 70:78C–83C.

64. Andrejak M, Andrejak M-T. Enalapril, captopril and cough. *Arch Intern Med.* 1988; 148:249–51.

65. Varonier HS, Panzoni R. The effect of inhalations of bradykinin in healthy and atopic (asthmatic) children. *Int Arch Allergy Appl Immunol.* 1968; 34:293–6.

66. Hargreaves MR, Benson MK. Inhaled sodium cromoglycate in angiotensin-converting enzyme inhibitor cough. *Lancet.* 1995; 345:13–6.

67. Packer M, Medina N, Yushak M. Relation between serum sodium concentration and the hemodynamic and clinical response to converting enzyme inhibition with captopril in severe heart failure. *J Am Coll Cardiol.*

1984; 3:1035–43.

68. Cooke HM, De Besse A. Angiotensin converting enzyme inhibitor-induced renal dysfunction: recommendations for prevention. *Int J Clin Pharmacol Ther.* 1994; 32:65–70.

69. Pouler H, Rousseau MF, Oakley C, et al. for the Xamoterol in Severe Heart Failure Study Group. Difference in mortality between patients treated with captopril or enalapril in the Xamoterol in Severe Heart Failure Study. *Am J Cardiol.* 1991; 68:71–4.

70. Pacher R, Globits S, Bergler-Klein J, et al. Clinical and neurohumoral response of patients with severe congestive heart failure treated with two different captopril dosages. *Eur Heart J.* 1993; 14:273–8.

71. Pflugfelder PW, Baird MG, Tonkon MJ, et al. for the Quinapril Heart Failure Trial Investigators. Clinical consequences of angiotensin-converting enzyme inhibitor withdrawal in chronic heart failure: a double-blind, placebo controlled study of quniapril. *J Am Coll Cardiol.* 1993; 22:1557–63.

72. Northridge DB, Dargie HJ. Quinapril in chronic heart failure. *Am J Hypertens.* 1990; 3:283S–287S.

73. Knapp LE, Frank GJ, McLain R, et al. The safety and tolerability of quinapril. *J Cardiovasc Pharmacol.* 1990; 15(suppl 2):S47–55.

74. Townend JN, West JN, Davies MK, et al. Effect of quinapril on blood pressure and heart rate in congestive heart failure. *Am J Cardiol.* 1992; 69:1587–90.

75. Canter D, Frank GJ, Knapp LE, et al. The safety profile of quinapril: is there a difference among ACE inhibitors? *Clin Cardiol.* 1990; 13(suppl 7):39–42.

76. Northridge DB, Rose E, Raftery ED, et al. A multicentre, double-blind, placebo-controlled trial of quinapril in mild, chronic heart failure. *Eur Heart J.* 1993; 14:403–9.

77. Brown EJ, Chew PH, MacLean A, et al. Effects of fosinopril on exercise tolerance and clinical deterioration in patients with chronic congestive heart failure not taking digitalis. *Am J Cardiol.* 1995; 75:596–600.

78. The Acute Infarction Ramipril Efficacy (AIRE) Study Investigators. Effect of ramipril on mortality and morbidity of survivors of acute myocardial infarction with clinical evidence of heart failure. *Lancet.* 1993; 342:821–8.

79. Aranow WS, Ahn C, Kronzon I. Prognosis of congestive heart failure in elderly patients with normal versus abnormal left ventricular systolic function associated with coronary artery disease. *Am J Cardiol.* 1990; 66:1257–9.

80. Creasey WA, Funke PT, McKinstry DN, et al. Pharmacokinetics of captopril in elderly healthy male subjects. *J Clin Pharmacol.* 1986; 26:264–8.

81. Kaiser G, Ackermann R, Dieterle W, et al. Pharmacokinetics and pharmacodynamics of the ace inhibitor benazepril hydrochloride in the elderly. *Eur J Clin Pharmacol.* 1990; 38:379–85.

82. Posvar EL, Sedman AJ. ACE inhibitors in the elderly. *Angiology.* 1991; 42:387–96.

83. Levinson B, Sugerman AA, Couchman T, et al. Advanced age per se has no influence on the kinetics of the active diacid of fosenopril. *J Clin Pharmacol.* 1986; 26:541. Abstract.

84. Giles TD. Clinical experience with lisinopril in congestive heart failure: focus on the older patient. *Drugs.* 1990; 38(suppl 2):17–22.

85. Gomez HJ, Smith SG, Moncloa F. Efficacy and safety of lisinopril in older patients with essential hypertension. *Am J Med.* 1988; 85(suppl 3B):35–7.

86. O'Neill CJA, Bowes SG, Sullens CM, et al. Evaluation of the safety of enalapril in the treatment of heart failure in the very old. *Eur J Clin Pharmacol.* 1988; 35:143–50.

87. Missouris CG, Buckenham T, Cappuccio F, et al. Renal artery stenosis: a common and important problem in patients with peripheral vascular disease. *Am J Med.* 1994; 96:10–4.

88. Vinson JM, Rich MW, Sperry JC, et al. Early readmission of elderly patients with congestive heart failure. *J Am Geriatr Soc.* 1990; 38:1290–5.

89. Navis GJ, de Jong PE, de Zeeuw D. Volume homeostasis, angiotensin converting enzyme inhibition, and lithium therapy. *Am J Med.* 1989; 86:621.

90. Baldwin CM, Safferman AZ. A case of lisinopril-induced lithium toxicity. *DICP Ann Pharmacother.* 1990; 24:946.

91. Douste-Blazey PH, Rostin M, Livarek B, et al. Angiotensin converting enzyme inhibitors and lithium treatment. *Lancet.* 1986; 1:1448. Letter.

92. Hall D, Zeitler H, Rudolph W. Counteraction of the vasodilator effects of enalapril by aspirin in severe heart failure. *J Am Coll Cardiol.* 1992; 20:1549–55.

93. Pitt B. Use of converting enzyme inhibitors in patients with asymptomatic left ventricular dysfunction. *J Am Coll Cardiol.* 1993; 22(suppl A):158A–161A.

94. Schwartz D, Kornowski R, Lehrman H, et al. Combined effect of captopril and aspirin in renal hemodynamics in elderly patients with congestive heart failure. *Clin Pharmacol.* 1992; 81:334–9.

95. Cleland JGF, Bulpitt CJ, Falk RH, et al. Is aspirin safe for patients with heart failure? *Lancet.* 1995; 346:215–9.

96. Beaune J and the Enalapril vs. Digoxin French Multicenter Study Group. Comparison of lisinopril versus digoxin for congestive heart failure during maintenance diuretic therapy. *Am J Cardiol.* 1989; 63:22D–25D.

97. Davies RF, Beanlands DS, Nadeau C, et al. Enalapril versus digoxin in patients with congestive heart failure: a multicenter study. *J Am Coll Cardiol.* 1991; 18:1602–9.

98. Kromer EP, Elsner D, Riegger GAJ. Digoxin, converting-enzyme inhibition (quinapril), and the combination in patients with congestive heart failure functional class II and sinus rhythm. *J Cardiovasc Pharmacol.* 1990; 16:9–14.

99. Packer M, Gheorghiade M, Young JB, et al. Withdrawal of digoxin from patients with chronic heart failure treated with angiotensin-converting-enzyme inhibitors. *N Engl J Med.* 1993; 329:1–7.

100. Kulick DL, Rahimtoola SH. Vasodilators have not been shown to be of value in all patients with chronic congestive heart failure due to left ventricular systolic dysfunction. *Am J Cardiol.* 1990; 66:435–8.

101. Loeb HS, Johnson G, Henrick A, et al. Effect of enalapril, hydralazine plus isosorbide dinitrate, and prazosin on hospitalization in patients with chronic congestive heart failure. *Circulation.* 1993; 87(suppl 6):78–87.

102. Schofield PM, Brooks NH, Lawrence GP, et al. Which vasodilator drug in patients with chronic heart failure? A randomised comparison of captopril and hydralazine.

Br J Clin Pharmacol. 1991; 31:25–32.

103. Fonarow GC, Chelimsky-Fallick C, Stevenson LW, et al. Effect of direct vasodilation with hydralazine versus angiotensin-converting enzyme inhibition with captopril on mortality in advanced heart failure: the Hy-C Trial. *J Am Coll Cardiol.* 1992; 19:842–50.

104. Van Vliet AA, Donker AJM, Nauta JJP, et al. Spironolactone in congestive heart failure refractory to high-dose loop diuretic and low-dose angiotensin-converting enzyme inhibitor. *Am J Cardiol.* 1993; 71:21A–28A.

105. Dahlstrom U, Karlsson E. Captopril and spironolactone therapy for refractory congestive heart failure. *Am J Cardiol.* 1993; 71:29A–33A.

106. Dunselman PHJM, van der Mark TW, Kuntze CEE, et al. Different results in cardiopulmonary exercise tests after long-term treatment with felodipine and enalapril in patients with congestive heart failure due to ischaemic heart disease. *Eur Heart J.* 1990; 11:200–6.

107. Packer M, O'Connor CM, Ghali JK, et al. for the Prospective Randomized Amlodipine Survival Evaluation Study Group. Effect of amlodipine on morbidity and mortality in severe chronic heart failure. *N Engl J Med.* 1996; 335:1107–14.

108. Crozier I, Ikram H, Awan N, et al. Losartan in heart failure: hemodynamic effects and tolerability. *Circulation.* 1995; 91:691–7.

109. Olsen SL, Gilbert EM, Renlund DG, et al. Carvedilol improves left ventricular function and symptoms in chronic heart failure: a double-blind randomized study. *J Am Coll Cardiol.* 1995; 25:1225–31.

This official ASHP practice standard was developed through the ASHP Commission on Therapeutics and approved by the ASHP Board of Directors on November 16, 1996.

Members of the 1996–1997 ASHP Commission on Therapeutics are Bruce Weiner, M.S., FASHP, Chair; Donna M. Kraus, Pharm.D., Vice Chair; Marianne Billeter, Pharm.D.; G. Dennis Clifton, Pharm.D.; Mathew A. Fuller, Pharm.D.; William C. Gong, Pharm.D., FASHP; Mary Beth Gross, Pharm.D.; Austin J. Lee, Pharm.D., FASHP; Christine A. Sorkness, Pharm.D.; Mary Ann Halloran, Student Member; Bruce E. Scott, M.S., FASHP, Board Liaison; and Leslie Dotson Jaggers, Pharm.D., Secretary.

The bibliographic citation for this document is as follows: American Society of Health-System Pharmacists. ASHP Therapeutic Guidelines on Angiotensin-Converting-Enzyme Inhibitors in Patients with Left Ventricular Dysfunction. *Am J Health-Syst Pharm.* 1997; 54:299–313.

ASHP Therapeutic Guidelines on Antimicrobial Prophylaxis in Surgery

The generally accepted principles of antimicrobial prophylaxis in surgery involve five considerations:

1. Surgical procedures for which prophylactic antimicrobials have been beneficial.
2. Timing of antimicrobial administration.
3. Duration of antimicrobial regimen.
4. Route of antimicrobial administration.
5. Selection of a particular antimicrobial agent.

Surgical Procedures

Antimicrobial prophylaxis is likely to be beneficial in surgical procedures associated with a high rate of infection (clean-contaminated or contaminated operations) and in any procedure where postoperative infection, however unlikely, may be severe or fatal. Antimicrobial prophylaxis is justified for surgical procedures that enter the gastrointestinal tract (colorectal operations and high risk gastroduodenal and biliary tract operations) and pose the risk of bacterial contamination, as well as in head and neck operations. The value of antimicrobial prophylaxis for abdominal hysterectomies and neurosurgical procedures is controversial.

Since most clean operations have a low rate of postoperative infection, the prophylactic use of antimicrobials is usually not justified. However, recent data on procedures that entail placement of prosthetic materials (e.g., cardiopulmonary bypass, vascular procedures, total hip replacement, and hip fracture repair), in which the few infections that do occur can be quite serious, justify the prophylactic use of antimicrobials. A recently published study suggests that prophylactic antibiotics may be beneficial in other clean procedures, although this suggestion is controversial.[1] For some clean procedures (aortic resections, total hip replacements, and hip fracture repairs), the value of prophylactic antimicrobials has been demonstrated by placebo-controlled trials.

Antimicrobial prophylaxis may be justified for any procedure if the patient is immunocompromised (e.g., malnourished, neutropenic, or receiving immunosuppressive agents).

Timing of Antimicrobial Administration

The timing of antimicrobial administration is important; antimicrobials given at inappropriate times can be ineffective for surgical prophylaxis. To be most effective in preventing postoperative infection, an antimicrobial must be present in the potentially contaminated tissues before bacteria enter the site (i.e., before the surgical incision) and must persist in tissues throughout the period of potential contamination. When antimicrobials are given after bacterial contamination, their ability to prevent infection is substantially reduced.

Ideally, antimicrobials should be given immediately after the patient arrives in the operating room. During cesarean section, however, antimicrobial prophylaxis is administered after cross-clamping of the umbilical cord. Administering prophylaxis at this time is effective, and it

minimizes neonatal exposure to antimicrobials. When antimicrobials are administered "on call" to the operating room, the time between administration and the start of the operation may be prolonged. This practice is not recommended.

If short-acting agents are used, they should be readministered if the operation extends beyond 3–4 hours. If an operation is expected to last more than 6–8 hours, it would be reasonable to administer an agent with a longer half-life and duration of action.

Duration of Antimicrobial Prophylaxis

The shortest duration of antimicrobial administration that is effective in preventing postoperative infection is not known; however, recent studies document that postoperative antimicrobial administration is not necessary for many operations.

Route of Antimicrobial Administration

Antimicrobials used for surgical prophylaxis may be administered intravenously, intramuscularly, orally, rectally, and topically (into the surgical wound). The preferred route of administration varies among surgeons; intravenous and intramuscular routes are used most often. Oral antimicrobials are often used for gut decontamination in elective colorectal operations.

For most elective operations, intramuscular and intravenous administration should be equivalent in terms of antimicrobial delivery to wound tissues. The antimicrobial agent should be given intravenously if the patient has an intravenous catheter in place. It is reasonable to wait to administer the agent until an intravenous line is placed in the operating room.

In situations where general anesthesia will interrupt bowel function or where nasogastric tubes may be placed, the absorption of orally administered antimicrobials may be unreliable. Orally administered antimicrobial agents are therefore not generally recommended for surgical prophylaxis.

Selection of Antimicrobial Agents

There is little evidence to suggest that the newer antimicrobials, with broader in vitro antibacterial spectra, result in lower rates of postoperative wound infection than older drugs whose spectra are narrower. The agent chosen should have antibacterial activity against the most common surgical wound pathogens. In clean operations, gram-positive cocci predominate. For clean-contaminated operations, the agent of choice should be effective against common pathogens found in the gastrointestinal or genitourinary tracts. For most operations, a first-generation cephalosporin such as cefazolin should be the agent of choice.

Specific recommendations for the selection of prophylactic antimicrobials for various surgical procedures are provided in Table 1. Recommendations for pediatric patients have been included where appropriate; however, these recommendations are based on data derived primarily from adult patients and from clinical experience. Few data exist on the use of antimicrobial prophylaxis for surgery in the pediatric population.

Cefazolin is most often recommended because of its relatively low cost and long duration of action and because it has activity against most pathogens commonly associated with clean and clean-contaminated operations. For clean operations where staphylococci are common pathogens, penicillinase-resistant penicillins (oxacillin and nafcillin) may be suitable alternatives. Vancomycin may sometimes be required in patients allergic to penicillins or cephalosporins or in cases involving a high number of methicillin-resistant staphylococci.

Numerous trials conducted in the 1970s and 1980s revealed no substantial differences in microbiological activity among the first-generation cephalosporins. In fact, the cephalothin disk has long served as the class disk for in vitro testing of all first-generation cephalosporins; individual agents have generally not been tested. Most clinical microbiological laboratories assumed that susceptibility or resistance to cephalothin extended to all drugs in its class.

During the past several years, however, two important findings have emerged that might affect the selection of cefazolin as the prophylactic agent in clean surgical procedures. First, several investigators demonstrated that there are marked differences in the rate and extent of hydrolysis when various cephalosporin antimicrobials are exposed to various staphylococcal β-lactamases.[2] Further, some strains of staphylococci produce β-lactamases capable of rapidly hydrolyzing cefazolin.[2]

In several studies, cefazolin was found to be less effective than cefamandole or cefuroxime in preventing deep wound infection in patients who had undergone heart surgery.[3] Although the data are conflicting, microbiologic and clinical studies such as these have called into question the prominence of cefazolin as the first-generation cephalosporin of choice. New studies may be needed to reevaluate the use of agents such as cephalothin, cefamandole, and cefuroxime, which are more resistant to β-lactamase.

A second factor influencing the selection of cefazolin is the recognition that methicillin- and oxacillin-resistant *Staphylococcus aureus* (MRSA) and methicillin-resistant, coagulase-negative staphylococci are resistant to all cephalosporins. These organisms are commonly associated with infection following cardiothoracic, orthopedic, vascular, and cerebrospinal fluid shunting procedures. This new finding may influence drug selection in hospitals where the incidence of such isolates is high.

Although prophylactic antimicrobials play an important part in reducing the incidence of postoperative wound infection, it is important to recognize that various other factors, such as the surgeon's experience, the length of the procedure, the hospital and operating-room environments, and the underlying medical condition of the patient, also have a strong impact on wound infection rates. These variables should be considered in evaluations of infection control problems.

At the present time, cefazolin remains the preferred first-generation cephalosporin for surgical prophylaxis. Recent data notwithstanding, the demonstrated cost-effectiveness of cefazolin must be weighed against the increased cost and broader spectrum of newer antimicrobials. The use of other first-generation cephalosporins such as cephalothin and cephradine, which, although they have a shorter duration of action, are more resistant to staphylococcal β-lactamases, should be evaluated.

Head and Neck Surgery

Elective surgical procedures of the head and neck can be categorized according to their risk of postoperative infection as either clean or clean-contaminated procedures. Clean procedures include parotidectomy, thyroidectomy, and submandibular-gland excision. Clean-contaminated procedures include all those involving an incision through the oral or pharyngeal mucosa. They vary from a tonsillectomy to complicated tumor-debulking procedures requiring massive reconstruction. Patient-specific criteria that might influence postoperative wound infection rates include age, nutritional status, and the presence of concomitant medical conditions such as diabetes mellitus. If the patient has cancer, the stage of the malignancy before operation and preoperative radiation therapy must also be assessed.[4-6]

The normal flora of the mouth and oropharynx are responsible for most infections that follow head and neck procedures. The predominant oropharyngeal organisms include various streptococci (including aerobic and anaerobic species), *Staph. aureus*, peptococcus, peptostreptococcus, and numerous anaerobic gram-negative bacteria including *Bacteroides* species, *Neisseria*, and *Veillonella*. Nasal flora include staphylococci, *Streptococcus pyogenes*, *Strep. pneumoniae*, *Branhamella*, and *Haemophilus* species.

Anaerobic bacteria are approximately 10 times more prevalent than aerobic bacteria in the oropharynx. As a result, bacteria isolated from patients with postoperative wound infections are primarily polymicrobial. Both aerobic and anaerobic bacteria are routinely cultured from infected wounds in more than 90% of cases.[7-10]

Johnson et al.[11] recently reviewed the need for gram-negative bacterial coverage in antimicrobial prophylaxis for clean-contaminated head and neck surgery. They concluded that clindamycin alone appears to be successful as a prophylactic agent and that broad-spectrum antimicrobials such as cefoxitin, while widely used for prophylaxis in this type of surgery, may be unnecessary. Since clindamycin does not offer any activity against aerobic gram-negative bacteria, the authors concluded that these bacteria are probably colonizers rather than pathogens in most patients.

The predominance of anaerobic bacteria in head and neck infections may explain why high dose cefazolin (2 g) has been shown to be effective whereas a 500-mg dose was not effective.[a] Cefazolin is known to inhibit many anaerobic bacteria at serum and tissue levels achieved with a 2-g dose.[12]

Clinical Trials. Systemic prophylactic antimicrobials have not proved effective in reducing wound infection rates among patients undergoing clean procedures of the head and neck. Johnson and Wagner[13] reviewed the records of 438 patients undergoing such procedures. Eighty percent of these patients had not received prophylactic antimicrobials, and the associated wound infection rate was 0.7%. The 20% of patients receiving antimicrobials had a similar rate of wound infection.

Patients undergoing clean-contaminated procedures of the head and neck or who received a placebo in double-blind clinical trials had wound infection rates between 24 and 87%. Patients in such studies who received antimicrobials had a dramatically lower incidence of postoperative wound infection. Brand et al.[14] enrolled 83 patients in a clinical trial; the treatment groups were as follows: cefazolin 500 mg every 8 hours for 1 day; cefazolin 500 mg every 8 hours for 5 days; gentamicin 1.7 mg/kg plus clindamycin 300

Table 1.
Recommendations for Antimicrobial Surgical Prophylaxis[a]

Type of Surgery	Recommended Antimicrobial Regimen	Comments
Head and neck procedures (clean-contaminated)	Cefazolin 2 g i.v. at induction of anesthesia and repeated twice at 8-hr intervals or clindamycin 600 mg plus gentamicin 1.7 mg/kg given i.v. at induction of anesthesia and repeated twice at 8-hr intervals	Clindamycin alone appears to be effective, but more data are needed
Gastrointestinal procedures		
Cholecystectomy	Cefazolin 1 g i.v. at induction of anesthesia	Broad-spectrum agents and multiple doses have not been found to be more effective than narrow-spectrum agents administered in a single dose
Gastroduodenal	Cefazolin 1 g i.v. at induction of anesthesia	Indicated only for procedures entering stomach
Colonic	Oral neomycin sulfate 1 g plus erythromycin base 1 g (after mechanical bowel preparation is completed) at 1300, 1400, and 2300 on day before surgery If oral route is contraindicated: cefoxitin, cefotetan, cefmeta-zole, cefotaxime, or ceftizoxime 2 g i.v. at induction of anesthesia	Mechanical bowel preparation with polyethylene, glycol-electrolyte lavage solution should always be performed for nonobstructed patients undergoing elective operations Cefoxitin should be repeated if procedure exceeds three hours
Rectal or colostomy closure	Combination of oral and injectable antimicrobials	
Appendectomy	Uncomplicated: cefoxitin, cefotetan, cefmetazole, cefotaxime, or ceftizoxime 1-2 g i.v. at induction of anesthesia Complicated: continue antimicro-bial for 3-5 days	
Obstetric/gynecologic procedures		
Cesarean section	Cefazolin 2 g i.v. as a single dose immediately after clamping of umbilical cord	Although controversial, recent data support prophylaxis in low-risk patients
Vaginal hysterectomy	Cefazolin 1 g i.v. at induction of anesthesia	Optional: 1-2 additional doses at 8-hr intervals
Abdominal hysterectomy	Cefazolin 1 g or cefotetan 1 g i.v. at induction of anesthesia	Probably most beneficial in risk patients
Neurosurgical procedures		
Elective craniotomy or laminectomy	Cefazolin or oxacillin or nafcillin 15 mg/kg up to 1 g i.v. at induction of anesthesia	Vancomycin 1 g i.v. should be substituted in hospitals with >10% prevalence of MRSA
CSF shunting	None	If prophylaxis is used, vancomycin 1 g i.v. at induction of anesthesia may be beneficial
Cardiothoracic procedures	Cefazolin 15 mg/kg (up to 1 g) q 8 hr or cefuroxime 50 mg/kg (up to 1.5 g) q 12 hr for 48-72 hr or until chest and mediastinal drainage tubes are removed	Cefamandole and cephalothin are effective alternatives
Orthopedic procedures		
Joint replacement	Cefazolin 15 mg/kg (up to 1 g) i.v. at induction of anesthesia and repeated twice at 8-hr intervals	Vancomycin is a suitable alternative
Hip-fracture repair	Cefazolin 1 g i.v. at induction of anesthesia and repeated q 8 hr for 48-72 hr	Vancomycin is a suitable alternative
Other clean orthopedic procedures	None	
Vascular procedures	Cefazolin 15 mg/kg (up to 1 g) i.v. at induction of anesthesia and repeated twice at 8-hr intervals	Vancomycin is a suitable alternative
Urologic procedures	Cefazolin 15 mg/kg (up to 1 g) i.v. at induction of anesthesia, trimethoprim 160 mg with sulfamethoxazole 800 mg p.o. 1-2 hr before surgery, or cephalexin or cephradine 500 mg p.o. 1-2 hr before surgery	Prophylaxis should be given to high-risk patients only (i.e., those with prolonged catheterization) or in hospitals where infection rates exceed 20%

[a]MRSA = methicillin-resistant *Staph. aureus*, CSF = cerebrospinal fluid.

mg every 8 hours for 1 day; and gentamicin plus clindamycin every 8 hours for 5 days. The wound infection rate in the combined cefazolin groups was 27%, while that of the gentamicin–clindamycin combined group was 7%. Because the numbers of patients were small, no statistical analysis was performed.

Mandell-Brown et al.[15] performed a double-blind trial with 101 patients who were divided into the following groups: placebo every 8 hours for four doses; cefazolin 500 mg every 8 hours for four doses; cefotaxime 2 g every 8 hours for four doses; and cefoperazone 2 g every 8 hours for four doses. Infection rates were 78% in the placebo group, 33% in the cefazolin group, 10% in the cefotaxime group, and 9% in the cefoperazone group. The difference between all antimicrobial groups and the placebo group was statistically significant. The hospital stay of infected patients was twice as long as that of noninfected patients.

Johnson et al.[16] performed a similar trial with cefotaxime and cefoperazone and attained similar results. Other studies have produced similar results.[7–28]

Two additional trials deserve mention. In a randomized trial, Johnson et al.[17] compared cefazolin 2 g (as opposed to previous studies using 500 mg) with moxalactam 2 g. Each drug was given 1 hour before surgery and three more times, for a total of four doses. Infection rates were 8.5% in the cefazolin group and 3.4% in the moxalactam group. The difference did not reach statistical significance. Because of this study, the *Medical Letter on Drugs and Therapeutics* continues to recommend a 2-g dose of cefazolin for clean-contaminated head and neck surgery.[18]

Gerard et al.[19] randomly assigned 113 patients to receive either amikacin plus clindamycin or ticarcillin–clavulanic acid. Infection rates were 10% in the amikacin–clindamycin group and 36% in the ticarcillin–clavulanic acid group. This difference was significant. Examination of the bacteria isolated from the ticarcillin–clavulanic acid group revealed a high prevalence of gram-negative and gram-positive anaerobic bacteria responsible for the wound infections. These results are difficult to reconcile, given the nearly complete in vitro coverage reported for ticarcillin–clavulanic acid against anaerobic bacteria.

Recommendations. *Clean head and neck surgical procedures.* Infection rates are generally less than 2%. Antimicrobial prophylaxis is not justified.

Clean-contaminated head and neck surgical procedures. Systemic antimicrobial prophylaxis is mandatory. Wound infection rates are extraordinarily high (24–87%) when antimicrobials are not used. Rates below 10% may be expected when appropriate antimicrobial prophylaxis is given. Several regimens have been demonstrated to be effective in clinical trials. All agents should be given in regimens of one to four doses. In no case should prophylaxis exceed 24 hours. Single-dose regimens might be preferable, particularly when cost and the possibility of resistance are considered; however, this approach remains controversial.[4]

Based on the marginal performance of ticarcillin–clavulanic acid in one clinical trial, the β-lactamase inhibitor combinations cannot be recommended at this time. The preferred regimens are clindamycin 600 mg (15 mg/kg for children) plus gentamicin 1.7 mg/kg given every 8 hours for 24 hours or cefazolin 2 g (20 mg/kg for children) every 8 hours for 24 hours.

Biliary Tract Surgery

Operations involving the biliary tract are among the most commonly performed abdominal procedures. They include cholecystectomies, explorations of the common bile duct, and choledochoenterostomies (e.g., choledochoduodenostomy). Endoscopic sphincterotomy and liver transplantation, although related, will not be considered here.

The postoperative wound infection rates after biliary tract operations have been reported to be between 7 and 20%.[29–35] The incidence of postoperative wound infections is related to the microbial status of the biliary tract at the time of operation. In the majority of patients, the biliary tract is sterile; the risk of infection is no higher than that of other clean operations (i.e., less than 5%). If bacteria colonize the biliary tract, the rate of infection may reach as high as 36%.[36] Appropriate use of antimicrobial prophylaxis in this setting therefore requires identification of patients likely to have bactibilia. High risk groups include patients over 70 years of age and those with obstructed biliary tracts, acute cholecystitis, or common-bile-duct stones without jaundice.[37,38] Some studies have shown that patients 60 years of age and above are at increased risk of infection.[39,40] Moreover, some patients with bactibilia do not fit into any of the categories described above.

The organisms most likely to be associated with wound infection after biliary tract surgery have been well characterized[33,36,39–46] and include *Escherichia coli*, *Klebsiella*, and enterococci. Other gram-negative bacilli, streptococci, and staphylococci are occasionally isolated. Anaerobes are infrequently isolated from the biliary tract; species of clostridia are most common. Bacteria that are isolated from bile during surgery are those most likely to be associated with subsequent wound infections.

Clinical Trials. Controlled clinical trials of the use of preoperative antimicrobials for prevention of infection following biliary tract operations have sought to answer three key questions:

1. Do antimicrobials prevent wound infections with biliary tract operations?
2. Are certain agents more effective than others?
3. What is the minimum duration of antimicrobial exposure necessary to prevent postoperative infection?

A recently published review and meta-analysis of 42 studies published between 1965 and 1988 demonstrated that patients who receive prophylactic antimicrobials for biliary tract surgery are less likely to develop infection than those who do not.[47] More than 4000 patients (both high and low risk) were included in this analysis. The overall incidence of postoperative infection was 15% in patients receiving no treatment and 9% less in those receiving antimicrobials (95% confidence interval, 7–11% reduction). Results for the control group were more favorable than those for the treatment group in only four of the 42 studies. A wide variety of antimicrobials, primarily cephalosporins, were used in these trials. The effectiveness of antimicrobial prophylaxis was demonstrated in both low and high risk patients.

Most recent antimicrobial prophylaxis trials involving biliary tract operations have focused on the relative effectiveness of different antimicrobials, usually cephalosporins. Significant differences among agents have been demonstrated in only two of 16 comparative studies. Meta-analysis of these comparative trials has demonstrated no significant differences between first-, second-, and third-generation cephalosporins.[47] When first-generation cephalosporins were compared with second- or third-generation cephalosporins,[45,48–52] only one trial demonstrated a significant difference between regimens.[52] In that study, the wound infection rate was 0% with cefotetan and 14% with cefazolin.

Second-generation cephalosporins have also been compared with second- or third-generation agents.[39,40,53–57] In the latter group, only one trial reported a significant difference.[57] These investigators studied more than 1400 patients and found wound infection rates of 3.3% with cefotaxime and 7.6% with cefoxitin. Other trials reported no significant differences between ampicillin and cefamandole,[44] cefonicid and mezlocillin,[58] and ceftriaxone and ciprofloxacin.[41]

The third major issue addressed by the clinical studies was the minimum duration of antimicrobial administration for prevention of postoperative wound infection. A number of different antimicrobials have been studied, including cefazolin,[33,58] cefonicid,[54,55,59] ceftriaxone,[48] cefotetan,[56] and cefotaxime.[57] Most of these studies compared a single preoperative antimicrobial dose with longer regimens. In all studies, the single-dose regimen was as effective as the multiple-dose regimen. Other trials have compared various single-dose regimens,[45,49,53] additionally demonstrating the effectiveness of single-dose cefotetan, cefazolin,[49] cefuroxime,[53] and moxalactam.[45]

Recommendations. The studies described above support the use of antimicrobial prophylaxis in all patients undergoing cholecystectomy. Although only patients with bactibilia are believed to be at increased risk of infection, it is difficult to identify these patients preoperatively, since they often do not fall into one of the recognized high risk categories.

The recommended regimen is a single 1-g dose of cefazolin, given intravenously within 30 minutes of the start of the operation. Clinical trial data demonstrate that first-generation cephalosporins are as effective as second- or third-generation agents and that a single preoperative dose is as effective as multiple doses.

Gastroduodenal Surgery

Common gastric operations for which antimicrobial prophylaxis may be considered include resection with or without vagotomy for gastric or duodenal ulcers, revision necessitated by development of strictures of the gastric outlet, resection for gastric carcinoma, and gastroplasty or gastric bypass for morbid obesity.

The risk of postoperative infection after gastroduodenal surgery varies markedly, depending on the type of operation performed and the patient's clinical status. Conditions with a relatively high risk of infection include gastric ulcer, gastric carcinoma, bleeding duodenal or gastric ulcers, and obstructing duodenal ulcers.[60] In one study, the wound infection rate was 4% after operations for duodenal ulcer, 29% for gastric ulcer, and 33% for gastric resection for cancer.[61] Infection rates in the placebo group in controlled studies have varied from 10 to 35%.[60,62,63] With gastric-bypass operations, a wound infection rate of 21% has been reported.[64] Another important factor associated with infection risk is the use of histamine H_2-receptor blockers or the presence of achlorhydria. Gastric bacterial counts are increased when H_2-receptor blockers are used; this may in-

crease the risk of postoperative infection.[65,66]

In healthy individuals, the stomach is usually colonized by relatively few organisms (fewer than 10^4/ml). Among the most common are nasopharyngeal commensals (streptococci, lactobacilli, diphtheroids, and micrococci).[67,68] Increased pH from the use of H_2-receptor blockers, gastric obstruction, or bleeding can increase bacterial concentrations to 10^6/ml, and increased gastric bacterial concentrations are related to an increased rate of infection.[63]

Wound infections after gastroduodenal surgery tend to be polymicrobial and usually involve coliforms, such as *E. coli*, and aerobic gram-positive cocci, such as enterococci.[61,69] In a study of patients undergoing gastric-bypass surgery, staphylococci were the most common organisms isolated from infected wounds, and gram-negative bacilli were isolated from two subphrenic abscesses.[64]

Clinical Trials. Relatively few studies have evaluated the effectiveness of antimicrobial prophylaxis for gastroduodenal operations. Of those published, most compared antimicrobials with placebo. Cephalosporins that have demonstrated efficacy over nonantimicrobial controls include cephaloridine,[63,70,71] cefazolin,[30,64] cefamandole,[61,72] and cefuroxime.[73,74] The latter two trials studied single doses of cefuroxime and involved relatively few patients. Pories et al.[64] demonstrated a reduction in wound infection rate from 21 to 4% with the use of antimicrobial prophylaxis for gastric-bypass surgery.

Few published studies have compared the effectiveness of the various antimicrobials used for gastroduodenal operations. Three studies reported no significant differences between cephalosporins and penicillins.[62,75,76] Another study, which included relatively few patients, demonstrated no significant difference between cefazolin and moxalactam.[50]

Recommendations. Prophylactic antimicrobials should be used when the stomach or duodenum is entered surgically, since such procedures place the patient at risk for postoperative infection. Antimicrobials are not needed when the lumen of the intestinal tract is not entered (e.g., selective vagotomy). Although some authors believe that antimicrobials are not necessary for patients undergoing gastric resection for nonobstructing ulcers, the widespread use of H_2-receptor blockers makes it likely that these patients will have high intraluminal bacterial concentrations, making antimicrobial prophylaxis advisable.

Most studies of antimicrobial prophylaxis with gastroduodenal operations have involved the cephalosporins. Although few comparative antimicrobial studies have been published, it appears that first-generation cephalosporins are as effective as second- or third-generation agents. Therefore, a first-generation agent such as cefazolin is preferred. Although the efficacy of single-dose prophylaxis in this setting has not been thoroughly studied, results of studies with cefuroxime suggest the effectiveness of a single preoperative dose. Given the cumulative experience of single-dose prophylaxis for abdominal operations, it is justified to recommend single-dose prophylaxis for gastroduodenal operations as well.

Colorectal Surgery

Wound infections are the most common complication following elective colorectal surgery. This complication causes extensive morbidity and mortality and increases hospital costs. Factors associated with an increased risk for postoperative wound infections include impaired host defenses, age greater than 60 years, hypoalbuminemia, poor preoperative bowel preparation, and bacterial contamination of the surgical wound.[77]

Colonic aspirates obtained from patients undergoing colorectal surgery yield large numbers of aerobic and anaerobic microorganisms. More than 20 different aerobic and 50 anaerobic bacteria have been identified in the lumen of the bowel. These microorganisms make up to 20–30% of the fecal mass. *E. coli*, the most commonly isolated gram-negative aerobe, is found in concentrations of 10^6–10^8 organisms per gram of fecal contents. The concentration of anaerobes is 1000–10,000 times greater. *Bacteroides fragilis* is the most frequently isolated of these organisms.

The goal of surgical prophylaxis for elective colorectal surgery is to reduce the risk of contamination of the operative wound by bacteria spilled from the colon and rectum at the time of surgery. Attaining this goal entails reduction in the concentration of the resident bacteria and eradication of any bacteria that may contaminate the surgical wound.

When no attempt is made to reduce the number of microorganisms present in the bowel, elective colorectal surgeries have been associated with infection rates as high as 40%.[78,79] Various methods of mechanical cleansing of the bowel have been devised to reduce these high concentrations of colorectal bacteria. Bartlett et al.[80] have shown that the use of a mechanical bowel preparation alone decreases the total number of bacteria but does not decrease the number of microorganisms per gram of stool in the colon at the time of operation. With conventional bowel-cleansing techniques alone, the wound infection rate is still 35–40%.[81,82] Until the mid-1980s, the conventional bowel-preparation technique required a minimum of 36–48 hours of enemas and oral cathartics in the immediate preoperative period. The goal was to reduce the concentration of bacteria, with the assumption that this was accomplished once the rectal effluent was clear. More recently, single-day (12 hours or less) orthograde lavage techniques using an isosmotic non-absorbable electrolyte solution[83,84] or mannitol solution[85,86] have been used.

Since 1939, when Garlock and Seely[87] documented the value of preoperative administration of oral sulfonamides in reducing the incidence of wound infections after colonic surgery, investigators have searched for the most effective method to reduce postoperative infection. Antimicrobial agents, combined with mechanical cleansing of the colonic lumen, have significantly reduced postoperative wound infection rates from 30–60% to less than 10% in clean-contaminated procedures.[88–97] Numerous studies have unequivocally shown this approach to be safe and effective,[98,99] and it has become the standard approach for prophylaxis in elective colorectal surgery.

Although the method of bowel cleansing has been narrowed to one or two options, the choice of antimicrobial regimen is still vigorously debated. Given the nature of the microorganisms present in the colon and rectum, it seems reasonable that any prophylactic regimen should use an agent or combination of agents that is active against both aerobic and anaerobic bacteria. In the United States, three such antimicrobial regimens have been extensively studied:

- Administration of one or more oral antimicrobials (erythromycin or neomycin) in doses high enough to decrease the resident colonic flora.

- Administration of injectable antimicrobials immediately before surgery to attain maximal tissue concentrations at the time the surgical wound is made.
- A combination of the first two techniques.

Various drug regimens have been studied and advocated for prophylaxis for colorectal surgery during the past two decades.[89] Many of these trials have presented inconsistent results. Problems in methodology have been well documented.[90–92]

Clinical Trials. With the exception of a few classic studies, only reports published after 1980 were included in this analysis. The studies reviewed were predominantly prospective, randomized, controlled trials in which criteria for wound infection were clearly defined. Only half of the trials were blinded. Most experts agree that the rate for postoperative wound infection following clean-contaminated colorectal surgical procedures should be less than 10% if an appropriate mechanical bowel-cleansing and antimicrobial regimen (active against aerobes and anaerobes) is used.[93–96] Therefore, studies that reported wound infection rates of greater than 15% when an antimicrobial regimen effective against both gram-negative aerobes and anaerobes was used were not evaluated for this review. Studies that did not discuss dosage and timing of antimicrobial administration and that had a placebo group were likewise excluded.

Preoperative oral antimicrobials. Washington et al.[97] were the first to document that the use of preoperative oral antimicrobials (neomycin and tetracycline) effective against both aerobes and anaerobes led to a dramatic reduction in the postoperative wound infection rate. Nichols et al.[98,99] and Clarke et al.[81] altered this approach, using neomycin and erythromycin in an attempt to increase effectiveness against anaerobic bacteria in the large bowel. Various agents, both singly and in combination, have been evaluated for prophylaxis for colorectal surgery.

Numerous studies using oral agents for prophylaxis have demonstrated that the combination of neomycin plus an effective anaerobic agent, generally erythromycin[81,100–109] or metronidazole,[86,105,110–116] (less commonly a tetracycline derivative[86,97,117] or clindamycin[111]), in conjunction with a bowel-cleansing technique reduced the incidence of postoperative wound infections to less than 10%. These results occurred in 19 (76%) of 25 studies evaluated.[81,86,97,100,104–108] Forty-eight percent of these investigations documented a postoperative wound infection rate that was less than 5%.[86,97,102–105,107–110,116]

The standard neomycin sulfate–erythromycin regimen (1 g of each drug orally at 1300, 1400, and 2300 1 day preoperatively, with surgery performed at 0800 the next morning) used in the United States has resulted in postoperative infectious wound complications of less than 5% in half of the trials evaluated. In 90% of the studies evaluated, infectious wound complication rates were less than 10%.[86,97,102,104,108]

When metronidazole was combined with an agent active against gram-negative aerobes, only 44% of the treatment regimens reported a reduction of the postoperative wound infection rate to 5% or less.[86,105,107,112,114] Only 63% of the trials that evaluated metronidazole reported the wound infection rate to be less than 10%.[86,105,107,111,112,114] The difference in postoperative wound infections with a metronidazole combination versus the neomycin–erythromycin regimen may be a result of the different doses of metronidazole (2 g, 1 g, 750 mg, and 200 mg) used in these studies, as well as the fact that most of these studies were carried out in Europe.

Other combination regimens have been used as well. Neither tetracycline nor its derivatives have been shown to be more effective than neomycin–erythromycin in reducing postoperative wound infections.[86,97,117] With metronidazole alone, the postoperative wound infection rate is between 10 and 15%.[110,115,116]

Thus, available data demonstrate that the standard oral regimen of neomycin (nonabsorbable antibiotic) and erythromycin (which is absorbed and attains measurable tissue levels) provides the most effective means of preventing wound infection following elective colorectal surgery in adults. The safety and efficacy of this regimen in the pediatric population have not been documented; consequently, preoperative oral antimicrobials are not used in infants or young children.

Preoperative and postoperative regimens of injectable antimicrobials. In the late 1970s and early 1980s, debate about antimicrobial use in colorectal surgery centered on the issue of oral versus injectable antimicrobials. The oral, nonabsorbable antimicrobials were administered to reduce intraluminal concentrations of bacteria, whereas injectable antimicrobials were given to ensure high tissue concentrations at the time of surgery. All studies of wound infection rates following elective colorectal surgery have used oral absorbable antimicrobials (erythromycin, tetracycline, doxycycline, or metronidazole) as part of the standard bowel preparation.

One early study evaluating the use of injectable agents alone was conducted by Polk and Lopez-Meyer,[78] who evaluated the use of intramuscular cephaloridine. The wound infection rate in the treatment group was significantly lower than that of the control group.

In almost half of the studies that used only the intravenous route, a cephalosporin was among the treatment regimens evaluated.[85,100,104,118–130] Other antimicrobials evaluated, singly or in combination, included aminoglycosides,[103,126,131–133] erythromycin,[132] ampicillin,[123,134] piperacillin, ticarcillin–clavulanic acid,[131,135] doxycycline,[127,136,137] lincosamides,[133] and metronidazole.[104,121,123,125–129,131–134,138]

When an injectable antimicrobial regimen (in conjunction with a mechanical bowel preparation) was used without any oral antimicrobial, only 26% of the studies evaluated reported postoperative infectious wound complication rates of 5% or less,[85,100,123,127–129,136,137] and only 65% of the treatment regimens reported infectious wound complication rates of less than 10%.[85,100,104,118,119,122,123,127–129,131–138] Those studies that evaluated injectable cephalosporins included first-,[116,117,128,129] second-,[85,100,118,120,121,123–125] and third-generation cephalosporins.[104,122,126]

The first-generation cephalosporins have produced inconsistent results and do not appear to be of benefit in preventing postoperative wound infections.[107,116,117,128,129,139,140] The postoperative wound infection rate with these agents is generally greater than 20%. These results are not surprising, considering the relative inactivity of these agents against the anaerobic bacteria commonly associated with postoperative wound infections after elective colorectal surgery.

Cephalosporins with short half-lives, such as cefoxitin and cefotaxime, are associated with higher postoperative wound infections if the surgical procedures extend longer than 4–5 hours and the drugs are administered every 6–8 hours.[130,141,142]

Evaluation of these studies seems to imply that the use of injectable antimicrobials, along with some mechanical bowel-cleansing procedure, is not as effective as an oral regimen in reducing postoperative wound infections. The use of an oral regimen effective against aerobes and anaerobes reduced postoperative wound infections to 5% or less in 48% of the treatment regimens evaluated. An injectable antimicrobial regimen produced a similar reduction in only 26% of the studies evaluated.

Combination of oral and injectable antimicrobials. Attempting to decrease the rate of postoperative wound infections further, investigators have evaluated the combination of oral and intravenous antimicrobial agents for elective colorectal surgery. In theory, the goals are to reduce bacterial concentrations in the lumen and to attain sufficient tissue concentrations of antimicrobial to prevent postoperative infections.

Although some of these trials have documented significantly lower postoperative wound infection rates,[124,130,140,143,144] results are not consistent.[100,101,113,122]

Various intravenous antimicrobials have been added to oral antimicrobial regimens for prophylaxis for elective colorectal surgery.[100,101,112,113,122,124,131,139,143–146] Postoperative wound infection rates were 5% or less in 57% of the treatment regimens evaluated. All treatment regimens evaluated reported postoperative wound infection rates under 10% after elective colorectal surgery. These outcomes are similar to those achieved by oral regimens alone. The cephalosporins have been studied more than any other class of intravenous antimicrobials.[100,101,112,124,131,139,143,144]

It has recently been suggested that further stratification of the types of operative procedures may result in significantly different postoperative wound infection rates.[77,124,144,147] Coppa et al.[124,144] presented data suggesting that operations involving the rectum are associated with a higher wound infection rate than operations involving the colon and that the use of a combination of oral and intravenous antimicrobials reduces the wound infection rate significantly more than does an oral regimen alone.

Other factors affecting postoperative wound infections after elective colorectal surgery include the length of the operative procedure[119,124,130,148] and the duration of antimicrobial administration after the surgical incision.[149–153] Unfortunately, the majority of studies do not report the duration of surgery. Kaiser et al.[130] reported a threefold increase in the incidence of postoperative wound infection when the operative procedure lasted longer than 4 hours. If the procedure was less than 4 hours, the infection rate was only 5%. In this study, cefoxitin, a short half-life cephalosporin, was given at 6-hour intervals.

Coppa and Eng[124] reported an unacceptably high postoperative wound infection rate with cefoxitin alone when the surgical procedure lasted more than 3.5 hours. When cefoxitin was combined with an oral antimicrobial regimen, the infection rate dropped to 6%; if the procedure lasted less than 3.5 hours, the infection rate was 4% when cefoxitin was used alone. Jones et al.[141] and Shatney[142] reported that cefotaxime (also a short half-life cephalosporin) resulted in unacceptable postoperative wound infection rates when used for prophylaxis after colorectal surgery. These data imply that if the surgical procedure lasts longer than 3.5–4 hours, a cephalosporin with a relatively long half-life (e.g., cefotetan, ceftizoxime, and cefmetazole) should be considered for prophylaxis. No published comparative trials have specifically addressed this issue.

Discussions of how many doses are needed to ensure

adequate prophylaxis also merit careful review.[149–153] Stone et al.[154] was one of the first to document that prolonged administration of antimicrobials (5 days) was no more beneficial than a shorter course of antimicrobials administered in the immediate operative period, as described by Polk and Lopez-Meyer.[78] This approach has now been confirmed by many other investigations. DiPiro et al.[149] recently reviewed 40 published clinical trials that evaluated single-dose systemic antimicrobial prophylaxis for several types of surgical procedures. Their review indicated that multiple-dose regimens were no more effective than single-dose prophylaxis. The authors stated that it was difficult to evaluate the literature on colorectal surgery because many studies combined a single intravenous dose of antimicrobial with an oral regimen.

In this review of the literature, five trials[85,104,118,119,136] evaluating colorectal surgery specifically were found to compare a single intravenous dose with multiple doses of an antimicrobial regimen. The postoperative wound infection rate for the single-dose studies was between 5 and 10% in three-quarters of the reported regimens, and no significant differences in the postoperative wound infection rate after colorectal surgery were noted between the single- and multiple-dose regimens. While these studies indicate that the number of doses of antimicrobial prophylaxis is not of clinical significance, it is important to note that neither intravenous regimen is as effective as an oral regimen alone.

The review of evaluable studies of antimicrobial prophylaxis for elective colorectal surgery supports the use of an oral antimicrobial regimen (i.e., one that is active against aerobes and anaerobes and that attains adequate antianaerobic tissue concentrations immediately before surgical incision) and an adequate bowel-cleansing preparation. The use of intravenous antimicrobials alone does not reduce postoperative infectious wound complications to the same extent as do the oral regimens. The question of whether the combination of intravenous and oral antimicrobials is more efficacious than oral agents alone remains to be answered.

A recent survey of 352 board-certified colorectal surgeons concerning the use of bowel preparations and antimicrobials for prophylaxis revealed that all of the responding surgeons used some sort of bowel-cleansing procedure plus an antimicrobial regimen.[155] The preferred method of bowel cleansing, used by 58% of respondents, was oral polyethylene glycol–electrolyte lavage. The next most common approach, used by 36% of these surgeons, was a 1–3-day bowel preparation consisting of cathartics and enemas. The preferred regimen for the prevention of surgical infectious complications was a combined oral and injectable antimicrobial regimen plus bowel cleansing (88%). The most common oral regimen used by these surgeons consisted of an oral aminoglycoside (neomycin, kanamycin, or gentamicin) plus erythromycin base (82%). The most common injectable antimicrobials used by these surgeons were the second-generation cephalosporins cefoxitin and cefotetan (74%).

Recommendations. *Mechanical bowel preparation.* Four liters of a polyethylene glycol–electrolyte lavage solution should be given over 3 hours, starting the morning of the day before surgery; the lavage solution should always be used in conjunction with one of the following antimicrobial regimens.

Antimicrobial regimen. Oral neomycin sulfate 1 g and erythromycin base 1 g should be given after the bowel preparation is complete at 19, 18, and 9 hours before surgery.

If the oral route is contraindicated, a single 2-g intravenous dose of a cephalosporin that is effective against both aerobic and anaerobic bacteria and has a half-life of 60 minutes or longer (cefotetan, cefmetazole, cefotaxime, or ceftizoxime) should be administered at induction of anesthesia. If a cephalosporin with a half-life of 60 minutes or less is used (the half-life of cefoxitin is less than 60 minutes) and surgery lasts longer than 3 hours, a second dose of the intravenous antimicrobial should be given. The choice of cephalosporin should be based on cost to the institution. If the patient is to undergo a colostomy closure or rectal procedure, a combination of oral and intravenous agents should be given, following the dosage recommendations described above. Infants and young children should not receive oral antimicrobials. Ampicillin (50 mg/kg every 6 hours) and gentamicin (2.5 mg/kg every 8–12 hours) for three doses beginning at induction of anesthesia are recommended.

Appendectomy

The incidence of infectious complications following appendectomy is extremely variable and depends on the appearance of the appendix at the time of surgery. In uncomplicated appendectomy (appendix is normal or acutely inflamed), the postoperative infection rate is reported to range between 0 and 30%.[156–158] In the studies evaluated for this review, the rate of surgical wound infection in uncomplicated appendectomy without antimicrobial prophylaxis ranged from 8 to 27%.[159–169] However, if the appendix is gangrenous, perforated, or abscessed (complicated appendicitis), wound infection rates approach 80% without antimicrobial prophylaxis.[162] The goal of antimicrobial administration in patients with uncomplicated and complicated appendicitis is to reduce postoperative wound infection rates to less than 10% and between 10 and 25%, respectively.[158,164]

Appropriate antimicrobial prophylaxis has reduced surgical wound infection rates to as low as 1% in both uncomplicated and certain complicated appendectomies. The majority of studies have shown that even when appropriate antimicrobials are used, infectious complications will occur in 10–25% of patients with a gangrenous or perforated appendix.[162,170,171]

The most common microorganisms cultured from wound infections after appendectomy are anaerobic organisms (especially *B. fragilis*) and aerobic gram-negative enteric organisms (predominantly *E. coli*). Aerobic and anaerobic streptococci, *Staphylococcus* species, and *Enterococcus* species have also been cultured frequently, although not nearly as often as the aerobic and anaerobic gram-negative organisms. *Pseudomonas* species, reported by some researchers[172,173] to be a major pathogen in this setting, was not noted to be a problem in the studies reviewed for this discussion; in all, only 16 patients had a *Pseudomonas* species isolated in the studies reviewed.[166,167,172,173]

With the exception of certain classic articles, only studies published after 1979 were considered for this review. All studies evaluated were prospective, randomized, and blinded. Only studies that reported specific criteria for postoperative infectious wound complications and presented a statistical analysis were considered for this review.

Time of administration was shown to be important in the studies reviewed. In two trials where antimicrobials were administered after the abdomen had been opened and the appendix visualized, the rates of wound infection tended to be higher than in studies where the antimicrobial was administered before the surgical incision was made.[161,174] To be most efficacious, drugs should be administered before incision. Therefore, in almost all studies evaluated for this review, the antimicrobial(s) were administered at induction of anesthesia.

Clinical Trials. Uncomplicated appendicitis. In studies involving patients with uncomplicated appendicitis, cefoxitin,[159,163,164,168] cefotaxime,[166,167] mezlocillin,[169] and clindamycin[162] were shown to be of approximately equal efficacy for prophylaxis; in all cases, the postoperative infectious wound complications were reduced to less than 10%. Overall, 80% of the treatment regimens evaluated noted a wound infection rate of 10% or less following appendectomy. Combination regimens including metronidazole[164-166] also resulted in a reduction in wound infections, but they were not shown to be more efficacious than single-drug therapy with cefoxitin or cefotaxime. Metronidazole as a single agent or the first-generation cephalosporins cefazolin[162] and cephalothin[160] were no more effective than placebo and resulted in more infectious complications than did other comparative regimens. These studies appear to indicate that first-generation cephalosporins are ineffective as prophylactic regimens for uncomplicated appendectomy.

Clindamycin,[162] while better than placebo, generally was associated with a higher rate of wound infection than cefoxitin (10% versus 0–7%, respectively).[159,163,164,168] Cefoxitin has been studied more extensively than the other cephalosporins. The use of a single 1-g intravenous dose was consistently shown to result in low rates of wound infection (less than 7%).[159,163,164,168] The studies were almost evenly split as to the duration of prophylaxis in the postoperative period. Five studies administered between two and 15 postoperative doses (>60% used two or three doses);[159,160,163,165,168] all reported infectious wound complication rates of less than 10%. The remaining six studies[161,162,164,166,167,169] administered a single preoperative dose; with one exception, wound complication rates were reduced to 10% or less.[161]

Evaluation of these studies indicates that the antimicrobial(s) used for prophylaxis in uncomplicated appendectomy should be active against aerobic bacteria. These data also support the use of a single preoperative dose.

Complicated appendicitis. The studies evaluating antimicrobial prophylaxis in complicated appendicitis (gangrenous, perforated, or involving an abscess) report postoperative wound infection rates from 0 to 80%.[162,164-169,172-176] The approach to management should comprise surgical and antimicrobial treatment of the contaminated area with the goal of preventing postoperative wound complications. The standard prophylaxis used for a clean or clean-contaminated surgical procedure is insufficient. Only five of 12 studies evaluated for this review included patients diagnosed as having complicated appendicitis.[172-176]

Use of the first-generation cephalosporins cefazolin and cephalothin has resulted in an unacceptably high (27–80%) incidence of postoperative infectious wound complications.[162,168] While studies using a second-generation[164,166,168,173,174,176] or third-generation[166,167,173,176] cephalosporin reported postoperative wound infection rates of 25% or less in more than three-quarters of the clinical trials evaluated, only half of the treatment regimens that used either a second-generation[164,173,176] or third-generation[167,173,176] cephalosporin reported reductions to less than 10%.

Combination therapies including metronidazole[164-166,175]

or clindamycin[164,172,173,175] plus an aminoglycoside have not been shown to be more efficacious than cefoxitin[164,168,174,177] in preventing wound infection, intra-abdominal infection, or both following appendectomy. A single study comparing ceftizoxime with cefoxitin showed no difference in the rate of infection between the two agents; wound infection rates were 0 and 3%, respectively.[176]

In more than 71% of the antimicrobial regimens evaluated, patients treated with a single dose had postoperative wound infection rates of 25% or greater.[162,169,174,175] Postoperative wound infection rates of this magnitude were found in only 8% of the treatment regimens of 3–5 days' duration.[166,168,172,173,176] Treating for longer than 5 days has not proved to be of any additional benefit.[164,165]

Of all the evaluable studies of the cephalosporins, cefoxitin 1–2 g intravenously every 6 hours is considered by many to be the preferred regimen for antimicrobial prophylaxis before appendectomy and for treatment afterward. Based on their activity against aerobes and anaerobes, ceftizoxime, cefotaxime, cefmetazole, cefotetan, or combinations of an aminoglycoside plus metronidazole or clindamycin seem reasonable alternatives.

Recommendations. No single agent is clearly preferable to any other agent for prophylaxis in uncomplicated appendicitis or for the treatment of complicated appendicitis. Given the lack of data supporting a single-agent regimen for children, pediatric surgeons continue to prefer the combination of ampicillin, gentamicin, and clindamycin.

Uncomplicated appendicitis. The recommended regimen is a cephalosporin having anaerobic and aerobic activity (cefoxitin, cefmetazole, ceftizoxime, cefotaxime, or cefotetan) given as a single 1–2-g intravenous dose at induction of anesthesia. If surgery lasts more than 3 hours, a second dose should be given. For pediatric patients, two doses of ampicillin, gentamicin, and clindamycin (5–15 mg/kg every 8 hours) should be given.

Complicated appendicitis. A cephalosporin having anaerobic and aerobic activity (cefoxitin, cefmetazole, ceftizoxime, cefotaxime, or cefotetan) should be given as a 1–2-g intravenous dose. The first dose should be administered at induction of anesthesia, and the regimen should be continued for 3–5 days. Alternatives include an aminoglycoside or aztreonam plus metronidazole or clindamycin. Additional options are imipenem or ticarcillin–clavulanate. For pediatric patients with complicated appendicitis, the regimen suggested for uncomplicated appendicitis should be continued for 3–5 days.

Cesarean Section

Approximately 1 million infants are born by cesarean section in the United States annually.[177] The rate of cesarean section has risen from 4.5 per 100 deliveries in 1965, to 16.5 in 1980, to 24.7 in 1988. Until 1986, repeat cesarean sections represented an increasingly large share of total cesareans, rising from approximately 25% of all cesareans in 1970 to more than 33% in 1986.[177] These increases now appear to have leveled off.

Postpartum infectious complications are common following cesarean section. Endometritis (infection of the uterine lining) has been reported to occur in high risk populations at a rate as high as 85%.[178] High risk patients are defined as women who have not received prenatal care, who are poorly nourished, who undergo multiple vaginal examinations, who have prolonged labor, and who have undergone frequent invasive monitoring. A majority of these women live in poverty. In contrast, patients in upper or middle socioeconomic populations, who tend to be better nourished and have received appropriate prenatal care, are at lower risk; the postpartum rate of endometritis in these patients ranges from 5 to 15%.

The factor most frequently associated with postcesarean section infectious morbidity is prolonged labor in the presence of ruptured membranes. Intact chorioamniotic membranes serve as a protective barrier against bacterial infection. Rupture of the membrane exposes the uterine surface to bacteria from the birth canal. The vaginal fluid with its bacterial flora is drawn up into the uterus when it relaxes between contractions during labor.[179] The flora include various aerobic and anaerobic streptococci, staphylococci, enteric gram-negative bacilli, and anaerobic gram-negative bacteria such as *Bacteroides bivius*, *B. fragilis*, and *Fusobacterium*.[180] In contrast, the organisms causing postcesarean section wound infections are *Staph. aureus* and other staphylococci, streptococci, and Enterobacteriaceae. Anaerobes are also present but less commonly than in endometritis.[180] In addition to rupture of membranes, frequent vaginal examinations and invasive fetal monitoring also carry vaginal organisms into the uterine cavity. Other risk factors include systemic illness, poor hygiene, obesity, and anemia.[180]

Although febrile morbidity, or temperature elevation in an asymptomatic patient, is often considered in evaluations of antimicrobial prophylaxis, it appears that this temperature elevation is often not associated with an identifiable infection source or with symptoms specific for infection. It may occur in women with normal physical examination results and sometimes disappears without treatment. In controlled trials, it occurs with equal frequency in the placebo and treatment groups.[180,181] Moreover, women exhibiting febrile morbidity appear not to be those who later develop clinical infection. The presence or absence of febrile morbidity is probably not an appropriate indication of the efficacy of antimicrobial prophylaxis and therefore will not be considered.

Most investigations documenting the efficacy of prophylactic antimicrobials in cesarean section have been conducted in high risk patients. Considerable controversy has existed regarding the necessity for prophylaxis in low risk women undergoing cesarean section.

Two early investigations documented significant reductions in postcesarean endometritis following low risk procedures with the use of prophylactic antimicrobials.[182,183] Some authorities have dismissed these benefits, arguing that limited morbidity, theoretical risks, and excess costs do not justify the use of prophylaxis in these patients.[184] From 1980 to 1982, Ehrenkranz et al.[185] undertook a large-scale prospective study of the efficacy of prophylaxis in more than 1800 low risk women who underwent cesarean section. Although the form of prophylaxis was not controlled and case controls were used, significant differences in endometritis and wound infection rates were found between women who did and did not receive prophylaxis. The investigators also found that primary cesarean section was associated with a fivefold higher rate of endometritis and that the odds of developing endometritis, wound infection, or both without timely antimicrobial prophylaxis was 3.7 to 1 in this cohort. Given their findings and assumptions regarding frequency of low risk cesarean sections and efficacy and safety of the three 1-g

doses of cefazolin used in the study, these authors concluded that more than $9 million could be saved annually by administration of prophylaxis to low risk patients. The savings estimated from the lower limit of the odds ratio (1.4) is still $3.6 million annually. Thus, brief antimicrobial prophylaxis may be appropriate for all cesarean sections.

Clinical Trials. There have been more than 40 placebo-controlled, prospective trials evaluating the efficacy of antimicrobials in cesarean section, most of which have been carried out in high risk populations. More than 50% of these trials demonstrated benefit in terms of reduction of serious infection, and approximately 75% revealed significant reductions in rates of postoperative endometritis.[186] The remaining 25% showed no statistical benefit in the prevention of serious infection or endometritis. Only approximately one in five of these trials demonstrated a statistically significant reduction in wound infection rates.[186]

A meta-analysis of these data by Enkin et al.[186] suggests a 75% reduction in serious infections and endometritis and a 65% reduction in wound infections for antimicrobial-treated patients compared with controls. These data are combined for high and low risk patients undergoing both emergency and elective procedures. When the data are cumulated via meta-analysis for the few trials of elective cesarean section, the summary odds ratios for endometritis (0.23, 95% confidence interval = 0.13–0.42) and wound infection (0.10, 95% confidence interval = 0.03–0.36) also support the use of prophylaxis in these procedures.

Timing of prophylaxis. Unlike other surgical procedures where antimicrobials are ideally administered just before incision, administration of antimicrobials in cesarean section is usually delayed until after cord clamping. This is done principally to avoid suppression of the normal flora of the infant and minimize the risk of neonatal sepsis.

Although toxicity in the infant is of potential concern, the majority of drugs used for this procedure (primarily β-lactams) have a documented record of safety in the treatment of infections in pregnancy, and many are used in the treatment of neonatal sepsis. The issue of timing was addressed in two controlled trials. Cunningham et al.[187] and Gordon et al.[188] demonstrated no difference in infectious complications, regardless of whether the antimicrobials were given preoperatively or after cord clamping. In the study by Cunningham et al.,[187] the infants who were not exposed to antimicrobial in utero underwent significantly fewer evaluations for neonatal sepsis. Thus, antimicrobials provide effective prophylaxis, even when given after clamping of the umbilical cord.

Duration of prophylaxis. Most recent trials of antimicrobial prophylaxis have assessed the value of a single dose versus multiple doses (usually up to 24 hours). Early studies used regimens that lasted as long as 5 or 6 days. Studies by D'Angelo and Sokol[189] and Scarpignato et al.[190] found that a 5-day course of cephalosporin prophylaxis was no more efficacious than a 24-hour course. Elliott et al.,[191] by contrast, found that 3 days of ampicillin were significantly more effective than three doses of ampicillin. The explanation for this difference is unclear.

Faro et al.[192] assessed the efficacy of several types of β-lactam antimicrobials given in various regimens to nearly 1600 patients. One group of patients was given three doses of cefazolin and the two other groups received a single dose of cefazolin, either 1 or 2 g. Results in patients receiving the single 2-g dose of cefazolin were statistically superior to those in patients receiving the other two cefazolin regimens.[192]

Based on the data from the studies by D'Angelo and Scarpignato and more recent studies that demonstrated comparable efficacy of single doses, it does not seem necessary to extend prophylaxis beyond a single dose.

Route of administration. Although the majority of studies have examined the effects of intravenous administration of antimicrobials, a few have evaluated the benefit of antimicrobial irrigations. Enkin et al.[186] summarized the data from six such trials. In one of these trials, Conover and Moore[193] found that intrauterine antimicrobial lavage was inferior to systemic administration of the same agents. None of the other trials demonstrated any difference in infectious morbidity. Therefore, given the adequate tissue penetration and demonstrated efficacy of injectable antimicrobials, irrigations of the uterine cavity are not warranted.

Selection of antimicrobials. Guidelines for selection of antimicrobial prophylaxis established by Ledger et al.[194] more than 15 years ago are still applicable. The antimicrobial selected must

- Have a spectrum of activity effective against those bacteria likely to cause infection.
- Be present in tissue at the operative site in concentrations potentially effective against the infecting pathogen.
- Have been demonstrated to be clinically effective.
- Not be considered for first-line therapy of infection.
- Be nontoxic.
- Not promote the emergence of resistance.
- Be cost effective.

Although more than 20 different drugs have been used alone or in combination for prophylaxis, most obstetricians currently use either a penicillin or a cephalosporin.[195] A recent large-scale study by Faro et al.,[192] involving more than 1500 high risk patients, indicates that several single-dose regimens, including cefazolin 2 g, cefotetan 1 g, and piperacillin 4 g, are comparably effective. This provides three disparate choices, with drugs that offer differing spectra of activity with roughly equivalent efficacy.

The earlier large-scale trials of Stiver et al.[196] and Rayburn et al.[197] offer a potential solution to this dilemma. Both studies involved hundreds of high risk patients and compared cefazolin (poor *Bacteroides* coverage) with cefoxitin or moxalactam (good *Bacteroides* coverage). The Stiver study was placebo controlled. In both of these studies, cefoxitin and moxalactam were slightly less effective than cefazolin.

In another study of nearly 350 high risk women undergoing cesarean section, a 2-g dose of cefoxitin or piperacillin was given immediately after cord clamping and at 4 and 8 hours after surgery.[198] Despite its superior in vitro activity against enterococci, *Pseudomonas aeruginosa,* and several enteric gram-negative bacillary species, piperacillin was found to be no more effective than cefoxitin.

Recommendations. Despite multiple clinical trials assessing the effectiveness of broad-spectrum antimicrobials or multiple doses of antimicrobials for prophylaxis in cesarean section, the data support the use of narrow-spectrum agents, such as first-generation cephalosporins, administered in a single dose immediately after clamping of the umbilical cord.[199,200] Given all of the above, it seems reasonable to use a single 2-g dose of cefazolin for all women undergoing cesarean section.

Hysterectomy

Hysterectomy is second only to cesarean section as the most frequently performed surgical procedure in the United States. Approximately 700,000 hysterectomies, or seven hysterectomies per 1000 women, are performed annually in this country. This rate has not changed substantially since the mid-1960s. The average hospital stay is now less than 6 days, a figure that has dropped by 50% in the past 25 years.[201]

Hysterectomy may be performed by a transvaginal or transabdominal approach. Uterine fibroid tumors account for 30% of all presurgical diagnoses leading to hysterectomy; the other most common diagnoses are endometriosis, uterine prolapse, cancer, and endometrial hyperplasia. The proportion of patients undergoing concurrent unilateral or bilateral oophorectomy increases with age; this procedure is done in approximately two-thirds of women over the age of 60 years who undergo hysterectomy.[201] Radical hysterectomy, which entails removal of the uterus, fallopian tubes, and ovaries as well as extensive stripping of the pelvic lymph nodes, is performed in patients with extension of cervical cancer.

Microbiology. The vagina is normally colonized with a wide variety of bacteria, including gram-positive and gram-negative aerobes and anaerobes. The normal flora of the vagina includes staphylococci, streptococci, enterococci, lactobacilli, diphtheroids, *E. coli,* anaerobic streptococci, *Bacteroides* species, and *Fusobacterium* species.[202-204] The vaginal flora changes during the menstrual cycle, which may affect the nature of postoperative infection.[202] Postoperative vaginal flora differs from preoperative flora; enterococci, gram-negative bacilli, and *Bacteroides* species increase postoperatively. Postoperative changes in flora may occur independently of prophylactic antimicrobial administration and are not by themselves predictive of postoperative infection.[203,205] Postoperative infections associated with vaginal hysterectomy are frequently polymicrobial, with enterococci, aerobic gram-negative bacilli, and *Bacteroides* species isolated most frequently. Postoperative wound infections following abdominal or radical hysterectomy are also polymicrobial; gram-positive cocci and enteric gram-negative bacilli predominate.[206,207]

Vaginal Hysterectomy. In a vaginal hysterectomy, the uterus and, occasionally, one or two fallopian tubes, the ovaries, or both, are removed through the vagina. No abdominal incision is made. Because the procedure is performed in an organ that is normally colonized with bacteria, it is associated with a higher risk of postoperative infection than is abdominal hysterectomy. The rate of postoperative infection (wound and pelvic sites) in women administered placebo or no prophylactic antimicrobials has generally fallen to between 17 and 40%, although it ranges from 12 to 78%.[208-261] A number of antimicrobial agents, including chloramphenicol, clindamycin, metronidazole, penicillin and tetracycline derivatives, streptomycin, and first-, second-, and third-generation cephalosporins, have been studied as perioperative prophylaxis for vaginal hysterectomy. Overall, the use of antimicrobials has markedly reduced the incidence of postoperative infection following vaginal hysterectomy to a generally acceptable rate of less than 10%.

The cephalosporins are used more frequently for prophylaxis in this procedure than any other class of drugs. Cefazolin has been associated with a postoperative infection rate ranging from 0 to 12%. Most recent studies have compared the efficacy of various second- and third-generation cephalosporins; postoperative infection rates have ranged between 0 and 16%. Studies directly comparing the newer second- or third-generation cephalosporins with cefazolin indicate that cefazolin is equivalent to the new agents in reducing the incidence of postoperative wound infections.[262–265]

The observation that *Bacteroides* species are commonly associated with infections following vaginal hysterectomy has prompted several investigators to study the efficacy of cephalosporins with enhanced anaerobic activity (cefmetazole, cefotetan, cefoxitin, ceftizoxime, and moxalactam) for perioperative prophylaxis. Postoperative infection rates associated with these agents have ranged from 0 to 15%.

The trend in recent years has been toward use of single-dose regimens of antimicrobials, administered immediately before surgery. Studies comparing single doses of one antimicrobial with multidose regimens of a different antimicrobial have shown the two regimens to be equally effective.

Abdominal Hysterectomy. Abdominal hysterectomy involves removal of the uterus and, in some cases, of one or both fallopian tubes, the ovaries, or both. Because bacterial contamination associated with this procedure is minimal, postoperative infection rates in women receiving no antimicrobial prophylaxis have generally been lower than those in women undergoing vaginal hysterectomy. The abdominal approach, however, takes more time, and this may predispose these patients to higher infection rates than patients undergoing vaginal hysterectomy with prophylaxis.[266] The need for antimicrobial prophylaxis in abdominal hysterectomy is controversial, although most obstetricians and gynecologists do currently employ prophylactic antimicrobials.

At least 25 placebo-controlled or no-antimicrobial-controlled studies have been performed in abdominal hysterectomy.[213,215,229,234–238,242,244,249,252,253,258,263,265,267–301] First- and second-generation cephalosporins and metronidazole have been studied more widely than any other agents. A meta-analysis recently demonstrated the general efficacy of antimicrobial prophylaxis for abdominal hysterectomy.[223] In this analysis, postoperative infection rates in the placebo group averaged 19.5%, whereas in women receiving prophylaxis the mean infection rate was 9.3%. A 24-hour regimen has been shown to be as effective as longer courses of prophylaxis, and many single-dose prophylaxis regimens have proved as effective as multiple-dose regimens.

The prophylactic efficacy of various cephalosporin regimens was recently compared. Few comparisons have been made of second- and third-generation cephalosporins versus cefazolin; however, a number of second-generation cephalosporins have been compared. Single doses of cefotetan or cefotaxime appear to be as effective as multiple doses of cefoxitin.

Radical Hysterectomy. Many factors increase the risk of postoperative infection in women undergoing radical hysterectomy, including extended length of surgery, blood loss and replacement, presence of malignancy, prior radiation therapy, obesity, and presence of indwelling drainage catheters.[216,224] Nonetheless, because of the low degree of contamination

associated with this procedure, the need for prophylaxis has not been definitively established. The use of prophylactic antimicrobials in radical hysterectomy was recently reviewed by Hemsell et al.[217]

Six prospective, placebo-controlled trials have evaluated the impact of antimicrobial prophylaxis on wound infection following radical hysterectomy.[216,217,225–227,302,303] Rates of infection in the placebo groups ranged from 17 to 87%, whereas corresponding infection rates in antimicrobial-treated patients ranged from 0 to 15%. The incidence of postoperative infection was reduced in antimicrobial-treated patients in all of these trials. In one study, prophylaxis with cefamandole given by injection and by intraperitoneal irrigation reduced postoperative infection rates to less than 4%.[225] It should be noted, however, that other authors have noted similarly low infection rates in uncontrolled patient series and have been unable to recommend routine prophylaxis for radical hysterectomy.[226]

The optimal agent for and duration of antimicrobial prophylaxis for radical hysterectomy have not been determined; however, 24-hour regimens of mezlocillin or cefoperazone–sulbactam appear to be as effective as other antimicrobial regimens.[217,226] Antimicrobial prophylaxis is indicated for radical hysterectomy, and a 24-hour regimen is probably sufficient.

Recommendations. Infection is common in women who have undergone vaginal or abdominal hysterectomy without antimicrobial prophylaxis. Antimicrobial prophylaxis is indicated for all types of hysterectomy. Cefazolin is the drug of choice for surgical prophylaxis in vaginal hysterectomy. Although there have been few comparative trials involving single-dose cefazolin, clinical experience and the drug's relatively long serum half-life (1.8 hours) indicate that this regimen is effective for most women. A second dose of cefazolin may be administered if surgery lasts more than 4 hours. Single-dose regimens with cephalosporins such as cefazolin and cefotetan have been demonstrated to be as effective as multiple doses for abdominal hysterectomy. Extending antimicrobial prophylaxis beyond 24 hours for uncomplicated hysterectomy is unnecessary.

Neurosurgery

Clean neurosurgical procedures are those where there is no break in surgical technique and no entry into the respiratory, gastrointestinal, and genitourinary tracts. Clean procedures usually carry a risk of postoperative wound infection of less than 5%, and in many hospitals the risk is 1–2%.[304] It is therefore understandable that the use of injectable antimicrobials in such procedures is quite controversial. In addition, it is difficult to design clinical trials that could distinguish between infection rates of 2 and 5%. A valid study would require placebo-controlled, randomized trials with at least 1000 patients in each study group.[305] Multicenter trials are usually required to accrue enough patients to avoid statistical errors.[306]

Among the clean neurosurgical procedures are elective craniotomies for the repair of aneurysms, correction of arteriovenous malformations, and removal of various types of brain tumors. There are major differences relating to such factors as immune status and nutrition between an individual who undergoes elective surgery for a nonmalignant condition and a patient with cancer; such variables make clinical trials difficult to assess. Some craniotomies for ruptured aneurysms must be done on an emergency basis, and meticulous preparation of the skin cannot be assured. Neurosurgical procedures following trauma occurring outside the hospital should never be included in comparative trials and would be considered contaminated surgery. Laminectomies (both with and without the use of the operating microscope) are performed by neurosurgeons, although in some centers this procedure is also performed by orthopedic surgeons. Many studies will include laminectomies as well as elective craniotomies in trials of clean neurosurgical procedures. The microscope introduces another variable (additional source of potential contamination) that should be considered.

Ventricular fluid-shunting procedures (ventriculoperitoneal shunts), performed to control increased intracranial pressure seen in patients with hydrocephalus, have also been included in some clinical trials of clean neurosurgical procedures. Since this procedure involves the placement of a foreign body (pressure-release valve and tubing) into the cranium, another variable is introduced. Most infectious disease consultants believe that such shunting operations should be studied as a separate entity.[307] Ventricular fluid-shunting procedures are also performed following serious head trauma and in some elective craniotomy procedures to drain cerebrospinal fluid and lower intracranial pressure. The shunts are left in place for varying lengths of time, ranging from 48 hours to 7 days. The rate of infection (usually ventriculitis) is generally reported to be between 5 and 20%.[308–310]

Data from most published clinical trials indicate that gram-positive bacteria are primarily associated with wound infections. *Staph. aureus* and coagulase-negative staphylococci are responsible for greater than 85% of such infections and are isolated in mixed cultures with other gram-positive bacteria in an additional 5–10% of cases. Gram-negative bacteria are isolated as the sole cause of postoperative neurosurgical wound infections in only 5–8% of cases.[311–317] Therefore, most clinical trials of antimicrobial prophylaxis use a drug with primary activity against staphylococci. Drugs most frequently studied include clindamycin, erythromycin, penicillinase-stable penicillins (oxacillin, nafcillin, and methicillin), first-generation cephalosporins, and vancomycin.

Clinical Trials. Before 1983, virtually all published reports of antimicrobials used prophylactically in clean neurosurgery cases were based on uncontrolled, nonrandomized, retrospective studies.[311–313,318–322] These reports seem to favor some type of prophylactic regimen. In 1980, Haines[323] published an excellent review of these reports. He concluded that a final recommendation regarding antimicrobial prophylaxis in clean neurosurgical procedures must await the results of controlled clinical trials. In 1984, Geraghty and Feely[315] published the results of a randomized, nonblinded, clinical trial of 402 cases. The control group had a wound infection rate of 3.5%, versus 0% in the antimicrobial group.

In 1986, Shapiro et al.[317] published a randomized, placebo-controlled, double-blind trial involving 148 neurosurgery cases. Operations included craniotomies, spinal surgery, and shunting procedures. The study was stopped prematurely because of an excess number of wound infections in the placebo group. The overall rate of infection was 2.8% in the antimicrobial group and 11.7% in the placebo group.

Other studies involving retrospective chart reviews with large number of patients have also been published.[314,318,324,325] A neurosurgery group in the Netherlands performed a prospective, double-blind, placebo-controlled study of cloxacillin in craniotomy patients.[326] Postoperative infection rates in the cloxacillin group were 3.9% (six of 156 patients) and in the placebo group 13% (20 of 154 patients). The difference was statistically significant ($p < 0.05$).

Bullock et al.,[327] from South Africa, conducted a double-blind, placebo-controlled study in 417 patients undergoing clean elective neurosurgical procedures. Although the wound infection rate was significantly lower in the antimicrobial group than in the placebo group (2 versus 5.8%), the results of this study are questionable because the drug selected was piperacillin. This choice is unusual for procedures where β-lactamase-producing staphylococci are the major bacteria causing wound infections. Piperacillin would not have stability against the β-lactamase produced by most staphylococci.

Blomstedt and Kytta,[328] in a randomized study, used vancomycin in patients undergoing craniotomy with and without bone flaps. In comparison with groups of patients not receiving antimicrobials, only those patients with the bone-flap procedures demonstrated a reduction in postoperative infections after receiving vancomycin.

Postoperative central nervous system (CNS) shunt infections are a major complication associated with mortality and serious morbidity. Infections following surgery include meningitis, ventriculitis, and, less frequently, wound infections.[329] In most cases, antimicrobial therapy without shunt removal is not effective in eradicating the infecting organism.[330–335] Therefore, shunt removal or replacement, in addition to injectable antimicrobial therapy, is the preferred therapeutic modality. Staphylococci account for 75–80% of CNS and wound infections following shunting procedures. Gram-negative bacteria are responsible for only 10–20% of such infections.[336–344]

Because CNS infections following shunting procedures are responsible for substantial mortality and morbidity, especially in children, the possible role of prophylactic antimicrobials in such procedures has been the subject of numerous clinical trials.[345–353] Unfortunately, the majority of such trials have been neither randomized nor controlled; many were retrospective. Reaching a conclusion about the effectiveness of prophylactic antimicrobials in shunting procedures is therefore difficult. Nonetheless, many neurosurgical services continue to use some type of prophylactic regimen.

Further confusion exists because more than 50% of the time the isolated pathogen is a member of the coagulase-negative group of staphylococci. The majority of such isolates are methicillin resistant, which would make injectable vancomycin the only effective agent. Several trials using either intraventricular or intravenous vancomycin failed to show a reduction in postoperative CNS infection rates.[328]

Recommendations. *Clean neurosurgical procedures: elective craniotomy and laminectomy.* Although the effectiveness of antimicrobials in lowering postoperative wound infection rates following elective craniotomy and laminectomy has not been demonstrated in a single, large, pivotal clinical trial, there is enough evidence to suggest that a single dose of an antimicrobial, directed toward *Staph. aureus*, can be recommended. A single dose of cefazolin (1 g intravenously at the induction of anesthesia) appears to be the best choice. Alternatively, a single dose of one of the β-lactamase-stable penicillins might also be used (1 g of intravenous oxacillin or nafcillin).

For elective procedures lasting longer than 3 hours, the dose of cefazolin should be repeated; for procedures lasting more than 2 hours in which oxacillin or nafcillin has been used, the dose should likewise be repeated. In hospitals where methicillin-resistant *Staph. aureus* prevalence rates exceed 10%, the use of injectable vancomycin in a single-dose regimen is probably justified. Large-scale, randomized trials are needed to verify the need for prophylactic antimicrobials in clean neurosurgical procedures.

Cerebrospinal fluid-shunting procedures. Meticulous surgical and aseptic technique and short operation time are important factors in lowering infection rates following shunt placement. The number of patients studied to date is small, and the results of trials do not lend support to the use of prophylactic antimicrobials. Therefore, antimicrobials cannot generally be recommended. However, clinicians must remember that the risk of Type II statistical errors in such studies is ever present.

Neurosurgeons who want to prescribe a single dose of an appropriate intravenous antimicrobial or to administer a dose of intraventricular antimicrobial through the shunt at the end of the procedure should be given the benefit of the doubt, provided that they understand the available research concerning such a practice. Unfortunately, because the majority of postoperative infections following shunting procedures are caused by methicillin-resistant, coagulase-negative staphylococci, the only reasonable drug at present is intravenous or intraventricular vancomycin.

Cardiothoracic Surgery

Approximately 600,000 cardiothoracic surgeries are performed annually in the United States.[354,355] Of these, 80% are coronary-artery bypass graft (CABG) procedures, and 20% are heart-valve replacements. A relatively small number involve heart or heart–lung transplants and repair of congenital heart defects in children. Risk factors that predispose to infection following cardiothoracic surgery have been reviewed elsewhere.[355–358]

The selection, use, and efficacy of prophylactic antimicrobials for cardiothoracic surgery have been sources of controversy since the first study in this area was published in 1961 by Kittle and Reed.[359] They found no advantage to the administration of penicillin and streptomycin in a retrospective review of patients undergoing extracorporeal circulation for valve repair. At that time, antimicrobial prophylaxis was frequently not initiated until after surgery, and many surgeons believed it to be of no value.[359]

In 1963, Slonim et al.[360] showed that patients undergoing open-heart surgery who had received penicillin and streptomycin had fewer infections than those who had received no antimicrobials. This evaluation, however, was performed retrospectively and was not randomized.

Two prospective, randomized, double-blind, placebo-controlled trials of cardiothoracic antimicrobial prophylaxis were published in the late 1960s.[361,362] These studies, which involved small numbers of patients who were primarily undergoing valve repair, found a modest benefit to the use of a semisynthetic penicillin or a combination of penicillin G and streptomycin in preventing postoperative wound infections.

The primary intent of early antimicrobial prophylaxis in open-heart surgery was to reduce the incidence of postoperative endocarditis following valve repair. Early studies showed that coagulase-positive and coagulase-negative staphylococci were the primary pathogens infecting prosthetic valves.[359–361] As a result, most early prophylactic regimens were directed against staphylococci, with semisynthetic penicillins and first-generation cephalosporins emerging as the drugs of choice.

With the advent of the CABG procedure and an expansion of the number of cardiothoracic procedures performed in the United States, the focus of prophylaxis has shifted to include a broader spectrum of gram-negative pathogens causing wound infections postoperatively, at the sternal incision and the saphenous vein harvest sites.[361–364]

Clinical Trials. In 1979, a prospective, randomized, double-blind, placebo-controlled trial of antimicrobial prophylaxis for CABG confirmed the benefit of using a semisynthetic penicillin to prevent postoperative wound infection.[365] This study was terminated early because of a high incidence of postoperative wound infections in the placebo group, a finding that validated the ongoing practice of administering prophylactic antimicrobials for cardiothoracic surgery. Austin et al.[366] also terminated a double-blind, placebo-controlled study of cephalothin prophylaxis after four of the first 15 patients developed *Staph. aureus* sternal wound infections. Penketh et al.[367] terminated a double-blind, placebo-controlled study evaluating cephradine after 12 of the first 22 placebo patients developed wound infections. Wound infection rates ranged from 9.1 to 54.5% in the placebo groups of these studies. Wound infection rates were reduced in all patient groups receiving antimicrobials; postoperative wound infection rates ranged from 0 to 6.7%. Postoperative wound infection rates since the routine administration of prophylactic antimicrobials for cardiothoracic surgeries have ranged from 0.8 to 25%.

The optimal duration of antimicrobial prophylaxis for cardiothoracic surgery was addressed by four different studies.[363,368–370] Cephalothin was the prophylactic cephalosporin in all four; in one study, it was combined with kanamycin. Doses and durations in the short groups ranged from a single 1-g-duration treatment dose of cephalothin to 2 g every 6 hours for 2 days. Long treatment regimens ranged from 2 g of cephalothin preoperatively followed by 1 g every 6 hours for 3 days to 2 g every 6 hours for 6 days. Two of the studies were performed before the development of the CABG procedure. Total wound infection rates were lower in the short-duration treatment groups in two of the four studies, although the differences were not statistically significant.

Cephalosporins were compared with antistaphylococcal penicillins as prophylactic agents in five studies. The antistaphylococcal penicillins were used in combination with another penicillin, an aminoglycoside, or both in four of the five studies.[371–375] Four of the five studies revealed fewer total wound infections in the cephalosporin-treated patients; however, none of the results reached statistical significance.

Cephalothin was compared with the second-generation cephalosporin cefamandole or ceforanide in five studies, while cephradine was compared with cefamandole in one of these studies. Results from the six studies varied; no agent showed a significant advantage over the others.

Recently published trials comparing cefazolin, cefamandole, and cefuroxime as prophylactic antimicrobials for cardiothoracic surgery have shown a trend toward statistical significance in favor of the second-generation cephalosporins.[376–380] Total wound infection rates (sternal plus leg wound infection) ranged from 2.5 to 16.7% in cefazolin-treated patients and from 0 to 13.5% in cefamandole- or cefuroxime-treated patients. Total wound infection rates were lower in patients receiving the second-generation cephalosporin in seven of the eight comparison groups. Sternal wound infection rates were also reduced in seven of the eight treatment groups receiving either cefamandole or cefuroxime. Leg wound infection rates were lower in five of the eight second-generation cephalosporin treatment groups. The study by Doebbeling et al.[380] demonstrated results that are contrary to those of the other studies, with cefuroxime-treated patients faring more poorly than cefazolin-treated patients with regard to sternal wound infections.

Two recent surveys by Woods et al.[381,382] of antimicrobial prophylaxis practice in cardiothoracic surgery have shown that the choice of antimicrobials used for prophylaxis has changed in recent years to include the use of second-generation cephalosporins.

Cefamandole was compared directly with cefuroxime in two studies. Cefuroxime was associated with lower wound infection rates at sternal and leg sites in both studies, although the differences were not statistically significant. In both trials the total wound infection rate was less than 4%, and the study lacked sufficient power to distinguish a difference between treatment groups.[383]

Cefazolin was compared with ceftriaxone in two studies.[384,385] Cefazolin was associated with lower sternal and lower total wound infection rates in both studies, although the studies lacked statistical power to distinguish a significant difference between the two treatment groups.

Six other prospective, randomized, controlled studies of cardiothoracic prophylaxis have been performed. Kini et al.[386] compared cephalothin and cefazolin and found no differences in total wound infection rates. Pien et al.[387] compared cephalothin with clindamycin and found a nonstatistically significant reduction in both sternal and leg wound infection rates in the clindamycin group. Geroulanos et al.[378] compared cefuroxime with ceftriaxone in 512 patients and found no differences in total wound infection rates. Kaiser et al.[377] compared cefazolin and cefamandole, both with the addition of gentamicin, and found a statistically significant reduction in sternal and total wound infection rates in the cefamandole–gentamicin group. Joyce and Szczepanski[388] compared penicillin G with vancomycin and found a significant reduction in total wound infections in the vancomycin group. Wilson et al.[389] evaluated 517 patients receiving teicoplanin, in two dosage regimens, or a combination of flucloxacillin and gentamicin. They found unacceptably high sternal wound infection rates in the teicoplanin treatment group, although patients in the flucloxacillin–gentamicin groups also experienced high sternal wound infection rates.

The postoperative infection rate in clean cardiothoracic surgeries is intrinsically low, and the degree of improvement of one regimen over another is relatively small. Antimicrobial prophylaxis in cardiothoracic surgery reduces the incidence of postoperative wound infection by fivefold when compared with placebo, to approximately 5%. On average, cefamandole and cefuroxime each reduced the incidence of wound infection by approximately 1.5-fold when compared with cefazolin. Wound infections were not reduced in studies comparing cephalothin with either cefamandole or ceforanide, or when cefazolin was compared with ceftriaxone. Additionally, no differences in outcome were seen in studies comparing cefamandole with cefuroxime. No differences were found between short (single-dose to 2-day) and long (3–6-day) regimens. No differences were found between antistaphylococcal penicillin regimens (often used in combination with aminoglycosides or other penicillins) and single-agent first- or second-generation cephalosporin regimens.

The reduction in morbidity and mortality associated with postoperative wound infection is the most important result of antimicrobial prophylaxis in surgery. Financial constraints have led many individuals to reevaluate the use of antimicrobial prophylaxis. When the costs associated with the management of postoperative infection are factored into these calculations, the cost-effectiveness of prophylaxis becomes evident.[390,391]

Recommendations. Cephalosporins, as single agents, are at least as effective as combination regimens of antistaphylococcal penicillins and aminoglycosides and are much easier to administer. Cephalothin and cefazolin have been the traditional cephalosporins of choice; however, cefamandole and cefuroxime have been shown to be slightly superior to cefazolin with regard to the overall incidence of postoperative wound infection. Further trials must be performed to confirm their superiority.

The frequency with which methicillin-resistant staphylococci have been recovered has increased steadily in recent years throughout the United States,[392,393] and one would predict that antistaphylococcal penicillins and cephalosporins might be ineffective in a patient colonized with this organism. Insufficient data exist regarding the prophylactic role of vancomycin in cardiothoracic surgery, either with or without an additional agent active against gram-negative pathogens.

It is recommended that cefazolin 1 g intravenously every 8 hours or cefuroxime 1.5 g intravenously every 12 hours be given for 48–72 hours or until chest and mediastinal drainage tubes are removed. Cefamandole and cephalothin are suitable alternatives.

Insufficient data are available to document the appropriateness of cephalosporins in infants less than 1 month of age. Ampicillin (50 mg/kg every 6 hours for a total of four doses) and gentamicin (2.5 mg/kg every 8 hours for a total of three doses) are generally used in this age group. Children older than 1 month should receive cefuroxime 50 mg/kg every 8 hours for three doses.

Orthopedic Surgery

Postoperative wound infection is one of the more frequent complications of orthopedic surgery, and it often yields devastating results. Although early studies did not support the routine use of prophylactic antimicrobials,[394,395] these studies were flawed by an improper choice of agent(s), inappropriate dosage or route of administration, or failure to institute therapy until well beyond the time of the initial surgical incision. Later work has established that antimicrobial prophylaxis is indicated in some types of orthopedic procedures.[396–405]

Antimicrobial prophylaxis will be discussed for total joint-replacement surgery, repair of hip fractures, and clean orthopedic procedures. Open (compound) fractures are often associated with extensive wound contamination and are virtually always managed empirically with antimicrobial therapy as well as surgical debridement. This practice is viewed as treatment rather than prophylaxis.[406] The issue of whether patients with prosthetic joints who undergo dental, gastrointestinal, or genitourinary procedures should receive prophylaxis to reduce the likelihood of prosthesis infection has not been sufficiently studied, and no formal recommendations can be made at this time.

Organisms that make up the skin flora are the most frequent causes of postoperative infections in orthopedic surgery.[396-398,404] Gram-positive organisms such as *Staph. aureus*, *Staph. epidermidis*, and various streptococci, including enterococci, are responsible for more than two-thirds of postoperative infections. Aerobic gram-negative bacilli (e.g., *E. coli* and *Proteus mirabilis*), anaerobes such as peptococci, and diphtheroids constitute the remainder of infecting organisms. The antimicrobials that have been studied most often for prophylaxis in orthopedic surgery include the antistaphylococcal penicillins and first-generation cephalosporins.

First-generation cephalosporins (particularly cefazolin) are the most suitable agents for orthopedic prophylaxis, given their expanded spectrum, which includes gram-negative bacilli (such as *E. coli*), ease of administration, low cost, and safety. Second- and third-generation cephalosporins offer no major advantages over first-generation agents. Agents in the two former groups are more expensive; furthermore, indiscriminate use is likely to promote resistance, particularly to nosocomial gram-negative bacilli. Therefore, the use of second- and third-generation cephalosporins as surgical prophylaxis in orthopedic surgery should be avoided. In patients with serious β-lactam allergy, vancomycin is a suitable alternative agent for surgical prophylaxis.

Total Joint Replacement. The incidence of deep sepsis complicating joint replacements of the hip, knee, elbow, and shoulder is low, ranging from 0.6 to 11%.[396] With the introduction of prophylactic antimicrobials and the use of "ultraclean" operating rooms, the incidence of infection has declined substantially, generally to less than 1%.[396,399,400] The two main types of infectious complications of total joint arthroplasty are superficial wound infections and deep infections of the prosthesis. Deep sepsis of the joint prosthesis may occur as an early (less than 1 year after the procedure) or late (occurring after the first year) complication of joint-replacement surgery. Infection after joint arthroplasty can be disastrous, frequently requiring removal of the prosthesis and a prolonged course of antimicrobials for effective cure.

Clinical trials. The majority of studies evaluating prophylactic antimicrobials in joint-replacement surgery have been conducted in patients undergoing total hip arthroplasty. Early double-blind, controlled trials demonstrated that 14 days of cloxacillin (given with probenecid) can significantly reduce the incidence of early and late infection.[397,398] Ericson et al.[397] reported 10 infections in 48 patients (17%) given placebo and none in those receiving cloxacillin after a 6-month period of followup. Carlsson et al.[398] found a 15% incidence of late, deep infection with no prophylaxis, compared with a 2% incidence with 2 weeks of cloxacillin prophylaxis in a total of 1065 hip-replacement procedures. Although these studies have been criticized because of the unusually high incidence of infection in the control group,[407] they demonstrate a clear-cut decrease in infectious complications with antistaphylococcal prophylaxis.

Hill et al.[399] evaluated the efficacy of prophylactic cefazolin in a double-blind, randomized, placebo-controlled trial involving 2137 hip replacements in 2097 patients. Cefazolin 1 g was given before surgery and continued every

6 hours for a total of 5 days. After a 2-year followup period, "hip infection" was encountered in 3.3% of patients given placebo and in 0.9% of patients who received cefazolin (*p* < 0.001). When these results were further analyzed for the type of operating-room environment, a significant difference was observed only when surgery was carried out in a conventional operating room. Antimicrobial prophylaxis did not significantly reduce infection when hip-replacement surgery was performed in a "hypersterile" (laminar airflow) operating room (1.3% with placebo versus 0.8% with cefazolin). This study was well designed in that sufficient numbers of patients were enrolled to avoid either Type I or II errors in terms of the efficacy of prophylaxis.

The impact of ultraclean operating rooms on deep sepsis following joint-replacement surgery was further evaluated by Lidwell et al.[400] in more than 8000 hip or knee operations. A significant decrease in deep infection was observed with the use of ultraclean operating rooms compared with conventional rooms (0.6 versus 1.5%, respectively). Although not strictly controlled in this study, the use of prophylactic antimicrobials (primarily flucloxacillin) was associated with a further reduction in the rate of deep infection of the prosthesis (*p* < 0.01).[400]

The issue of duration of prophylaxis was addressed by Pollard et al.,[401] who compared three 1-g intramuscular doses of cephaloridine with a 2-week course of flucloxacillin (500 mg intramuscularly for 24 hours, then orally thereafter) in a randomized trial of 297 patients. Wound infection developed in 1.7% of these patients; deep infections, 1.3%. Both occurred with equal frequency in the two treatment groups.

Taken together, the above studies suggest that a short course of antimicrobial prophylaxis can significantly reduce the incidence of postoperative infection in joint-replacement surgery, particularly of late, deep-seated infection. Although infectious complications are infrequent, the consequences of an infected joint prosthesis can be devastating. The use of ultraclean operating rooms has been shown to reduce the incidence of deep sepsis significantly after joint-replacement surgery, regardless of whether antimicrobials are also given.[399,400] Because such operating environments are not widely available, prophylactic administration of antimicrobials with activity directed primarily against *Staph. aureus* is indicated in patients undergoing joint-replacement surgery.

Recommendations. All patients undergoing total hip, elbow, knee, and shoulder arthroplasty should be given cefazolin 1 g intravenously immediately before surgery. Treatment should be continued every 8 hours for a total of three doses. A longer prophylactic regimen does not further reduce the incidence of infection but may increase the likelihood of adverse effects. Patients with β-lactam allergy should be given vancomycin 15 mg/kg intravenously just before surgery. Therapy should be continued every 12 hours for two additional doses.

Repair of Hip Fractures. Because repair of hip fractures often involves internal fixation using foreign bodies such as nails, screws, plates, and wires, postoperative infection can produce extensive morbidity. Consequently, antimicrobial prophylaxis has become an accepted practice, even though the incidence of infection following hip fracture repairs is less than 5%.

Clinical trials. The value of antimicrobial prophylaxis in hip fracture repair was studied in three double-blind, randomized, placebo-controlled trials. Boyd et al.[402] found postoperative wound infections in seven of 145 patients

(4.8%) receiving placebo and in one of 135 patients (0.8%) given nafcillin 0.5 g intramuscularly every 6 hours for 2 days ($p = 0.04$; one-tailed t test). The authors failed to detect a difference in the incidence of infected wound hematomas between the two groups.[402] It has been argued that had Boyd et al. used a two-tailed test, the p value would become 0.08, which is not statistically significant.[407] Given the authors' hypothesis that antimicrobial prophylaxis is likely to result only in a reduction in postoperative infection (as opposed to a possible increase in the incidence of infection), the use of a one-tailed test seems appropriate.

In another study involving 307 patients, Burnett et al.[403] reported major postoperative wound infections in 4.7% of patients given placebo versus 0.7% of those given cephalothin 1 g intravenously on call to the operating room and every 4 hours for 72 hours thereafter ($p < 0.05$). Burnett et al. observed a trend toward colonization with cephalothin-resistant organisms in patients who received this drug as a prophylactic measure.

Tengve and Kjellander[404] compared no antimicrobial prophylaxis with cephalothin 2 g intravenously, preoperatively and intraoperatively and continued every 6 hours for 2 days in 140 patients undergoing repair of trochanteric femur fractures. Patients receiving cephalothin were switched to cephalexin 1 g orally every 6 hours once they were able to take medication by mouth. Postoperative wound infections occurred in 12 of 71 patients (16.9%) given no prophylaxis and in one of 56 patients (1.8%) given cephalothin. The validity of this study may be questionable because of the small number of patients enrolled and the unusually high incidence of wound infections occurring in the control group. Nonetheless, results from the above three studies, taken together, support the efficacy of short-term prophylactic antimicrobials in reducing the incidence of postoperative wound infection in patients undergoing hip fracture repair. The long-term benefits of prophylaxis have not been determined.

Recommendations. Patients undergoing repair of hip fractures, particularly those in whom nails, plates, or screws are to be used, should receive short-term prophylaxis using an agent with activity directed primarily against staphylococci. Cefazolin 1 g intravenously should be initiated before surgery and continued every 8 hours for no more than 48–72 hours. Although cephalothin was used in two of the three studies cited above, cefazolin is preferred because it achieves better bone penetration[406] and higher and more sustained serum concentrations, causes less venous irritation, is more convenient to administer, and, in many cases, is more cost effective. Second- and third-generation cephalosporins should not be used as prophylaxis in hip fracture repairs. Patients with allergy to β-lactams should receive vancomycin at the dosages recommended for joint-replacement surgery.

Clean Orthopedic Procedures. The necessity for prophylactic antimicrobials for clean orthopedic procedures is not well established.[405,408] Included in this category are knee, hand, and foot surgery and laminectomy, with and without fusion. These procedures are considered clean and do not normally involve the implantation of foreign materials. The risk of infection and long-term sequelae is quite low. The risk of infection must be weighed against the cost and the potentially toxic effects of antimicrobial therapy before prophylaxis can be routinely recommended.

Clinical trials. The most extensive investigation of the efficacy of antimicrobial prophylaxis in clean orthopedic

procedures was performed in the early 1970s by Pavel et al.[405] In a randomized, double-blind, prospective study, these authors compared the efficacy of cephaloridine with that of placebo in reducing postoperative wound infection in more than 1500 patients. The incidence of infection was 5% with placebo and 2.8% with perioperative cephaloridine ($p = 0.025$). It was not until more than 1500 cases were assessed that a statistically significant difference between the treatment and control groups was seen.[405] Drug fever (loosely defined as fever occurring in any patient on the days he or she received the study drug) was noted in 34 antimicrobial-treated patients and in 14 patients in the placebo group ($p = 0.06$).

Given the small difference in infection rates between the groups and the lack of significant long-term sequelae associated with these procedures, many authorities have questioned the necessity for prophylactic antimicrobials. Attempts to correlate the incidence of infection with specific types of clean orthopedic procedures or with certain patient characteristics (e.g., age and disease state) have been unsuccessful. While one recent study suggested that prophylaxis (with cefamandole) is more effective than placebo when procedures last longer than 2 hours,[408] these results were not supported by those observed by Pavel et al.,[405] whose series was much larger.

Recommendations. Antimicrobial prophylaxis is not recommended for patients undergoing clean orthopedic procedures. The low incidence of infection, coupled with the absence of serious morbidity as a consequence of postoperative infection, does not justify the expense and potential for toxicity associated with routine use of antimicrobial prophylaxis in this setting.

Vascular Surgery

Infection following peripheral vascular surgery often is associated with extensive morbidity and mortality. Postoperative infection is particularly devastating if it involves the vascular graft material. As a result, antimicrobial prophylaxis is widely used with surgical revascularization.[409]

Clinical Trials. In the first controlled study of antimicrobial prophylaxis in peripheral vascular surgery, Kaiser and colleagues[410] administered cefazolin intravenously on call and then every 6 hours for four doses. If the surgical procedure was longer than 4 hours, an additional 500-mg dose was administered. Only two of 225 patients (0.9%) who were given prophylaxis developed wound infection, compared with 16 of 237 (6.8%) in the control group. This difference was statistically significant. Four deep graft infections were observed in the control group; none occurred in the patients who received cefazolin. No infections were observed among 103 patients who underwent brachiocephalic procedures. Cefazolin-susceptible *Staph. aureus* was the predominant pathogen; however, gram-negative aerobic bacilli, coagulase-negative staphylococci, and enterococci were also isolated.

In a subsequent trial,[411] intravenous cephradine, topical cephradine, or both were compared with placebo in patients undergoing peripheral vascular surgery. Patients were randomly divided into four groups in the following manner:

- Group 1, no antimicrobial.
- Group 2, topical cephradine instilled in the incision before closure.

- Group 3, a 24-hour perioperative course of intravenous cephradine.
- Group 4, topical and intravenous cephradine.

Groups 2–4 had significantly fewer wound infections than did the control group. No infections were noted in patients receiving an intravenous or a topical drug; however, three of 51 patients in Group 4 became infected. Thirteen of those patients receiving no antimicrobial (24.5%) developed wound infections. Ten of 16 infected patients grew *Staph. aureus. E. coli* and other gram-negative bacilli infrequently were associated with infection.

Patients undergoing vascular-access surgery for hemodialysis also benefit from the administration of antistaphylococcal antimicrobials. Perioperative cefamandole (1 g intravenously before surgery and every 6 hours for three doses) was compared with placebo in patients receiving placement of polytetrafluoroethylene vascular-access grafts.[412] Two of 19 cefamandole-treated patients became infected, compared with eight of 19 placebo patients. This difference was statistically significant.

The duration of antimicrobial prophylaxis was investigated by Hasselgren et al.[413] Cefuroxime 1.5 g intravenously every 8 hours was administered for either 1 or 3 days after surgery. A control group received placebo. The incidence of wound infection in control patients was 16.7%, versus 3.8 and 4.3% in the 1- and 3-day groups, respectively. The difference in the incidence of infection between the latter two groups was not significant, and the authors concluded that no benefit is derived from continuing prophylaxis for more than 24 hours in patients undergoing surgery of the lower abdominal vasculature. *Staph. aureus* was the dominant pathogen; however, *Staph. epidermidis* and occasional aerobic gram-negative bacilli were also isolated.

Recommendations. Prophylactic antimicrobials are efficacious in decreasing the rate of infection after vascular procedures involving the lower abdominal vasculature and procedures required for dialysis access. Patients undergoing brachiocephalic procedures do not appear to benefit from antimicrobial prophylaxis. Considering that second-generation cephalosporins (cefamandole and cefuroxime) have not been shown to be superior to first-generation agents (cefazolin and cephradine), the latter are recommended. Because of its long half-life, cefazolin is recommended over shorter-acting agents. Cefazolin 1 g (30 mg/kg for children) intravenously should be administered at the induction of anesthesia and every 8 hours for 24 hours. Prolongation of prophylaxis for more than 24 postoperative hours is unnecessary. For patients with a history of an accelerated reaction to β-lactam agents, vancomycin is recommended.

Urological Surgery

The potential benefit of antimicrobial prophylaxis in urological surgery has been investigated in many clinical trials, particularly in patients undergoing transurethral resection of the prostate.[414–428] Many patients with resection of bladder tumors[429] have also been studied. A wide range of antimicrobial regimens, including cephalosporins,[415,417,419,421,423,425,426,429] aminoglycosides,[414,420,427,428] carbenicillin,[416,418] trimethoprim–sulfamethoxazole,[419,422] and nitrofurantoin,[424] has been used in these trials.

The most common infectious complication after urological procedures is bacteriuria, the incidence of which

has varied from 0 to 54% in reported studies. More serious infection, including bacteremia, is rare after transurethral resection of the prostate. In general, *E. coli* is most commonly isolated in patients with postoperative bacteriuria; however, other gram-negative bacilli and enterococci also cause infection.

Considering that bacteriuria is the most common postoperative infection after urological surgery, it is important to emphasize certain points. First, to determine the effectiveness of antimicrobial prophylaxis, one must be certain that the urine was sterile before surgery. Patients with preoperative bacteriuria must be considered infected, and the use of antimicrobials becomes therapeutic rather than prophylactic. Second, since these patients are routinely catheterized, one must question whether postoperative bacteriuria has been caused by the catheter or the surgical procedure. Furthermore, the length of postoperative catheterization, mode of irrigation (closed versus open), and other factors must be incorporated into the analysis of the effectiveness of antimicrobial prophylaxis.

A review of the literature reveals that antimicrobials generally have not been found to decrease the incidence of postoperative bacteriuria when infection rates are less than 15%.[415–418] When the incidence of infection is greater than 20%, however, a marked antimicrobial effect has been observed.[420–422,424–428] Considering the low rate of serious postoperative infection, it is not surprising that prophylactic antimicrobials have not been shown to decrease the incidence of bacteremia.

The results of these studies suggest that no single antimicrobial regimen is superior to another. Broad-spectrum antimicrobials, such as aminoglycosides or second- and third-generation cephalosporins, are no more effective than first-generation cephalosporins or oral agents (trimethoprim–sulfamethoxazole and nitrofurantoin). Although a large number of the trials continued prophylaxis for up to 3 weeks postoperatively,[414,416,418,420–422,424,426] the most recent studies suggest that continuation of prophylaxis after the preoperative dose is unnecessary.[425,427,428]

Recommendations. Considering the low risk of serious infection after urological surgery, antimicrobial prophylaxis should be considered only in those patients considered to be at high risk of postoperative bacteriuria (e.g., those with prolonged postoperative catheterization) or in hospitals with infection rates of greater than 20%. Low risk patients do not appear to benefit from the use of perioperative antimicrobials. If oral antimicrobials are used, a single dose of trimethoprim–sulfamethoxazole or cephalexin (or cephradine) 500 mg within 2 hours of surgery should be administered. If an injectable agent is recommended, cefazolin 1 g intravenously (30 mg/kg for pediatric patients), administered at the induction of anesthesia, is recommended. Continuation of antimicrobial prophylaxis postoperatively is not recommended.

References

1. Platt R, Zaleznik DF, Hopkins CC, et al. Perioperative antibiotic prophylaxis for herniorrhaphy and breast surgery. *N Engl J Med*. 1990; 322:153–60.
2. Kernodle DS, Classen DC, Burke JP, et al. Failure of cephalosporins to prevent *Staphylococcus aureus* surgical wound infection. *JAMA*. 1990; 263:961–6.
3. Ariano RE, Zhanel GG. Antimicrobial prophylaxis in

coronary bypass surgery: a critical appraisal. *DICP.* 1991; 25:478–84.

4. Robbins KT, Favrot S, Hanna D, et al. Risk of wound infection in patients with head and neck cancer. *Head Neck.* 1990; (Mar/Apr):143–8.

5. Tabet JC, Johnson JT. Wound infection in head and neck surgery: prophylaxis, etiology and management. *J Otolaryngol.* 1990; 3:143–8.

6. Tramont EC. Host defense mechanisms. In: Mandell GL, Douglas RG, Bennett JE, eds. Principles and practice of infectious disease. 3rd ed. New York: Churchill; 1990:33–6.

7. Becker GD, Welch WD. Quantitative bacteriology of closed-suction wound drainage in contaminated surgery. *Laryngoscope.* 1990; 100:403–6.

8. Johnson JT, Yu VL. Role of aerobic gram-negative rods, anaerobes, and fungi in wound infection after head and neck surgery: implications for antibiotic prophylaxis. *Head Neck.* 1989; (Jan/Feb):27–9.

9. Rubin J, Johnson JT, Wagner RL, et al. Bacteriologic analysis of wound infection following major head and neck surgery. *Arch Otolaryngol Head Neck Surg.* 1988; 114:969–72.

10. Brown BM, Johnson JT, Wagner RL. Etiologic factors in head and neck wound infections. *Laryngoscope.* 1987; 97:587–90.

11. Johnson JT, Yu VL, Myers EN, et al. An assessment of the need for gram-negative bacterial coverage in antibiotic prophylaxis for oncological head and neck surgery. *J Infect Dis.* 1987; 155:331–3.

12. Atkinson BA. Species incidence, trends of susceptibility to antibiotics in the United States, and minimum inhibitory concentration. In: Lorian V, ed. Antibiotics in laboratory medicine. Baltimore: Williams & Wilkins; 1980:607–722.

13. Johnson JT, Wagner RL. Infection following uncontaminated head and neck surgery. *Arch Otolaryngol Head Neck Surg.* 1987; 113:368–9.

14. Brand B, Johnson JT, Myers EN, et al. Prophylactic perioperative antibiotics in contaminated head and neck surgery. *Otolaryngol Head Neck Surg.* 1982; 90:315–8.

15. Mandell-Brown M, Johnson JT, Wagner RL. Cost-effectiveness of prophylactic antibiotics in head and neck surgery. *Otolaryngol Head Neck Surg.* 1984; 92:520–3.

16. Johnson JT, Yu VL, Myers EN, et al. Efficacy of two third-generation cephalosporins in prophylaxis for head and neck surgery. *Arch Orolaryngol.* 1984; 110:224–7.

17. Johnson JT, Yu VL, Myers EN, et al. Cefazolin vs moxalactam? A double blind randomized trial of cephalosporins in head and neck surgery. *Arch Otolaryngol Head Neck Surg.* 1986; 112:151–3.

18. Antimicrobial prophylaxis in surgery. *Med Lett Drugs Ther.* 1989; 31:105–8.

19. Gerard M, Meunier F, Dor P, et al. Antimicrobial prophylaxis for major head and neck surgery in cancer patients. *Antimicrob Agents Chemother.* 1988; 32:1557–9.

20. Cuchural GJ, Tally FP, Macobus NV, et al. Comparative activities of new beta-lactam agents against members of the *Bacteroides fragilis* group. *Antimicrob Agents Chemother.* 1990; 34:479–80.

21. Dor P, Klastersky J. Prophylactic antibiotics in oral pharyngeal and laryngeal surgery for cancer: a double-

blind study. *Laryngoscope.* 1973; 83:1992–8.

22. Dor P, Klastersky J. Etude comparative de la ticarcillin et de la carbenicillin comme traitement prophylactique associé à la chirurgie carcinologique cervico-faciale. *Acta Chir.* 1976; 75:129–33.

23. Mombelli G, Coppens L, Dor P, et al. Antibiotic prophylaxis in surgery for head and neck cancer. Comparative study of short and prolonged administration of carbenicillin. *J Antimicrob Chemother.* 1981; 7:665–7.

24. VanLaethem Y, Lagast H, Klastersky J. Anaerobic infections in cancer patients—comparison between therapy oriented strictly against anaerobes or both anaerobes and aerobes. *J Antimicrob Chemother.* 1982; 10:137–40.

25. Johnson JT, Meyers EN, Thearle PB, et al. Antimicrobial prophylaxis for contaminated head and neck surgery. *Laryngoscope.* 1984; 94:46–51.

26. Saginur R, Odell PF, Poliquin JF. Antibiotic prophylaxis in head and neck cancer surgery. *J Otolaryngol.* 1988; 17:78–80.

27. Robbins KT, Byers RM, Fainstein V, et al. Wound prophylaxis with metronidazole in head and neck surgical oncology. *Laryngoscope.* 1988; 98:803–6.

28. Gehanno P, Noisy N, Guedon C. Cefotaxime in the prophylaxis of otorhinolaryngological cancer surgery. *Drugs.* 1988; 35(Suppl 2):111–5.

29. Polk HC. Diminished surgical infection by systemic antibiotic administration in potentially contaminated operations. *Surgery.* 1974; 75:312–4.

30. Stone HH, Hooper CA, Kolb LD, et al. Antibiotic prophylaxis in gastric, biliary and colonic surgery. *Ann Surg.* 1976; 184:443–52.

31. Renvall S, Nikoski J, Aho AJ. Wound infection in abdominal surgery. *Acta Chir Scand.* 1980; 146:25–30.

32. Cunha BA, Pyrtek LJ, Quintiliani R. Prophylactic antibiotic in cholecystectomy. *Lancet.* 1978; 2:207–8.

33. Strachan CJL, Black J, Powis SJA, et al. Prophylactic use of cephazolin against wound sepsis after cholecystectomy. *Br Med J.* 1977; 1:1254–6.

34. McLeish AR, Keighley MRB, Bishop HM. Selecting patients requiring antibiotics in biliary surgery by immediate gram stains of bile at surgery. *Surgery.* 1977; 81:473–7.

35. Reiss R, Eliasive A, Deutsch A. Septic complication and bile culture in 800 consecutive cholecystectomies. *World J Surg.* 1982; 6:195–9.

36. Cainzos M, Potel J, Puente JL. Prospective randomized controlled study of prophylaxis with cefamandole in high risk patients undergoing operations upon the biliary tract. *Surg Gynecol Obstet.* 1985; 160:27–32.

37. Elliot DW. Biliary tract surgery. *South Med J.* 1977; 70(Suppl 1):31–4.

38. Chetlin SH, Elliott DW. Preoperative antibiotics in biliary surgery. *Arch Surg.* 1973; 107:319–23.

39. Berne TV, Yellin AE, Appleman MD, et al. Controlled comparison of cefmetazole with cefoxitin for prophylaxis in elective cholecystectomy. *Surg Gynecol Obstet.* 1990; 170:137–40.

40. Wilson SE, Hopkins JA, Williams RA. A comparison of cefotaxime versus cefamandole in prophylaxis for surgical treatment of the biliary tract. *Surg Gynecol Obstet.* 1987; 164:207–12.

41. Kujath P. Brief report: antibiotic prophylaxis in biliary tract surgery. *Am J Med.* 1989; 87(Suppl 5A):255–7.

42. Nanavati AL, Singer JA. Routine bile cultures during cholecystectomy. *Infect Surg*. 1977; 6:523–6.

43. Garibaldi RA, Skolnck D, Maglio S, et al. Post-cholecystectomy wound infection. *Ann Surg*. 1986; 204:650–4.

44. Levi JU, Martinez OV, Hutson DG, et al. Ampicillin versus cefamandole in biliary tract surgery. *Am Surg*. 1984; 50:412–7.

45. Kellum JM, Duma RJ, Gorbach SL, et al. Single-dose antibiotic prophylaxis for biliary surgery. *Arch Surg*. 1987; 122:918–22.

46. Muller EL, Pitt HA, Thompson JE, et al. Antibiotics in infections of the biliary tract. *Surg Gynecol Obstet*. 1987; 165:285–92.

47. Meijer WS, Schmitz PIM, Jeeke J. Meta-analysis of randomized, controlled clinical trials of antibiotic prophylaxis in biliary tract surgery. *Br J Surg*. 1990; 77: 282–90.

48. Kellum JM, Gargano S, Gorbach SL, et al. Antibiotic prophylaxis in high-risk biliary operations: multicenter trial of single preoperative ceftriaxone versus multidose cefazolin. *Am J Surg*. 1984; 148:15–21.

49. Drumm J, Donovan IA, Wise R. A comparison of cefotetan and cephazolin for prophylaxis against wound infection after elective cholecystectomy. *J Hosp Infect*. 1985; 6:227–80.

50. Plouffe JF, Perkins RL, Fass RJ, et al. Comparison of the effectiveness of moxalactam and cefazolin in the prevention of infection in patients undergoing abdominal operations. *Diagn Microbiol Infect Dis*. 1985; 3:25–31.

51. Crenshaw CA, Glanges E, Webber CE, et al. A prospective randomized, double blind study of preventive cefamandole therapy in patients at high risk for undergoing cholecystectomy. *Surg Gynecol Obstet*. 1981; 153:546–52.

52. Leaper DJ, Cooper MJ, Turner A. A comparative trial between cefotetan and cephazolin for wound sepsis prophylaxis during elective upper gastrointestinal surgery with an investigation of cefotetan penetration into the obstructed biliary tree. *J Hosp Infect*. 1986; 7:269–76.

53. Hurlow RA, Strachan CJL, Wise R, et al. A comparative study of the efficacy of cefuroxime for preventing wound sepsis after cholecystectomy. International Congress and Symposium series: Royal Society of Medicine; 1981:1–8.

54. Maki DG, Lammers JL, Aughey DR. Comparative studies of multidose cefoxitin vs single dose cefonicid for surgical prophylaxis in patients undergoing biliary tract operations or hysterectomy. *Rev Infect Dis*. 1984; 6(Suppl):887–95.

55. Roufail WM. Comparison of cefonicid and cefoxitin for prophylaxis in biliary tract surgery. *Adv Ther*. 1985; 2:225–32.

56. Fabian TC, Zellner SR, Gazzaniga A, et al. Multicenter open trial of cefotetan in elective biliary surgery. *Am J Surg*. 1988; 155:77–80.

57. Garcia-Rodriguez JA, Puig-LaCalle J, Arnau C, et al. Antibiotic prophylaxis with cefotaxime in gastroduodenal and biliary surgery. *Am J Surg*. 1989; 158:428–32.

58. Lewis RT, Allan CM, Goodall RG, et al. A single preoperative dose of cefazolin prevents postoperative sepsis in high-risk biliary surgery. *Dis Colon Rectum*. 1984; 27:44–7.

59. Targarona EM, Garau J, Munoz-Ramos C, et al. Single-dose antibiotic prophylaxis in patients at high risk for infection in biliary surgery: a prospective and randomized study comparing cefonicid with mezlocillin. *Surgery*. 1990; 107:327–34.

60. Nichols RL, Webb WR, Jones JW, et al. Efficacy of antibiotic prophylaxis in high risk gastroduodenal operations. *Am J Surg*. 1982; 143:94–8.

61. Stone HH. Gastric surgery. *South Med J*. 1977; 70 (Suppl 1):35–7.

62. Morris DL, Yound D, Burdon DW, et al. Prospective randomized trial of single dose cefuroxime against mezlocillin in elective gastric surgery. *J Hosp Infect*. 1984; 5:200–4.

63. Lewis RT, Allan CM, Goodall RG, et al. Discriminate use of antibiotic prophylaxis in gastroduodenal surgery. *Am J Surg*. 1979; 138:640–3.

64. Pories WJ, Van Rij AM, Burlingham BT, et al. Prophylactic cefazolin in gastric bypass surgery. *Surgery*. 1981; 90:426–32.

65. Ruddell WSJ, Axon ATR, Findlay JM, et al. Effect of cimetidine on the gastric bacterial flora. *Lancet*. 1980; 1:672–4.

66. LoCiero J, Nichols RL. Sepsis after gastroduodenal operations; relationship to gastric acid, motility, and endogenous microflora. *South Med J*. 1980; 73:878–80.

67. Gorbach SL, Plaut AG, Nahas L, et al. Studies of intestinal microflora: II. Microorganisms of the small intestine and their relations to oral fecal flora. *Gastroenterology*. 1967; 53:856–67.

68. Gorbach SL. Intestinal microflora. *Gastroenterology*. 1971; 60:1110–29.

69. Lewis RT, Allan CM, Goodall RG, et al. Cefamandole in gastroduodenal surgery: a controlled prospective, randomized, double-blind study. *Can J Surg*. 1982; 25:561–3.

70. Polk HC, Lopez-Mayor JF. Postoperative wound infection: a prospective study of determinant factors and prevention. *Surgery*. 1969; 66:97–103.

71. Evans C, Pollock AV. The reduction of surgical wound infections by prophylactic parenteral cephaloridine. *Br J Surg*. 1973; 60:434–7.

72. Stone HH, Haney BB, Kolb LD, et al. Prophylactic and preventive antibiotic therapy. *Ann Surg*. 1979; 189:691–9.

73. Mitchell NJ, Evans DS, Pollock D. Pre-operative, single-dose cefuroxime antimicrobial prophylaxis with and without metronidazole in elective gastrointestinal surgery. *J Antimicrob Chemother*. 1980; 6:393–9.

74. Hares MM, Hegarty MA, Warlow J, et al. A controlled trial to compare systemic and intra-incisional cefuroxime prophylaxis in high risk gastric surgery. International Congress and Symposium series: Royal College of Medicine. 1981:9–15.

75. Brown JJ, Mutton TP, Wasilauskas BL, et al. Prospective, randomized, controlled trial of ticarcillin and cephalothin as prophylactic antibiotics for gastrointestinal operations. *Am J Surg*. 1982; 143:343–8.

76. Polk HC, Trachtenberg L, George CD. A randomized, double-blind trial of single dose piperacillin versus multidose cefoxitin in alimentary tract operations. *Am J Surg*. 1986; 152:517–21.

77. Svensson LG. Prophylactic antibiotic administration. *S Afr J Surg*. 1985; 23:55–62.

78. Polk H, Lopez-Meyer J. Postoperative wound infec-

tion: a prospective study of determinant factors and prevention. *Surgery*. 1969; 66:97–103.

79. Burton RC. Postoperative wound infection in colon and rectal surgery. *Br J Surg*. 1973; 60:363–8.

80. Bartlett J, Condon R, Gorbach S, et al. Veterans Administration Cooperative Study on bowel preparation for elective colorectal operations: impact of oral antibiotic regimen on colonic flora, wound irrigation cultures and bacteriology of septic complications. *Ann Surg*. 1978; 188:249–54.

81. Clarke J, Condon R, Bartlett J, et al. Preoperative oral antibiotics reduce septic complications of colon operations: results of a prospective randomized, double-blind clinical study. *Ann Surg*. 1977; 186:251–9.

82. Nichols RL. Prophylaxis for elective bowel surgery. In: Wilson SE, Williams RA, Finegold S, eds. Intra-abdominal infections. New York: McGraw Hill; 1982:267–85.

83. Davis G, Santa Ana C, Morawiski S, et al. Development of a lavage solution associated with minimal water and electrolyte absorption or secretion. *Gastroenterology*. 1980; 78:991–5.

84. Beck D, Harford F, DiPalma JA. Comparison of cleansing methods in preparation for colon surgery. *Dis Colon Rectum*. 1985; 28:491–5.

85. Jagelman D, Fazio V, Lavery I, et al. Single dose piperacillin versus cefoxitin combined with 10 percent mannitol bowel preparation as prophylaxis in elective colorectal operations. *Am J Surg*. 1987; 154:478–81.

86. Wolff B, Beart R, Dozios R, et al. A new bowel preparation for elective colon and rectal surgery: a prospective, randomized clinical trial. *Arch Surg*. 1988; 123:895–900.

87. Garlock JH, Seely GP. The use of sulfanilamide in surgery of the rectum and colon. *Surgery*. 1939; 5:787–90.

88. Baum M, Anish D, Chalmers T, et al. A survey of clinical trials of antibiotic prophylaxis in colon surgery: evidence against further use of no treatment controls. *N Engl J Med*. 1981; 305:795–9.

89. Bartlett S, Burton R. Effects of prophylactic antibiotics on wound infection after elective colon and rectal surgery. *Am J Surg*. 1983; 145:300–9.

90. Chodak GW, Plaut ME. Use of systemic antibiotics for prophylaxis in surgery. *Arch Surg*. 1977; 112:326–34.

91. Berger SA, Nager H, Weitzman S. Prophylactic antibiotics in surgical procedures. *Surg Gynecol Obstet*. 1978; 146:469–75.

92. Evans M, Pollock AV. The inadequacy of published random control trials of antibacterial prophylaxis in colorectal surgery. *Dis Colon Rectum*. 1987; 30:743–6.

93. National Research Council, National Academy of Sciences. Postoperative wound infections: the influence of ultraviolet irradiation on the operating room and on various other factors. *Ann Surg*. 1965; 160(Suppl):1–192.

94. Cruse PJ, Foord R. The epidemiology of wound infection: a ten-year prospective study of 62,939 wounds. *Surg Clin North Am*. 1980; 60:27–40.

95. Nichols RL. Prophylaxis for intraabdominal surgery. *Rev Infect Dis*. 1984; 6(Suppl 1):276–82.

96. Condon RE. Preoperative antibiotic bowel preparation. *Drug Ther*. 1983; Jan:29–37.

97. Washington J, Dearing W, Judd E, et al. Effect of preoperative antibiotic regimen on development of infection after intestinal surgery. *Ann Surg*. 1974; 180:567–72.

98. Nichols R, Condon R, Gorbach S, et al. Efficacy of preoperative antimicrobial preparation of the bowel. *Ann Surg*. 1972; 176:227–32.

99. Nichols R, Broldo P, Condon R, et al. Effect of preoperative neomycin–erythromycin intestinal preparation on the incidence of infectious complications following colon surgery. *Ann Surg*. 1973; 178:453–62.

100. Stellato T, Danziger L, Gordon N, et al. Antibiotics in elective colon surgery: a randomized trial of oral, systemic, and oral/systemic antibiotics for prophylaxis. *Am Surg*. 1990; 56:251–4.

101. Maki D, Aughey D, Lammers J. Study of cefazolin, cefoxitin, and ceftizoxime for prophylaxis of colorectal surgery. Paper presented at 24th Interscience Conference on Antimicrobial Agents and Chemotherapy. Washington, DC: 1984 Oct 10.

102. Petrelli N, Contre C, Herrera L, et al. A prospective randomized trial of perioperative prophylactic cefamandole in elective colorectal surgery for malignancy. *Dis Colon Rectum*. 1988; 31:427–9.

103. Felip JF, Bonet EB, Eisman FI, et al. Oral is superior to systemic antibiotic prophylaxis in operations upon the colon and rectum. *Surg Gynecol Obstet*. 1984; 158:359–62.

104. Kling PA, Dahlgren S. Oral prophylaxis with neomycin and erythromycin in colorectal surgery; more proof for efficacy than failure. *Arch Surg*. 1989; 124:705–7.

105. Lewis RT, Goodall RG, Marien B, et al. Is neomycin necessary for bowel preparation in surgery of the colon? Oral neomycin plus erythromycin versus erythromycin–metronidazole. *Dis Colon Rectum*. 1989; 32:265–70.

106. Keithly MR, Arabi Y, Alexander-Williams J, et al. Comparison between systemic and oral antimicrobial prophylaxis in colorectal surgery. *Lancet*. 1979; 1:894–7.

107. Lewis RT, Allan CM, Goodall RG, et al. Are first-generation cephalosporins effective for antibiotic prophylaxis in elective surgery of the colon? *Can J Surg*. 1983; 26:504–7.

108. Edmondson HT, Rissing JP. Prophylactic antibiotics in colon surgery: cephaloridine vs erythromycin and neomycin. *Arch Surg*. 1983; 118:227–1.

109. Wapnick S, Gunito R, Leveen HH, et al. Reduction of postoperative infection in elective colorectal surgery with preoperative administration of kanamycin and erythromycin. *Surgery*. 1979; 85:317–21.

110. Hagen TB, Bergan T, Liavag I. Prophylactic metronidazole in elective colorectal surgery. *Acta Chir Scand*. 1980; 146:71–5.

111. Gahhos FN, Richards GK, Hinchey EJ, et al. Elective colon surgery: clindamycin versus metronidazole prophylaxis. *Can J Surg*. 1982; 25:613–6.

112. Dion YM, Richards GK, Prentis JJ, et al. The influence of oral metronidazole versus parenteral preoperative metronidazole on sepsis following colon surgery. *Ann Surg*. 1980; 192:221–6.

113. Beggs FD, Jobanputra RS, Holmes JT. A comparison of intravenous and oral metronidazole as prophylactic in colorectal surgery. *Br J Surg*. 1982; 69:226–7.

114. Goldring J, McNaught W, Scott A, et al. Prophylactic oral antimicrobial agents in elective colonic surgery: a

controlled trial. *Lancet.* 1975; 2:997–9.

115. Willis A, Fergunson I, Jones P, et al. Metronidazole in prevention and treatment of *Bacteroides* infections in elective colonic surgery. *Br Med J.* 1977; 1:607–10.

116. Bjerkesett T, Digranes A. Systemic prophylaxis with metronidazole (Flagyl) in elective surgery of the colon and rectum. *Surgery.* 1980; 87:560–6.

117. Hojer H, Wehherfors J. Systemic prophylaxis with doxycycline in surgery of the colon and rectum. *Ann Surg.* 1978; 187:362–8.

118. Periti P, Mazzei T, Tonelli F. Single dose cefotetan vs multiple dose cefoxitin-antimicrobial prophylaxis in colorectal surgery: results of a prospective, multicenter, randomized study. *Dis Colon Rectum.* 1989; 32:121–7.

119. Jagelman D, Fabian T, Nichols R, et al. Single dose cefotetan versus multiple dose cefoxitin as prophylaxis in colorectal surgery. *Am J Surg.* 1988; 155:71–6.

120. Hoffman C, McDonald P, Watts J. Use of perioperative cefoxitin to prevent infection after colonic and rectal surgery. *Ann Surg.* 1981; 193:353–6.

121. Morton A, Taylor E, Wells G. A multicenter study to compare cefotetan alone with cefotetan and metronidazole as prophylaxis against infection in elective colorectal operations. *Surg Gynecol Obstet.* 1989; 169:4–45.

122. Hinchey E, Richards G, Lewis R, et al. Moxalactam as single agent prophylaxis in the prevention of wound infection following colon surgery. *Surgery.* 1987; 101:15–9.

123. Madsen M, Toftgaard C, Graversen H, et al. Cefoxitin for one day vs ampicillin and metronidazole for three days in elective colorectal surgery: a prospective, randomized, multicenter study. *Dis Colon Rectum.* 1988; 31:774–7.

124. Coppa G, Eng K. Factors involved in antibiotic selection in elective colon and rectal surgery. *Surgery.* 1988; 104:853–8.

125. Cunliffe WJ, Carr N, Schofield PF. Prophylactic metronidazole with and without cefuroxime in elective colorectal surgery. *J R Coll Surg Edinb.* 1985; 30:123–5.

126. McCulloch PG, Blamey SL, Finlay IG, et al. A prospective comparison of gentamicin and metronidazole and moxalactam in the prevention of septic complications associated with elective operations of the colon and rectum. *Surg Gynecol Obstet.* 1986; 162:521–30.

127. Roland M. Prophylactic regimens in colorectal surgery: an open randomized consecutive trial of metronidazole used alone or in combination with ampicillin or doxycycline. *World J Surg.* 1986; 10:1003–8.

128. McDermott F, Polyglase A, Johnson W, et al. Prevention of wound infection in colorectal resections by preoperative cephazolin with and without metronidazole. *Aust NZ J Surg.* 1981; 51:351–3.

129. Panichi G, Pantosto A, Giunchi G, et al. Cephalothin, cefoxitin, or metronidazole in elective colorectal surgery? A single-blind randomized trial. *Am J Surg.* 1979; 137:68–74.

130. Kaiser A, Herrington J, Jacobs J, et al. Cefoxitin vs erythromycin, neomycin and cefazolin in colorectal surgery: importance of the duration of the operative procedure. *Ann Surg.* 1983; 198:525–30.

131. Blair J, McLeod R, Cohen Z, et al. Ticarcillin/clavulanic acid (Timentin) compared to metronidazole/netilmicin

in preventing postoperative infection after elective colorectal surgery. *Can J Surg.* 1987; 30:120–2.

132. Bell GA, Smith JA, Murphy J. Prophylactic antibiotics in elective colon surgery. *Surgery.* 1983; 93:204–8.

133. Lozano F, Alonso AG, Almazan A, et al. A comparison of three different prophylactic parenteral antibiotic regimens in colorectal surgery: a prospective study. *Int Surg.* 1985; 70:227–31.

134. Juul PZ. Klaaborg KE, Kronborg O. Single or multiple doses of metronidazole and ampicillin in elective colorectal surgery: a randomized trial. *Dis Colon Rectum.* 1987; 30:526–8.

135. University of Melbourne Colorectal Group. A comparison of single dose Timentin with mezlocillin for prophylaxis of wound infection in elective colorectal surgery. *Dis Colon Rectum.* 1989; 32:940–3.

136. Goransson G, Nilsson–Ehle I, Olsson S, et al. Single versus multiple dose doxycycline prophylaxis in elective colorectal surgery. *Acta Chir Scand.* 1984; 150:245–9.

137. Bergman L, Solhaug JH. Single-dose chemoprophylaxis in elective colorectal surgery. *Ann Surg.* 1987; 205:77–81.

138. Olsen PR, Andersen HH, Hebjorn M, et al. The prophylaxis of metronidazole in colorectal surgery. *Dan Med Bull.* 1983; 30:345–8.

139. Condon RE, Bartlett JG, Nichols RL, et al. Preoperative prophylactic cephalothin fails to control septic complications of colorectal operations: results of a controlled clinical trial. *Am J Surg.* 1979; 137:68–74.

140. Stone HH, Hooper CA, Kolb LD, et al. Antibiotic prophylaxis in gastric, biliary, and colonic surgery. *Ann Surg.* 1976; 184:443–50.

141. Jones RN, Wojeski W, Bakke J, et al. Antibiotic prophylaxis to 1,036 patients undergoing elective surgical procedures. A prospective randomized comparative trial of cefazolin, cefoxitin, and cefotaxime in a prepaid medical practice. *Am J Surg.* 1987; 153:341–6.

142. Shatney CH. Antibiotic prophylaxis in elective gastrointestinal tract surgery: a comparison of single dose preoperative cefotaxime and multiple dose cefoxitin. *J Antimicrob Chemother.* 1984; 14(Suppl B):241–5.

143. Condon RE, Bartlett J, Greenlee H, et al. Efficacy of oral and systemic antibiotic prophylaxis in colorectal operations. *Arch Surg.* 1983; 118:496–502.

144. Coppa G, Eng K, Gouge T, et al. Parenteral and oral antibiotics in elective colorectal surgery: a prospective randomized trial. *Am J Surg.* 1983; 145:62–5.

145. Jagelman DG, Fazio VW, Lavery IC, et al. A prospective, randomized double-blind study of 10% mannitol mechanical bowel preparation combined with oral neomycin and short-term, perioperative, intravenous Flagyl as prophylaxis in elective colorectal resections. *Surgery.* 1985; 98:861–5.

146. Barbar MS, Hirxberg BC, Rice C, et al. Parenteral antibiotics in elective colon surgery? A prospective, controlled clinical study. *Surgery.* 1979; 86:23–9.

147. Galandiuk S, Polk HC, Jagelman DG, et al. Reemphasis of priorities in surgical antibiotic prophylaxis. *Surg Gynecol Obstet.* 1989; 169:219–22.

148. Shapiro M, Munoz A, Tasger I, et al. Risk factors for infection at the operative site after abdominal or vaginal hysterectomy. *N Engl J Med.* 1982; 307:1661–6.

149. DiPiro JT, Cheung RP, Bowden TA, et al. Single dose

systemic antibiotic prophylaxis of surgical wound infections. *Am J Surg.* 1986; 152:552–9.

150. Hall JC, Watts MK, O'Brien P, et al. Single dose antibiotic prophylaxis in contaminated abdominal surgery. *Arch Surg.* 1989; 124:244–7.

151. Kasier AB. Antimicrobial prophylaxis in surgery. *N Engl J Med.* 1986; 315:1129–38.

152. Lambert WG, Mullinger BM. Single dose cefuroxime in the prophylaxis of abdominal wound sepsis. *Curr Med Res Opin.* 1980; 6:404–6.

153. DiPiro JT, Welage LS, Levine BA, et al. Single dose cefmetazole versus multiple dose cefoxitin for prophylaxis in abdominal surgery. *J Antimicrob Chemother.* 1989; 23(Suppl D):71–7.

154. Stone H, Haney B, Kolb L, et al. Prophylactic and preventative antibiotic therapy: timing, duration and economics. *Ann Surg.* 1979; 189:691–9.

155. Solla J, Rothenberger D. Preoperative bowel preparation: a survey of colon and rectal surgeons. *Dis Colon Rectum.* 1990; 33:154–9.

156. Gilmore OJ, Martin TD. Aetiology and prevention of wound infection in appendectomy. *Br J Surg.* 1974; 62:567–72.

157. Pinto DJ, Sanderson PJ. Rational use of antibiotic therapy after appendectomy. *Br Med J.* 1980; 280:275–7.

158. Keighley MR. Infection: prophylaxis. *Br Med Bull.* 1988; 44:374–402.

159. Winslow RE, Rem D, Harley JW. Acute nonperforating appendicitis: efficacy of brief antibiotic prophylaxis. *Arch Surg.* 1983; 118:651–5.

160. Keiser TA, Mackenzie RL, Feld LN. Prophylactic metronidazole in appendectomy: a double-blind controlled trial. *Surgery.* 1983; 93:201–3.

161. Ahmed ME, Ibrahim SZ, Arabi YE, et al. Metronidazole prophylaxis in acute mural appendicitis: failure of a single intra-operative infusion to reduce wound infection. *J Hosp Infect.* 1987; 10:260–4.

162. Donovan IA, Ellis D, Gatehouse D, et al. One-dose antibiotic prophylaxis against wound infection after appendectomy: a randomized trial of clindamycin, cefazolin sodium and a placebo. *Br J Surg.* 1979; 66: 193–6.

163. O'Rourke MGE, Wynne MJ, Morahan RJ, et al. Prophylactic antibiotics in appendectomy: a prospective double blind randomized study. *Aust NZ J Surg.* 1984; 54:535–41.

164. Lau WY, Fan ST, Chu KW, et al. Cefoxitin versus gentamicin and metronidazole in prevention of postappendectomy sepsis: a randomized, prospective trial. *J Antimicrob Chemother.* 1986; 18:613–9.

165. Lau WY, Fan ST, Yiu TF, et al. Prophylaxis of postappendectomy sepsis by metronidazole and ampicillin; a randomized, prospective and double blind trial. *Br J Surg.* 1983; 70:155–7.

166. Lau WY, Fan ST, Yiu TF, et al. Prophylaxis of postappendectomy sepsis by metronidazole and cefotaxime; a randomized, prospective and double blind trial. *Br J Surg.* 1983; 70:670–2.

167. Lau WY, Fan ST, Chu KW, et al. Randomized, prospective, and double-blind trial of new beta-lactams in the treatment of appendicitis. *Antimicrob Agents Chemother.* 1985; 28:639–42.

168. Panichi G, Pantosti AL, Marsiglio F. Cephalothin or cefoxitin in appendectomy? *J Antimicrob Chemother.* 1980; 6:801–4. Letter.

169. McIntosh GS, Jacob G, Townell NH, et al. Prevention of post-appendectomy sepsis by mezlocillin and metronidazole: a prospective randomized, double-blind trial. *J Antimicrob Chemother.* 1984; 14:537–42.

170. Jensen NG, Bach–Nilsen P, Damgaard B, et al. A Danish multicenter study; cefoxitin versus ampicillin vs. metronidazole in perforated appendicitis. *Br J Surg.* 1984; 71:144–6.

171. Stone HH. Bacterial flora of appendicitis in children. *J Pediatr Surg.* 1976; 11:37–42.

172. Berne TV, Appleman MD, Chenella FC, et al. Surgically treated gangrenous or perforated appendicitis: a comparison of aztreonam and clindamycin versus gentamicin and clindamycin. *Ann Surg.* 1987; 205: 133–7.

173. Berne TV, Yellin AW, Appleman MD, et al. Antibiotic management of surgically treated gangrenous or perforated appendicitis; comparison of gentamicin and clindamycin versus cefamandole versus cefoperazone. *Am J Surg.* 1982; 144:8–13.

174. Corder AP, Bates T, Prior JE, et al. Metronidazole v. cefoxitin in severe appendicitis: a trial to compare a single intraoperative dose of two antibiotics given intravenously. *Postgrad Med J.* 1983; 59:720–3.

175. Flannigan GM, Clifford RP, Carver RA, et al. Antibiotic prophylaxis in acute appendicitis. *Surg Gynecol Obstet.* 1983; 156:209–22.

176. Bennin RS, Thompson JE, Baron EJ, et al. Gangrenous and perforated appendicitis with peritonitis: treatment and bacteriology. *Clin Ther.* 1990; 12(Suppl B):I–XIV.

177. Taffel SM, Placek PJ, Meien M. 1988 U.S. C-section rate at 24.7 per 100 births—a plateau? *N Engl J Med.* 1990; 323:199–200.

178. Amstey MT, Sheldon GW, Blyth JF. Infectious morbidity after primary cesarean section in a private institution. *Am J Obstet Gynecol.* 1980; 136:205–10.

179. Faro S. Infectious disease relations to cesarean section. *Obstet Gynecol Clin North Am.* 1989; 16:363–71.

180. Faro S. Antibiotic prophylaxis. *Obstet Gynecol Clin North Am.* 1989; 16:279–89.

181. Hemsell DL. Infections after gynecologic surgery. *Obstet Gynecol Clin North Am.* 1989; 16:381–400.

182. Duff P, Smith PN, Keiser JF. Antibiotic prophylaxis in low-risk cesarean section. *J Reprod Med.* 1982; 27: 133–8.

183. Apuzzio JJ, Reyelt C, Pelosi MA, et al. Prophylactic antibiotics for cesarean section: comparison of high- and low-risk patients for endometritis. *Obstet Gynecol.* 1982; 59:693–8.

184. Duff P. Prophylactic antibiotics for cesarean delivery: a simple cost effective strategy for prevention of postoperative morbidity. *Am J Obstet Gynecol.* 1987; 157:794–8.

185. Ehrenkranz NJ, Blackwelder WC, Pfaff SJ, et al. Infections complicating low-risk cesarean sections in community hospitals: efficacy of antimicrobial prophylaxis. *Am J Obstet Gynecol.* 1990; 162:337–43.

186. Enkin M, Enkin E, Chalmers I, et al. Prophylactic antibiotics in association with cesarean section. In: Chalmers I, Enkin M, Keiser MJNC, eds. Effective care in pregnancy and childbirth. Vol 1. London: Oxford University; 1989:1246–69.

187. Cunningham FG, Leveno KJ, DePalma RT, et al. Perioperative antimicrobials for cesarean delivery:

before or after cord clamping. *Obstet Gynecol.* 1983; 62:151–4.

188. Gordon HP, Phelps D, Blanchard K. Prophylactic cesarean section antibiotics: maternal and neonatal morbidity before and after cord clamping. *Obstet Gynecol.* 1979; 53:151–6.

189. D'Angelo LJ, Sokol RJ. Short- versus long-course prophylactic antibiotic treatment in cesarean section patients. *Obstet Gynecol.* 1980; 55:583–6.

190. Scarpignato C, Caltabiano M, Condemi V, et al. Short term vs long term cefuroxime prophylaxis in patients undergoing emergency cesarean-section. *Clin Ther.* 1982; 5:186–91.

191. Elliott JP, Freeman RK, Dorchester W. Short versus long course of prophylactic antibiotics in cesarean section. *Am J Obstet Gynecol.* 1982; 143:740–4.

192. Faro S, Martens MG, Hammill HA, et al. Antibiotic prophylaxis: is there a difference? *Am J Obstet Gynecol.* 1990; 162:900–9.

193. Conover WB, Moore TR. Comparison of irrigation and intravenous antibiotic prophylaxis at cesarean section. *Obstet Gynecol.* 1984; 63:787–91.

194. Ledger WJ, Gee C, Lewis WP. Guidelines for antibiotic prophylaxis in gynecology. *Am J Obstet Gynecol.* 1975; 121:1038–45.

195. Galask R. Changing concepts in obstetric antibiotic prophylaxis. *Am J Obstet Gynecol.* 1987; 157:491–5.

196. Stiver HG, Forward KR, Livingstone RA, et al. Multicenter comparison of cefoxitin vs cefazolin for prevention of infectious morbidity after nonelective cesarean section. *Am J Obstet Gynecol.* 1985; 145: 158–63.

197. Rayburn W, Varner M, Galask R, et al. Comparison of moxalactam and cefazolin as prophylactic antibiotics during cesarean section. *Antimicrob Agents Chemother.* 1985; 27:337–9.

198. Benigno BB, Ford LC, Lawrence WD, et al. A double-blind, controlled comparison of piperacillin and cefoxitin in the prevention of post-operative infection in patients undergoing cesarean section. *Surg Gynecol Obstet.* 1986; 162:1–7.

199. Crombleholme WR. Use of prophylactic antibiotics in obstetrics and gynecology. *Clin Obstet Gynecol.* 1988; 31:466–72.

200. Jakobi P, Weissmann A, Zimmer EZ, et al. Single dose cefazolin prophylaxis for cesarean section. *Am J Obstet Gynecol.* 1988; 158:1049–52.

201. Faro S. Antibiotic prophylaxis. *Obstet Gynecol Clin North Am.* 1989; 16:279–89.

202. Hemsell DL. Infections after gynecologic surgery. *Obstet Gynecol Clin North Am.* 1989; 16:381–400.

203. Crombleholme WR. Use of prophylactic antibiotics in obstetrics and gynecology. *Clin Obstet Gynecol.* 1988; 31:466–72.

204. Hirsch HA. Prophylactic antibiotics in obstetrics and gynecology. *Am J Med.* 1985; 78(Suppl 6B):170–6.

205. Gibbs RS. Obstetrics and gynecology. In: Conte JE, Jacob LS, Polk HC, eds. Antibiotic prophylaxis in surgery. Philadelphia: Lippincott; 1984:137–55.

206. Ohm MJ, Galask RP. The effect of antibiotic prophylaxis on patients undergoing total abdominal hysterectomy. II. Alterations of microbial flora. *Am J Obstet Gynecol.* 1976; 125:448–52.

207. Grossman JH, Adams RL. Vaginal flora in women undergoing hysterectomy with antibiotic prophylaxis.

Obstet Gynecol. 1979; 53:23–9.

208. Hamod KA, Spence MR, Roshenshein NB, et al. Single and multidose prophylaxis in vaginal hysterectomy: a comparison of sodium cephalothin and metronidazole. *Am J Obstet Gynecol.* 1980; 136:976–9.

209. Polk BF, Shapiro M, Goldstein P, et al. Randomized clinical trial of perioperative cefazolin in preventing infection after hysterectomy. *Lancet.* 1980; 1:437–40.

210. Benigno BB, Evard J, Faro S, et al. A comparison of piperacillin, cephalothin, and cefoxitin in the prevention of postoperative infections in patients undergoing vaginal hysterectomy. *Surg Gynecol Obstet.* 1986; 163:421–7.

211. Pokras R. Hysterectomy: past, present and future. *Stat Bull.* 1989; Oct–Dec:12–21.

212. Bartlett JG, Onderdonk AB, Durde E. Quantitative bacteriology of the vaginal flora. *J Infect Dis.* 1977; 136:271–5.

213. Grossman J, Greco T, Minkin MJ, et al. Prophylactic antibiotics in gynecologic surgery. *Obstet Gynecol.* 1979; 53:537–44.

214. Levison ME, Corman LC, Carrington ER, et al. Quantitative microflora of the vagina. *Am J Obstet Gynecol.* 1977; 127:80–5.

215. Ohm MJ, Galask RP. The effect of antibiotic prophylaxis on patients undergoing vaginal operations. II. Alterations of microbial flora. *Am J Obstet Gynecol.* 1975; 123:597–604.

216. Marsden DE, Cavanagh D, Wisniewski BJ, et al. Factors affecting the incidence of infectious morbidity after radical hysterectomy. *Am J Obstet Gynecol.* 1985; 152:817–21.

217. Hemsell D, Bernstein S, Bawdon R, et al. Preventing major operative site infection after radical hysterectomy and pelvic lymphadenectomy. *Gynecol Oncol.* 1989; 35:55–60.

218. Hemsell D, Menon M, Friedman A. Ceftriaxone or cefazolin prophylaxis for the prevention of infection after vaginal hysterectomy. *Am J Surg.* 1984; 148:22–6.

219. Hemsell D, Johnson E, Bawdon R, et al. Ceftriaxone and cefazolin prophylaxis for hysterectomy. *Surg Gynecol Obstet.* 1985; 161:197–203.

220. Soper D, Yarwood R. Single-dose antibiotic prophylaxis in women undergoing vaginal hysterectomy. *Obstet Gynecol.* 1987; 879–82.

221. Hemsell D, Hemsell P, Nobles B, et al. Moxalactam versus cefazolin prophylaxis for vaginal hysterectomy. *Am J Obstet Gynecol.* 1983; 147:379–85.

222. Shapiro M, Munoz A, Tager I, et al. Risk factors for infection at the operative site after abdominal or vaginal hysterectomy. *N Engl J Med.* 1982; 107:1661–6.

223. Wtteewall-Evelaar E, Koreks M, Verbrugh H. The value of prophylaxis in abdominal hysterectomies: meta-analysis. Paper presented at the 29th Interscience Conference on Antimicrobial Agents and Chemotherapy, Houston, TX: 1989 Sep 18.

224. Mann W, Orr J, Shingleton H, et al. Perioperative influences on infectious morbidity in radical hysterectomy. *Gynecol Oncol.* 1981; 11:207–12.

225. Miyazawa K, Hernandez E, Dillon MB. Prophylactic topical cefamandole in radical hysterectomy. *Int J Gynaecol Obstet.* 1987; 25:133–8.

226. Bendvold E, Kjorstad KE. Antibiotic prophylaxis for radical hysterectomy. *Gynecol Oncol.* 1987; 28: 201–4.

227. Micha JP, Kucera PR, Birkett JP, et al. Prophylactic mezlocillin in radical hysterectomy. *Obstet Gynecol.* 1987; 69:251–4.

228. Goosenberg J, Emich JP Jr, Schwarz RH. Prophylactic antibiotics in vaginal hysterectomy. *Am J Obstet Gynecol.* 1969; 105:503–6.

229. Allen J, Rampone J, Wheeless C. Use of a prophylactic antibiotic in elective major gynecologic operations. *Obstet Gynecol.* 1972; 39:218–24.

230. Ledger WJ, Sweet RL, Headington JT. Prophylactic cephaloridine in the prevention of postoperative pelvic infections in premenopausal women undergoing vaginal hysterectomy. *Am J Obstet Gynecol.* 1972; 115:766–74.

231. Breeden JT, Mayo JE. Low dose prophylactic antibiotics in vaginal hysterectomy. *Obstet Gynecol.* 1974; 43:379–85.

232. Ohm MJ, Galask RP. The effect of antibiotic prophylaxis on patients undergoing vaginal operations. I. The effect of morbidity. *Am J Obstet Gynecol.* 1975; 123:590–6.

233. Glover MW, Van Nagell JR Jr. The effect of prophylactic ampicillin on pelvic infection following vaginal hysterectomy. *Am J Obstet Gynecol.* 1976; 126:385–8.

234. Swartz WH, Tenaree P. T-tube suction drainage and/or prophylactic antibiotics. A randomized study of 451 hysterectomies. *Obstet Gynecol.* 1976; 47:665–70.

235. Lett WJ, Ansbacher R, Davison BL, et al. Prophylactic antibiotics for women undergoing vaginal hysterectomy. *J Reprod Med.* 1977; 19(Aug):51–4.

236. Jennings RH. Prophylactic antibiotics in vaginal and abdominal hysterectomy. *South Med J.* 1978; 71:251–4.

237. Homan J, McGowan J, Thompson J. Perioperative antibiotics in major elective gynecologic surgery. *South Med J.* 1978; 71:417–20.

238. Roberts JM, Homesley HD. Low-dose carbenicillin prophylaxis for vaginal and abdominal hysterectomy. *Obstet Gynecol.* 1978; 52:83–7.

239. Mendelson J, Portnoy J, De Saint Victor JR, et al. Effect of single and multidose cephradine prophylaxis on infectious morbidity of vaginal hysterectomy. *Obstet Gynecol.* 1979; 53:31–5.

240. Mickal A, Curole D, Lewis C. Cefoxitin sodium: double-blind vaginal hysterectomy prophylaxis in premenopausal patients. *Obstet Gynecol.* 1980; 56:222–5.

241. Hemsell DL, Cunningham FG, Kappus S, et al. Cefoxitin for prophylaxis in premenopausal women undergoing vaginal hysterectomy. *Obstet Gynecol.* 1980; 56:629–34.

242. Polk B, Tager I, Shapiro M, et al. Randomized clinical trial of perioperative cefazolin in preventing infection after hysterectomy. *Lancet.* 1980; 1:437–40.

243. Ledger WJ, Child MA. The hospital care of patients undergoing hysterectomy: an analysis of 12,026 patients from the Professional Activity Study. *Am J Obstet Gynecol.* 1973; 117:423–30.

244. Agalle PC, Urban RB, Homesley HD, et al. Single dose carbenicillin versus T-tube drainage in patients undergoing vaginal hysterectomy. *Surg Gynecol Obstet.* 1981; 153:351–2.

245. Karhunen M, Koskela O, Hannelin M. Single dose of tinidazole in prophylaxis of infections following hysterectomy. *Br J Obstet Gynaecol.* 1980; 87:70–2.

246. Rapp RP, Van Nagell JR, Donaldson ES, et al. A double-blind randomized study of prophylactic antibiotics in vaginal hysterectomy. *Hosp Formul.* 1982; 1:524–9.

247. Jacobson JA, Hebertson R, Kasworm E. Comparison of ceforanide and cephalothin prophylaxis for vaginal hysterectomies. *Antimicrob Agents Chemother.* 1982; 22:643–7.

248. Stage AH, Glover DD, Vaughan JE. Low-dose cephradine prophylaxis in obstetric and gynecologic surgery. *J Reprod Med.* 1982; 27:113–9.

249. Vincelette J, Finkelstein F, Aoki FY, et al. Double-blind trial of perioperative intravenous metronidazole prophylaxis for abdominal and vaginal hysterectomy. *Surgery.* 1983; 93:185–9.

250. Hemsell DL, Heard ML, Nobles BJ, et al. Single-dose cefoxitin prophylaxis for premenopausal women undergoing vaginal hysterectomy. *Obstet Gynecol.* 1984; 63:285–90.

251. Roy S, Wilkins J. Single dose cefotaxime versus 3 to 5 dose cefoxitin for prophylaxis of vaginal or abdominal hysterectomy. *J Antimicrob Chemother.* 1984; 14(Suppl B):217–21.

252. Savage EW, Thadepalli H, Rambhatla K, et al. Minocycline prophylaxis in elective hysterectomy. *J Reprod Med.* 1984; 29:81–7.

253. Maki DG, Lammers JL, Aughey DR. Comparative studies of multiple dose cefoxitin vs. single dose cefonicid for surgical prophylaxis in patients undergoing biliary tract operations or hysterectomy. *Rev Infect Dis.* 1984; 6(Suppl 4):887–95.

254. Blanco JD, Lipscomb KA. Single-dose prophylaxis in vaginal hysterectomy: a double blind, randomized comparison of ceftazidime versus cefotaxime. *Curr Ther Res.* 1984; 36:389–93.

255. McDonald PJ, Sanders T, Higgins G, et al. Antibiotic prophylaxis in hysterectomy: cefotaxime compared to ampicillin–tinidazole. *J Antimicrob Chemother.* 1985; 14(Suppl B):223–30.

256. Hemsell DL, Hemsell PG, Nobles BJ. Doxycycline and cefamandole prophylaxis for premenopausal women undergoing vaginal hysterectomy. *Surg Gynecol Obstet.* 1985; 161:462–4.

257. Benson WL, Brown RL, Schmidt PM. Comparison of short and long courses of ampicillin for vaginal hysterectomy. *J Reprod Med.* 1985; 30:874–6.

258. Hemsell DL, Johnson ER, Bawdon RE, et al. Ceftriaxone and cefazolin prophylaxis for hysterectomy. *Surg Gynecol Obstet.* 1985; 161:197–203.

259. Forney JP, Morrow CP, Townsend DE, et al. Impact of cephalosporin prophylaxis on colonization: vaginal hysterectomy morbidity. *Am J Obstet Gynecol.* 1976; 125:100–5.

260. Rapp RP, Connors JE, Hager WD, et al. Comparison of single-dose moxalactam and a three-dose regimen of cefoxitin for prophylaxis in vaginal hysterectomy. *Clin Pharm.* 1986; 5:988–93.

261. Brautigam HH, Knothe H, Rangoonwala R. Impact of cefotaxime and ceftriaxone on the bowel and vaginal flora after single dose prophylaxis in vaginal hysterectomy. *Drugs.* 1988; 35(Suppl 2):163–8.

262. Faro S, Pastorek JG, Aldridge KE, et al. Randomized double blind comparison of mezlocillin versus cefoxitin prophylaxis for vaginal hysterectomy. *Surg Gynecol*

Obstet. 1988; 166:431–5.

263. Gordon SF. Results of a single center study of cefotetan prophylaxis in abdominal or vaginal hysterectomy. *Am J Obstet Gynecol.* 1988; 158:710–4. (Erratum published in *Am J Obstet Gynecol.* 1989; 160:1025.)

264. Roy S, Wilkins J, Hemsell DL, et al. Efficacy and safety of single dose ceftizoxime vs. multiple dose cefoxitin in preventing infection after vaginal hysterectomy. *J Reprod Med.* 1988; 33(1 Suppl):149–53.

265. Mercer LJ, Murphy HJ, Ismail MA, et al. A comparison of cefonicid and cefoxitin for preventing infections after vaginal hysterectomy. *J Reprod Med.* 1988; 33:223–6.

266. Berkeley AS, Orr JW, Cavanagh D, et al. Comparative effectiveness and safety of cefotetan and cefoxitin as prophylactic agents in patients undergoing abdominal or vaginal hysterectomy. *Am J Surg.* 1988; 155:81–5.

267. Davey PG, Duncan ID, Edward D, et al. Cost–benefit analysis of cephradine and mezlocillin prophylaxis for abdominal and vaginal hysterectomy. *Br J Obstet Gynaecol.* 1988; 95:1170–7.

268. Mozzillo N, Dionigi R, Ventriglia L. Multicenter study of aztreonam in the prophylaxis of colorectal, gynecologic and urologic surgery. *Chemotherapy.* 1989; 35(Suppl 1):58–71.

269. The Multicenter Study Group. Single dose prophylaxis in patients undergoing vaginal hysterectomy: cefamandole versus cefotaxime. *Am J Obstet Gynecol.* 1989; 160:1198–201.

270. Roy S, Wilkins J, Galaif E, et al. Comparative efficacy and safety of cefmetazole or cefoxitin in the prevention of postoperative infection following vaginal and abdominal hysterectomy. *J Antimicrob Chemother.* 1989; 23(Suppl D):109–17.

271. Friese S, Willems FTC, Loriaux SM, et al. Prophylaxis in gynaecological surgery: a prospective randomized comparison between single-dose prophylaxis with amoxycillin/clavulanate and the combination of cefuroxime and metronidazole. *J Antimicrob Chemother.* 1989; 24(Suppl B):213–6.

272. Willis A, Bullen C, Ferguson I, et al. Metronidazole in the prevention and treatment of *Bacteroides* infection in gynaecological patients. *Lancet.* 1974; 2:1540–3.

273. Mayer W, Gordon M, Rothbard MJ. Prophylactic antibiotics. Use in hysterectomy. *NY State J Med.* 1976; 76:2144–7.

274. Ohm MJ, Galask RP. The effect of antibiotic prophylaxis on patients undergoing total abdominal hysterectomy. II. Alterations of microbial flora. *Am J Obstet Gynecol.* 1976; 125:448–54.

275. Mathews D, Ross H. Randomized controlled trial of a short course of cephaloridine in the prevention of infection after abdominal hysterectomy. *Br J Obstet Gynecol.* 1978; 85:381–5.

276. Appelbaum P, Moodley J, Chatterton S, et al. Metronidazole in the prophylaxis and treatment of anaerobic infection. *S Afr Med J.* 1978; 1:703–6.

277. Wheeless CR Jr, Dorsey JH, Wharton LR Jr. An evaluation of prophylactic doxycycline in hysterectomy patients. *J Reprod Med.* 1978; 21:146–50.

278. Duff P. Antibiotic prophylaxis for abdominal hysterectomy. *Obstet Gynecol.* 1982; 60:25–9.

279. Walker EM, Gordon AJ, Warren RE, et al. Prophylactic single dose metronidazole before abdominal hysterectomy. *Br J Obstet Gynaecol.* 1982; 89:957–61.

280. Manthorpe T, Justesen T. Metronidazole prophylaxis in abdominal hysterectomy. A double blind controlled trial. *Acta Obstet Gynecol Scand.* 1982; 61:243–6.

281. Ohm MJ, Galask RP. The effect of antibiotic prophylaxis on patients undergoing total abdominal hysterectomy. I. Effect on morbidity. *Am J Obstet Gynecol.* 1976; 125:442–7.

282. Hemsell DL, Reisch J, Nobles B, et al. Prevention of major infection after elective abdominal hysterectomy. Individual determination required. *Am J Obstet Gynecol.* 1983; 147:520–3.

283. Kvist-Poulsen H, Borel J. T-tube suction drainage and/or prophylactic two dose metronidazole in abdominal hysterectomy. *Acta Obstet Gynecol Scand.* 1984; 63:711–4.

284. Berkeley AS, Haywork SD, Hirsch JC, et al. Controlled, comparative study of moxalactam and cefazolin for prophylaxis of abdominal hysterectomy. *Surg Gynecol Obstet.* 1985; 161:457–61.

285. Gonen R, Hakin M, Samberg I, et al. Short term prophylactic antibiotic for elective abdominal hysterectomy: how short? *Eur J Obstet Gynecol Reprod Biol.* 1985; 20:229–34.

286. Senior C, Steirad J. Are preoperative antibiotics helpful in abdominal hysterectomy? *Am J Obstet Gynecol.* 1986; 154:1004–8.

287. Evaldson GR, Lindgren S, Malmborg AS, et al. Single dose intravenous tinidazole prophylaxis in abdominal hysterectomy. *Acta Obstet Gynecol Scand.* 1986; 65:361–5.

288. Tuomala RE, Fischer SG, Munoz A, et al. A comparative trial of cefazolin and moxalactam as prophylaxis for preventing infection after abdominal hysterectomy. *Obstet Gynecol.* 1985; 66:372–6.

289. Periti P, Mazzei T, Periti E. Prophylaxis in gynaecological and obstetric surgery: a comparative randomized multicentre study of single dose cefotetan versus two doses of cefazolin. *Chemioterapia.* 1988; 7:245–52.

290. Hemsell DL, Martin JN Jr, Pastorek JG II, et al. Single dose antimicrobial prophylaxis at abdominal hysterectomy. Cefamandole vs. cefotaxime. *J Reprod Med.* 1988; 33:939–44.

291. Scarpignato C, Labruna C, Condemi V, et al. Comparative efficacy of two different regimens of antibiotic prophylaxis in total abdominal hysterectomy. *Pharmatherapeutica.* 1980; 2:450–5.

292. Wijma J, Kauer F, Van Saene H, et al. Antibiotics and suction drainage as prophylaxis in vaginal and abdominal hysterectomy. *Obstet Gynecol.* 1987; 70:384–8.

293. Eron LJ, Gordon SF, Harvey LK, et al. A trial using early preoperative administration of cefonicid for antimicrobial prophylaxis with hysterectomies. *DICP.* 1989; 23:655–8.

294. Hemsell DL, Johnson ER, Bawdon RE, et al. Cefoperazone and cefoxitin prophylaxis for abdominal hysterectomy. *Obstet Gynecol.* 1984; 63:467–72.

295. Tchabo JG, Cutting ME, Butler C. Prophylactic antibiotics in patients undergoing total vaginal or abdominal hysterectomy. *Int Surg.* 1985; 70:349–52.

296. Hemsell DL, Hemsell PG, Heard ML, et al. Preoperative cefoxitin prophylaxis for elective abdominal hysterectomy. *Am J Obstet Gynecol.* 1985; 153:225–6.

297. Hemsell DL, Johnson ER, Heard MC, et al. Single dose

piperacillin versus triple dose cefoxitin prophylaxis at vaginal and abdominal hysterectomy. *South Med J.* 1989; 82:438–42.

298. Orr JW Jr, Sisson PF, Barrett JM, et al. Single center study results of cefotetan and cefoxitin prophylaxis for abdominal or vaginal hysterectomy. *Am J Obstet Gynecol.* 1988; 158:714–6.

299. Orr JW Jr, Varner RE, Kilgore LC, et al. Cefotetan versus cefoxitin as prophylaxis in hysterectomy. *Am J Obstet Gynecol.* 1986; 154:960–3.

300. Berkeley AS, Freedman KS, Ledger WJ, et al. Comparison of cefotetan and cefoxitin prophylaxis for abdominal and vaginal hysterectomy. *Am J Obstet Gynecol.* 1988; 158:706–9.

301. Periti P, Mazzei T, Lamanna S, et al. Single dose ceftriaxone versus multidose cefotaxime antimicrobial prophylaxis in gynecologic and obstetrical surgery. Preliminary results of a multicenter prospective randomized study. *Chemioterapia.* 1984; 3:299–304.

302. Sevin B, Ramos R, Lichtinger M, et al. Antibiotic prevention of infection complicating radical abdominal hysterectomy. *Obstet Gynecol.* 1984; 64:539–45.

303. Rosenshein NB, Ruth JC, Villar J, et al. A prospective randomized study of doxycycline as a prophylactic antibiotic in patients undergoing radical hysterectomy. *Gynecol Oncol.* 1983; 15:201–6.

304. Ehrenkranz NJ. Surgical wound infection occurrence in clean operations. Risk stratification for interhospital comparisons. *Am J Med.* 1981; 50:909–14.

305. Freiman JA, Chalmers TC, Smith H, et al. The importance of beta, the type II error and sample size in the design and interpretation of the randomized control trial. *N Engl J Med.* 1978; 299:690–4.

306. Barza M. Guidelines for reports of clinical studies. *Antimicrob Agents Chemother.* 1989; 33:1829–30.

307. Fan-Harvard P, Nahata MC. Treatment and prevention of infections of cerebrospinal fluid shunts. *Clin Pharm.* 1987; 6:866–80.

308. Keucher TR, Mealey J. Long term results after ventriculoatrial and ventriculoperitoneal shunting for infantile hydrocephalus. *J Neurosurg.* 1979; 50:179–86.

309. Yogev R, Davis T. Neurosurgical shunt infections—a review. *Childs Brain.* 1980; 6:74–80.

310. Renier D, Lacombe J, Pierre-Kahn A, et al. Factors causing acute shunt infection—computer analysis of 1174 patients. *J Neurosurg.* 1984; 61:1072–8.

311. Wright RL. Postoperative craniotomy infections. Springfield, IL: Charles C Thomas; 1966:26–31.

312. Horwitz NH, Curtin JA. Prophylactic antibiotics and wound infections following laminectomy for lumbar disc disease. A retrospective study. *J Neurosurg.* 1975; 43:727–31.

313. Savitz MH, Malis LI. Prophylactic clindamycin for neurosurgical patients. *NY State J Med.* 1976; 76:64–7.

314. Haines SJ, Goodman ML. Antibiotic prophylaxis of postoperative neurosurgical wound infection. *J Neurosurg.* 1982; 56:103–5.

315. Geraghty J, Feely M. Antibiotic prophylaxis in neurosurgery. A randomized controlled trial. *J Neurosurg.* 1984; 60:724–6.

316. Mollman HD, Haines SJ. Risk factors for postoperative neurosurgical wound infection. A case-control study. *J Neurosurg.* 1986; 64:902–6.

317. Shapiro M, Wald U, Simchen E, et al. Randomized clinical trial of intra-operative antimicrobial prophylaxis of infection after neurosurgical procedures. *J Hosp Infect.* 1986; 8:283–95.

318. Wright RL. Postoperative craniotomy infections. Springfield, IL: Charles C Thomas; 1970:26–39.

319. Tenney JH, Vlahov D, Saleman M, et al. Wide variation in risk of wound infection following clean neurosurgery. Implication for perioperative antibiotic prophylaxis. *J Meirpsirg.* 1986; 62:243–7.

320. Wright RL. Septic complication of neurosurgical spinal procedures. Springfield, IL: Charles C Thomas; 1970:26–39.

321. Savitz MH, Malis LI, Meyers BR. Prophylactic antibiotics in neurosurgery. *Surg Neurol.* 1974; 2:95–100.

322. Malis LI. Prevention of neurosurgical infection by intraoperative antibiotics. *Neurosurgery.* 1979; 5: 339–43.

323. Haines SJ. Systemic antibiotic prophylaxis in neurological surgery. *Neurosurgery.* 1980; 6:355–61.

324. Quarterly GRC, Polyzoidis K. Intraoperative antibiotic prophylaxis in neurosurgery: a clinical study. *Neurosurgery.* 1981; 8:669–71.

325. Savitz MH, Katz SS. Prevention of primary wound infection in neurosurgical patients: a 10-year study. *Neurosurgery.* 1986; 18:685–8.

326. Van Ek B, Dijkmans BA, Van Dulken H, et al. Antibiotic prophylaxis in craniotomy: a prospective, double-blind, placebo controlled study. *Scan J Infect Dis.* 1988; 20:633–9.

327. Bullock R, Van Dellen JR, Ketelbey W, et al. A double-blind, placebo controlled trial of perioperative prophylactic antibiotics for elective neurosurgery. *J Neurosurgery.* 1988; 69:687–91.

328. Blomstedt GC, Kytta J. Results of a randomized trial of vancomycin prophylaxis in craniotomy. *J Neurosurgery.* 1988; 69:216–20.

329. Fan-Harvard P, Nahata MC. Treatment and prevention of infections of cerebrospinal fluid shunts. *Clin Pharm.* 1987; 6:866–80.

330. O'Brien M, Parent A, Davis B. Management of ventricular shunt infections. *Childs Brain.* 1979; 5:304–9.

331. Schoenbaum SC, Gardner P, Shillito J. Infection of cerebrospinal fluid shunts: epidemiology, clinical manifestations and therapy. *J Infect Dis.* 1975; 131:534–52.

332. Walters BC, Hoffman HJ, Hendrick EB, et al. Cerebrospinal fluid shunt infection. Influences on initial management and subsequent outcome. *J Neurosurg.* 1984; 60:1014–21.

333. Wilson HD, Bean JR, James HE, et al. Cerebrospinal fluid antibiotic concentrations in ventricular shunt infections. *Childs Brain.* 1978; 4:74–82.

334. James HE, Walsh JW, Wilson HD, et al. The management of cerebrospinal fluid shunt infections. A clinical experience. *Acta Neurochir.* 1981; 59:157–66.

335. Mates S, Glaser J, Shapiro K. Treatment of cerebrospinal fluid shunt infections with medical therapy alone. *Neurosurgery.* 1982; 11:781–3.

336. George R, Leibrock L, Epstein M. Long-term analysis of cerebrospinal fluid shunt infections—a 25-year experience. *J Neurosurg.* 1979; 51:804–11.

337. Bayston R. Hydrocephalus shunt infections and their treatment. *J Antimicrob Chemother.* 1985; 15:259–61.

338. Renier D, Lacombe J, Pierre-Kahn A, et al. Factors causing acute shunt infection—computer analysis of 1174 patients. *J Neurosurg.* 1984; 61:1072–8.

339. Forrest DM, Cooper DG. Complications of ventric-

uloatrial shunts. A review of 455 cases. *J Neurosurg.* 1968; 29:506–12.

340. Odio C, McCracken JC, Nelson JD. CSF shunt infections in pediatrics—a seven-year experience. *Am J Dis Child.* 1984; 138:1103–8.

341. Petrak RM, Pottage JC, Harris AA, et al. *Haemophilus influenzae* meningitis in the presence of a cerebrospinal fluid shunt. *Neurosurgery.* 1986; 18:79–81.

342. Sells CJ, Shurtleff DB, Coeser JD. Gram-negative cerebrospinal fluid shunt associated infections. *Pediatrics.* 1977; 59:614–8.

343. Shapiro S, Boaz J, Kleiman M, et al. Origins of organisms infecting ventricular shunts. *Neurosurgery.* 1988; 22:868–72.

344. Gardner P, Leipzig TJ, Sadigh M. Infections of mechanical cerebrospinal fluid shunts. *Curr Clin Top Infect Dis.* 1988; 9:185–214.

345. Wang EL, Prober CG, Hendrick BE. Prophylactic sulfamethoxazole and trimethoprim in ventriculoperitoneal shunt surgery. A double-blind, randomized, placebo-controlled trial. *JAMA.* 1984; 251:1174–7.

346. Blomstedt GC. Results in trimethoprim–sulfamethoxazole prophylaxis in ventriculostomy and shunting procedures. *J Neurosurg.* 1985; 62:694–7.

347. Djindjian M, Fevrier MJ, Ottervbein G, et al. Oxacillin prophylaxis in cerebrospinal fluid shunt procedures: results of a randomized open study in 60 hydrocephalic patients. *Surg Neurol.* 1986; 25:178–80.

348. Blum J, Schwarz M, Voth D. Antibiotic single-dose prophylaxis of shunt infections. *Neurosurg Rev.* 1989; 12:239–44.

349. Shurtleff DB, Stuntz JT, Hayden PW. Experience with 1201 cerebrospinal fluid shunt procedures. *Pediatric Neurosci.* 1985–86; 12:49–57.

350. Shmidt K, Gjerris F, Osgaard O, et al. Antibiotic prophylaxis in cerebrospinal fluid shunting: a prospective randomized trial in 152 hydrocephalic patients. *Neurosurgery.* 1985; 17:1–5.

351. Griebel R, Khan M, Tan L. CSF shunt complications: an analysis of contributory factors. *Childs Nerv Syst.* 1985; 1:77–80.

352. Lambert M, MacKinnon AE, Vaishnav A. Comparison of two methods of prophylaxis against CSF shunt infection. *Z Kinderchir.* 1984; 39(Suppl):109–10.

353. Odio C, Mohs E, Sklar FH, et al. Adverse reactions to vancomycin used as prophylaxis for CSF shunt procedures. *Am J Dis Child.* 1984; 138:17–9.

354. Coronary bypass surgery charges, 1982–3 and 1986. *Stat Bull.* 1989; Jan–Mar:2–15.

355. National Heart Lung and Blood Advisory Council. Fifteenth report of the National Heart, Lung, and Blood Advisory Council: Progress and Challenge. Washington, DC: U.S. Department of Health and Human Services; 1988.

356. Beam T Jr. Perioperative prevention of infection in cardiac surgery. *Antibiot Chemother.* 1985; 33:114–39.

357. Bor D, Rose R, Modlin J, et al. Mediastinitis after cardiovascular surgery. *Rev Infect Dis.* 1983; 5:885–97.

358. Nagachinta T, Stephens M, Reitz B, et al. Risk factors for surgical-wound infection following cardiac surgery. *J Infect Dis.* 1987; 156:967–73.

359. Kittle C, Reed W. Antibiotics and extracorporeal circulation. *J Thorac Cardiovasc Surg.* 1961; 41:34–48.

360. Slonim R, Litwak R, Gadboys H, et al. Antibiotic prophylaxis of infection complicating open-heart operations. *Antimicrob Agents Chemother.* 1963; 3:731–5.

361. Goodman J, Schaffner W, Collins H, et al. Infection after cardiovascular surgery. *N Engl J Med.* 1968; 278:117–23.

362. Fekety F, Cluff L, Sabiston D, et al. A study of antibiotic prophylaxis in cardiac surgery. *J Thorac Cardiovasc Surg.* 1969; 57:757–63.

363. Conte J, Cohen S, Roe B, et al. Antibiotic prophylaxis and cardiac surgery: a prospective double-blind comparison of single-dose versus multi-dose regimens. *Ann Intern Med.* 1972; 76:943–9.

364. Firor W. Infection following open-heart surgery, with special reference to the role of prophylactic antibiotics. *J Thorac Cardiovasc Surg.* 1967; 53:371–8.

365. Fong I, Baker C, McKee D. The value of prophylactic antibiotics in aorta-coronary bypass operations. *J Thorac Cardiovasc Surg.* 1979; 78:908–13.

366. Austin T, Coles J, Burnett R, et al. Aorta-coronary bypass procedures and sternotomy infections: a study of antistaphylococcal prophylaxis. *Can J Surg.* 1980; 23:483–5.

367. Penketh A, Wansbrough-Jones M, Wright E, et al. Antibiotic prophylaxis for coronary artery bypass graft surgery. *Lancet.* 1985; 1:1500.

368. Goldman D, Hopkins C, Karchmer A, et al. Cephalothin prophylaxis in cardiac valve surgery; a prospective, double-blind comparison of two-day and six-day regimens. *J Thorac Cardiovasc Surg.* 1977; 73:470–9.

369. Austin T, Coles J, McKechnie P, et al. Cephalothin prophylaxis and valve replacement. *Ann Thorac Surg.* 1977; 23:333–6.

370. Hillis D, Rosenfeldt F, Spicer W, et al. Antibiotic prophylaxis for coronary bypass grafting. *J Thorac Cardiovasc Surg.* 1983; 86:217–21.

371. Hill D, Yates A. Prophylactic antibiotics in open heart surgery. *Aust N Z J Med.* 1975; 81:414–7.

372. Myerowitz P, Caswell K, Lindsay W, et al. Antibiotic prophylaxis for open-heart surgery. *J Thorac Cardiovasc Surg.* 1977; 73:625–9.

373. Cooper D, Norton R, Mobin M, et al. A comparison of two prophylactic antibiotic regimes for open-heart surgery. *J Cardiovasc Surg (Torino).* 1980; 21:279–86.

374. Bailey J, Perciva H. Cefamandole as a prophylactic in cardiac surgery. *Scand J Infect Dis.* 1980; (Suppl 25):112–7.

375. Ghoneim A, Tandon A, Ionescu M. Comparative study of cefamandole versus ampicillin plus cloxacillin: prophylactic antibiotics in cardiac surgery. *Ann Thorac Surg.* 1982; 33:152–8.

376. Slama T, Sklar S, Misinski J, et al. Randomized comparison of cefamandole, cefazolin and cefuroxime prophylaxis in open-heart surgery. *Antimicrob Agents Chemother.* 1986; 29:744–7.

377. Kaiser A, Petracek M, Lea J, et al. Efficacy of cefazolin, cefamandole, and gentamicin as prophylactic agents in cardiac surgery. *Ann Surg.* 1987; 206:791–7.

378. Geroulanos S, Oxelbark S, Donfried B, et al. Antimicrobial prophylaxis in cardiovascular surgery. *Thorac Cardiovasc Surg.* 1987; 35:199–205.

379. Conklin C, Gray R, Neilson D, et al. Determinants of wound infection incidence after isolated coronary ar-

tery bypass surgery in patients randomized to receive prophylactic cefuroxime or cefazolin. *Ann Thorac Surg.* 1988; 46:172–7.

380. Doebbeling B, Pfaller M, Kuhns K, et al. Cardiovascular surgery prophylaxis: a randomized, controlled comparison of cefazolin and cefuroxime. *J Thorac Cardiovasc Surg.* 1990; 99:981–9.

381. Woods M, Rahija M. Survey of antimicrobial prophylaxis in cardiovascular surgery. Poster presented at the 43rd ASHP Annual Meeting. Denver, CO: 1986 Jun 5.

382. Woods M, LeBlanc K, Gersema L. Antibiotic prophylaxis in open heart surgery: results of a second survey. *Hosp Pharm.* 1990; 25:641–3.

383. Gentry L, Zeluff B, Cooley D. Antibiotic prophylaxis in open-heart surgery: a comparison of cefamandole, cefuroxime and cefazolin. *Ann Thorac Surg.* 1988; 46:167–71.

384. Beam T, Raab T, Spooner J, et al. Single-dose antimicrobial prophylaxis in open heart surgery. *Eur J Clin Microbiol.* 1984; 3:598–604.

385. Soteriou M, Recker F, Geroulanos S, et al. Perioperative antibiotic prophylaxis in cardiovascular surgery: a prospective randomized comparative trial of cefazolin versus ceftriaxone. *World J Surg.* 1989; 13:798–802.

386. Kini P, Fernandez J, Causay R, et al. Double-blind comparison of cefazolin and cephalothin in open-heart surgery. *J Thorac Cardiovasc Surg.* 1978; 76:506–9.

387. Pien F, Michael N, Mamiya R, et al. Comparative study of prophylactic antibiotics in cardiac surgery: clindamycin versus cephalothin. *J Thorac Cardivasc Surg.* 1979; 77:908–13.

388. Joyce F, Szczepanski K. A double-blind comparative study of prophylactic antibiotic therapy in open heart surgery: penicillin G versus vancomycin. *Thorac Cardiovasc Surg.* 1986; 34:100–3.

389. Wilson A, Treasure T, Gruneberg R, et al. Antibiotic prophylaxis in cardiac surgery: a prospective comparison of two dosage regimens of teicoplanin with a combination of flucloxacillin and tobramycin. *J Antimicrob Chemother.* 1988; 21:213–23.

390. Boyce J, Potter-Bynoe G, Dziobek L. Hospital reimbursement patterns among patients with surgical wound infections following open heart surgery. *Infect Control Hosp Epidemiol.* 1990; 11:89–93.

391. Roach A, Kernodle D, Kaiser A. Selecting cost-effective antimicrobial prophylaxis in surgery: Are we getting what we pay for? *DICP.* 1990; 24:183–5.

392. Preheim L, Rimland D, Bittner M. Methicillin-resistant *Staphylococcus aureus* in Veterans Administration Medical Centers. *Infect Control.* 1987; 8:191–4.

393. Thornsberry C. Methicillin-resistant staphylococci. *Clin Lab Med.* 1989; 9:255–67.

394. Olix ML, Klug TJ, Coleman CR, et al. Prophylactic penicillin and streptomycin in elective operations on bones, joints, and tendons. *Surg Forum.* 1960; 10: 818–9.

395. Schonholtz GJ, Borgia CA, Blair JD. Wound sepsis in orthopedic surgery. *J Bone Joint Surg.* 1962; 44A: 1548–52.

396. Fitzgerald RH. Infections of hip prostheses and artificial joints. *Infect Dis Clin North Am.* 1989; 3:329–38.

397. Ericson C, Lidgren L, Lindberg L. Cloxacillin in the prophylaxis of postoperative infections of the hip. *J Bone Joint Surg.* 1973; 55A:808–13.

398. Carlsson AS, Lidgren L, Lindberg L. Prophylactic antibiotics against early and late deep infections after total hip replacements. *Acta Orthop Scand.* 1977; 48:405–10.

399. Hill C, Mazas F, Flamant R, et al. Prophylactic cefazolin versus placebo in total hip replacement. *Lancet.* 1981; 1:795–7.

400. Lidwell OM, Lowbury EJL, Whyte W, et al. Effect of ultraclean air in operating rooms on deep sepsis in the joint after total hip or knee replacement: a randomized study. *Br Med J.* 1982; 285:10–4.

401. Pollard JP, Hughes SPF, Scott JE, et al. Antibiotic prophylaxis in total hip replacement. *Br Med J.* 1979; 1:707–9.

402. Boyd RJ, Burke JF, Colton T. A double-blind clinical trial of prophylactic antibiotics in hip fractures. *J Bone Joint Surg.* 1973; 55A:1251–8.

403. Burnett JW, Gustilo RB, Williams DN, et al. Prophylactic antibiotics in hip fractures. *J Bone Joint Surg.* 1980; 62A:457–62.

404. Tengve B, Kjellander J. Antibiotic prophylaxis in operations on trochanteric femoral fractures. *J Bone Joint Surg.* 1978; 60A:97–9.

405. Pavel A, Smith RL, Ballard A, et al. Prophylactic antibiotics in clean orthopedic surgery. *J Bone Joint Surg.* 1974; 56A:777–82.

406. Eron LJ. Prevention of infection following orthopedic surgery. *Antibiot Chemother.* 1985; 33:140–64.

407. Norden CW. A critical review of antibiotic prophylaxis in orthopedic surgery. *Rev Infect Dis.* 1983; 5:928–32.

408. Henley MB, Jones RE, Wyatt RWB, et al. Prophylaxis with cefamandole nafate in elective orthopedic surgery. *Clin Orthop.* 1986; 209:24–54.

409. Burnakis TG. Surgical antimicrobial prophylaxis: principles and guidelines. *Pharmacotherapy.* 1984; 4:248–71.

410. Kaiser AB, Clayson KR, Mulherin JL, et al. Antibiotic prophylaxis in vascular surgery. *Ann Surg.* 1978; 188:283–9.

411. Pitt HA, Postier RG, Macgowan WA, et al. Prophylactic antibiotics in vascular surgery. Topical, systemic, or both. *Ann Surg.* 1980; 192:356–64.

412. Bennion RS, Hiatt JR, Williams RA, et al. A randomized, prospective study of perioperative antimicrobial prophylaxis for vascular access surgery. *J Cardiovasc Surg.* 1985; 26:270–4.

413. Hasselgren P-O, Ivarson L, Risberg B, et al. Effects of prophylactic antibiotics in vascular surgery. A prospective, randomized double-blind study. *Ann Surg.* 1984; 200:86–92.

414. Gibbons RP, Stark RA, Gorrea RJ, et al. The prophylactic use—or misuse—of antibiotics in transurethral prostatectomy. *J Urol.* 1978; 119:381–3.

415. Ferrie B, Scott R. Prophylactic cefuroxime in transurethral resection. *Urol Res.* 1984; 12:279–81.

416. Upton JD, Das S. Prophylactic antibiotics in transurethral resection of bladder tumors: are they necessary? *Urology.* 1986; 27:421–3.

417. Houle AM, Mokhless I, Sarto N, et al. Perioperative antibiotic prophylaxis for transurethral resection of the prostate; is it justifiable? *J Urol.* 1989; 142:317–9.

418. Fair WR. Perioperative use of carbenicillin in transurethral resection of the prostate. *Urology.* 1986; 27(Suppl 2):15–8.

419. Shah P, Williams G, Chaudary M, et al. Short-term antibiotic prophylaxis and prostatectomy. *Br J Urol.* 1981; 53:339–43.

420. Morris MJ, Golovsky D, Guinness MDG, et al. The value of prophylactic antibiotics in transurethral prostatic resection: a controlled trial, with observations on the origin of postoperative infection. *Br J Urol.* 1976; 48:479–84.

421. Gonzalez R, Wright R, Blackard CE. Prophylactic antibiotics in transurethral prostatectomy. *J Urol.* 1976; 116:203–5.

422. Hills NH, Bultitude MI, Eykyn S. Co-trimoxazole in prevention of bacteriuria after prostatectomy. *Br Med J.* 1976; 2:498–9.

423. Dorflinger T, Madsen PO. Antibiotic prophylaxis in transurethral surgery. *Urology.* 1984; 24:643–6.

424. Matthew AD, Gonzales R, Jeffords D, et al. Prevention of bacteriuria after transurethral prostatectomy with nitrofurantoin macrocrystals. *J Urol.* 1978; 120:442–3.

425. Childs SJ, Wells WG, Mirelman S. Antibiotic prophylaxis for genitourinary surgery in community hospitals. *J Urol.* 1983; 130:305–8.

426. Nielsen OS, Maigaard S, Frimodt-Moller N, et al. Prophylactic antibiotics in transurethral prostatectomy. *J Urol.* 1981; 126:60–2.

427. Charton M, Vallancien G, Veillon B, et al. Antibiotic prophylaxis or urinary tract infection after transurethral resection of the prostate: a randomized study. *J Urol.* 1987; 138:87–9.

428. Ramsey E, Sheth NK. Antibiotic prophylaxis in patients undergoing prostatectomy. *Urology.* 1983; 21:376–8.

429. DeBessonet DA, Merlin AS. Antibiotic prophylaxis in elective genitourinary tract surgery: a comparison of single-dose pre-operative cefotaxime and multiple-dose cefoxitin. *J Antimicrob Chemother.* 1984; 14 (Suppl B):271–5.

---

^aDosages of ampicillin sodium, ampicillin trihydrate, cefamandole nafate, cefazolin sodium, cefmetazole sodium, cefoperazone sodium, cefotaxime sodium, cefotetan disodium, cefoxitin sodium, ceftizoxime sodium, cefuroxime sodium, cephalexin hydrochloride, cephalothin sodium, clindamycin phosphate, gentamicin sulfate, moxalactam disodium, nafcillin sodium, oxacillin sodium, piperacillin sodium, and vancomycin hydrochloride are expressed in terms of base. Salt forms are specified in the text and table only when dosage is expressed in terms of salt.

Approved by the ASHP Commission on Therapeutics and the ASHP Board of Directors, April 22, 1992.

This document was written by the ASHP Commission on Therapeutics Task Force on Antimicrobial Prophylaxis in Surgery: Steven L. Barriere, Pharm.D., Specialist in Infectious Diseases, Department of Pharmaceutical Services, and Adjunct Professor of Medicine and Pharmacology, School of Medicine, University of California at Los Angeles Center for the Health Sciences, Los Angeles; John Connors, Pharm.D., Assistant Professor of Pharmacy Practice, Philadelphia College of Pharmacy and Science, Philadelphia, PA; Larry H. Danziger, Pharm.D., Assistant Professor of Pharmacy, College of Pharmacy, University of Illinois, Chicago; Joseph T. DiPiro, Pharm.D., Professor of Pharmacy and Surgery, Medical College of Georgia, Augusta; John F. Flaherty, Pharm.D., Associate Professor of Clinical Pharmacy, School of Pharmacy, University of California, San Francisco; B. Joseph Guglielmo, Pharm.D., Professor of Clinical Pharmacy, School of Pharmacy, University of California, San Francisco; Bruce Kreter, Pharm.D., Associate Director for Antiinfective Clinical Research, Bristol-Myers Squibb, Princeton, NJ; and Robert P. Rapp, Pharm.D., Professor and Chair, Division of Pharmacy Practice and Science, College of Pharmacy, University of Kentucky, Lexington.

The contributions of John M. Benson, Pharm.D., Douglas Fish, Pharm.D., and Paul O. Gubbins, Pharm.D., in the preparation of these guidelines are acknowledged.

The recommendations in this document do not indicate an exclusive course of treatment to be followed. Variations, taking into account individual circumstances, may be appropriate.

The bibliographic citation for this document is as follows: American Society of Hospital Pharmacists. ASHP therapeutic guidelines on antimicrobial prophylaxis in surgery. *Clin Pharm.* 1992; 11:483–513.

ASHP Therapeutic Guidelines on Nonsurgical Antimicrobial Prophylaxis

Antimicrobial prophylaxis is indicated in selected patients to prevent certain infections that are not a direct result of a surgical procedure. Of the medical indications for antimicrobial prophylaxis, many have a sound basis, but others are based primarily on anecdotal information or cautious medical practice.

In general, antimicrobial prophylaxis should be directed at individuals who are (1) classified as being at risk for developing an infection because of certain physical characteristics and (2) in a situation where temporary exposure to a particular pathogen is likely. This paper reviews the persons at risk for these infections, indications for antimicrobial prophylaxis, the efficacy of prophylaxis, and current recommendations regarding patient eligibility and drug selection, as determined by the ASHP Commission on Therapeutics Task Force on Nonsurgical Antimicrobial Prophylaxis.

Prophylaxis of Bacterial Endocarditis

The recommendations of the American Heart Association (AHA) regarding prophylaxis of bacterial endocarditis were last updated in 1984. Although these guidelines tend to serve as standards for medical, dental, and medicolegal purposes, there is insufficient evidence that prophylaxis is entirely beneficial. While there is unquestionable support for prophylaxis in patients with certain underlying cardiac conditions, the risk–benefit ratio of prophylaxis for other conditions is unclear.

Although there may be some question about the usefulness of prophylaxis, the rationale for prevention is clear: Endocarditis carries a significant risk of severe morbidity and mortality. In some cases, morbidity may continue beyond the actual period of active endocardial infection.

Persons at Risk. Cardiac abnormalities or conditions that may predispose patients to bacterial endocarditis include prosthetic cardiac valves, congenital cardiac malformations, valvular disease, and a history of endocarditis.[1–3] Many surgeons have now adopted valve repair, rather than valve replacement with a prosthesis, as the procedure of choice for many patients.[4] Patients with prosthetic heart valves, surgically repaired valves, or surgically constructed systemic pulmonary shunts are at the greatest risk for endocarditis and, therefore, should receive the highest attention as candidates for antimicrobial prophylaxis.

Prosthetic heart valve endocarditis (PVE) accounts for up to 33% of the reported cases of infective endocarditis.[5] The risks for development of PVE vary according to the valve site. For example, mitral valve and aortic valve replacement are associated with risks of about 0.4 and 2%, respectively.[6]

Antimicrobial prophylaxis of endocarditis is also highly recommended for patients with a history of rheumatic heart disease. Rheumatic heart disease constitutes about 25% of the underlying cardiac disease involved in endocarditis.[7] The mitral valve is the valve most commonly damaged by the rheumatic process (85% of patients). The overall incidence of endocarditis in patients with chronic rheumatic heart disease is approximately 0.4%, about the same as in patients with PVE involving a mitral valve prosthesis.[6]

Congenital heart malformations account for 4–26% of cases of endocarditis. Lesions that produce high pressure gradients, including patent ductus arteriosus, ventricular septal defect, tetralogy of Fallot, pulmonary stenosis, and coarctation of the aorta, commonly predispose patients to infective endocarditis.[5] Other high risk conditions that warrant prophylaxis include bicuspid aortic valve, cyanotic congenital heart disease, and mitral insufficiency.[6]

Patients with previous episodes of endocarditis are also considered to be at relatively high risk for endocarditis. Valvular damage from previous infections predisposes the patient to subsequent development of endocarditis. While the overall recurrence rate for endocarditis is 2.5–10%, the incidence of reinfection in intravenous drug abusers has been reported to be as high as 41%.[5]

There has been considerable discussion about the need for antimicrobial prophylaxis in patients with mitral valve prolapse (MVP). Despite the high prevalence of MVP (4000–6000 cases per 100,000 population), the prevalence of endocarditis (1.1 cases per 100,000 population) is relatively low. Currently, the AHA recommends that only patients with MVP and valvular insufficiency receive antimicrobial prophylaxis. Kaye[7] suggested that prophylaxis is indicated whenever both MVP and a systolic murmur are present.[7] Von Reyn et al.,[8] Clemons et al.,[9] Devereux et al.,[10] and MacMahon et al.[11] concluded that while the overall relative risk of endocarditis in patients with MVP is very low, the risk is greatest in men older than 45 years and in patients with MVP and a systolic murmur.

Other cardiac conditions have not been clearly identified as placing patients at risk for endocarditis and do not appear to merit prophylaxis. These conditions include isolated secundum atrial septal defect, secundum atrial septal defect repaired without a patch 6 or more months earlier, patent ductus arteriosus ligated and divided 6 or more months earlier, and prior coronary artery bypass graft surgery.

Special considerations must be undertaken when prescribing therapy for the prevention of bacterial endocarditis in patients with a history of rheumatic fever. These patients often receive secondary antimicrobial prophylaxis to prevent colonization or infection of the upper respiratory tract by group A streptococci and subsequent recurrent attacks of rheumatic fever. The secondary prophylactic therapy often continues into adulthood and may have to be continued for life in patients with a history of rheumatic carditis.[12]

Indications for Prophylaxis. A number of medical, dental, and surgical procedures have been identified that may predispose patients to endocarditis. These procedures generally carry a high risk of associated transient bacteremia. Because viridans streptococci are still the organisms that most commonly cause endocarditis, prophylaxis for all dental procedures (including routine professional cleaning) that are likely to cause gingival bleeding is recommended for patients at risk.[1] The risk is higher for patients undergoing oral surgery, including dental extractions, because of the potentially larger bacterial inoculum and the increased risk of transient bacteremia (40–60%). The risk associated with such procedures as routine professional dental cleaning or the injection of a local anesthetic into the gums is less well defined. Prophylaxis for procedures involving the lower respiratory tract, such as surgery, biopsy, and rigid bronchoscopy, appears to be justified because of the bacteremia associated with them.

Prophylaxis during procedures involving the upper gastrointestinal tract has been an area of debate.[2,7,13] There is controversy because bacteremia occurs in only a small percentage of patients (except for those undergoing esophageal dilation and sclerotherapy of esophageal varices)[13] and because the organisms cultured from the blood of these patients are usually not those that cause endocarditis.[7,13] It has been suggested that prophylaxis should be eliminated or made optional for most gastrointestinal procedures (except for patients with prosthetic valves).[2,7,13]

The AHA has made no definite recommendations with respect to several lower gastrointestinal and genitourinary procedures that infrequently or rarely lead to endocarditis, including percutaneous liver biopsy, upper gastrointestinal tract endoscopy or proctosigmoidoscopy without biopsy, barium enema, uncomplicated vaginal delivery, and brief ("in-and-out") bladder catheterization with sterile urine. These procedures should probably be listed as ones for which prophylaxis is not recommended except for patients with prosthetic heart valves.[7]

Efficacy of Prophylaxis. Bacterial endocarditis may still occur in patients receiving appropriate prophylaxis. Well-defined studies evaluating the effectiveness of prophylaxis in preventing this infection are lacking, primarily because of the large number of subjects that would be required for statistical significance of the results to be established. However, an effort has been made by the AHA Committee on Rheumatic Fever, Endocarditis, and Kawasaki Disease to record occurrences of antimicrobial prophylaxis failure.

Durack et al.[14] analyzed 52 case studies submitted to this national registry. The following underlying heart diseases or conditions were associated with prophylaxis failure: MVP (33%), congenital heart disease (29%), rheumatic heart disease (21%), prosthetic valves (19%), and other valvular disease (10%). Of the 52 patients, 4 (8%) had more than one abnormality, and only 1 (2%) had no known heart disease. These findings confirm those of Clemons et al.,[9] who also reported that MVP may be a risk factor for endocarditis. Ninety-two percent of cases of prophylaxis failure described by Durack et al. occurred after a dental procedure. Only 12% of the patients had received antimicrobial prophylaxis according to the guidelines of the AHA and the American Dental Association, which were available when the patients were treated. These findings suggest that more rigid adherence to the guidelines may reduce the risk of prophylaxis failure. Durack et al. encouraged the continued reporting of prophylaxis failures.

It is unlikely that the efficacy of antimicrobial therapy to prevent endocarditis will ever be adequately evaluated. Guidelines for current practice will, therefore, continue to be dependent on results of animal studies and case reports.

Recommendations. Recommendations regarding prophylactic therapy for each risk group are listed in Table 1. Some recommendations differ from current AHA guidelines. It has been suggested that oral amoxicillin given 1 hour before procedures and repeated 6 hours later could serve as the standard prophylactic regimen for nearly all procedures. In cases of penicillin allergy, erythromycin or vancomycin could be substituted—the latter when risk of the growth of methicillin-resistant organisms is high. This simplified version of the AHA recommendations would, in most cases, alleviate the need for complicated and costly intravenous administration.[15] The AHA is revising its 1984 statement; it is anticipated that the amoxicillin regimen will be included in the next AHA statement.

In patients for whom prophylaxis of recurrent rheumatic fever is indicated, the most common regimen is penicillin G benzathine intramuscularly every 4 weeks. Patients receiving secondary therapy for rheumatic fever prophylaxis require additional short-term antimicrobial treatment before surgical and dental procedures to prevent the possible development of bacterial endocarditis, since antimicrobial regimens used to prevent recurrences of acute rheumatic fever are inadequate for the prevention of bacterial endocarditis.[12] Because viridans streptococci that are relatively resistant to penicillin may be present in the oral cavity of patients receiving monthly injections of penicillin G benzathine,[16] erythromycin or an intravenous regimen of ampicillin plus gentamicin should be considered.

Prophylaxis of Recurrent Urinary Tract Infections

Recurrent urinary tract infections (UTIs) are often categorized as either relapsed infections or reinfections. Those UTIs classified as relapsing are recurrent infections caused by the same bacterial strain (implying failure of the initial antimicrobial regimen). Reinfections, on the other hand, are recurrent infections caused by a strain different from the original pathogen. Reinfection is the cause of most recurrent UTIs in women and usually reflects some underlying host defect. It is for this type of patient that prophylaxis is of greatest benefit in preventing recurrent UTIs.

Persons at Risk. In premenopausal women, a number of risk factors may be predisposing to recurrent UTIs. For unknown reasons, the urethral and vaginal squamous epithelium of some women is more susceptible to attachment by *Escherichia coli*, increasing the likelihood for colonization and UTIs in these individuals.[17] Many women develop recurrent UTIs within 24 hours after sexual intercourse. This is believed to occur secondary to trauma to the urethra, which allows a small bacterial inoculum to enter the bladder.[18] The use of a diaphragm contraceptive has been associated with increased vaginal colonization with *E. coli*.[19] Finally, voluntary retention of urine for more than an hour after the urge to urinate is first experienced may lead to ureteral reflux and possibly to UTIs.[20]

It is often assumed that anatomical abnormalities of the urinary tract are a frequent cause of recurrent UTIs. In fact, most adult women with recurrent UTIs have normal genitourinary tracts and will not benefit from roentgenographic studies of the upper and lower urinary tracts. On the other hand, recurrent UTIs in men and children are frequently associated with anatomical or functional abnormalities of the urinary tract.[21,22]

All men and children with recurrent UTIs should, therefore, undergo radiographic studies to detect possible renal abnormalities. In addition, men with chronic bacterial prostatitis frequently develop relapsing UTIs caused by

Table 1.
Recommendations for Antimicrobial Prophylaxis

Infection	Indication(s)	Eligible Patients	Recommended Regimen[a]	Alternative Regimen(s)[a]
Bacterial endocarditis	Dental procedures that cause gingival bleeding, oral or respiratory tract surgery	Standard risk[b]	Oral: PCN VK 2 g 1 hr before procedure, then 1 g 6 hr later. For children of <27 kg, half the adult dose. Intravenous: PCN G 50,000 units/kg (max., 2 million units) i.v. or i.m. 0.5–1 hr before procedure, then 25,000 units/kg (max., 1 million units) 6 hr later	Amoxicillin 50 mg/kg (max., 3 g) p.o. 1 hr before procedure, then 25 mg/kg (max., 1.5 g) 6 hr later. Or erythromycin 20 mg/kg (max., 1 g) p.o. 1–2 hr before procedure, then 10 mg/kg (max., 500 mg) p.o. 6 hr later. Or vancomycin 20 mg/kg (max., 1 g) i.v. over 60 min given more than 1 hr before procedure.
		Special risk[c]	Ampicillin 50 mg/kg (max., 2 g) i.m. or i.v. plus gentamicin 1.5–2 mg/kg i.m. or i.v. 0.5 hr before procedure, followed by a second dose of each 8 hr later or PCN VK 1 g p.o. 6 hr later	Amoxicillin, erythromycin, or vancomycin as above
	Certain gastrointestinal and genitourinary tract procedures[d]	Standard and special risk	Ampicillin 50 mg/kg (max., 2 g) i.m. or i.v. plus gentamicin 1.5–2 mg/kg 0.5–1 hr before procedure and repeated 8 hr later	Amoxicillin p.o. as above, or vancomycin 20 mg/kg (max., 1 g) i.v. over 60 min plus gentamicin 1.5–2 mg/kg i.m. or i.v. given 1 hr before procedure and repeated 8–12 hr later
	Low-risk procedures[e]	Standard risk	None	. . .
		Special risk	Amoxicillin 50 mg/kg (max., 3 g) p.o. 1 hr before procedure, then 25 mg/kg (max., 1.5 g) 6 hr later	Erythromycin p.o. as above, or single-dose vancomycin
Rheumatic fever	Group A streptococcal pharyngitis	History of rheumatic fever	PCN G benzathine 1.2 million units every 4 wk	PCN VK 250 mg p.o. b.i.d., sulfadiazine 500–1000 mg p.o. q.d., or erythromycin 250 mg p.o. b.i.d.
Recurrent urinary tract infections	Postcoital urinary tract infections	History of postcoital urinary tract infections	TMP–SMX 80–400 mg p.o. × 1 dose after intercourse	Nitrofurantoin 50 mg p.o. × 1 dose
	Prevention of reinfection	Frequent (>3/yr) urinary tract infections		
		Prophylaxis	TMP–SMX 80–400 mg p.o. 3–7×/wk	Trimethoprim 50 mg p.o. h.s.
		Self-treatment of symptomatic infections	TMP–SMX 160–180 mg p.o. b.i.d. × 3 days or 320–1600 mg as a single dose	Trimethoprim 100 mg p.o. b.i.d., amoxicillin 500 mg p.o. t.i.d., or nitrofurantoin 100 mg p.o. q.i.d. × 3 days
	Chronic bacterial prostatitis	Elderly men with recurrent urinary tract infections	TMP–SMX 160–800 mg p.o. b.i.d. × 12 wk	Norfloxacin 400 mg p.o. b.i.d., or ciprofloxacin 250 mg p.o. b.i.d.
	Suppression of persistent bacteriuria	Those with frequent (>3/yr) symptomatic urinary tract infections	TMP–SMX 80–400 mg p.o. q.d. indefinitely	Nitrofurantoin 100 mg p.o. q.d. indefinitely, or methenamine mandelate 1 g p.o. q.i.d., or methenamine hippurate 1 g p.o. b.i.d.
Tuberculosis	Recent exposure (<2 mo) to an active case of pulmonary tuberculosis	All children, adults with skin-test reactivity (5-mm induration)	INH 10–15 mg/kg/day (max., 300 mg) p.o. × 6–12 mo plus pyridoxine 15–50 mg p.o. daily	Rifampin 15–20 mg/kg (max., 600 mg) p.o. with or without ethambutol hydrochloride 15 mg/kg p.o. daily
	Recent (<2 yr) skin-test conversion (≥10-mm induration)	All patients	INH as above	As above
	Skin-test reactivity of unknown duration	Stable lesions on chest roentgenogram or compromised immune system[f]	INH as above	As above

Continued on next page

Table 1 (continued)

Infection	Indication(s)	Eligible Patients	Recommended Regimen[a]	Alternative Regimen(s)[a]
		No risks, age <35 yr	INH as above or close follow-up	As above
		No risks, age >35 yr	No prophylaxis	. . .
Meningitis	Cerebrospinal fluid leakage for ≥7 days	Closed head trauma, basilar skull fracture	No prophylaxis—monitor for signs of CNS infection	. . .
HIV infection	Accidental exposure to blood products or secretions	Health-care workers after needle-stick injury or possibly after mucous membrane or open-skin exposure	Prophylaxis has not been proved to be beneficial	Zidovudine 200 mg p.o. q4h × 4–6 wk
Influenza A infection	Epidemiologic or virologic evidence of outbreak in the environment	Unvaccinated elderly patients, immunocompromised patients, and health-care workers	Amantadine hydrochloride 100 mg p.o. b.i.d. (reduce dose for renal dysfunction) × 4–6 wk; immunize unvaccinated patients	None
Recurrent genital herpes simplex type 2 infection	An unacceptably high rate (four or more bouts/yr) of recurrent infection, immunocompromised state	Patients with prior infection by herpes simplex virus type 2	Acyclovir 200 mg p.o. t.i.d. × 1 yr; some patients may require higher dosages (e.g., 400 mg p.o. b.i.d.)	None
Traveler's diarrhea	Travel to underdeveloped countries in Latin America, Africa, the Middle East, and Asia	Elderly patients and those traveling for a prolonged period of time are at higher risk	Dietary restriction; treat symptomatic cases as symptoms occur	Doxycycline 100 mg p.o., TMP–SMX 160–800 mg p.o., TMP 200 mg p.o., or norfloxacin 200 mg p.o. daily; BSS 2.4 g/d, divided q.i.d. Children: TMP–SMX 4–20 mg/kg p.o. b.i.d. (symptomatic only)
Malaria	Before travel to countries endemic for the disease (in the Middle East, Southeast Asia, India, South and Central America, Oceania, and sub-Saharan Africa)	Travelers to areas with no or few cases of chloroquine-resistant *Plasmodium falciparum* infection	Chloroquine 5 mg/kg (max., 300 mg) p.o. weekly, beginning 1–2 wk before travel and continuing for 6 wk after travel	Doxycycline 100 mg p.o. q.d. beginning 1–2 days before travel. Children: hydroxychloroquine 5 mg/kg p.o. weekly
		Travelers to areas with many cases of chloroquine-resistant *Plasmodium falciparum* infection	Chloroquine as above; may also add pyrimethamine–sulfadoxine 25–500 mg p.o. weekly (some recommend using in symptomatic patients only). Children: 1/8 tablet (<1 yr), 1/4 tablet (1–2 yr), or 1/2 tablet (>2 yr)	Doxycycline as above
	Prophylaxis after travel	After prolonged stay in an area endemic for *P. vivax* or *P. ovale*	Primaquine 0.3 mg/kg (max., 15 mg) p.o. q.d. × 14 days, or 0.9 mg/kg (max., 45 mg) weekly × 8 wk	None
Haemophilus influenzae carrier state	Exposure to one or more index cases of invasive *H. influenzae* infection	Persons who had household or close contact with an index case within past 2 wk who will be in contact with other children at risk,[g] children exposed in a day-care center to 1 or more index cases in	Rifampin 20 mg/kg (max., 600 mg) p.o. q.d. × 4 days Infants <1 mo old should receive 10 mg/kg	None

Continued on next page

Table 1 *(continued)*

Infection	Indication(s)	Eligible Patients	Recommended Regimen[a]	Alternative Regimen(s)[a]
		past 2 mo, children with index cases who will be in contact with children at risk		
		Adults who had household or close contact with an index case diagnosed in past 2 wk who will not be exposed to other children at risk, children exposed at school to 1 index case diagnosed in past 2 mo, persons exposed to index case more than 2 mo ago	No prophylaxis	
Neisseria meningitidis carrier state	Household or intimate (exposure to oral secretions) contact with an index case of meningococcal meningitis, index cases after treatment	All age groups	Rifampin 10 mg/kg (max., 600 mg) p.o. b.i.d. × 2 days	Ciprofloxacin, minocycline, and ceftriaxone
	Day-care center or other closed-population contacts (e.g., military recruits).	All age groups	Rifampin as above	As above
Methicillin-resistant *Staphylococcus aureus* carrier state	Individuals documented as being colonized with methicillin-resistant *Staph. aureus* (in nares, axillae, perineum, etc.)	Health-care workers (physicians, nurses) and high-risk patients (patients with indwelling devices such as intravenous catheters, dialysis catheters or shunts, and prosthetic heart valves)	Single site: mupirocin ointment applied q.i.d. × 5 days. Multiple sites: rifampin 300 mg p.o. plus TMP–SMX 150–800 mg × 7–14 days, or until eradication. Antibacterial soaps should also be used daily	Single site: bacitracin ointment or systemic therapy. Multiple sites: ciprofloxacin 750 mg p.o. b.i.d. or fusidic acid
Perinatal group B streptococcal infection	Low-birth-weight infants (≤2500 g), prolonged (>18-hr) rupture of membranes, maternal intrapartum fever	Mothers with cervical or vaginal colonization with group B streptococci, and their newborns	Mothers: during labor, ampicillin 2 g i.v. and 1 g i.v. q4h until delivery. Infants: after birth, ampicillin 50 mg/kg i.m. q12h × 4 doses	Cefazolin (?)
Nosocomial bacterial pneumonia	Trauma patients, organ transplant recipients, other intensive-care patients for whom a limited duration of ventilation is anticipated	Intensive-care patients requiring mechanical ventilation	None	Aminoglycoside–polymyxin B–amphotericin B combination administered as a solution orally and as a paste to the buccal mucosa, plus 4–7 days of treatment with a systemic antimicrobial (penicillin G, cefotaxime)
Gram-negative bacterial infection or sepsis	Onset of granulocytopenia	Those with a total granulocyte count of <500/cu mm	TMP–SMX 160–800 mg p.o. b.i.d. until resolution of neutropenia	Norfloxacin 400 mg p.o. b.i.d., or ciprofloxacin 500 mg p.o. b.i.d.
Pneumocystis carinii pneumonia	History of *P. carinii* pneumonia, AIDS, ARC; human immunodeficiency virus-positive with T4 lymphocyte count of ≤200 cu mm or T4 lymphocytes accounting for <20% of total lymphocytes	Human immunodeficiency virus-infected patients and other patients (e.g., transplant) who are profoundly immunocompromised	Aerosolized pentamidine isethionate 300 mg/mo or divided and given semimonthly	TMP–SMX 160–800 mg p.o. b.i.d.

Continued on next page

Table 1 (continued)

Infection	Indication(s)	Eligible Patients	Recommended Regimen[a]	Alternative Regimen(s)[a]
Opportunistic infections (bacterial, viral, fungal, protozoal)	Bone marrow or organ transplant recipients	Cytomegalovirus- and herpes simplex virus-seronegative and graft from cytomegalovirus-seronegative donor	TMP–SMX 160–800 mg p.o. b.i.d. plus clotrimazole troches p.o. 3–4× daily for 3–4 mo (organ) or until engraftment (marrow)	Norfloxacin or ciprofloxacin plus nystatin suspension, low-dose amphotericin B
		Cytomegalovirus- or herpes simplex virus-seropositive or graft from cadaver or cytomegalovirus-positive donor	As above, plus acyclovir 200–400 mg p.o. q.i.d. (herpes simplex virus) or 800 mg p.o. q.i.d. (cytomegalovirus) for 3–4 mo (organ) to 1 yr (marrow)	Ganciclovir (?)

[a] PCN VK = penicillin V potassium, PCN G = penicillin G, TMP–SMX = trimethoprim–sulfamethoxazole, INH = isoniazid, BSS = bismuth subsalicylate. Dosages of penicillin V potassium, ampicillin sodium, gentamicin sulfate, amoxicillin trihydrate, penicillin G benzathine, vancomycin hydrochloride, ciprofloxacin hydrochloride, chloroquine hydrochloride, primaquine phosphate, doxycycline hyclate, and hydroxychloroquine sulfate are expressed in terms of the base. Salt forms are specified in the table only when dosage is expressed in terms of the salt.

[b] Congenital cardiac malformations, surgically constructed systemic–pulmonary shunts, rheumatic and other acquired valvular dysfunction, idiopathic hypertrophic subaortic stenosis, previous history of bacterial endocarditis, mitral valve prolapse with insufficiency.

[c] Prosthetic valves, including biosynthetic valves.

[d] Cystoscopy, prostatic surgery, vaginal hysterectomy, gallbladder surgery, esophageal dilation, sclerotherapy for esophageal varices, colonoscopy, upper gastrointestinal tract endoscopy with biopsy, proctosigmoidoscopic biopsy.

[e] Percutaneous liver biopsy, upper gastrointestinal tract endoscopy or proctosigmoidoscopy without biopsy, barium enema, uncomplicated vaginal delivery, brief bladder catheterization with sterile urine.

[f] Diabetes mellitus, therapy with prednisone 15 mg/day or equivalent for two or more weeks, other immunosuppressive therapy, HIV-positive patients, end-stage renal disease, Hodgkin's lymphoma or leukemia, significant malnutrition. Note: The amount of objective data justifying use of INH prophylaxis in many of these conditions is minimal.

[g] Children less than two years of age and unvaccinated children two to four years of age.

persistence of the pathogen in the prostatic secretory system. The pathogenesis of recurrent UTIs in men with chronic bacterial prostatitis is unclear. Bacteria enter the prostate via the urethral lumen. The prostate has a high lipid content, which limits penetration of many antimicrobials. Recurrent prostatitis is, therefore, often caused by the same pathogen(s) once antimicrobials are discontinued. Therapy with antimicrobials that enter the prostate is necessary.

Indications for Prophylaxis. All patients with risk factors for recurrent UTIs are candidates for prophylaxis. The decision to initiate prophylaxis should be based on the number of UTIs per year and such factors as the patient's desire to receive continuous low-dose antimicrobial therapy versus therapy for each symptomatic UTI.

Efficacy of Prophylaxis. Several methods for the prophylaxis of recurrent UTIs have been explored. Continuous low-dose antimicrobial treatment is usually successful in preventing recurrent UTIs but requires daily administration and is effective only during the period of administration. In addition, patients may still develop recurrent UTIs with resistant organisms. Postcoital prophylaxis is effective in women who are susceptible to recurrent infection associated with sexual intercourse.[23] Urination soon after intercourse decreases the frequency of UTIs in women who are at increased risk and should be encouraged.

Intermittent, self-initiated antimicrobial treatment of symptomatic infections may be tried in well-motivated individuals. Patients keep prescriptions at home and fill them at the first sign of symptoms, thereby reducing drug costs, the incidence of adverse effects, and the potential for infection by resistant bacteria.[24]

Recommendations. In general, long-term prophylactic therapy should be considered for patients with three or more

symptomatic reinfections per year. The prophylactic regimen chosen depends on the physician and the patient's preference. For continuous low-dose therapy in women, trimethoprim–sulfamethoxazole three to seven times weekly or trimethoprim once daily may be used. The latter regimen has no advantage over the combination therapy unless the patient has a sulfa allergy. Prophylaxis with norfloxacin also appears to be effective, although more expensive.[25] Nitrofurantoin is another alternative but should be avoided in patients with impaired renal function.

Continuous low-dose therapy should be continued for 6 months. Many patients have sterile urine after 6 months of continuous therapy, but a substantial number become reinfected and require longer treatment. In those patients, therapy can be continued for up to 2 years. For postcoital prophylaxis, single-dose regimens with amoxicillin, trimethoprim–sulfamethoxazole, or nitrofurantoin have been successful. This practice may be continued for 6–18 months. Most patients revert to multiple recurrence once prophylaxis is discontinued.

A number of intermittent, self-initiated treatment regimens have been used (Table 1). Single-dose therapy with trimethoprim–sulfamethoxazole taken at onset of acute urinary symptoms is the most popular.[24] Alternatively, a 3-day regimen of trimethoprim–sulfamethoxazole, trimethoprim, amoxicillin, or nitrofurantoin may be used.[26]

Men with chronic bacterial prostatitis require long-term antimicrobial therapy. Even 12 weeks of treatment with trimethoprim–sulfamethoxazole results in a cure in only 30–40% of patients. Quinolone antimicrobials such as norfloxacin and ciprofloxacin are newer alternatives that may improve response rates because of their improved penetration of prostatic fluid.

Continuous suppressive therapy may be considered for men and women in whom sterilization of the urine cannot be achieved. The goal for these patients is to keep the degree of bacteriuria at a minimum, thereby reducing the frequency of symptomatic infection. Commonly used regimens include single daily doses of trimethoprim–sulfamethoxazole or nitrofurantoin and therapy with methenamine with or without ascorbic acid. Suppressive therapy does not sterilize the urinary tract; when the medication is discontinued, the patient frequently develops bacteriuria and recurrent symptoms.

Antimicrobial prophylaxis has little impact on the incidence of UTIs in patients with indwelling urinary catheters. A minimal period of catheterization, aseptic technique in catheter care, and the use of condom catheters in male patients (whenever possible) should be part of routine care in these patients; antimicrobial therapy is appropriate only for symptomatic episodes of bacteriuria.

Prophylaxis of Tuberculosis

Clinical infection with *Mycobacterium tuberculosis* may be prevented by administering bacillus Calmette Guerin (BCG) vaccine or antimicrobials. The use of BCG vaccine is not addressed in this paper; interested readers are referred to a recent review.[27]

The majority of new cases of tuberculosis in the United States each year occur in patients in whom the primary infection with *M. tuberculosis* occurred at an earlier date. Approximately 22,000 cases of tuberculosis are diagnosed annually among a group of 10,000,000 Americans considered to have subclinical infection with *M. tuberculosis*.[28] Prevention of the reactivation of tuberculosis is the basis for the (1) widespread periodic screening of patients at risk for exposure to *M. tuberculosis* and (2) use of antimicrobial prophylaxis in patients with positive skin-test results.

Official recommendations regarding candidates for prophylactic therapy of tuberculosis were issued by the American Thoracic Society and the Centers for Disease Control in 1986.[29] These guidelines are based on the relative risks of developing active tuberculosis and experiencing clinically important isoniazid toxicity. Before initiating isoniazid therapy in accordance with these guidelines, it is important for the clinician to detect bacteriologically positive or roentgenographically progressive tuberculosis. These patients should be treated with multiple-drug regimens designed for the therapy of active disease. In addition, patients with relative contraindications to isoniazid therapy should be identified. Contraindications include

- Previous isoniazid-associated hepatitis.
- History of severe adverse reactions (fever, rash, and arthritis) to isoniazid.
- Acute or chronic active hepatic disease (note that hepatitis B surface-antigen positivity is not a contraindication unless associated with chronic active hepatitis).

Persons at Risk. Those at greatest risk for clinical tuberculosis can be categorized as (1) individuals who have recently (within 1 or 2 years) been infected with *M. tuberculosis* and (2) patients with past exposure who have not received antimicrobial prophylaxis and have a compromised immune system. Category 1 patients are at highest risk; category 2 patients are susceptible to reactivation of latent disease. It is toward these two categories of patients that prophylaxis should be directed.

Indications for Prophylaxis. Household members and other close contacts of potentially infectious tuberculosis patients who do not receive prophylaxis have a relatively high risk of developing active tuberculosis (2–4% during the first year). This is particularly true for persons with a positive tuberculin skin-test result (induration of 5 mm or more). For recent contacts who do not have tuberculin skin-test reactivity, the clinician may still choose to administer isoniazid for 3 months, followed by repeat tuberculin skin testing. This approach is especially important for children. If the 3-month followup tuberculin skin-test result is negative, isoniazid therapy can be discontinued.[29]

Since the greatest risk of active disease is present during the first 2 years of primary infection, all newly infected persons known to have developed tuberculin skin-test reactivity within the past 2 years should be given isoniazid if no contraindications exist. There is no upper age limit.

Preventive therapy should also be given to patients with (1) tuberculin skin-test reactivity of unknown duration when associated with chest roentgenographic findings consistent with stable, nonprogressive parenchymal lesions of previous tuberculosis and (2) negative results in sputum bacteriologic tests. In addition, patients with previously diagnosed but inadequately treated tuberculosis should be considered for preventive therapy with isoniazid, even if they are older than 35 years.

A number of medical conditions are thought to increase the risk of recrudescence of tuberculosis due to suppression of the immune system. These conditions include diabetes mellitus, silicosis, prolonged use of adrenocorticosteroids (prednisone 15 mg or more per day or an equivalent dosage of another adrenocorticosteroid for 2 or more weeks), use of immunosuppressive therapy, human immunodeficiency virus (HIV) infection, end-stage renal disease, Hodgkin's disease or leukemia, and malnutrition. Individuals with positive tuberculin skin-test results who are considered to be immunocompromised for these or other reasons may be treated with isoniazid regardless of age if they have not previously received preventive therapy.

Finally, any person with tuberculin skin-test reactivity who is under 35 years of age should be considered for preventive isoniazid therapy or monitored closely for signs of active disease, even if none of the risk factors described above is present.

While isoniazid is inexpensive, it cannot be used in all individuals with tuberculin skin-test reactivity or exposure to persons with active tuberculosis. Several factors are associated with increased risk for isoniazid toxicity and should be carefully assessed by the clinician who is considering the initiation of isoniazid prophylaxis: age greater than 35 years, daily use of alcohol, and the presence of chronic liver disease. Although no harmful effects of isoniazid on the fetus have been clearly documented, isoniazid prophylaxis is not routinely recommended during pregnancy and should be postponed until after delivery. Isoniazid may be present in detectable amounts in breast milk.

Efficacy of Prophylaxis and Recommendations. Isoniazid is the only drug proved to be effective for the prophylaxis of tuberculosis (Table 1). It is administered as a single daily dose of 300 mg in adults and 10–15 mg/kg/day (maximum dose, 300 mg) in children for 24–52 weeks. Early trials of isoniazid demonstrated the efficacy of a 52-week regimen.

Because it is generally recognized that compliance with a regimen is inversely related to its duration, shorter regimens of isoniazid have been investigated. The International Union Against Tuberculosis published data indicating that a 12-week regimen of preventive therapy eliminates no more than one-third of the cases of tuberculosis that would occur without treatment.[30] Two-thirds of the cases were prevented with a 24-week regimen—only slightly less than the proportion prevented by the traditional 52-week regimen. Moreover, the 24-week regimen prevented the greatest number of cases of tuberculosis per case of isoniazid-associated hepatitis observed. On the basis of these data, many clinicians now endorse the 24-week regimen for widespread use.

Since peripheral neuropathy secondary to isoniazid therapy is considered to be a result of altered pyridoxine metabolism and excretion, the use of pyridoxine in conjunction with isoniazid has been recommended for patients at risk for neuropathy or pyridoxine deficiency, such as those who are very young, very old, malnourished, diabetic, or alcoholic.

On rare occasions, isoniazid cannot or should not be used in patients who otherwise meet the criteria for receiving preventive therapy. If a patient has been infected with an isoniazid-resistant organism, the use of rifampin with or without isoniazid or ethambutol has been suggested.[29] For individuals who are unable to take isoniazid because of adverse effects or allergy, rifampin or rifampin–ethambutol may be tried. These agents should be given at full dosages for 12 months.

Prophylaxis for Closed Head Trauma with Cerebrospinal Fluid Leakage

Persons at Risk and Indications for Prophylaxis. Persons who suffer closed head trauma with subsequent cerebrospinal fluid (CSF) leakage are at risk for central nervous system infection due to CSF exposure to potentially pathogenic microorganisms located in the nasopharynx, nasal sinus passages, and auditory canals. Patients with concomitant basilar skull fracture and leakage lasting more than 7 days are at increased risk for infection. Bacterial meningitis is a possible infectious complication in patients with closed head trauma and CSF leakage. The exact incidence of meningitis in this clinical situation is unknown; depending on the patient series, 0–25% of adults with CSF rhinorrhea and 0–18% of adults with CSF otorrhea have developed meningitis.[31–34] The predominant pathogens in meningitis are *Streptococcus pneumoniae* and other streptococci, *Haemophilus influenzae*, and *Staphylococcus aureus*.

Efficacy of Prophylaxis. The prophylactic use of antimicrobials in patients with closed head trauma with CSF leakage remains controversial. No placebo-controlled trials assessing the prophylactic value of antimicrobials in these patients have been reported. MacGee et al.[33] pooled their data on 58 cases with those on 344 other cases from the literature in an attempt to determine this value. In patients with CSF rhinorrhea, 6.1% receiving no prophylaxis developed meningitis; 4.2, 23.3, and 18.8% of patients receiving chloramphenicol or penicillin plus streptomycin, penicillin alone, or sulfadiazine alone, respectively, developed meningitis. The incidence of meningitis in patients with CSF otorrhea was lower; 4.5% of patients receiving no antimicrobials and 7% of patients receiving penicillin alone developed meningitis. Of patients with CSF otorrhea receiving chloramphenicol or penicillin plus streptomycin or sulfadiazine alone, none developed meningitis. Thus, it appears that the incidence of meningitis after closed head trauma with CSF leakage is very low and may actually increase if certain antimicrobial regimens are used. In fact, Ignelzi and VanderArk[32] found that prophylactic antimicrobials contributed to shifts to more resistant pathogens colonizing the nasopharynx.

Conclusions based on the analysis of pooled data are inherently suspect. In the patient series compiled by MacGee et al.,[33] variables included type of head injury, time of onset of CSF leakage, antimicrobial regimen used, and occurrence of surgical repair of leaks. It does appear that the incidence of meningitis after closed head trauma with CSF leakage is very low. Because most cases of CSF leakage resolve spontaneously in a week or less, the period of increased risk is short.

Recommendations. Prophylactic antimicrobials cannot be routinely recommended for patients with closed head trauma with CSF leakage. Management of these patients consists of close clinical observation for signs or symptoms of meningitis and prompt initiation of appropriate antimicrobials should such signs or symptoms become manifest.

Prophylaxis after Occupational Exposure to HIV

Persons at Risk and Indications for Prophylaxis. Anyone exposed through certain routes to contact with blood or blood-contaminated body fluids from HIV-infected patients is at risk for HIV infection. The major routes of exposure—sexual intercourse, intravenous drug abuse, and blood transfusion—are well known, as are the major risk groups—homosexual or bisexual males, intravenous drug abusers, hemophiliacs, and the sexual partners of any of the preceding.

Health-care workers involved in the care of HIV-infected patients constitute a group with a small but noteworthy risk. The rate of seroconversion after a single exposure to HIV ranges from 0 to 2.7%. In health-care workers who have received needle-stick injuries resulting in the injection of contaminated blood, the seroconversion rate is 0.4% (five infections resulting from more than 1200 documented needle-stick episodes).[35–37] Seroconversion can also occur, although rarely, after the exposure of wounds or sores in mucous membranes or skin to contaminated fluids. Thus, the risk of seroconversion and infection, even after documented needle-stick injury, is low. Other variables, including the duration of exposure and volume of contaminated fluid contacted, are likely to influence transmission.

Efficacy of Prophylaxis and Recommendations. Zidovudine has been the only antiviral agent shown in placebo-controlled clinical trials to reduce HIV-associated morbidity and mortality in previously infected patients.[38] Although animal studies have shown that administration of zidovudine after retroviral inoculation can prevent infection, no such data exist for humans.

Until June 1989, health-care workers could participate in a placebo-controlled double-blind trial of the efficacy of zidovudine for postexposure prophylaxis.[37] Eighty-four patients were enrolled in the study before it was terminated; 49 received zidovudine 200 mg orally every 4 hours for 6 weeks and 35 received placebo. None developed HIV seropositivity during the 6-month followup period.[36] This finding is not surprising given the low incidence of seroconversion in this population. The data from this small study are insufficient to permit evaluation of the safety and efficacy of zidovudine for this indication. Without this information, it would appear that routine prophylaxis with zidovudine cannot be advocated; in addition, the high cost of zidovudine must be considered. However, programs of prophylaxis for occupationally exposed patients are in place at San Francisco General Hospital and the National Institutes of Health (NIH). These programs and associated legal and ethical issues were discussed by Henderson and Gerberding.[39] Protection is best achieved by observing universal precautions in the handling of blood and other body fluids.

Prophylaxis of Influenza A Infection

Persons at Risk. Persons at increased risk for contracting serious influenza infection during outbreaks include patients with chronic illnesses (e.g., diabetes mellitus, pulmonary disease, and cardiovascular disease), patients whose immune systems have been weakened by disease or drugs, persons whose occupations put them in contact with many influenza patients (health-care workers and public servants), and the elderly. Without prophylaxis, these persons are at increased risk for influenza and resultant complications.

Indications for Prophylaxis. If there is epidemiologic or virologic evidence of an influenza A outbreak in the environment (hospital, community, or nursing home), elderly patients, immunocompromised patients, patients with chronic diseases, and health-care workers who have not yet been immunized should receive prophylactic therapy. The variability in antigenic serotype of strains producing outbreaks suggests that previously vaccinated individuals may also benefit from prophylactic therapy.[40,41]

Efficacy of Prophylaxis. Immunization of high risk patients with influenza vaccine is the primary means of preventing infection. However, several controlled clinical trials have shown amantadine hydrochloride 100 mg orally twice daily to be 70–90% effective in preventing influenza A.[42–45] Amantadine has no appreciable activity against influenza B. Since influenza vaccine is not 100% effective (it tends to be less effective in certain high risk groups), combination prophylaxis with the vaccine and amantadine may be indicated in some patients.[40,41] Reports of infections with amantadine-resistant strains of influenza A support this practice.[46,47]

Recommendations. During an outbreak, all persons at risk should receive amantadine unless there are contraindications. The unvaccinated elderly, patients with chronic heart and pulmonary conditions, and immunocompromised patients should receive the vaccine as well. Other hospitalized patients, health-care workers, and public servants may receive amantadine alone. The dosage of amantadine hydrochloride is 100 mg orally twice daily; elderly patients and patients with renal dysfunction should receive dosages adjusted in accordance with package insert recommendations. Amantadine prophylaxis should begin as soon as there is epidemiologic or virologic evidence of an influenza A outbreak and should continue for as long as the virus can be isolated in the community (usually 4–6 weeks). Persons vaccinated during an influenza outbreak should also receive amantadine for at least 2 weeks thereafter to allow sufficient time for immunity to develop.

Prophylaxis of Recurrent Genital Herpes Simplex Virus Type 2 Infection

Persons at Risk. After primary genital infection with herpes simplex virus (HSV) type 2, the virus establishes itself in a latent form in neural tissue. Under certain conditions (e.g., anxiety, premenstrual syndrome, and immunosuppression), persons with latent infection may develop clinically active disease due to viral reactivation. Therefore, anyone who has experienced primary genital infection with HSV type 2 is at risk for recurrent disease. Reactivation of latent genital herpes virus infection causes both physical and emotional pain and increases the likelihood of viral transmission to sexual partners. Although the rate of recurrence appears to diminish over time, the mean number of recurrences is about four per year.[48]

Indications for Prophylaxis. Antiviral prophylaxis of genital HSV type 2 infection is indicated for any patient in whom the recurrence rate is unacceptably high to the patient or clinician—often defined arbitrarily as six or more episodes per year in immunocompetent patients. Immunocompromised patients, such as transplant recipients and HIV-infected persons who have a history of HSV type 2 infection, should probably receive antiviral prophylaxis routinely. Acyclovir should be administered to pregnant women only when its use is essential, despite reports that this practice is safe.

Efficacy of Prophylaxis. Prophylactic acyclovir has been shown to reduce both the frequency and severity of recurrent episodes of genital herpes infection.[49–52] Depending on the patient series, 65–85% of patients experienced no recurrences while receiving acyclovir for up to 4 months. Protection from recurrent infection is realized only during the period of acyclovir therapy. Patients who do experience recurrences while receiving acyclovir have milder symptoms, a shorter duration of viral shedding, and more rapid resolution of symptoms. Acyclovir 200 mg orally three to five times daily (average, three times daily) is effective in preventing episodes of recurrent genital herpes. Doses can be administered less frequently. A dosage of 400 mg twice daily was as effective as 200 mg four times daily and is associated with a higher rate of compliance.[50] A single daily dose of 800 mg may also be as effective as 400 mg twice daily.[53]

Recommendations. Patients who have at least six episodes of HSV type 2 reactivation per year and who experience marked pain and emotional stress should receive acyclovir orally for 1 year (Table 1). Since the frequency of recurrence seems to decrease,[53] most clinicians advocate the discontinuation of acyclovir prophylaxis after 1 year so that the risk for and frequency of further episodes can be determined.

International Travel

Approximately 8 million Americans travel to other countries each year. International travel places a person at risk for acquiring infections that are not normally encountered at home. Special precautions, including the use of prophylactic antimicrobials, may be of benefit.

Prophylaxis of Traveler's Diarrhea

Traveler's diarrhea frequently starts during the first week of travel to another country. The syndrome is characterized by a twofold increase in the frequency of unformed bowel movements, often accompanied by such symptoms as abdominal cramping, nausea, fever, chills, urgency, and malaise. The duration of the syndrome is variable; without treatment, most individuals recover fully within 3–5 days, and 60% recover within the first 48 hours. A few individuals may, however, remain ill for as long as 3 weeks. Complications from traveler's diarrhea are rare.

Persons at Risk. Risk factors for traveler's diarrhea include young age, low experience in traveling to an area, high socioeconomic status, and a prolonged stay. The illness is believed to result from the ingestion of contaminated food or water. The contamination is generally fecal and consists of a variety of microorganisms, including enterotoxigenic *E. coli*, *Campylobacter* spp., *Shigella* spp., *Salmonella* spp., *Vibrio* spp., *Giardia* spp., *Entamoeba* spp., rotaviruses, and the Norwalk agent. Foods often cited as being risky include fresh fruits that are not peeled, vegetables, soil-contaminated leafy greens, raw seafood, and improperly stored or cooked meats.[54]

Indications for Prophylaxis. Travel to certain less-developed countries is associated with a high incidence of diarrhea. Travelers to such countries would appear to benefit most from antimicrobial prophylaxis. The incidence of traveler's diarrhea is highest among persons traveling to Latin America (70%), Africa (54–62%), the Middle East, and Asia and lowest among travelers to industrialized countries such as Canada and northern European nations.[55-61]

Efficacy of Prophylaxis. Dietary discretion. Travelers are advised to avoid tap water, ice, unbottled beverages, fruits that cannot be peeled, uncooked or cold meats and fish, and uncooked ground-grown vegetables.[62] Although these dietary recommendations are not easy to comply with, they may reduce the incidence of traveler's diarrhea.

Antimicrobial prophylaxis. Bismuth subsalicylate has been shown to reduce the incidence and severity of traveler's diarrhea by up to 60% among students traveling to Mexico.[63] The frequency of administration may be important: 2.4 g/day divided into four doses may be more effective than the same daily dosage divided into two doses.[64] Although some persons may develop discoloration of the tongue, bismuth subsalicylate is generally well tolerated. Individuals taking other salicylic acid-containing products, as well as all children, should avoid this drug lest salicylism develop.

Various antimicrobials, including trimethoprim–sulfamethoxazole,[65] doxycycline,[66] trimethoprim,[65,67] ciprofloxacin,[68] and norfloxacin,[69] have been shown to decrease the incidence of diarrhea in persons traveling for short periods (less than 3 weeks). The effectiveness of prophylaxis lasts only as long as the antimicrobial is taken.[67] Antimicrobial prophylaxis of traveler's diarrhea may be limited by toxicity of the agent, superinfection with resistant bacteria, fungal infection, and emergence of resistant strains.[62,70] Trimethoprim–sulfamethoxazole is the only antimicrobial that has been used extensively in children because of contraindications for other agents.[71]

Recommendations. Practitioners are sometimes pressured by international travelers to prescribe antimicrobials that will prevent diarrhea. However, traveler's diarrhea, even when untreated, is most often mild and ephemeral. These antimicrobials place the otherwise healthy person at unnecessary risk of toxicity, superinfection, and the emergence of resistant organisms. An NIH consensus panel recommended that travelers who are otherwise healthy not take antimicrobials for the prevention of traveler's diarrhea.[55] Rather, travelers should be encouraged to practice dietary precautions; if symptoms of diarrhea occur, antimicrobial treatment may then be instituted.

Prophylaxis of Malaria

Malaria is one of the greatest health risks faced by international travelers. There are 200–300 million new cases of malaria around the globe each year and 2 million to 3 million deaths.

Persons at Risk and Indications for Prophylaxis. Malaria is endemic in the Middle East, Southeast Asia, the Indian subcontinent, South America, Central America, Oceania, and sub-Saharan Africa. The relative risk of acquiring malaria in the countries of these regions is reported each year by the Centers for Disease Control.[72] The risk of acquiring malaria depends to a great degree on the itinerary. Although *Plasmodium vivax* causes most cases, *Plasmodium falciparum* is responsible for most fatalities.[73,74]

Efficacy of Prophylaxis. Protective clothing and repellents. All persons traveling to areas where malaria is endemic should be encouraged to avoid exposure to mosquitoes. Protective measures include wearing long pants and long shirt sleeves, remaining inside well-screened areas, and using insect repellents and pesticides. The most effective repellents contain at least 30% N,N-diethylmetatoluamide (DEET). Repellents with high concentrations of DEET have a longer effect but should be used cautiously on small children because of potential neurotoxicity.[75]

Antimicrobial prophylaxis. Chloroquine alone is generally the preferred agent for travelers, especially in areas where chloroquine-resistant *P. falciparum* (CRPF) is rare or unreported; resistance of *P. falciparum* to chloroquine is an increasing problem. Chloroquine phosphate can prevent the erythrocytic stages of sensitive *Plasmodium* species but is inactive against the sporozoite and hepatic stages. Chloroquine is active against *P. malariae*, *P. ovale*, and *P. vivax*.

Pyrimethamine–sulfadoxine is no longer routinely recommended for persons traveling to areas where CRPF is endemic because of the high risk of a fatal reaction.[76] Instead, chloroquine alone is recommended. Travelers should report to a medical facility at the first symptom of a flu-like illness for evaluation and possible treatment of CRPF infection.[62,72,73,77,78]

Travelers to areas where prompt medical attention is not available should carry a therapeutic dose of pyrimethamine–sulfadoxine to be taken at the first symptom and should seek medical attention as soon as possible.[79] Prophylactic pyrimethamine–sulfadoxine may be considered for travelers at high risk for CRPF infection.[73] Patients should discontinue pyrimethamine–sulfadoxine and seek medical attention at the first sign of skin rash, pruritus, genital lesions, or sore throat as a definite risk for Stevens-Johnson syndrome and agranulocytosis exists. The efficacy of alternative regimens for the prevention of CRPF infection such as doxycycline, chloroguanide (proguanil), and mefloquine has not been fully established.[80]

Recommendations. The necessity for and type of antimicrobial prophylaxis of malaria depend on the traveler's itinerary (Table 1).[72] If prophylactic antimicrobials are determined to be necessary, treatment should begin before the trip begins. After a traveler returns from prolonged visits to areas where *P. vivax* or *P. ovale* is endemic, prophylactic therapy with primaquine phosphate is recommended because the hepatic stage of the parasite may persist for years if untreated.

Prophylaxis to Eliminate *Haemophilus influenzae* Carrier States

H. influenzae continues to be a prominent bacterial pathogen in the pediatric population. Despite advances in antimicrobial therapy, meningitis due to *H. influenzae* type b infection is still frequently associated with substantial morbidity. Vaccination against this organism produces variable immunologic responses in children less than 2 years old and does little to eliminate nasopharyngeal carriage of the organism. Therefore, antimicrobial prophylaxis continues to be important in controlling the spread of this disease.

Persons at Risk. Children under 4 years of age are the single largest risk group, accounting for 95% of all invasive *H. influenzae* type b infections.[81] Children at high risk for secondary infection include all those less than 2 years of age and unvaccinated children 2–4 years of age. The goal of antimicrobial prophylaxis is, therefore, to eradicate the nasopharyngeal carrier state in high risk children, as well as in persons likely to transmit the organism to these children. Because vaccine does not reliably prevent nasopharyngeal carriage, vaccination status is of minimal importance in determining whether someone should receive a prophylactic antimicrobial.

Indications for Prophylaxis. High risk children who have had recent (within 2 weeks) close contact with an index patient with invasive *H. influenzae* type b disease are estimated to have a 100–600 times higher risk of becoming infected than members of the general population.[81,82] Close contact may be defined as household contact or contact for more than 4 hours a day or 25 hours a week. Adult contacts in the household are also likely to harbor the organism and should receive prophylaxis if they may come in contact with another child at high risk. The risk of school and day-care contacts of an index patient becoming infected is much less (approximately 20 times higher than in the general population), although the risk is higher for small groups (fewer than 10 children) and when more than one index patient has been identified.[83]

Efficacy of Prophylaxis. Rifampin 20 mg/kg/day for 4 days (maximum daily dose, 600 mg) is effective in eradicating *H. influenzae* type b from the nasopharynx. Success rates in excess of 95% have been reported.[84] Whether antimicrobial prophylaxis can successfully prevent transmission and infection is less clear. While it appears that antimicrobials do prevent secondary infection in household contacts, their benefit for contacts in schools or day-care centers where a single index case is isolated is questionable.[85,86] Antimicrobial prophylaxis for the latter kinds of contacts is advocated

by the Centers for Disease Control but not by the American Academy of Pediatrics. The decision to use antimicrobial prophylaxis in school and day-care contacts should probably be based on supplementary criteria, such as the size of the group and the number of index cases.

Recommendations. The ultimate decision regarding indications for prophylaxis should be made by local health departments. Rifampin prophylaxis should definitely be provided to (1) all persons who have had household or other close contact with an index patient within the past 2 weeks and who are likely to be exposed to high risk children, (2) all children who were exposed in a day-care center to more than one index patient diagnosed during the past 2 months, and (3) children with index cases who will be in contact with high risk children after treatment. Rifampin should probably be given to all children who have had day-care contact with one index patient diagnosed within the past 2 months.

Prophylaxis appears unnecessary in (1) all adults who have had household or other close contact with an index patient diagnosed within the past 2 weeks if exposure to other high risk children is not anticipated, (2) all children who were exposed during school to one index case diagnosed within the past 2 months, and (3) persons who were exposed to an index case more than 2 months ago. Ceftriaxone is an alternative to rifampin in pregnant women but has not undergone extensive study.

Antimicrobial Prophylaxis to Eliminate *Neisseria meningitidis* Carrier State

N. meningitidis remains a common cause of bacterial meningitis in the United States and other countries. Routine administration of a meningococcal polysaccharide vaccine to civilians in this country has not been advocated because of the low risk for infection and the lack of protection against serogroup B. Therefore, antimicrobial prophylaxis has maintained an important role in preventing the spread of meningococcal disease.

Persons at Risk. Meningococcal disease is ubiquitous. Outbreaks in contained populations, such as those of military camps and small communities, have been reported. Children less than 5 years of age constitute the group at highest risk for endemic disease, while adults and children are affected with equal frequency during epidemics.[87–89]

Indications for Prophylaxis. Intimate contact (e.g., household contact and exposure to oral secretions) with a person with meningococcal meningitis poses the highest risk: The infection rate for these persons is 300–1000 times higher than in the general population.[89] In localized outbreaks, less intimate contact, such as with day-care center attendees or fellow military recruits, may be risky—especially the latter when serotype B is determined to be the cause. Patients recovering from meningococcal meningitis frequently continue to harbor organisms in the nasopharynx and should also receive prophylaxis to eradicate the organism from this site.

Efficacy of Prophylaxis. Sulfadiazine, rifampin, and minocycline have all demonstrated efficacy in eliminating the nasopharyngeal carriage of meningococcus as well as in reducing the rate of secondary infection.[90–92] Rifampin 10 mg/kg twice daily for 2 days (maximum daily dose, 600 mg) is the current treatment of choice. Reports of resistance with sulfadiazine and an unacceptably high incidence of adverse effects with minocycline have relegated these agents to second-line status. Recent failures with rifampin and the emergence of rifampin-resistant strains have led to studies with newer antimicrobials such as ciprofloxacin and ceftriaxone.[93,94] Both appear to be at least as effective as rifampin in eradicating nasopharyngeal colonization, although the length of followup monitoring in some studies might have been too brief to detect recurrence.

Recommendations. Prophylaxis is definitely recommended for members of households with an index case, intimate contacts or day-care-center contacts of an index patient, and the index patient after he or she has undergone systemic antimicrobial treatment (Table 1). Prophylaxis should probably be given to casual contacts in contained groups. Alternatives to rifampin are ciprofloxacin, minocycline, sulfadiazine, and possibly ceftriaxone. Ciprofloxacin is contraindicated in children less than 18 years of age because of the potential for arthropathy with its use.

Antimicrobial Prophylaxis to Eliminate Methicillin-Resistant *Staphylococcus aureus* Carrier State

Methicillin-resistant *Staph. aureus* infections create a dilemma for hospital physicians and infection control specialists. Treatment of these infections involves the use of expensive, potentially toxic antimicrobials; lasting eradication of the carrier state is difficult to accomplish because of reacquisition of the organism or development of resistance. While antimicrobials help to eliminate the carrier state, they are useful on a large scale only when combined with surveillance and isolation techniques. In many institutions where these infections are endemic, antimicrobial prophylaxis has little impact on overall incidence. However, where the incidence is still low, attempts at eradication in carriers are still indicated.

Persons at Risk. Persons at particular risk for methicillin-resistant *Staph. aureus* infection are similar to those at risk for methicillin-sensitive staphylococcal infection, namely hospitalized patients and individuals with indwelling devices such as intravenous catheters, peritoneal dialysis catheters, and prosthetic heart valves.[95–98] Approximately 40–50% of normal individuals are colonized with *Staph. aureus*, usually in the anterior nares, axillae, and perineum. Patients, nurses, physicians, and individuals with skin disorders like eczema or seborrhea are even more likely to be carriers of staphylococci and should be examined for such carriage in the event of an outbreak. Intravenous drug users appear to be particularly likely to be colonized.[97]

Indications for Prophylaxis. The goal of antimicrobial prophylaxis is to eliminate carriage of methicillin-resistant *Staph. aureus* in persons at risk as well as in individuals likely to come in close contact with them. Eradication of the carriage of methicillin-sensitive staphylococci is also important in many individuals (e.g., hemodialysis patients)[98] but is not discussed here, since most of the agents used to eradicate resistant strains from carriers are also effective in eradicating sensitive strains. After documentation of a case of colonization or infection with resistant *Staph. aureus*, surveillance cultures of samples from patients and health-care workers should be performed. Culture-positive individuals should be

isolated or removed from the hospital setting as soon as possible and eradication of *Staph. aureus* attempted.

Efficacy of Prophylaxis. Topical antimicrobials, such as chlorhexidine, bacitracin, and tetracycline, have been of only limited value in eradicating methicillin-resistant *Staph. aureus* carriage.[97] Systemically admininistered vancomycin does not reach sufficiently high concentrations in skin and nasal mucosa to be effective. The use of rifampin alone or in combination with another antimicrobial, such as trimethoprim–sulfamethoxazole, fusidic acid, or ciprofloxacin, appears to be most effective.[99–104] These therapies are often supplemented with topical application of agents to the nares and baths with antimicrobial soaps. Successful eradication of resistant *Staph. aureus* with intranasal mupirocin, a topical antimicrobial, has been reported, but evidence of resistance has raised concern.[105]

Recommendations. No particular antimicrobial regimen appears to be universally effective in eradicating methicillin-resistant *Staph. aureus* from the skin and nares. If colonization is confined to the nares, local application of mupirocin four times daily for 5 days would appear to be an appropriate initial regimen. If multiple sites are colonized or topical agents have failed, systemic therapy with rifampin plus trimethoprim–sulfamethoxazole or ciprofloxacin (both given twice daily) may be used (Table 1). The optimal duration of therapy may range from 5 to 21 days. Since the recurrence of colonization is usually associated with reexposure to rather than regrowth of this organism, it is unlikely that a longer course of therapy offers additional benefit.

Antimicrobial Prophylaxis to Prevent Perinatal Infection with Group B Streptococci

Group B streptococci are the pathogens most frequently implicated in neonatal sepsis in the United States and are directly implicated in 20% of all episodes of peripartum sepsis.[106] Two distinct disease types, early and late onset, have been described. Early-onset sepsis, which occurs during the first week of life and results from intrauterine infection, is more common than late-onset disease and is associated with a higher infant mortality rate.[107] It is estimated that 0.2–0.3% of all neonates in the United States develop sepsis involving group B streptococci; the fatality rate is 25%. Survivors have a 30–50% likelihood of permanent neurological sequelae.[106,107]

Persons at Risk. Because group B streptococci are transmitted from mother to neonate during delivery, infants born to mothers with cervical or vaginal colonization are at greatest risk for sepsis. Approximately 20% of all pregnant women in the United States are colonized with these organisms, which may be identified by routine prenatal surveillance cultures or coagglutination tests performed during labor. Of infants born to colonized mothers, 50–70% become colonized themselves; 1–2% develop sepsis (5–10 times the rate in the general population and 30–60 times the rate for infants born to mothers who are not colonized).[107]

Indications for Prophylaxis. The subset of neonates whose mothers are colonized by group B streptococci and who have certain other risk factors is at highest risk for group B streptococcus sepsis and, therefore, constitutes the group most likely to benefit from antimicrobial prophylaxis. The other risk factors include low birth weight (less than or equal to 2500 g), prolonged interval between membrane rupture and birth (more than 18 hours), and maternal fever during labor. Neonates with colonized mothers and one or more of the other risk factors account for 4–5% of all live births, 63% of all cases of group B streptococcus sepsis, and 95% of all deaths from this infection. The benefits of antimicrobial prophylaxis in this group clearly outweigh the risks of adverse effects from penicillin administration.[107]

Efficacy of Prophylaxis. A number of studies have documented the efficacy of penicillin or ampicillin, administered during the peripartum period, in preventing transmission of group B streptococci from mother to infant.[108,109] More recent studies have confirmed the efficacy of ampicillin in preventing group B streptococcus sepsis in infants with colonized mothers and one or more other risk factors.[110–112] In one study, ampicillin (as the sodium salt) 2 g was administered intravenously to mothers at the onset of labor, followed by 1 g intravenously every 4 hours until delivery; in addition, the neonates received ampicillin (as the sodium salt) 50 mg/kg intramuscularly every 12 hours for 48 hours.[110] No cases of group B streptococcus infection developed in the mothers or their infants. It is not known whether a similar response would have been observed had only mothers or infants alone been treated.

Recommendations. Peripartum administration of ampicillin or penicillin to mothers and infants considered, on the basis of the criteria described above, to be at high risk for group B streptococcus infection appears to be justifiable (Table 1). A history of penicillin allergy should be excluded before antimicrobials are given. A vaccine against these organisms is needed, along with more sensitive rapid diagnostic methods for detecting colonization in women who do not undergo routine prenatal screening.

Prophylaxis of Nosocomial Pneumonia

Bacterial pneumonia, UTIs, wound infections, and bacteremia compose the majority of infections acquired by hospitalized patients. Of these, nosocomial pneumonia is associated with the greatest morbidity and mortality. Nosocomial pneumonia is frequently caused by gram-negative aerobic bacilli, which colonize the upper respiratory tract soon after hospital admission.[113] Antimicrobial prophylaxis has, therefore, been directed primarily toward these organisms (selective decontamination).

Patients at Risk. Patients requiring prolonged mechanical ventilation in an intensive-care unit (ICU) are at greatest risk for nosocomial pneumonia. The reported incidence of nosocomial pneumonia in intubated patients ranges from 5 to 60%.[113–116] It has been estimated that 60% of critically ill patients develop pneumonia within 5 days of the start of mechanical ventilation.[113] Other risk factors for infection include advanced age and the presence of underlying disease states. From the wide range of the reported incidence of nosocomial pneumonia, it would appear that some institutions may benefit more from antimicrobial prophylaxis than others.

Indications for Prophylaxis. Patients who would be expected to benefit most from prophylaxis would be those in whom prolonged but not indefinite ventilation is anticipated. Trauma patients constitute one such group and have been studied extensively;[117–122] organ recipients may also benefit from prophylaxis while in the ICU.[123]

Efficacy of Prophylaxis. Several European studies have shown that selective decontamination may successfully prevent nosocomial pneumonia. The most successful approach involves three components:

1. Oral administration of nonabsorbable antimicrobials, such as aminoglycosides, polymyxin in B, and amphotericin B, to reduce the gastrointestinal population of organisms that may migrate to the upper and lower respiratory tracts.
2. Application to the oral mucosa of a paste containing the same antimicrobials to prevent upper respiratory tract colonization.
3. Brief (4–7 days) administration of an intravenous antimicrobial to treat any "incubating" pneumonia that may have been acquired at the time of admission.[119–122]

These procedures are apparently remarkably effective in reducing the incidence of nosocomial pneumonia. However, the lack of studies in the United States, the continued question of the development of infection with resistant organisms, and the minor impact of prophylaxis on mortality have led to only cautious optimism by many clinicians.[124]

Recommendations. Until prospective studies are performed in the United States, no definite recommendations for routine antimicrobial prophylaxis of nosocomial pneumonia in mechanically ventilated patients can be made.

Antimicrobial Prophylaxis for Granulocytopenic Patients

The goal of antimicrobial prophylaxis in granulocytopenic patients is to prevent infection, the cause of death in 50–80% of these patients. Prophylaxis is primarily directed toward gram-negative aerobic bacilli colonizing the alimentary and respiratory tracts; infections with these bacteria are associated with the greatest risk of morbidity and mortality due to endotoxic shock. The gastrointestinal tract is the major source of gram-negative bacterial infections. These infections frequently are the result of bacteremias that arise because of mucosal damage caused by antineoplastic therapy or the disease state itself.

Patients at Risk. Patients with acute leukemia who are expected to experience granulocytopenia (usually defined as less than 500 granulocytes/cu mm) for a prolonged time (more than 7 days) as a result of antineoplastic therapy are at particular risk for infection. Patients with solid tumors or lymphomas usually are not subjected to such profound and extended granulocytopenia by their antineoplastic regimens. In these patients, a benefit from prophylactic antimicrobials may not be as readily demonstrated.

The degree of granulocytopenia also appears to be an important prognostic indicator in these patients. Antimicrobial prophylaxis has shown benefit in preventing infection in patients with severe granulocytopenia (less than 100 granulocytes/cu mm). In contrast, while some studies have shown a beneficial effect of antimicrobial prophylaxis in patients who have a granulocyte count of less than 1000/cu mm, an equal number have not.

Indications for Prophylaxis. Patients with acute leukemia who receive antineoplastic therapy that results in a granulocyte count of less than 500/cu mm for 7 days or longer should receive antimicrobial prophylaxis. In addition, prophylaxis is possibly useful in selected granulocytopenic patients with lymphomas or solid tumors, although evidence supporting this measure has not been conclusive and specific guidelines are not available.

Efficacy of Prophylaxis. *Oral nonabsorbable antimicrobials.* Some prospective controlled evaluations of prophylactic regimens of oral vancomycin, gentamicin, colistin, polymyxin B, and neomycin have demonstrated benefit while others have not.[125] Concurrent administration of these drugs has led to suppression of all of the organisms normally colonizing the alimentary canal, resulting in colonization by resistant organisms. For example, combination therapy with gentamicin has resulted in the emergence of gentamicin-resistant flora, obviating its future use in systemic therapy of the patient's febrile episodes.[126]

Patient compliance is also a major problem with these regimens. In addition to being expensive, these drugs are unpalatable and often cause nausea, vomiting, and diarrhea. Many granulocytopenic patients undergoing antineoplastic therapy have mucositis, anorexia, and nausea and are, therefore, unable or unwilling to take these antimicrobials.

Oral absorbable antimicrobials. Such agents as trimethoprim–sulfamethoxazole, norfloxacin, and ciprofloxacin have been used to achieve a selective antimicrobial effect by reducing the aerobic bacterial flora of the colon without suppressing the anaerobic flora. This practice theoretically preserves resistance to colonization by undesirable aerobic gram-negative bacilli, an effect known as colonization resistance.

Trimethoprim–sulfamethoxazole is by far the most frequently studied antimicrobial for this indication. Investigators have shown that prophylaxis with trimethoprim–sulfamethoxazole significantly decreases the number of days the patient is febrile, the number of days intravenous antimicrobials are required, the number of infections, and the number of gram-negative rod bacteremias compared with control patients and patients given a placebo, various nonabsorbable antimicrobials, and nalidixic acid.[127,128] No significant beneficial effects on overall death rates have been observed, however.

There are major concerns about the use of trimethoprim–sulfamethoxazole in these patients. Some studies have demonstrated a significant increase in the mean duration of granulocytopenia, presumably because of the myelosuppressive effect of the drug.[127,128] Organisms resistant to trimethoprim–sulfamethoxazole have been isolated; one report cited the isolation of a self-transferable plasmid.[129,130] An increase in opportunistic fungal infections (some fatal) has also been reported.[131,132] Therefore, alternatives to the use of trimethoprim–sulfamethoxazole appear necessary for prophylaxis in some individuals.

Nalidixic acid has been proposed as an alternative means of prophylaxis. However, studies have shown nalidixic acid to be inferior to trimethoprim–sulfamethoxazole for this purpose, and it should not be considered for use in granulocytopenic patients.[131,133]

Preliminary studies have suggested that fluoroquinolones such as norfloxacin and ciprofloxacin provide the best currently available alternative to trimethoprim–sulfamethoxazole for antimicrobial prophylaxis in granulocytopenic patients. Advantages of these agents include easier tolerance, fewer adverse effects (resulting in good compliance), and fewer problems with resistance.

Norfloxacin and ciprofloxacin have both been shown to decrease significantly infections caused by gram-negative bacilli compared with other prophylactic regimens.[134,135] Norfloxacin has also been shown to delay significantly the onset of the patient's first fever and to reduce the duration of fever compared with a placebo.[136] Again, however, therapy with these agents has not resulted in a reduced overall mortality rate. In fact, prophylaxis associated with the quinolones is associated with an increased incidence of infections by gram-positive bacteria, especially streptococci. It is unclear whether this problem is due to the limited spectrum of activity of the quinolones against gram-positive bacteria or to a general increase in infections in granulocytopenic patients caused by gram-positive organisms such as staphylococci.

There is no evidence to support the use of oral antifungal agents (e.g., clotrimazole, amphotericin B, nystatin, and ketoconazole), either alone or in combination with antimicrobial drugs, to decrease the incidence of fungal infections in these patients, except perhaps in the granulocytopenic patient who has received a bone marrow transplant.

Recommendations. Although there is controversy, current literature on balance supports the use of trimethoprim–sulfamethoxazole or a quinolone for prophylaxis in eligible granulocytopenic patients. Ciprofloxacin and norfloxacin have not been directly compared in a clinical trial. Quinolones should be avoided in children because of their deleterious effects on cartilage formation.

Prophylaxis should be started when antineoplastic therapy is begun. Prophylactic therapy may be started even if patients have an ongoing infection or are febrile. The prophylaxis should be continued until the granulocytopenia is resolved (granulocyte count, greater than 500/cu mm). Some authors suggested stopping prophylactic antimicrobials when systemic antimicrobial treatment is required, regardless of the degree of granulocytopenia.

Prophylaxis for *Pneumocystis carinii* Pneumonia in HIV-Infected Persons

Persons at Risk. Nearly everyone has at some point been exposed to *P. carinii*, an organism ubiquitous in the environment. Once exposed, a person has a lifelong risk of developing clinical disease should his or her cell-mediated immune system become compromised. Although any patient with compromised cell-mediated immunity may develop *P. carinii* pneumonia (PCP), HIV-infected persons have the greatest risk and are, therefore, the most important candidates for antimicrobial prophylaxis.[137]

Indications. PCP is the most common opportunistic infection diagnosed in persons with acquired immunodeficiency syndrome (AIDS); 80% develop PCP at some time during their illness. Although 75% of patients survive the initial episode, the organism is not completely eradicated from the lungs. About 20% of patients develop recurrences of the disease within 6 months, which may ultimately prove to be fatal: PCP is the primary cause of death in 25% of persons with AIDS.[137] Because of the frequency and mortality rate of

PCP among people with AIDS, prophylaxis is indicated for (1) HIV-positive persons if the T4 lymphocyte count is less than 200–300/cu mm or if T4 lymphocytes account for fewer than 20% of the total number of lymphocytes counted and (2) persons with AIDS or AIDS-related complex, regardless of their history of *P. carinii* pneumonia.[137,138]

Efficacy of Prophylaxis. While zidovudine appears to reduce the incidence of PCP in HIV-infected persons,[38] specific prophylaxis directed at *P. carinii* can play a major role. Among 60 HIV-infected patients with newly diagnosed Kaposi's sarcoma, trimethoprim 160 mg–sulfamethoxazole 800 mg twice daily prevented the development of PCP in the 30 patients receiving the drug, while more than half of the 30 patients receiving a placebo developed clinical disease.[139] However, 50% of those patients receiving trimethoprim–sulfamethoxazole experienced adverse effects.

Since persons with AIDS have such a high rate of adverse reactions to sulfa drugs, alternative treatments for PCP prophylaxis are being sought. They include intravenous pentamidine, aerosolized pentamidine (at various doses and dosage intervals), pyrimethamine–sulfadoxine, and dapsone. Open trials with these agents (aerosolized pentamidine, in particular) suggest that they are effective in preventing PCP in HIV-positive individuals. Data are not yet available from the comparative controlled studies being conducted by the AIDS Clinical Trials Groups (ACTG).

Recommendations. Kovacs and Masur[140] summarized existing data and offered recommendations on rational therapy to prevent PCP in HIV-infected persons. Although data from ACTG studies using trimethoprim–sulfamethoxazole as a control are not yet available, most clinicians now advocate aerosolized pentamidine as first-line therapy for PCP prophylaxis. Aerosolized pentamidine isethionate 300 mg administered monthly via a Respirgard II nebulizer recently received FDA-approved labeling for PCP prophylaxis.[137] However, patients receiving pentamidine by inhalation will remain at risk for extrapulmonary infection with *P. carinii*.[141] Therefore, prophylaxis with oral trimethoprim–sulfamethoxazole is an important, less expensive alternative for patients who can tolerate it.

Antimicrobial Prophylaxis in Transplant Patients

Patients who have received organ or bone marrow transplants are at substantial risk for infection. Immunosuppressive therapies used to suppress the host immune response and prevent organ rejection and graft-versus-host disease predispose the patient to infection by a number of opportunistic pathogens. In addition, bone marrow transplant patients are severely neutropenic in the early postengraftment period and are, therefore, at increased risk for bacterial infection.

Pathogens. Routine antimicrobial prophylaxis should be directed at those pathogens most likely to cause infection and for which infection is associated with a high degree of morbidity or mortality. These pathogens may be classified as bacterial, viral, fungal, and protozoal.

Bacteria. Bacterial pathogens such as *Listeria*, *Nocardia*, and *Legionella* species are rarely pathogenic for normal hosts but may cause infections in transplant patients.

Like other opportunistic pathogens, they are most likely to cause infection from 1 to more than 6 months after the transplantation procedure.[142,143] In contrast, other more common bacterial species, such as gram-negative bacilli and gram-positive cocci, may cause infection in the early posttransplant period. Colonization of the upper respiratory tract may lead to pneumonia in intubated patients, early pyelonephritis due to gram-negative bacilli most commonly involves the transplanted kidney and may lead to rejection, and neutropenic marrow transplant recipients are at risk for intravenous catheter sepsis and primary bacteremia from organisms colonizing the skin and gastrointestinal tract.[142,143] Encapsulated bacteria such as pneumococci can also cause infection in the late posttransplant period.

Viruses. Herpesviruses [herpes simplex virus (HSV), herpes zoster virus (HZV), and cytomegalovirus (CMV)] can also infect transplant patients. Clinical infections by HSV and HZV are most commonly due to reactivation of latent infection and are usually mucocutaneous or cutaneous. Among solid organ transplant recipients, the most severe cases of CMV infection (usually pneumonia) occur in seronegative patients who acquire the virus through the graft or blood products;[144] among marrow recipients, disease most commonly occurs in patients who were previously seropositive.[145] Both the organ donor and recipient should undergo serologic screening for CMV whenever possible. HSV reactivation usually develops within the first month after transplantation, whereas CMV pneumonia and HZV infection are most prevalent during months 1–4 and 2–6, respectively.

Fungi and protozoans. Fungal infections in transplant patients are usually due to *Candida* or *Aspergillus* species and, to a lesser extent, *Cryptococcus neoformans*. Colonization of the skin and upper respiratory tract with *Candida* species occurs frequently. Infections involving *Candida* or *Aspergillus* species occur primarily in the first or second month after transplantation. In contrast, respiratory tract infections by *Cryptococcus* species occur later.

Other common opportunistic pathogens in transplant patients are *P. carinii* and *Toxoplasma gondii*. Once thought to be protozoan, *P. carinii* has been reclassified as a fungus. *P. carinii* pneumonia usually occurs either within the first 1–4 months after transplantation or later in patients receiving high-dose immunosuppression therapy for chronic rejection. Toxoplasmosis usually occurs due to reactivation of latent disease and can develop at any time during immunosuppression.

Because of the array of pathogens that can infect transplant patients, prophylactic regimens may consist of antimicrobials directed at some or all of these organisms.

Patients at Risk. All patients receiving organ or bone marrow transplants are at risk for infection, especially in the first 6 months after the procedure. In general, because of their concurrent neutropenia, marrow recipients are at higher risk of infection by aerobic bacteria and *Candida* species. CMV-seronegative patients who receive a graft or blood products from a seropositive donor are at greatest risk for severe CMV infection.

Other factors that contribute to a patient's relative risk of infection include the degree of immunosuppression, viral seropositivity before transplantation, the requirement for intubation, the presence of graft-versus-host disease, how such disease is treated, and the underlying disease state that led to the transplant (e.g., diabetes).[146]

Indications for Prophylaxis. Antimicrobial prophylaxis is indicated for all transplant recipients during the early posttransplant period—when high-dose immunosuppressive therapies are used and the risk of infection is greatest.[147] Patients who require pulse immunosuppressive therapy for impending rejection may benefit from additional prophylaxis. Prophylactic regimens for recipients of solid organs may differ from those given to bone marrow recipients. For example, renal transplant patients require prophylaxis of UTIs, which may be continued indefinitely. In general, a triad of prophylactic antimicrobials that are active against bacteria, fungi, and viruses is given to transplant patients.[147] However, other infection control measures, such as pretransplant serologic screening, hand washing, and isolation techniques, are of equal importance in reducing the incidence of infection.

Efficacy of Prophylaxis. Antimicrobial prophylaxis has been directed primarily at eradicating aerobic gram-negative bacteria while sparing the anaerobic flora of the gastrointestinal tract. As a result, many investigators have studied and confirmed the ability of trimethoprim–sulfamethoxazole therapy to reduce the incidence of bacterial infections as well as infections by *P. carinii*.[148,149] Other strategies, such as the use of nonabsorbable oral antimicrobials and of the quinolones, have also been attempted, notably in kidney and bone marrow recipients, but have not shown clear superiority over trimethoprim–sulfamethoxazole.[143]

Antifungal prophylaxis has been most successful in preventing infections due to *Candida* species by eliminating oropharyngeal colonization.[150–153] Either topical nystatin or clotrimazole appears to be effective in this regard; clotrimazole may have a slight advantage because of its greater palatability and lower cost.[153] While ketoconazole has been shown to be effective in some studies, it costs more than the other agents, has a potential for interaction with cyclosporine and for inducing resistance to subsequent amphotericin B therapy, and has been associated with an increased incidence of infections by other filamentous fungi.[151,152] Whether fluconazole will have fewer problems associated with its use and will become an attractive alternative is uncertain. In bone marrow recipients who are unable to tolerate topical antifungals because of nausea or mucositis, low-dose intravenous amphotericin B may be indicated. The use of efficient air filters to reduce spore counts has been the most effective means of prophylaxis of infection by *Aspergillus* species.[132]

Acyclovir reduces the incidence of infection by HSV and HZV in seropositive transplant patients.[154–157] Recent data suggest that high-dose oral acyclovir may also be effective in preventing infection by CMV, especially in seronegative recipients who receive a kidney from a seropositive donor.[158] Use of intravenous immune globulin or CMV immune globulin in selected individuals may also be of benefit in preventing CMV infection, but controlled studies are necessary to define the indications for this costly intervention.

Recommendations. Organ recipients should receive trimethoprim–sulfamethoxazole for at least 1 year after surgery and acyclovir for 1–4 months. Longer courses of acyclovir may be given to patients receiving a cadaveric kidney or a kidney from a CMV-positive donor (Table 1). Acyclovir prophylaxis may not be cost effective if the recipient has CMV-negative serum and receives an organ

from a CMV-negative donor. In addition, patients should receive clotrimazole troches or nystatin suspension for at least 3 months.

Bone marrow recipients should receive an antimicrobial (usually trimethoprim–sulfamethoxazole or a quinolone) and an antifungal (usually clotrimazole or nystatin) as prophylaxis until successful engraftment has occurred, as documented by an increasing white blood cell count. Patients should also receive antimicrobial prophylaxis during episodes of graft-versus-host disease. Prophylaxis with acyclovir is also recommended for these patients, but the duration of therapy is controversial; it ranges from 1 to 12 months depending on the institution.

References

1. Shulman ST, Amren DP, Bisno AL, et al. Prevention of bacterial endocarditis: a statement for health professionals by the Committee on Rheumatic Fever and Infective Endocarditis of the Council on Cardiovascular Disease in the Young. *Circulation*. 1984; 70:1123–7A.

2. The antibiotic prophylaxis of infective endocarditis: report of a working party of the British Society for Antimicrobial Chemotherapy. *Lancet*. 1982; 2:1323– 6.

3. Prevention of bacterial endocarditis. *Med Lett Drugs Ther*. 1986; 29:22. Editorial.

4. Durack DT. Current practices in endocarditis prophylaxis: search for compromise. Paper presented at 29th Interscience Conference on Antimicrobial Agents and Chemotherapy. Houston, TX: 1989 Sep 19.

5. Okawa JH, Kaye D. Endocarditis: epidemiology, pathophysiology, management and prophylaxis. *Cardiovasc Clin*. 1985; 15(2):335–57.

6. Durack DT. Current issues in prevention of infective endocarditis. *Am J Med*. 1985; 78(Suppl 613):149–56.

7. Kaye DP. Prophylaxis for infective endocarditis: an update. *Ann Intern Med*. 1986; 104:419–23.

8. Von Reyn CF, Levy BS, Arbeit RD, et al. Infective endocarditis: an analysis based on strict case definition. *Ann Intern Med*. 1981; 94:505.

9. Clemons JD, Horwitz RI, Jaffe CC, et al. A controlled evaluation of the risk of bacterial endocarditis in persons with mitral valve prolapse. *N Engl J Med*. 1982; 307:776–81.

10. Devereux RB, Hawkins J, Kramer-Fox R, et al. Complications of mitral valve prolapse: disproportionate occurrences in men and older patients. *Am J Med*. 1986; 81:751–8.

11. MacMahon SW, Hickey AJ, Wilcken DEL, et al. Risk of infective endocarditis in mitral valve prolapse with and without precordial systolic murmurs. *Am J Cardiol*. 1987; 59:105–8.

12. Dajani AS, Bisno AL, Chung KJ, et al. Prevention of rheumatic fever: a statement for health professionals by the Committee on Rheumatic Fever, Endocarditis and Kawasaki Disease of the Council on Cardiovascular Disease in the Young, American Heart Association. *Pediatr Infect Dis J*. 1989; 8:263–6.

13. Rossiter SJ, Stinson EB, Oyer PE, et al. Prosthetic valve endocarditis: comparison of heterograft tissue valves and mechanical valves. *J Thorac Cardiovasc Surg*. 1978; 76:795–803.

14. Durack DT, Bisno AL, Kaplan EL. Apparent failures of endocarditis prophylaxis: an analysis of 52 cases

submitted to a national registry. *JAMA*. 1983; 250:2318–22.

15. Durack DT. Prophylaxis of infective endocarditis. In: Mandell GL, Douglas RG, Bennett JE, eds. Principles and practice of infectious diseases. New York: John Wiley; 1989.

16. Committee on Rheumatic Fever and Bacterial Endocarditis of the Council on Cardiovascular Diseases in the Young, American Academy of Pediatrics. Prevention of bacterial endocarditis. *Pediatrics*. 1985; 75(3):603–7.

17. Fowler JE Jr, Stamey TA. Studies of introital colonization in women with recurrent urinary infections. VII. The role of bacterial adherence. *J Urol*. 1977; 117:472–6.

18. Nicolle LE, Harding GKM, Preiksaitis J, et al. The association of urinary tract infection with sexual intercourse. *J Infect Dis*. 1982; 145:579–83.

19. Fihn SD, Latham RH, Roberts P, et al. Association between diaphragm use and urinary tract infection. *JAMA*. 1985; 254:240–5.

20. Adatto K, Doebele KG, Galland L, et al. Behavioral factors and urinary tract infection. *JAMA*. 1979; 241:2525–6.

21. McCracken GH. Diagnosis and management of acute urinary tract infections in children. *Pediatr Infect Dis J*. 1987; 6:107–12.

22. Lipsky BA. Urinary tract infections in men: epidemiology, pathophysiology, diagnosis, and treatment. *Ann Intern Med*. 1989; 110:138–50.

23. Vosti KL. Recurrent urinary tract infections. Prevention by prophylactic antibiotics after sexual intercourse. *JAMA*. 1975; 231:934–40.

24. Wong ES, McKevitt M, Running K, et al. Management of recurrent urinary tract infections with patient-administered single-dose therapy. *Ann Intern Med*. 1985; 102:302–7.

25. Nicolle LE, Harding GKM, Thompson M, et al. Prospective, randomized, placebo-controlled trial of norfloxacin for the prophylaxis of recurrent urinary tract infection in women. *Antimicrob Agents Chemother*. 1989; 33:1032–5.

26. Johnson JR, Stamm WE. Urinary tract infections in women: diagnosis and management. *Ann Intern Med*. 1989; 111:906–17.

27. Immunization Practices Advisory Committee and the Advisory Committee for Elimination of Tuberculosis. Use of BCG vaccines in the control of tuberculosis: a joint statement. *MMWR*. 1988; 37(43):663–4.

28. Supplement on future research in tuberculosis. Improving methods for prevention of disease among the infected. *Am Rev Respir Dis*. 1986; 134(2):413–4.

29. American Thoracic Society and Centers for Disease Control. Treatment of tuberculosis and tuberculosis infection in adults and children: joint statement. *Am Rev Respir Dis*. 1986; 134(2):355–63.

30. International Union Against Tuberculosis. Efficacy of various durations of isoniazid preventive therapy for tuberculosis: five years of followup in the IUAT trial. *Bull WHO*. 1982; 60(4):555–64.

31. Einhorn A, Mizrahi EM. Basilar skull fractures in children: the incidence of CNS infection and the use of antibiotics. *Am J Dis Child*. 1978; 132:1121–4.

32. Ignelzi RJ, VanderArk GD. Analysis of the treatment of basilar skull fractures with and without antibiotics.

J Neurosurg. 1975; 43:721–6.

33. MacGee EE, Cauthen JC, Brackett CE. Meningitis following acute traumatic cerebrospinal fluid fistula. *J Neurosurg*. 1970; 33:312–6.

34. Leech PJ, Paterson A. Conservative and operative management for cerebrospinal fluid leakage after closed head injury. *Lancet*. 1973; 1:1013–6.

35. Beecher CE, Cone JE, Gerberding J. Occupational infection with human immunodeficiency virus (HIV): risks and risk reduction. *Ann Intern Med*. 1989; 110:653–6.

36. Centers for Disease Control. Public Health Service statement on occupational exposure to human immunodeficiency virus, including considerations regarding zidovudine post-exposure use. *MMWR*. 1990; 39:1–14.

37. LaFon SW, Lehrman S, Barry DW. Prophylactically administered Retrovir in health care workers potentially exposed to the human immunodeficiency virus. *J Infect Dis* 1988; 158:503.

38. Fischl MA, Richman DD, Grieco MH, et al. The efficacy of azidothymidine (AZT) in the treatment of patients with AIDS and AIDS-related complex. *N Engl J Med*. 1987; 317:189–91.

39. Henderson DK, Gerberding JL. Prophylactic zidovudine after occupational exposure to the human immunodeficiency virus: an interim analysis. *J Infect Dis*. 1989; 160:321–7.

40. Centers for Disease Control. Recommendations of the Immunization Practices Advisory Committee: prevention and control of influenza. *MMWR*. 1988; 37:361–73.

41. Betts RF. Amantadine and rimantadine for the prevention of influenza A. *Semin Respir Dis*. 1989; 4:304–10.

42. Delker LL, Moser RH, Nelson JD, et al. Amantadine: does it have a role in the prevention and treatment of influenza? A National Institutes of Health Consensus Development Conference. *Ann Intern Med*. 1980; 92:256–8.

43. Douglas RG Jr. Amantadine as an antiviral agent in influenza. *N Engl J Med*. 1982; 307:617–8.

44. Monto AS, Gunn RA, Bandyk MG, et al. Prevention of Russian influenza by amantadine. *JAMA*. 1979; 241:1003–7.

45. Dolin R, Reichman RC, Madore HP, et al. A controlled trial of amantadine and rimantadine in the prophylaxis of Influenza A infections. *N Engl J Med*. 1982; 307:580–4.

46. Hayden FG, Belshe RB, Clover RD, et al. Emergence of apparent transmission of rimantadine-resistant influenza A virus in families. *N Engl J Med*. 1989; 321:1696–1702.

47. Belshe RB, Burk B, Newman F, et al. Resistance of influenza A virus to amantadine and rimantadine: results of one decade of surveillance. *J Infect Dis*. 1989; 159:430–5.

48. Centers for Disease Control. Sexually transmitted diseases treatment guidelines. *MMWR*. 1989; 38(Suppl): 5–8.

49. Gold D, Corey L. Acyclovir prophylaxis for *Herpes simplex* virus infection. *Antimicrob Agents Chemother*. 1987; 31:361–7.

50. Kinghorn GR. Long-term suppression with oral acyclovir of recurrent herpes simplex virus infections in otherwise healthy patients. *Am J Med*. 1988; 85(Suppl 2A):25–9.

51. Mertz GJ, Jones CC, Mills J, et al. Long-term acyclovir suppression of frequently recurring genital herpes simplex virus infection. *JAMA*. 1988; 260:201–6.

52. Strauss SE, Croen KD, Sawyer MH, et al. Acyclovir suppression of frequently recurring genital herpes: efficacy and diminishing need during successive years of treatment. *JAMA*. 1988; 260:2227–30.

53. Mostow SR, Mayfield JL, Marr JJ, et al. Suppression of recurrent genital herpes by single daily dosages of acyclovir. *Am J Med*. 1988; 85(Suppl 2A):30–3.

54. MacDonald KL, Cohen ML. Epidemiology of travelers' diarrhea: current perspectives. *Rev Infect Dis*. 1986; 8(Suppl 2):S117–21.

55. Travelers' diarrhea. Consensus conference. *JAMA*. 1985; 253:2700–4.

56. Shore EG, Dean AG, Holik KJ, et al. Enterotoxigenic-producing *Escherichia coli* and diarrheal disease in adult travelers: a prospective study. *J Infect Dis*. 1974; 129:577–82.

57. Merson MH, Morris GK, Sack DA, et al. Travelers' diarrhea in Mexico: a prospective study of physicians and family members attending Congress. *N Engl J Med*. 1975; 294:1299–305.

58. Ericsson CD, Pickering LK, Sullivan P, et al. The role of location of food consumption in the prevention of travelers' diarrhea in Mexico. *Gastroenterology*. 1980; 79:812–6.

59. Sack RB, Froehlich JL, Zulich AW, et al. Prophylactic doxycycline for travelers' diarrhea: results of prospective double-blind study of Peace Corps volunteers in Mexico. *Gastroenterology*. 1979; 76:1368–73.

60. Echeverria P, Sack RB, Blacklow NR, et al. Prophylactic doxycycline for travelers' diarrhea in Thailand: further supportive evidence of *Aeromonas hydrophila* as an enteric pathogen. *Am J Epidemiol*. 1984; 120:912–21.

61. Taylor DN, Echeverria P, Blaser MJ, et al. The polymicrobial aetiology of travelers' diarrhoea. *Lancet*. 1985; 1:381–3.

62. Hill DR, Pearson RD. Health advice for international travel. *Ann Intern Med*. 1988; 108:839–52.

63. DuPont HL, Sullivan P, Evans DG, et al. Prevention of travelers' diarrhea (emporiatric enteritis): prophylactic administration of subsalicylate bismuth. *JAMA*. 1980; 243:237–41.

64. Steffen R, Heusser R, DuPont HL. Prevention of travelers' diarrhea by nonantibiotic drugs. *Rev Infect Dis*. 1986; 8(Suppl 2):S151–9.

65. DuPont HL, Galindo E, Evans DG, et al. Prevention of travelers' diarrhea with trimethoprim–sulfamethoxazole and trimethoprim alone. *Gastroenterology*. 1983; 84:75–80.

66. Sack RB. Antimicrobial prophylaxis of travelers' diarrhea: a summary of studies using doxycycline or trimethoprim and sulfamethoxazole. *Scand J Gastroenterol*. 1983; 84(Suppl):111–7.

67. Sack RB. Antimicrobial prophylaxis of travelers' diarrhea: a selected summary. *Rev Infect Dis*. 1986; 8(Suppl 2):S160–6.

68. Pichler H, Diridl G, Wolf D. Ciprofloxacin versus placebo in the treatment of acute bacterial diarrhea. Paper presented at 14th International Congress of Chemotherapy. Kyoto, Japan: 1985 Jun 23–28.

69. Johnson PC, Ericsson CD, Morgan DR, et al. Prophylactic norfloxacin for acute travelers' diarrhea. *Clin*

70. Suarez J, Salamone FR. Management and prevention of bacterial diarrhea. *Clin Pharm*. 1988; 7:746–59.

71. Nahlen BL, Parsonnet J, Preblud SR, et al. International travel and the child younger than two years: recommendations for prevention of travelers' diarrhea and malaria chemoprophylaxis. *Pediatr Infect Dis J*. 1989; 8:735–9.

72. Centers for Disease Control. Health information for international travel. Washington, DC: U.S. Government Printing Office, 1987; HHS publication (CDC) 85-8280.

73. Recommendations for the prevention of malaria in travelers. *MMWR*. 1988; 37:277–84.

74. Lobel HO, Campbell CC, Roberts JM. Fatal malaria in US civilians. *Lancet*. 1985; 1:873. Letter.

75. Roland EH, Jan JE, Rigg JM. Toxic encephalopathy in a child after brief exposure to insect repellents. *Can Med Assoc J*. 1985; 132:155–6.

76. Miller KD, Lobel HO, Satriale RF, et al. Severe cutaneous reactions among American travelers using pyrimethamine–sulfadoxine (Fansidar) for malaria prophylaxis. *Am J Trop Med Hyg*. 1986; 35:451–8.

77. Drugs for parasitic infections. *Med Lett Drugs Ther*. 1988; 30:15–24.

78. World Health Organization. Vacation certificate requirements and health advice for international travel. Geneva: World Health Organization; 1988:46–52.

79. Miller KD, Lobel HO, Papaioanou M, et al. Failures of combined chloroquine and Fansidar prophylaxis in American travelers to East Africa. *J Infect Dis*. 1986; 154:689–91.

80. Krogstad DJ, Herwaldt BL. Chemoprophylaxis and treatment of malaria. *N Engl J Med*. 1988; 319: 1538–40.

81. Band JD, Fraser JW, Ajello MA. Prevention of *Hemophilus influenzae* type b disease. *JAMA*. 1984; 251:2381–6.

82. Peter G. Treatment and prevention of *Hemophilus influenzae* type b meningitis. *Pediatr Infect Dis J*. 1987; 6:787–90.

83. Granoff DM, Ward JI. Current status of prophylaxis for *Hemophilus influenzae* infections. In: Remington JS, Swartz MN, eds. Current clinical topics in infectious diseases. New York: McGraw-Hill; 1985: 290–315.

84. Murphy TV, Clements JF, Breedlove JA, et al. Risk of subsequent disease among day-care contacts of patients with systemic *Hemophilus influenzae* type b disease. *N Engl J Med*. 1987; 316:5–10.

85. Broome CV, Mortimer EA, Katz SL, et al. Use of chemoprophylaxis to prevent the spread of *Hemophilus influenzae* b in day-care facilities. *N Engl J Med*. 1987; 316:1226–8.

86. Immunization Practices Advisory Group. Update: prevention of *Hemophilus influenzae* type b disease. *MMWR*. 1986; 35:170–80.

87. Broome CV. The carrier state: *Neisseria meningitidis*. *J Antimicrob Chemother*. 1986; 18(Suppl A):25–34.

88. McCormick JB, Bennett JV. Public health considerations in the management of meningococcal disease. *Ann Intern Med*. 1975; 83:883–6.

89. Band JD, Chamberland ME, Platt T, et al. Trends in meningococcal disease in the United States, 1975–1980. *J Infect Dis*. 1983; 148:754–8.

90. Kuhns DM, Nelson CT, Feldman HA, et al. The prophylactic value of sulfadiazine in the control of meningococcic meningitis. *JAMA*. 1943; 123:335–9.

91. Meningococcal Disease Surveillance Group. Analysis of endemic meningococcal disease by serogroup and evaluation of chemoprophylaxis. *J Infect Dis*. 1976; 134:201–4.

92. Immunization Practices Advisory Committee. Meningococcal vaccine. *MMWR*. 1985; 34:255–9.

93. Schwartz B, Al-Tobaiqi A, Al-Ruwais A, et al. Comparative efficacy of ceftriaxone and rifampin in eradicating pharyngeal carriage of group A *Neisseria meningitidis*. *Lancet*. 1988; 1:1239–42.

94. Gaunt PN, Lambert BE. Single dose ciprofloxacin for the eradication of pharyngeal carriage of *Neisseria meningitidis*. *J Antimicrob Chemother*. 1988; 21: 489–96.

95. Casewell MW, Hill RLR. The carrier state: methicillin-resistant *Staphylococcus aureus*. *J Antimicrob Chemother*. 1985; 18(Suppl A):1–12.

96. Fekety R. The management of the carrier of methicillin-resistant *Staphylococcus aureus*. In: Remington JS, Swartz MN, eds. Current clinical topics in infectious diseases. New York: McGraw-Hill; 1988:169–80.

97. Brumfitt W, Hamilton-Miller J. Methicillin-resistant *Staphylococcus aureus*. *N Engl J Med*. 1989; 320: 1188–96.

98. Chow JW, Yu VL. *Staphylococcus aureus* nasal carriage in hemodialysis patients: its role in infection and approaches to prophylaxis. *Arch Intern Med*. 1989; 149:1258–62.

99. Wheat LJ, Kohler RB, White AL, et al. Effect of rifampin on nasal carriage of coagulase-positive staphylococci. *J Infect Dis*. 1981; 144:177.

100. McAnally TB, Lewis MR, Brown DR. Effect of rifampin and bacitracin on nasal carriers of *Staphylococcus aureus*. *Antimicrob Agents Chemother*. 1984; 25:422–6.

101. Ellison RT, Judson FN, Peterson LC, et al. Oral rifampin and trimethoprim/sulfamethoxazole therapy in asymptomatic carriers of methicillin-resistant *Staphylococcus aureus*. *West J Med*. 1984; 140:735– 40.

102. Roccaforte JS, Bittner MJ, Stumpf CA, et al. Attempts to eradicate methicillin-resistant *Staphylococcus aureus* colonization with the use of trimethoprim–sulfamethoxazole, rifampin, and bacitracin. *Am J Infect Control*. 1988; 16:141–6.

103. Hospital Infection Society and British Society for Antimicrobial Therapy. Guidelines for the control of epidemic methicillin-resistant *Staphylococcus aureus*. *J Hosp Infect*. 1985; 7:193–201.

104. Smith SM, Eng RHK, Tecson-Tumang F. Ciprofloxacin therapy for methicillin-resistant *Staphylococcus aureus* infections or colonization. *Antimicrob Agents Chemother*. 1989; 33:181–4.

105. Casewell MW, Hill RLR. Elimination of nasal carriage of *Staphylococcus aureus* with mupirocin: a controlled trial. *J Antimicrob Chemother*. 1986; 17:365–72.

106. Walsh JA, Hutchins S. Group B streptococcal disease: its importance in the developing world and prospect for prevention with vaccines. *Pediatr Infect Dis J*. 1989; 8:271–6.

107. Boyer KM, Gotoff SP. Antimicrobial prophylaxis of neonatal group B streptococcal sepsis. *Clin Perinatol*. 1988; 15:831–50.

108. Yow MD, Mason EO, Leeds LJ, et al. Ampicillin prevents intrapartum transmission of group B streptococcus. *JAMA*. 1979; 241:1245–7.

109. Easmon CSF, Hastings MJG, Deeley J, et al. The effect of intrapartum chemoprophylaxis on the vertical transmission of group B streptococci. *Br J Obstet Gynaecol*. 1983; 90:633–5.

110. Boyer KM, Gotoff SP. Prevention of early-onset neonatal group B streptococcal disease with selective intrapartum chemoprophylaxis. *N Engl J Med*. 1986; 314:1665–9.

111. Boyer KM, Gadzala CA, Burd LI, et al. Selective intrapartum chemoprophylaxis of neonatal group B streptococcal early-onset disease. *J Infect Dis*. 1983; 148:795–816.

112. Teres FO, Matorras R, Perea AG, et al. Prevention of neonatal group B streptococcal sepsis. *Pediatr Infect Dis J*. 1987; 6:874.

113. Kerver AJH, Rommes JH, Mevissen-Verhage EAE, et al. Colonization and infection in surgical intensive care patients—a prospective study. *Intensive Care Med*. 1987; 13:347–51.

114. Septimus EJ. Nosocomial bacterial pneumonias. *Semin Respir Infect*. 1989; 4:245–52.

115. Craven DE, Kunches LM, Kilinsky V, et al. Risk factors for pneumonia and fatality in patients receiving continuous mechanical ventilation. *Am Rev Respir Dis*. 1986; 133:792–6.

116. Fagon J-Y, Chastre J, Domart Y, et al. Nosocomial pneumonia in patients receiving continuous mechanical ventilation: prospective analysis of 52 episodes with use of a protected specimen brush and quantitative culture techniques. *Am Rev Respir Dis*. 1989; 139:877–84.

117. Stoutenbeek CP, van Saene HKF, Miranda DR, et al. Nosocomial gram-negative pneumonia in critically ill patients: a 3-year experience with a novel therapeutic regimen. *Intensive Care Med*. 1986; 12:419–23.

118. Van Uffelen R, Rommes JH, van Saene HKF. Preventing lower airway colonization and infection in mechanically ventilated patients. *Crit Care Med*. 1987; 15:99–102.

119. Unertl K, Ruckdeschl G, Selman HK, et al. Prevention of colonization and respiratory infections in long-term ventilated patients by local antimicrobial prophylaxis. *Intensive Care Med*. 1987; 13:106–13.

120. Stoutenbeek CP, van Saene HKF, Miranda DR, et al. The effect of oropharyngeal decontamination using topical nonabsorbable antibiotics in the incidence of nosocomial respiratory tract infections in multiple trauma patients. *J Trauma*. 1987; 27:357–64.

121. Ledingham IM, Alcock SR, Eastaway AT, et al. Triple regimen of selective decontamination of the digestive tract, systemic cefotaxime, and microbiological surveillance for prevention of acquired infection in intensive care. *Lancet*. 1988; 1:785–90.

122. Kerver AJH, Rommes JH, Mevissen-Verhage AE, et al. Prevention of colonization and infection in critically ill patients: a prospective study. *Crit Care Med*. 1988; 16:1087–93.

123. Weisner RH, Hermans PE, Rakela J, et al. Selective bowel decontamination to decrease gram-negative aerobic bacterial and *Candida* colonization and prevent infection after orthotopic liver transplantation. *Transplantation*. 1988; 45:570–4.

124. Weinstein RA. Selective intestinal decontamination—an infection control measure whose time has come? *Ann Intern Med.* 1989; 110:853–5.

125. Infectious Disease Society of America. Guidelines for use of antimicrobial agents in neutropenic patients with unexplained fever. *J Infect Dis.* 1990; 161:381–96.

126. Verhoef J, Rozenberg-Arska M, Dekker A. Prevention of infection in the neutropenic patient. *Rev Infect Dis.* 1989; 11(Suppl. 7):S1545–50.

127. Dekker AW, Rozenberg-Arska M, Sixma JJ, et al. Prevention of infection with trimethoprim/sulfamethoxazole plus amphotericin B in patients with acute nonlymphocytic leukemia. *Ann Intern Med.* 1981; 95:555–9.

128. Pizzo PA, Robichaud KH, Edwards BK, et al. Oral antibiotic prophylaxis in patients with cancer: a double-blind randomized placebo-controlled trial. *J Pediatr.* 1983; 102:125–33.

129. Murray BE, Rensimer ER, DuPont HL. Emergence of high-level trimethoprim resistance in fecal *Escherichia coli* during oral administration of trimethoprim or trimethoprim/sulfamethoxazole. *N Engl J Med.* 1982; 306:130–5.

130. Wilson JM, Guiney DG. Failure of oral trimethoprim/sulfamethoxazole prophylaxis in acute leukemia. *N Engl J Med.* 1982; 306:16–20.

131. Wade JC, DeJongh CA, Newman KA, et al. Selective antimicrobial modulation as prophylaxis against infection during granulocytopenia: trimethoprim/sulfamethoxazole vs. nalidixic acid. *J Infect Dis.* 1983; 147:624–34.

132. Gualtieri RJ, Donowitz GR, Kaiser DL, et al. Double-blind randomized study of prophylactic trimethoprim/sulfamethoxazole in granulocytopenic patients with hematologic malignancies. *Am J Med.* 1983; 74:934–40.

133. Bow EJ, Rayner E, Scott BA, et al. Selective gut decontamination with nalidixic acid or trimethoprim/sulfamethoxazole for infection prophylaxis in neutropenic cancer patients: relationship of efficacy to antimicrobial spectrum and timing of administration. *Antimicrob Agents Chemother.* 1987; 31:551–7.

134. Winston DJ, Ho WG, Nakao SL, et al. Norfloxacin versus vancomycin/polymyxin for prevention of infections in granulocytopenic patients. *Am J Med.* 1985; 80:884–90.

135. Dekker AW, Rozenberg-Arska M, Verhoef J. Infection prophylaxis in acute leukemia: a comparison of ciprofloxacin with trimethoprim/sulfamethoxazole and colistin. *Ann Intern Med.* 1987; 106:7–12.

136. Karp JE, Merz WG, Hendricksen C, et al. Oral norfloxacin for prevention of gram-negative bacterial infections in patients with acute leukemia and granulocytopenia. *Ann Intern Med.* 1987; 106:1–7.

137. Montgomery AB. Prophylaxis of *Pneumocystis carinii* pneumonia in patients infected with the human immunodeficiency virus type 1. *Semin Respir Infect.* 1989; 4:311–7.

138. Phair J, Muno A, Detels R, et al. The risk of *Pneumocystis carinii* pneumonia among men infected with human immunodeficiency virus type 1. *N Engl J Med.* 1990; 322:161–5.

139. Fischl MA, Dickinson GM, LaVoie L. Safety and efficacy of sulfamethoxazole and trimethoprim chemoprophylaxis for *Pneumocystis carinii* pneumonia. *JAMA.* 1988; 259:1185–9.

140. Kovacs JA, Masur H. *Pneumocystis carinii* pneumonia: therapy and prophylaxis. *J Infect Dis.* 1988; 158:254–9.

141. Hardy WD, Northfelt DW, Drake TA. Fatal, disseminated pneumocystosis in a patient with acquired immunodeficiency syndrome receiving prophylactic aerosolized pentamidine. *Am J Med.* 1989; 87:329–31.

142. Meyers JD. Infection in recipients of bone marrow transplants. In: Remington JS, Swartz MN, eds. Current clinical topics in infectious diseases. New York: McGraw-Hill; 1985:261–92.

143. Wade JC, Schimpff SC. Epidemiology and prevention of infection in the compromised host. In: Rubin RH, Young LS, eds. Clinical approach to infection in the compromised host. 2nd ed. New York: Plenum; 1988:5–40.

144. Peterson PK, Ferguson R, Fryd DS, et al. Infectious diseases in hospitalized renal transplant patients: a prospective study of a complex and evolving problem. *Medicine.* 1982; 61:360–72.

145. Meyer JD. Prevention of cytomegalovirus infection after marrow transplantation. *Rev Infect Dis.* 1989; 11(Suppl 7):S1691–705.

146. Rubin RH, Tolkoff-Rubin NE. Opportunistic infections in renal allograft recipients. *Transplant Proc.* 1988; 20(Suppl 8):12–8.

147. Simmons RL, Migliori RJ. Infection prophylaxis after successful organ transplantation. *Transplant Proc.* 1988; 20(Suppl 8):7–11.

148. Tolkoff-Rubin NE, Cosimi AB, Russell PS, et al. A controlled study of trimethoprim–sulfamethoxazole prophylaxis of urinary tract infection in renal transplant patients. *Rev Infect Dis.* 1982; 4:614–8.

149. Gurwith MJ, Brunton JL, Lank BA, et al. A prospective controlled investigation of prophylactic trimethoprim–sulfamethoxazole in hospitalized granulocytopenic patients. *Am J Med.* 1979; 66:248–56.

150. Owens NJ, Nightingale CH, Schweizer RT, et al. Prophylaxis of oral candidiasis with clotrimazole troches. *Arch Intern Med.* 1984; 144:290–3.

151. Hansen RM, Reinerio N, Sohnle PG, et al. Ketoconazole in the prevention of candidiasis in patients with cancer: a prospective, randomized, controlled, double-blind study. *Arch Intern Med.* 1987; 147:710–2.

152. Shepp DH, Kosterman A, Siegel MS, et al. Comparative trial of ketoconazole and nystatin for prevention of fungal infection in neutropenic patients treated in a protective environment. *J Infect Dis.* 1985; 152:1257–63.

153. Gombert ME, duBouchet L, Aulicino TM, et al. A comparative trial of clotrimazole troches and oral nystatin suspension in recipients of renal transplants: use in prophylaxis of oropharyngeal candidiasis. *JAMA.* 1987; 258:2553–5.

154. Saral R, Burns WH, Laskin OL, et al. Acyclovir prophylaxis of *Herpes simplex* virus infections: a randomized, double-blind, controlled trial in bone marrow transplant recipients. *N Engl J Med.* 1981; 305:63–7.

155. Gluckman E, Lotsberg J, Devergie A, et al. Prophylaxis of herpes infections after bone marrow transplantation by oral acyclovir. *Lancet.* 1983; 2:706–8.

156. Wade JC, Newton B, Flournoy N, et al. Oral acyclovir

for prevention of *Herpes simplex* virus reactivation after marrow transplantation. *Ann Intern Med.* 1984; 100:823–8.

157. Seale L, Jones CJ, Kathpalia S, et al. Prevention of herpes virus infections in renal allograft recipients by low-dose oral acyclovir. *JAMA.* 1985; 254:3435–8.

158. Balfour HH, Chace BA, Stepleton JT, et al. A randomized, placebo-controlled trial of oral acyclovir for the prevention of cytomegalovirus disease in recipients of renal allografts. *N Engl J Med.* 1989; 20:1381–7.

Approved by the ASHP Commission on Therapeutics and by the ASHP Board of Directors, May 1990.

This document was written by the ASHP Commission on Therapeutics Task Force on Nonsurgical Antimicrobial Prophylaxis: Steven C. Ebert, Pharm.D., Chairman, Assistant Professor, School of Pharmacy, University of Wisconsin, Madison, WI; S. Diane Goodwin, Pharm.D., Clinical Research Pharmacist, Center for AIDS Research, Duke University Medical Center, Durham, NC; Michael J. Rybak, Pharm.D., Associate Professor, College of Pharmacy and Allied Health Professions, Wayne State University and Detroit Receiving Hospital, Detroit, MI; Elaine Bailey, Pharm.D., Infectious Diseases Pharmacotherapy Fellow, College of Pharmacy and Allied Health Professions, Wayne State University and Detroit Receiving Hospital, Detroit, MI; Tom A. Larson, Pharm.D., Associate Professor, College of Pharmacy, University of Minnesota, Minneapolis, MN; Patricia Colaizzi, Pharm.D., Manager, Pharmacotherapeutic Services, McFaul & Lyons Inc., Trenton, NJ; Thomas C. Hardin, Pharm.D., Clinical Coordinator, Pharmacy Service, Audie L. Murphy Veterans Hospital, San Antonio, TX; and Paul Hale, Ph.D., Manager of Scientific Affairs, Hoechst-Roussel Pharmaceuticals Inc., Somerville, NJ.

The assistance of Alan W. Hopefl, Pharm.D., Joan E. Kapusnik-Uner, Pharm.D., Patricia Orlando, Pharm.D., Mary Pasko, Pharm.D., Michael D. Reed, Pharm.D., and Kathleen Reilly, Pharm.D., in reviewing this document is acknowledged. The document was also reviewed by representatives of the Infectious Diseases Society of America, the American Thoracic Society, and the American Heart Association.

The recommendations in this document do not indicate an exclusive course of treatment to be followed. Variations, taking into account individual circumstances, may be appropriate.

The bibliographic citation for this document is as follows: American Society of Hospital Pharmacists. ASHP therapeutic guidelines on nonsurgical antimicrobial prophylaxis. *Clin Pharm.* 1990; 9:423–45.

ASHP Residency Accreditation Regulations and Standards

Definitions of Pharmacy Residencies and Fellowships

Pharmacy residencies (originally termed "internships") began in the early 1930s, primarily for the purpose of training pharmacists for the management of pharmacy services in hospitals. The first nonacademic residency program is believed to have been conducted by Harvey A. K. Whitney at the University of Michigan Hospital.[1] Approximately 10 years later, the first residency program combined with formal graduate studies was created.[2] Developments in these programs eventually led the American Society of Hospital Pharmacists to establish, in 1948, standards for pharmacy internships in hospitals.[3] Those standards defined an internship as "a period of organized training in an accredited hospital pharmacy under the direction and supervision of personnel qualified to offer such training."

Two types of internships were recognized, nonacademic and academic. The nonacademic internship consisted of a period of training in a hospital pharmacy. The academic internship consisted of training in a hospital pharmacy and study in an accredited graduate school associated with a school of pharmacy and leading to a Master of Science degree.

In 1962, following several revisions in the standards, ASHP established an accreditation process and accreditation standards for residencies in hospital pharmacy.[4,5] In this action, the term "internship" was replaced by "residency." A residency was defined as "a postgraduate program of organized training . . ." (and further detailed within the various standards). In 1985, the concept that a resident's training should be *directed* was incorporated into the definition.[6-9] It was also acknowledged that a residency is practice oriented and that it is possible for a residency to focus on a defined (specialized) area.

During the early 1970s, numerous residencies developed in *clinical* practice, leading to the establishment, in 1980, of accreditation standards for clinical pharmacy and specialized residency training.[10,11] In 1986, the American Pharmaceutical Association published a compilation of programmatic essentials for community pharmacy residencies.[12] In that same year, the American College of Apothecaries published specific guidelines for the accreditation of community pharmacy residencies.[13]

Paralleling these developments and fostered by a growing sophistication and clinical thrust in institutional pharmacy practice, postgraduate research-oriented programs (generally termed "fellowships") developed in the 1970s. These programs were conducted primarily in colleges of pharmacy and in academically based health centers to educate and train individuals to conduct pharmacy research. A 1981 survey of fellowship programs reported the existence of 58 fellowships in 19 topic areas.[14] Two-thirds of these fellowships had existed for 3 years or less. The oldest program had existed for less than 9 years. The ASHP Research and Education Foundation initiated clinical fellowships in 1978 and defined a pharmacy fellowship as "a directed, but highly individualized program [that] emphasizes research. The focus of a pharmacy fellowship is to develop the participant's (the fellow's) ability to conduct research in his or her area of specialization."[15,16]

ASHP publishes an annual directory of ASHP-accredited residency programs. In 1985, there were 184 accredited programs.[17] The American College of Clinical Pharmacy publishes an annual listing of residencies and fellowships conducted by its members. In 1985, ACCP reported the availability of 51 such residencies and 83 such fellowships.[18] Another source reported 115 known fellowships in 1986.[19] In that year, there were 12 clinical fellowships sponsored by the ASHP Research and Education Foundation in nine areas of specialization.

By 1986, a lack of conformity had arisen in the use of the terms "residency" and "fellowship," and considerable potential existed for program applicants to be misinformed or misled regarding program purposes and content. In 1986, at the recommendation of the ASHP Commission on Credentialing, ASHP invited six other national pharmacy organizations to discuss the issue and develop consensus definitions for the terms. The definitions and interpretations that follow resulted from that conference. These definitions and interpretations are viewed as accurate for current residencies and fellowships yet sufficiently broad and flexible to allow the development of new types of programs. Education, practice, and research developments may generate changes in residencies and fellowships and ultimately stimulate revisions in the definitions and interpretations.

Residency

Definition. A pharmacy residency is an organized, directed, postgraduate training program in a defined area of pharmacy practice.

Interpretation. Residencies exist primarily to train pharmacists in professional practice and management activities. Residencies provide experience in integrating pharmacy services with the comprehensive needs of individual practice settings and provide indepth experiences leading to advanced practice skills and knowledge. Residencies foster an ability to conceptualize new and improved pharmacy services. Within a given residency program, there is considerable consistency in content for each resident. In addition, accreditation standards and program guidelines produced by national pharmacy associations provide considerable program content detail and foster consistency among programs.

A residency is typically 12 months or longer in duration, and the resident's practice experiences are closely directed and evaluated by a qualified practitioner–preceptor. A residency may occur at any career point following an entry-level degree in pharmacy. Individuals planning practice-oriented careers are encouraged to complete all formal academic education before entry into a residency.

Fellowship

Definition. A pharmacy fellowship is a directed, highly individualized, postgraduate program designed to prepare the participant to become an independent researcher.

Interpretation. Fellowships exist primarily to develop competency in the scientific research process, including conceptualizing, planning, conducting, and reporting research. Under the close direction and instruction of a qualified researcher–preceptor, the participant (the fellow) receives a highly individualized learning experience that utilizes research interests and knowledge needs as a focus for his or her education and training. A fellowship graduate should be capable of conducting collaborative research or functioning as a principal investigator.

Fellowships are typically offered through colleges of pharmacy, academic health centers, or specialized healthcare institutions. Fellowships are usually offered for predetermined, finite periods of time, often exceeding 12 or even 24 months. Individuals planning research-oriented careers should expect to complete formal education in research design and statistics either before or during a fellowship. A fellowship candidate is expected to possess basic practice skills relevant to the knowledge area of the fellowship. Such skills may be obtained through practice experience or through an appropriate residency and should be maintained during the program.

References

1. Niemeyer G. Ten years of the American Society of Hospital Pharmacists, 1942–1952: education and training. *Bull Am Soc Hosp Pharm.* 1952; 9:363–75.

2. American Society of Hospital Pharmacists. Approval program for internships in hospital pharmacy. *Bull Am Soc Hosp Pharm.* 1955; 12:309–13.

3. American Society of Hospital Pharmacists. Standards for internships in hospital pharmacies. *Bull Am Soc Hosp Pharm.* 1948; 5:233–4.

4. American Society of Hospital Pharmacists. Minimum standard for pharmacy internship in hospitals. *Bull Am Soc Hosp Pharm.* 1955; 12:288–90.

5. American Society of Hospital Pharmacists. Accreditation standard for residency in hospital pharmacy. *Am J Hosp Pharm.* 1963; 20:378–80.

6. American Society of Hospital Pharmacists. Accreditation standard for pharmacy residency in a hospital. *Am J Hosp Pharm.* 1971; 28:189–90.

7. American Society of Hospital Pharmacists. Accreditation standard for pharmacy residency in a hospital. *Am J Hosp Pharm.* 1973; 30:1129.

8. American Society of Hospital Pharmacists. ASHP accreditation standard for pharmacy residency in a hospital (with guide to interpretation). *Am J Hosp Pharm.* 1979; 36:74–80.

9. American Society of Hospital Pharmacists. ASHP accreditation standard for hospital pharmacy training (with guide to interpretation). *Am J Hosp Pharm.* 1985; 42:2008–18.

10. American Society of Hospital Pharmacists. ASHP accreditation standard for residency training in clinical pharmacy (with guide to interpretation). *Am J Hosp Pharm.* 1980; 37:1223–8.

11. American Society of Hospital Pharmacists. ASHP accreditation standard for specialized residency training (with guide to interpretation). *Am J Hosp Pharm.* 1980; 37:1229–32.

12. American Pharmaceutical Association, Academy of Pharmacy Practice. APhA community pharmacy residency program: programmatic essentials. *Am Pharm.* 1986; NS26:35–43.

13. American College of Apothecaries. Guidelines for accreditation of community pharmacy residencies. Memphis, TN: American College of Apothecaries; 1986.

14. Kaul AF, Powell SH, Cyr DA. Postgraduate pharmacy fellowships. *Drug Intell Clin Pharm.* 1981; 15:981–5.

15. ASHP Commission on Credentialing. Statement of definition of pharmacy fellowships and residency. Bethesda, MD: American Society of Hospital Pharmacists; 1981.

16. McConnell W. Fellowship program in critical care pharmacy. In: Majerus TC, Dasta JF, eds. Practice of critical care pharmacy. Rockville, MD: Aspen Systems; 1985:59–68.

17. American Society of Hospital Pharmacists. Residency directory. Accredited pharmacy residency programs and programs participating in the 1986 ASHP resident matching program. Bethesda, MD: American Society of Hospital Pharmacists; 1985.

18. American College of Clinical Pharmacy. Residency and fellowship programs offered by members of the American College of Clinical Pharmacy, 1986–87. Kansas City, MO: American College of Clinical Pharmacy; 1986.

19. Kaul AF, Janosik JE, Powell SH. Postgraduate pharmacy fellowships (1985–86). *Drug Intell Clin Pharm.* 1986; 20:203–8.

Developed by an ad hoc consortium made up of representatives from the American Association of Colleges of Pharmacy (AACP), the American College of Apothecaries (ACA), the American College of Clinical Pharmacy (ACCP), the American Pharmaceutical Association (APhA), the American Society of Consultant Pharmacists (ASCP), the American Society of Hospital Pharmacists (ASHP), and the National Association of Retail Druggists (NARD); the consortium was convened by ASHP and met on August 4, 1986. Approved by the ASHP Board of Directors, November 20, 1986, and subsequently approved by ACCP, APhA, ASCP, ACA, and AACP.

The bibliographic citation for this document is as follows: American Society of Hospital Pharmacists. Definitions of pharmacy residencies and fellowships. *Am J Hosp Pharm.* 1987; 44:1142–4.

Guidelines for Clinical Fellowship Training Programs

Definition

A clinical fellowship is a directed, highly individualized postgraduate training program designed to prepare the participant to become an independent researcher.

Introduction

Fellowships exist primarily to develop competency in the scientific research process, including conceptualizing, planning, conducting, and reporting research. Under the close direction and instruction of a qualified researcher–preceptor, the participant (the fellow) receives a highly individualized learning experience, utilizing the fellow's research interests and knowledge needs as a focus for his or her education and training. A fellowship graduate should be capable of conducting collaborative research or functioning as a principal investigator. Fellowships are typically offered through colleges of pharmacy, academic health centers, or specialized health-care institutions.

Fellowships are usually offered for predetermined, finite periods of time, often exceeding 12 or even 24 months. Individuals planning research-oriented careers should expect to complete formal education in research design and statistics either before or during a fellowship. A fellowship candidate is expected to possess basic practice skills relevant to the knowledge area of the fellowship. Such skills may be obtained through practice experience or an appropriate residency and should be maintained during the program.

Guidelines

Training Program Requirements

1. Commitment of a minimum of 75% of fellowship training time to research activities over a 1–2-year period. A 2-year research fellowship is preferable.
2. Administrative institutional support for the preceptor's research program and the fellowship training program.
3. Availability of graduate level coursework in the area of the fellowship.
4. Ready access to laboratory, medical library, and computer facilities.
5. Availability of personnel to teach laboratory-based and clinical research skills.
6. Availability of facilities to conduct research in patients, healthy volunteers, and/or animal/organ/tissue models.

Preceptor Qualifications

1. A clinical scientist with an established record of research accomplishments, which may be exemplified by
   a. Fellowship training or equivalent experience.
   b. Principal or primary investigator on research grants.
   c. Published research papers in peer-reviewed pharmacy/medical literature where the preceptor is the primary or senior author.
2. Active collaborative research relationships with other scientists.
3. Expertise in pharmacotherapeutics in the area of specialization.
4. Established relationships with physicians in the area of specialization.

Fellowship Applicant Requirements

1. Pharm.D. or equivalent experience.
2. Residency or equivalent experience.
3. High level of motivation for a research career.

Fellowship Experiences—Initiation and Completion of Original Research Project

1. Development of scientific hypothesis and experimental methods to test hypothesis.
2. Preparation and submission of a grant proposal.
3. Submission of a protocol to the institutional review board.
4. Laboratory training related to the field of specialization.
5. Experience in statistical analysis of data.
6. Preparation and submission of abstracts and manuscripts for publication.
7. Formal presentation of research at peer-reviewed scientific meetings.

Developed by the American Association of Colleges of Pharmacy and the American College of Clinical Pharmacy and endorsed by the American Society of Hospital Pharmacists.

The bibliographic citation for this document is as follows: American Society of Hospital Pharmacists. Guidelines for clinical fellowship training programs. *Am J Pharm Educ*. 1988; 52:427–8.

ASHP Regulations on Accreditation of Pharmacy Residencies

Preamble

Hospital pharmacists have, from the beginning of their formal association, recognized the need for perpetuating and improving their practice through organized training programs. Early in its history, ASHP supported the development of training programs in hospital pharmacy and promulgated standards for residency in hospital pharmacy.

In recent years, the nature of pharmacy practice in hospitals and other organized health-care settings has changed dramatically, primarily because of the increasing complexity of the total health-care delivery system. The provision of health care has become increasingly more organized. Since the division of labor is a fundamental objective of organization, it is obvious that as health care becomes more organized, the demand for specialized manpower will be greater.

The practice of pharmacy in an organized and highly complex system of health-care delivery, although grounded on a common knowledge base, includes an increasing number of differentiated functions, some of which are highly specialized. Economy and efficiency dictate that each of these functions be performed by personnel best suited to the job.

The Society recognizes the need for at least the following professional manpower categories in institutional pharmacy practice:

- Generalists.
- Clinical practitioners.
- Specialized practitioners.
- Managers and administrators.
  (The Society believes that, as time goes on, the distinction between a "generalist" and a "clinical practitioner" will diminish but that for the next few years there will continue to exist several recognized categories of pharmacists, such as those whose practice is oriented more toward the clinical elements of pharmacy practice and those whose responsibilities center primarily on drug distribution, technology, and other "non-clinical" activities.)

The Society believes that residency training programs have proved to be the best source of highly qualified hospital pharmacy manpower and that it has an obligation to support residencies in each of the manpower categories through the development of training standards and a program of accreditation. To ensure adherence to the principles and philosophy of such standards, an accreditation program is established by the Society.

Definition

For the purpose of accreditation, a pharmacy residency is defined as a postgraduate program of organized training that meets the requirements set forth and approved by ASHP in the "Accreditation Standard for Hospital Pharmacy Residency Training," "Accreditation Standard for Clinical Pharmacy Residency Training," "Accreditation Standard for Specialized Pharmacy Residency Training," "Accreditation Standard for Nuclear Pharmacy Residency Training," or "Accreditation Standard for Advanced Residency Training in Hospital Pharmacy Administration," with the respective Guides to Interpretation.

Authority

The program for accreditation of pharmacy residency programs in hospitals and other organized health-care settings is established by authority of the Board of Directors of ASHP under the direction of the Commission on Credentialing. All matters of policy relating to the accreditation program considered by the Commission on Credentialing will be submitted for approval to the Board of Directors of the Society. The Commission on Credentialing shall review and evaluate applications and survey reports submitted and shall be specifically delegated by the Board of Directors to take final action on all applications for accreditation, in accordance with the policies and procedures set forth herein. The minutes of all transactions of the Commission on Credentialing shall be submitted to the Board of Directors for its review.

Policies

The following policies shall apply to the accreditation program:

1. **Initial Evaluation of Residency Programs.**
   a. The accreditation program shall be conducted as a service of ASHP to any hospital or other organized health-care setting (hereafter referred to as the institution) voluntarily requesting evaluation of its program.
   b. To be eligible for accreditation, a program must have been in operation for 1 year and have at least one graduate. (If accreditation is granted, it shall be retroactive to the date on which a valid and complete application, including all requested supporting documents, is received by the Society's Director of Accreditation Services.)
   c. Program evaluation shall be by a site survey for which an appropriate fee, established by the Board of Directors, shall be assessed to the institution.
   d. Programs shall be reviewed by an accreditation survey team consisting of at least two individuals, one of whom shall be the Society's Director of Accreditation Services or his designee. The other may be a member of the Commission on Credentialing or an individual designated by the Director of Accreditation Services who is not from the same geographic area as the institution being surveyed and who has no conflict of interest with respect to the institution.
2. **Certificate of Accreditation.**
   a. A certificate of accreditation will be issued for a period not to exceed 6 years; however, the certificate remains the property of ASHP and shall be returned to the Society at any time accreditation is withdrawn.

b. Any reference by an institution to accreditation by the Society in certificates, catalogs, bulletins, communications, or other form of publicity shall state only the following: "(Name of Institution) is accredited for pharmacy residency in (category) by the American Society of Hospital Pharmacists."

3. **_Continuing Evaluation of Accredited Programs._**

a. The Society regards evaluation of accredited residency programs as a continuous process; accordingly, the Commission on Credentialing shall request directors of accredited programs to submit periodic written status reports to assist the Commission in evaluating the continued conformance of individual programs to the Accreditation Standard. Written reports shall be required from program directors at least every 2 years.

b. Accredited programs shall be reexamined by site visit at least every 6 years.

c. Any major change in the organization of a program will be considered justification for reevaluation.

d. A survey fee, as established by the ASHP Board of Directors, shall be assessed to the institution for reaccreditation site visits.

4. **_Withdrawal of Accreditation._**

a. Accreditation of a pharmacy residency program may be withdrawn by the Society for any of the reasons stated below:

1. Accredited programs that no longer meet the requirements of the Accreditation Standard shall have accreditation withdrawn. In the event that the Accreditation Standard is revised, all accredited programs will be expected to meet the revised Standard within 1 year.

2. Accredited programs without a resident in training for a period of 2 consecutive years shall have accreditation withdrawn.

3. Accreditation shall be withdrawn if the director of an accredited program is replaced by another individual whose qualifications do not meet the requirements of the Accreditation Standard.

4. Accreditation shall be withdrawn if the institution makes false or misleading statements about the status, condition, or category of its accreditation.

b. If accreditation is withdrawn, the institution shall submit a new application and undergo reevaluation to regain accreditation.

c. Accreditation shall not be withdrawn without first notifying the institution of the specific reasons why its program does not meet the requirements of the Accreditation Standard. In these instances, the institution shall be granted an appropriate period of time to correct the deficiencies.

d. The institution shall have the right to appeal the decision of the Commission on Credentialing.

Accreditation Procedures

1. **_Application for Accreditation._**

a. Application forms may be requested from the American Society of Hospital Pharmacists,

Director of Accreditation Services, 7272 Wisconsin Avenue, Bethesda, MD 20814. These forms should be filled out in duplicate. One copy of the application should be signed by the administrator and the director of pharmacy of the institution and submitted, along with the supporting documents specified in the application instructions, to the Society's Director of Accreditation Services. The duplicate copy should be retained for the applicant's files.

b. The Director of Accreditation Services will acknowledge receipt of the application and review it to make a preliminary judgment about conformance to the basic requirements of the Accreditation Standard. If the Director thinks that the program fails to meet the criteria of the Accreditation Standard in some fundamental way, he will notify the signatories of the application accordingly and advise against scheduling a site visit until the problems have been corrected. The applicant is not bound, however, to accept the Director's advice to delay the site visit.

2. **_The Site Visit._**

a. At a mutually convenient time, the Society will send a survey team to review the pharmacy service and the residency program. Instructions for preparation for the site visit (e.g., list of documents to be made available to the survey team and suggested itinerary for the surveyors) will be sent to the director of pharmacy well in advance. Normally, the site visit is conducted in 2 working days.

b. After concluding its onsite evaluation, the survey team will present a verbal report of its findings to the institution administrator and director of pharmacy.

3. **_The Survey Report._**

a. Following the site visit, the survey team will prepare a written report that will be sent to the institution administrator and the director of pharmacy for review of factual accuracy and comment. Any written comments that either person wishes to make must be submitted to the Director of Accreditation Services within 30 days of receiving the report. Any comment respecting the factual accuracy of the report must specifically set forth the facts contested, the reasons for the disagreement, and the institution's contentions with respect to the facts.

b. The institution's residency accreditation application file, including the surveyor's report, plus any written comments received from the institution, will be reviewed by the Commission at its next meeting. The Commission will resolve any factual issues at that time.

c. Notice of action taken by the Commission will be sent to the institution administrator and director of pharmacy, along with a list of any deficiencies that the Commission considered in arriving at its decision and recommendations for overcoming those deficiencies. The report will indicate that the Commission has acted either (1) to accredit or reaccredit the program for a period not to exceed 6 years or (2) to withhold or withdraw accreditation.

4. ***Appeal of Commission Decision.***

   a. *Notification of intent to appeal.* In the event the Commission shall fail to accredit or reaccredit a program, the institution administrator may appeal the decision of the Commission to an appeal board on the grounds that the decision of the Commission was arbitrary, prejudiced, biased, capricious, or based on incorrect application of the Standards to the institution. The institution administrator must notify the Director of Accreditation Services, in writing by registered or certified mail within 10 days after receipt of the Commission's decision, of the institution's intent to appeal. The institution administrator must state clearly on what grounds the appeal is being made. The institution shall then have an additional 30 days to prepare for its presentation to an appeal board.

   b. *Appeal board.* On receipt of an appeal notice, the Director of Accreditation Services shall proceed to constitute an ad hoc appeal board. The appeal board shall consist of one member of the Society's Board of Directors, to be appointed by the President of ASHP, who shall serve as Chairman and two preceptors of accredited pharmacy residency programs, neither of whom is a member of the Commission on Credentialing, one to be named by the appellant and one by the Chairman of the Commission. A hospital administrator shall also be appointed by the President of ASHP in an ex officio, nonvoting capacity. The Director of Accreditation Services shall serve as Secretary of the appeal board. As soon as appointments to the appeal board have been made, the Director of Accreditation Services will immediately forward copies of all of the written documentation considered by the Commission in rendering its decision to the appeal board members.

   c. *The hearing.* The appeal board shall have convened in no less than 30 days or more than 60 days from the date of receipt by the Director of Accreditation Services of an appeal notice. The Director of Accreditation Services shall notify appellants and appeal board members, at least 30 days in advance, of the date, time, and place of the hearing. The institution filing the appeal may be represented at the hearing by one or more appropriate officials and shall be given the opportunity at such hearing to present written or written and oral evidence and argument tending to refute or overcome the findings and decision of the Commission on Credentialing. The Director of Accreditation Services shall represent the Commission at the hearing.

   The appeal board shall advise the appellant institution of the board's decision, in writing by registered or certified mail, within 10 days of the date of the hearing. The decision of the appeal board shall be final and binding on both the appellant and ASHP.

   d. *Appeal board expenses.* The appellant shall be responsible for all expenses incurred by its own representatives at the appeal board hearing and shall pay all reasonable travel, living, and incidental expenses incurred by its appointee to the appeal board. Expenses incurred by the other board members and the Director of Accreditation Services shall be borne by ASHP.

Approved by the ASHP Board of Directors, September 21, 1981. Developed by the ASHP Commission on Credentialing. Supersedes the previous regulations on accreditation approved on November 8, 1962, and revised April 11, 1970, November 19, 1973, November 16, 1977, and March 20, 1980. Minor changes in these regulations were made in 1981.

The bibliographic citation for this document is as follows: American Society of Hospital Pharmacists. ASHP regulations on accreditation of pharmacy residencies. *Am J Hosp Pharm.* 1985; 42:2005–7.

ASHP Accreditation Standard for Residency in Pharmacy Practice (with Emphasis on Pharmaceutical Care)

Introduction

Definition. A residency in pharmacy practice is defined as an organized, directed, postgraduate training program that centers on development of the knowledge, attitudes, and skills needed to pursue rational drug therapy.[1]

Purpose. The purpose of this Standard is to establish criteria for the training and education of pharmacists in the fundamentals of exemplary contemporary pharmacy practice in organized health-care systems. Its contents outline specific elements of the knowledge and skills needed to achieve a basic level of practice competence and serve as a foundation for further training in specialized residencies and fellowships. It is expected, therefore, that a residency developed under this Standard will build on the practice experience and education obtained through internships, clerkships, externships, or other forms of academic instruction.

Philosophy. It is essential for pharmacy graduates to obtain the level of knowledge and skills needed to become competent in pharmacy practice. Pharmacy practice residencies serve as one of the best means by which to achieve that objective. Residencies in pharmacy practice provide residents with opportunities to conceptualize, integrate, and transform accumulated experiences and knowledge into improved drug therapy. A pharmacy practice residency instills a philosophy of practice that embraces the concept that pharmacists must be responsible and accountable for optimal drug therapy outcomes.

Application of the Standard. The interpretive narrative following each requirement of the Standard is intended to illustrate how the Standard will be interpreted by accreditation review teams and the American Society of Hospital Pharmacists Commission on Credentialing in the evaluation of residency programs in pharmacy practice.

A fundamental principle of this Standard is that a residency in pharmacy practice is structured to ensure the achievement of certain predetermined competencies. While the Standard requires a minimum of 1-year, full-time practice commitment or equivalent for the residency, there is no set way in which this time is to be assigned. Principle IVB of this Standard specifies those areas in which the resident's competence must be developed, and these must serve as the principal determinants by which programs are structured. The amount of time required to accomplish a minimum level of competence in each of these areas will likely vary from one resident to another; therefore, the resident's academic accomplishments, prior experience, and personal professional career goals should be considered in structuring each individual's program.

The "ASHP Accreditation Standard for Residency in Pharmacy Practice (with Emphasis on Pharmaceutical Care)" sets forth the basic criteria to be used in the evaluation of programs that apply for accreditation by ASHP. The accreditation program is conducted under the authority of the ASHP Board of Directors. The document "ASHP Regulations on Accreditation of Pharmacy Residencies"[2] sets forth the policies governing the accreditation program and describes the procedures to be followed in applying for accreditation of pharmacy residency programs.

Throughout this Standard, where the auxiliary verbs *shall* and *must* are used, an absolute requirement is implied. The use of *should* and *may* denotes a recommended guideline for compliance.

Part I—Qualifications of the Training Site

Principle IA

Residencies in pharmacy practice shall be conducted only in those practice settings where the governing bodies, personnel, and staff have committed to seek excellence in patient care, have sought and accepted outside appraisal, and have demonstrated substantial conformance with professionally developed and nationally applied practice and operational standards.

Requirements

1. A hospital that offers, or that participates in offering, a residency in pharmacy practice shall be accredited by the Joint Commission on Accreditation of Healthcare Organizations (JCAHO) or the American Osteopathic Association.
2. Other practice settings that offer a residency in pharmacy practice shall have demonstrated substantial conformance with applicable professionally developed and nationally applied standards.

Interpretation. The most recent evaluation report, including specific evaluative comments regarding pharmacy services and all other drug-related matters, will serve as evidence that this requirement has been met and shall be made available to the accreditation survey team.

Principle IB

Two or more practice sites, or a sponsoring organization working in cooperation with one or more practice sites, may jointly provide a residency in pharmacy practice.

Requirements

1. A residency in pharmacy practice is dependent on the availability of a broad range of patient categories and professional practice experience. It is appropriate for two or more practice sites, or a sponsoring organization (e.g., college of pharmacy) and one or more practice sites, to collaborate in conducting a pharmacy practice residency program.
2. A college of pharmacy that participates in offering a residency in pharmacy practice shall be accredited by

the American Council on Pharmaceutical Education (ACPE).

Interpretation. Application for accreditation of a multisite residency in pharmacy practice must be submitted in the name of the principal practice site (i.e., the practice site where the majority of the residency program is centered). In the case of a sponsoring organization (e.g., college of pharmacy) that has a contractual arrangement with one or more practice settings to provide for residency training, the application for accreditation must be completed by both the sponsoring organization and the principal practice site.

Further qualifications for an accredited multisite pharmacy practice residency program are set forth in Part II of this Standard.

Part II—Qualifications of the Residency Program Director and Preceptors

Principle II

Directors and preceptors of residencies in pharmacy practice shall be individuals who maintain high professional ideals, who have distinguished themselves in practice, and who have the desire and aptitude to teach.

Requirements

1. The director of pharmacy or designee shall serve as the residency program director.

Interpretation. The director of pharmacy services in the facility where the residency is conducted has ultimate responsibility for the residency program. In many instances, the director of pharmacy serves as the residency program director; however, the director of pharmacy may choose to appoint another pharmacist on staff to serve as residency program director. In these instances, the individual to whom coordination and oversight for the program have been delegated must be accountable to the director of pharmacy. The residency program director is responsible for ensuring that the overall program goals and specific learning objectives are met, training schedules are maintained, appropriate preceptorship for each rotation or period of training is provided, and resident evaluations based on the preestablished learning objectives are routinely conducted.

2. The residency program director must have demonstrated a sustained contribution and commitment to pharmacy practice. This may be characterized by the following:
   - A progressive, documented record demonstrating improvements in and contributions to pharmacy practice.
   - Formal recognition by peers as a model practitioner.
   - A demonstrated ability to teach.
   - Demonstrated and documented evidence of the ability to direct and manage a pharmacy practice residency.
   - A sustained record of contributing to the total body of knowledge in pharmacy practice through publications or formal presentations at professional meetings.

Interpretation. Evaluation of the residency program director's qualifications shall be based on professional education and the degree to which the individual's professional accomplishments satisfy this requirement. The residency program director should have completed an ASHP-accredited residency and hold an advanced degree in pharmacy or have obtained equivalent qualifications.

3. Multisite residency programs shall have one designated residency program director, whose appointment shall be agreed to in writing by each participating practice site.

Interpretation. The residency program director for multisite residencies is the individual held accountable for the conduct and quality of the residency program.

If a department of pharmacy and college of pharmacy constitute the two organizations providing for residency training, then the director of pharmacy shall be the residency program director, or, the director may choose, in cooperation with the dean, to delegate oversight for the program to a qualified individual within the pharmacy department or the college of pharmacy, provided that a clear line of accountability is established for the program between the director of pharmacy and this individual.

In multisite, college-sponsored programs, the directors of pharmacy, in cooperation with the dean, must appoint one of the directors as the residency program director or, as noted above, may delegate oversight for the program.

4. The residency program director shall have considerable latitude in delegating preceptorial responsibilities for specific segments of the residency program to other pharmacy practitioners. Preceptors must have demonstrated competence in the respective area of practice.

Interpretation. Each rotation or period of training must have a qualified pharmacist preceptor. Evaluation of a preceptor's qualifications shall be based on professional education and experience in the area of practice for which he or she shall serve as preceptor. All preceptors should have completed an ASHP-accredited residency and hold the doctor of pharmacy degree or have obtained equivalent qualifications; further, all are expected to practice routinely in the area in which they serve as preceptor.

Part III—Selection and Qualifications of the Resident

Principle III

The applicant must be a highly motivated pharmacist who desires to obtain advanced education and training leading to an enhanced level of professional practice.

Requirements

1. The applicant shall be a graduate of an accredited college of pharmacy; the doctor of pharmacy degree is preferred. Further, the applicant shall be licensed, or be eligible for licensure, in the state or jurisdiction in which the residency program is located.

Interpretation. The applicant must be a graduate of a college of pharmacy accredited by ACPE or otherwise be eligible for licensure. A residency in pharmacy practice is predicated on prior clerkship and externship experiences. For this reason, the residency applicant should have completed a comprehensive clerkship and externship program, such as is required in contemporary clinically based pharmacy curricula.

This Standard imposes no absolute requirement concerning the type of pharmacy degree the applicant must possess. However, in meeting the requirements for training set forth in Part IV of this Standard, it is clear that the doctor of pharmacy degree provides the applicant with the level of knowledge and skills needed to meet these requirements and that, over time, this degree is expected to serve as a prerequisite for applicants. It is the residency program director's responsibility to assess applicants' baseline knowledge and skills and to ascertain that they qualify for admission.

It is permissible to admit a resident on a part-time basis who is concurrently enrolled in a postbaccalaureate doctor of pharmacy degree program or master's degree program, provided that a clear distinction can be made between academic components (such as clerkships) and residency experiences. In each area of pharmacy practice, the residency experience must follow the clerkship in that area; dual credit is not allowed. ASHP assumes no authority for evaluation of an academic program taken concurrently with a residency training program.

Nothing in this Standard shall prevent individual practice sites from establishing more stringent entry-level requirements.

2.   The residency program director shall establish a formal procedure for evaluating applicants' qualifications.

Interpretation. Typical admission criteria should include, but not be limited to, evaluation of academic transcripts and submission of formal letters of recommendation from applicants' faculty or former faculty, including those who provided clinical training, and from former employers. Personal interviews should be conducted.

3.   Final acceptance of the applicant shall be the responsibility of the director of pharmacy.

Interpretation. The director of pharmacy is ultimately responsible for the pharmacy practice residency program. In multisite residencies or those provided by a sponsoring organization and one or more practice sites, a mechanism shall be in place that permits the individuals who have responsibility for coordinating the residency program to agree cooperatively on selection of applicants.

Part IV—Residency Training Program and Pharmacy Service

Principle IVA

The training and education of residents in the provision of pharmaceutical care shall be of paramount importance in the overall structure and organization of a pharmacy practice residency.

Requirement

1.   The pharmacy practice site shall conduct the residency in such a way as to ensure that any services the resident is required to provide complement, rather than compete with, the educational and experiential objectives of the program.

Interpretation. A residency in pharmacy practice involves active participation by the resident in the provision of pharmaceutical care. This is best achieved when the resident is directly involved in making judgments in such activities as providing patient services, participating in management operations, and working on assigned projects. Having responsibility for these services adds understanding, confidence, and purpose to the resident's academic knowledge.

A substantial portion of this participation must, of necessity, involve hands-on experience, since only through actual provision of care and involvement in other decision-making processes can the resident be expected to gain an understanding of the knowledge, skills, and judgments required to carry out these activities. Through actual experience the resident learns how these activities interrelate and are best coordinated with other disciplines involved with drug use throughout the practice site. Moreover, the residency program should concentrate on developing each resident's ability to conceptualize, integrate, and transform accumulated experiences and knowledge into improved drug therapy in cooperation with other health-care practitioners.

A residency is a full-time obligation; hence, the resident shall manage activities external to the residency so as not to interfere with the goals and objectives of the program as defined in this Standard.

Principle IVB

The residency in pharmacy practice shall be predicated on the knowledge, attitudes, and skills required for contemporary pharmacy practice. The practice site offering the residency shall provide an exemplary training environment; further, the scope of pharmacy services at the site must be adequate to make possible the attainment of the residency program objectives set forth below.

Requirements

1.   An accredited residency in pharmacy practice shall develop the resident's competence to provide pharmaceutical care. It is expected that residents shall receive training and develop competence in each of the following areas of pharmacy practice:
    - Acute patient care.
    - Ambulatory patient care.
    - Drug information and drug use policy development.
    - Practice management.
2.   The pharmacy service shall be an integral part of the health-care delivery system at the practice site where the residency program is offered, be organized in accordance with the principles of sound management under the direction of a legally qualified pharmacist, and have sufficient personnel, facilities, and other resources to carry out a broad scope of pharmacy services. It shall comply with all applicable federal, state, and local laws, codes, statutes, and regulations governing pharmacy practice.

Interpretation. The scope of pharmacy services routinely provided to patients at the practice site must be sufficiently broad to provide residents with the training and experience needed to fulfill the objectives established for the program. Implicit in this requirement is that any practice site that proposes to offer a pharmacy practice residency must offer a level of service sufficient in scope and quality to create an environment throughout the site that is conducive to the support of such a program.

The practice site must meet the requirements of the "ASHP Guidelines: Minimum Standard for Pharmacies in Institutions"[3] and "ASHP Guidelines on Pharmaceutical Services for Ambulatory Patients,"[4] requirements established for accreditation by JCAHO or other acceptable professionally developed and nationally applied criteria, and any additional or more stringent requirements set forth elsewhere in this Standard. It is not acceptable to simulate residency experiences to substitute for nonexistent pharmacy services, nor is it acceptable to substitute academic courses for segments of the program that clearly require practice experience.

It is expected that the resident will, during the training, become accountable and accept responsibility for pursuing optimal clinical outcomes of patients' drug therapy. There is a fine line between the amount of preceptor supervision required during the resident's training and the degree of autonomy needed to achieve this objective. Hence, pharmacy preceptors and the resident must work together closely to ensure that this fundamental element of the training program is met without compromising patient care through inadequate supervision.

At the completion of a pharmacy practice residency, the resident must demonstrate competence in each of the following areas:

Acute patient care. A pharmacy practice residency must provide for a broad experience in the application and management of drugs in the treatment of inpatients; therefore, the pharmacy must provide a level of service commensurate with the needs of patients served. The "ASHP Statement on the Pharmacist's Clinical Role in Organized Health-Care Settings"[5] and the "ASHP Technical Assistance Bulletin on Assessment of Departmental Directions for Clinical Practice in Pharmacy"[6] provide guidance in determining the extent to which pharmacy provides these services to inpatients.

It is essential that the pharmacy staff and residents work cooperatively with other health-care providers to determine desired therapeutic outcomes and thoroughly monitor patients' drug therapy. Pharmacists and the residents to whom they provide guidance must be held responsible and accountable for pursuing optimal drug therapy outcomes. To provide pharmaceutical care, pharmacists and residents must have access to patients' charts (or database) and opportunity for chart notation. The document "ASHP Guidelines for Obtaining Authorization for Documenting Pharmaceutical Care in Patient Medical Records"[7] provides assistance in this area. It is expected that these services extend to a broad range of categories of inpatients (e.g., internal medicine, surgery, pediatrics, critical care, and, depending on the practice site, a variety of medical and surgical subspecialties). Mechanisms must be in place to identify those inpatients who might benefit most from pharmaceutical care.

Further, established standards require that pharmacists must be responsible around-the-clock for the procurement, preparation, distribution, and control of all drugs used, including those that are investigational, within the practice site. Pharmacists and residents have responsibility for devel-

oping and implementing safeguards to ensure that the integrity and identity of all drugs are maintained up to the point of administration to patients. This includes procedures for storing and dispensing controlled substances, emergency drugs, and drug samples. The following documents shall provide guidance in developing drug distribution and control systems for inpatients: "ASHP Guidelines: Minimum Standard for Pharmacies in Institutions"[3] and several other ASHP documents including, but not limited to, the "ASHP Statement on the Pharmacist's Responsibility for Distribution and Control of Drugs,"[8,a] the "ASHP Statement on Unit Dose Drug Distribution,"[9] the "ASHP Statement on the Pharmacist's Role with Respect to Drug Delivery Systems and Administration Devices,"[10] the "ASHP Guidelines for the Use of Investigational Drugs in Organized Health-Care Settings,"[11] the "ASHP Technical Assistance Bulletin on Hospital Drug Distribution and Control,"[12] the "ASHP Technical Assistance Bulletin on Institutional Use of Controlled Substances,"[13] the "ASHP Technical Assistance Bulletin on Handling Cytotoxic and Hazardous Drugs,"[14] and the "ASHP Technical Assistance Bulletin on Surgery and Anesthesiology Pharmaceutical Services."[15]

Ambulatory patient care. The responsibility and accountability for pursuing optimal drug therapy in ambulatory patients continues to rest with pharmacists and residents and is reflective of the continuum of service that is pharmaceutical care. The pharmacy must provide a level of service that is commensurate with the needs of patients served. Pharmaceutical services should extend to all ambulatory care practice settings served by the health-care facilities offering residency training. These practice settings include, but are not limited to, ambulatory care clinics, home health-care programs, ambulatory managed care settings, outpatient pharmacy operations, and extended or long-term care ambulant patient programs.

The pharmacy staff and residents should work cooperatively with other health-care providers to determine therapeutic outcomes, select appropriate prescription and non-prescription drugs to be used in patients' treatment plans, and establish mechanisms for routine monitoring of the drug therapy of patients served in these settings. One principal objective of the provision of pharmaceutical care to ambulatory patients should be the prevention or resolution of drug-related problems, including treatment failures and drug-related morbidity. Thus, pharmaceutical care should be directed toward disease prevention and wellness promotion, in addition to treatment of disease.

The "ASHP Guidelines on Pharmaceutical Services for Ambulatory Patients"[4] and the "ASHP Statement on the Pharmacist's Clinical Role in Organized Health-Care Settings"[5] shall guide programs in providing the level of pharmaceutical care that is commensurate with the needs of patients served in these practice settings.

Drug information and drug use policy development. The practice site shall provide an organized program of drug information services, the purpose of which shall be to assist all professionals at the site in pursuing the goal of safe, appropriate, and cost-effective drug therapy for the patients they serve. These services shall be conducted in such a way that pharmacy practice residents receive instruction in the theory, organization, and practical applications of such services. Hence, a member of the pharmacy staff who has sufficient training and experience in providing drug information services and who meets the intent of Principle II, Requirement 4, of the Standard shall be assigned to coordinate these services and serve as the preceptor for this area of training. Compliance with this aspect of the Standard does not require the existence of a full-time, staffed drug information center.

Essential drug information services that must be provided by pharmacy staff and the residents include, but are not limited to, the following:

- Developing and maintaining a formulary; guidance is provided in the "ASHP Statement on the Pharmacy and Therapeutics Committee,"[16,b] the "ASHP Statement on the Formulary System,"[17,c] the "ASHP Technical Assistance Bulletin on Drug Formularies,"[18] and the "ASHP Technical Assistance Bulletin on the Evaluation of Drugs for Formularies."[19]
- Publishing periodic newsletters or bulletins for the medical and other health-care staff on timely drug-related matters and drug use policies.
- Preparing drug therapy monographs based on an analytical review of pertinent drug literature, including a comparative therapeutic and economic assessment of each new agent for presentation to and use by members of the pharmacy and therapeutics (P&T) committee in evaluating drugs being considered for formulary addition or deletion.
- Establishing and maintaining a system for retrieving drug information from the literature.
- Responding to drug information inquiries from physicians, nurses, pharmacists, and other health-care professionals at the practice site and maintaining written documentation of responses provided to such requests.
- Conducting educational programs about drugs, drug therapy, and other drug-related matters for health-care providers.
- Participating in the development or modification of policies related to drugs, drug use evaluation, adverse drug reaction monitoring and reporting, and appropriate methods of assessing ongoing compliance with such policies; guidance is provided in the "ASHP Guidelines on the Pharmacist's Role in Drug Use Evaluations"[20] and the "ASHP Guidelines on Adverse Drug Reaction Monitoring and Reporting."[21]

A drug information service must be supported by an adequate departmental library that includes textbooks and periodicals in appropriate pharmaceutical and biomedical subject areas. "Online" services, including an abstract service and computerized drug information reference system, should also be available.

Pharmacy staff and residents, in cooperation with the medical staff and administration, must develop and promulgate policies concerning drug use at the practice site and have evaluation systems in place to assess ongoing compliance with those policies. A member of the pharmacy staff shall be a member of and actively participate in all committees of the medical staff or practice site (e.g., P&T committee, quality-assurance committee, and institutional review board) responsible for establishing policies concerning drugs, drug therapy, drug delivery devices, and any other drug-related matters. Pharmacy practice residents must be active participants in drug use policy development activities.

Practice management. The focus of a pharmacy practice residency is centered on refining the knowledge and skills needed to pursue optimal drug therapy outcomes; therefore, a resident must be knowledgeable about the many integrated facets of a pharmacy service that, in essence, are directed toward that same objective. Hence, training in management, which provides overall direction and integration of pharmacy services, is viewed as an essential component of a pharmacy practice residency. It is intended that each resident shall

- Gain a thorough understanding of the department head's philosophy of comprehensive pharmaceutical services.
- Develop problem-solving abilities.
- Improve communications skills.
- Learn to make judgments, set priorities, and assume responsibility concerning management of pharmaceutical care resources at the practice site.
- Gain an understanding of policies concerning application and use of drugs and drug delivery systems.
- Learn the elements of a thorough quality improvement program that relates both to the quality of drugs prepared or packaged and to the quality of pharmaceutical care provided, including but not limited to inpatient and outpatient pharmacy services and drug information.[22]
- Engage in routine discussions with members of the management team concerning key health-care policy matters that may affect pharmacy.

A fundamental purpose of training in this area is to help each resident understand how all components of the pharmacy service are integrated in the provision of pharmaceutical care.

Essential aspects of administration and facilities needed in any practice site, and particularly in one offering a pharmacy practice residency, are outlined in the "ASHP Guidelines: Minimum Standard for Pharmacies in Institutions."[3] Key elements of management that the resident should also be knowledgeable about include

- The table of organization delineating the reporting lines of pharmacy service personnel and corresponding written position descriptions.
- Departmental objectives that are clearly defined and documented and whose intent and substance are familiar to all staff members; as a department head in the institution, the pharmacy director is responsible for determining departmental objectives, with corresponding timetables when appropriate, and these should be in accord with the established goals of the practice site.
- Pertinent legal and regulatory requirements that must be met and documentation pertaining to compliance with such requirements that must be maintained.
- Written policies and procedures for the pharmacy service, which must be kept current and supported by appropriate administrative mechanisms to ensure routine compliance.
- Application of computer technology to pharmacy operations.

The pharmacy service must have a sufficient complement and diversity of professional and technical staff to ensure that the department can provide the level of service required within the practice site and to which it is committed. While this Standard imposes no fixed ratio of full-time staff to residents, the number of pharmacists on staff must be adequate to provide supervision and guidance to the resident in each of the required areas of training outlined in Principle IVB, Requirement 1.

All staff pharmacists shall be currently licensed to practice in one of the jurisdictions of the United States. Professional staff members, including residents, should seek professional enrichment and must demonstrate their interest in maintaining competency. Ways in which these objectives may be met include, but are not limited to, the following: attending continuing-education programs, reading professional literature, and participating in local, state, or national professional organizations.

The supportive staff complement should be sufficient to handle all technical functions that can be appropriately assigned to them. The "ASHP Technical Assistance Bulletin on Outcome Competencies and Training Guidelines for Institutional Pharmacy Technician Training Programs"[23] provides examples of functions that should be routinely delegated to technicians. It should be the goal of the department that all technical personnel have completed a formally organized training program.

3. The resident shall complete an appropriate project.

Interpretation. An investigation of some particular pharmacy issue must be completed as one requirement for the residency. It may be in the form of original research, a problem-solving exercise, or development, enhancement, or evaluation of some aspect of pharmacy services. The residency director may require the resident to undertake one major project or several short-term projects.

Final reports, following an accepted manuscript style, shall be submitted by the resident before completion of the program, and the residency director shall require a formal presentation by the resident of the results obtained.

All such projects shall be directed toward useful outcomes and should not merely be academic exercises for the sole purpose of satisfying this requirement.

Part V—Evaluation of Resident and Residency Program

Principle V

The residency program must be evaluated to assess the training environment and the performance of residents and preceptors.

Requirements

1. A plan for each resident shall be developed and documented at the beginning of the program. The plan shall relate to practice skills required in contemporary pharmacy practice and shall describe the competencies to be attained in the residency program.

Interpretation. Each incoming resident shall be evaluated in an attempt to assess the individual's strengths and weaknesses. Based on this evaluation, a written plan shall be developed by the residency program director in consultation with the resident. The relative emphasis in specific areas of training may vary according to each resident's individualized plan. This plan shall be evaluated regularly and modified accordingly.

2. Each resident's activities shall be scheduled in advance and planned to make possible the attainment of the predetermined program goals and learning objectives.

Interpretation. The program director shall develop, in cooperation with the resident, a training schedule designed to achieve the predetermined goals and learning objectives for the residency program, which is in concert with the mission and needs of the department. The schedule shall be written in sufficient detail to give each resident a clear understanding of assignments and activities and must reflect the predetermined goals and learning objectives the program director expects each resident to achieve.

3. Learning objectives that relate specifically to the knowledge, skills, and attitudes required in contemporary pharmacy practice shall be developed and documented for each period of training. These objectives shall describe the terminal competencies to be attained, shall relate directly to the program plan established for each resident as reflected in Requirement 1 above, and shall be provided to and reviewed with the resident at the beginning of each period of training.

Interpretation. Learning objectives serve as a guide for the residents, the preceptors, and any other individuals who may share responsibility for specific rotations, developing and supervising experiences, and evaluating achievement. These objectives shall be fundamentally the same for each resident, although the relative emphasis on specific areas may vary according to the resident's previous practice experience and individualized program plan. The learning objectives should stress outcomes rather than the process by which those outcomes are achieved.

4. Continuous feedback to and communication with the resident shall be provided by the preceptor during each training segment, and a final evaluation, based on preestablished learning objectives, shall be conducted after every period of training; further, the resident shall assess each period of training and corresponding preceptor.

Interpretation. Periodic evaluation throughout the training segment is an essential means by which to provide residents with an assessment of ongoing performance. Therefore, both during and at the end of each period of training, the preceptor must evaluate the resident based on preestablished learning objectives for that training segment. All *final* evaluations must be documented, reviewed with the resident by the preceptor, and signed by the program director. An assessment of the resident's communication skills (oral and written) and ability to interrelate with other health-care professionals is also required. When deficiencies are noted, appropriate remedial action must be taken.

The resident shall provide overall assessment of the period of training and the preceptor responsible for the training segment; this shall be documented and reviewed by the resident with the program director and preceptor.

5. Each resident shall undertake periodic written self-evaluation; it shall be reviewed with the resident by the residency program director.

Interpretation. Written self-evaluation reports shall be required of each resident by the residency program director and must be completed at least quarterly during the training program. The purpose of these reports shall be to assist the resident in identifying any unmet objectives that were established for the period of time covered by the report.

Part VI—Experimentation and Innovation

Principle VI

Experimentation and innovation in developing and implementing postgraduate residency training programs shall be encouraged.

Requirement

1.   Experimental and innovative approaches to developing and implementing residency training programs and alternative methods for meeting this Standard should be pursued; these activities must be adequately planned and coupled with an appropriate evaluation system.

Interpretation. The intent is to provide programs with an opportunity to explore new mechanisms for meeting this Accreditation Standard that will maintain excellence in established program areas.

Particular areas of experimentation and innovation include, but are not limited to, structure and process of training segments, scheduling, program length, and affiliation with academic programs or differentiated practice sites. Program directors and preceptors desiring to explore program alternatives or methods that depart from current requirements in the Standard should provide assurances that quality in the training program is not adversely affected; further, consultation with the ASHP Accreditation Services staff is strongly encouraged.

Part VII—Certificate

Principle VII

The pharmacy practice residency graduate's completion of the program shall be attested to by the accredited practice site(s).

Requirements

1.   The practice site(s) and, if applicable, the sponsoring organization (e.g., college of pharmacy) shall recognize those pharmacists who have completed successfully the residency in pharmacy practice by awarding an appropriate certificate of residency.

Interpretation. It is the program director's prerogative and responsibility to award the certificate of residency. In accrediting a residency program, ASHP does not certify the individual resident. Reference may be made in the residency certificate to its ASHP-accredited status, in accordance with the provisions of the "ASHP Regulations on Accreditation of Pharmacy Residencies."[2]

2.   No certificate shall be issued to any individual who has failed to complete the practice site's prescribed program or to meet the intent of this Standard.

Interpretation. In issuing a certificate of residency to a pharmacist, the practice site attests that the individual has achieved the predetermined goals and objectives of the pharmacy practice residency program. If the site knowingly issues an unearned certificate of residency, its accreditation by ASHP shall be subject to revocation.

References

1.   American Society of Hospital Pharmacists.   Definitions of pharmacy residencies and fellowships. *Am J Hosp Pharm.* 1987; 44:1141–4.
2.   American Society of Hospital Pharmacists. ASHP regulations on accreditation of pharmacy residencies. *Am J Hosp Pharm.* 1985; 42:2005–7.
3.   American Society of Hospital Pharmacists. ASHP guidelines: minimum standard for pharmacies in institutions. *Am J Hosp Pharm.* 1985; 42:372–5.
4.   American Society of Hospital Pharmacists. ASHP guidelines on pharmaceutical services for ambulatory patients. *Am J Hosp Pharm.* 1991; 48:311–5.
5.   American Society of Hospital Pharmacists. ASHP statement on the pharmacist's clinical role in organized health-care settings. *Am J Hosp Pharm.* 1989; 46:2345–6.
6.   American Society of Hospital Pharmacists. ASHP technical assistance bulletin on assessment of departmental directions for clinical practice in pharmacy. *Am J Hosp Pharm.* 1989; 46:339–41.
7.   American Society of Hospital Pharmacists. ASHP guidelines for obtaining authorization for documenting pharmaceutical care in patient medical records. *Am J Hosp Pharm.* 1989; 46:338–9.
8.   American Society of Hospital Pharmacists. ASHP statement on the pharmacist's responsibility for distribution and control of drugs. *Am J Hosp Pharm.* 1991; 48:1782.
9.   American Society of Hospital Pharmacists. ASHP statement on unit dose drug distribution. *Am J Hosp Pharm.* 1989; 46:2346.
10.   American Society of Hospital Pharmacists. ASHP statement on the pharmacist's role with respect to drug delivery systems and administration devices. *Am J Hosp Pharm.* 1989; 46:2342–3.
11.   American Society of Hospital Pharmacists. ASHP guidelines for the use of investigational drugs in organized health-care settings. *Am J Hosp Pharm.* 1991; 48:315–9.
12.   American Society of Hospital Pharmacists. ASHP technical assistance bulletin on hospital drug distribution and control. *Am J Hosp Pharm.* 1980; 37:1097–103.
13.   American Society of Hospital Pharmacists. ASHP technical assistance bulletin on institutional use of controlled substances. *Am J Hosp Pharm.* 1987; 44:580–9.
14.   American Society of Hospital Pharmacists. ASHP technical assistance bulletin on handling cytotoxic and hazardous drugs. *Am J Hosp Pharm.* 1990; 47:1033–49.
15.   American Society of Hospital Pharmacists. ASHP technical assistance bulletin on surgery and anesthesiology pharmaceutical services. *Am J Hosp Pharm.* 1991; 48:319–25.
16.   American Society of Hospital Pharmacists. ASHP statement on the pharmacy and therapeutics committee. *Am J Hosp Pharm.* 1984; 41:1621.

17. American Society of Hospital Pharmacists. ASHP statement on the formulary system. *Am J Hosp Pharm.* 1983; 40:1384–5.

18. American Society of Hospital Pharmacists. ASHP technical assistance bulletin on drug formularies. *Am J Hosp Pharm.* 1991; 48:791–3.

19. American Society of Hospital Pharmacists. ASHP technical assistance bulletin on the evaluation of drugs for formularies. *Am J Hosp Pharm.* 1988; 45:386–7.

20. American Society of Hospital Pharmacists. ASHP guidelines on the pharmacist's role in drug use evaluation. *Am J Hosp Pharm.* 1988; 45:385–6.

21. American Society of Hospital Pharmacists. ASHP guidelines on adverse drug reaction monitoring and reporting. *Am J Hosp Pharm.* 1989; 46:336–7.

22. Coe CP. The elements of quality in pharmaceutical care. Bethesda, MD: American Society of Hospital Pharmacists; 1992.

23. American Society of Hospital Pharmacists. ASHP technical assistance bulletin on outcome competencies and training guidelines for institutional pharmacy technician training programs. *Am J Hosp Pharm.* 1982; 39:317–20.

[a]The "ASHP Statement on the Pharmacist's Responsibility for Distribution and Control of Drug Products" was approved by the ASHP Board of Directors November 20, 1991, and by the ASHP House of Delegates June 1, 1992. This document now supersedes Reference 8.

[b]The "ASHP Statement on the Pharmacy and Therapeutics Committee" was approved by the ASHP Board of Directors November 20, 1991, and by the ASHP House of Delegates June 1, 1992. This document now supersedes Reference 16.

[c]The "ASHP Guidelines on Formulary System Management" was approved by the Board of Directors November 20, 1991 (*Am J Hosp Pharm.* 1992; 49:648–52).

Approved by the ASHP Board of Directors, September 27, 1991. Developed by the ASHP Commission on Credentialing. Supersedes the "ASHP Accreditation Standard for Hospital Pharmacy Residency Training," approved April 25, 1985, and the "ASHP Accreditation Standard for Residency Training in Clinical Pharmacy Practice," approved April 28, 1988.

The bibliographic citation for this document is as follows: American Society of Hospital Pharmacists. ASHP accreditation standard for residency in pharmacy practice (with emphasis on pharmaceutical care). *Am J Hosp Pharm.* 1992; 49:146–53.

ASHP Accreditation Standard for Specialized Pharmacy Residency Training (with Guide to Interpretation)

Introduction

Definition. A specialized pharmacy residency is defined as an organized, directed, postgraduate training program that centers on the development of the knowledge, attitudes, and skills needed to provide pharmaceutical care in a specialized area of pharmacy practice.[1]

Purpose. The purpose of this Standard is to establish criteria for the training and education of pharmacists in the delivery of exemplary pharmaceutical care in specialized areas of pharmacy practice. The Accreditation Standard for Specialized Pharmacy Residency Training, together with the Supplemental Standards and Learning Objectives for each specialized area in which residency training is offered, sets forth the basic criteria to be used in the evaluation of programs applying for accreditation by the American Society of Hospital Pharmacists (ASHP).

Philosophy. Specialized pharmacy residency programs should be designed to develop expert knowledge and skills in the respective specialized area of pharmacy practice, far beyond that which might be expected from a residency in pharmacy practice. On the other hand, a specialized residency will not, per se, develop the broad skills and practice competence that a residency in pharmacy practice affords. Further, specialized pharmacy residency programs should develop professional practice patterns, habits, and a level of accountability far exceeding that obtained through clerkships or other forms of academic instruction. Although a specialized pharmacy residency program may include the requirement for the resident to complete a research project or a series of problem-solving tasks, specialized pharmacy residencies are not intended to prepare residents to become clinical scientists or clinical researchers. A specialized residency differs from a pharmacy fellowship in that the latter concentrates primarily on developing a set of skills in clinical research, whereas the primary objective of a residency is to develop professional practice skills.

Application of the Standard. The interpretive narrative following each requirement of the Standard is intended to illustrate how the Standard will be interpreted by the accreditation review teams and the ASHP Commission on Credentialing in the evaluation of specialized pharmacy residency programs.

A fundamental principle of this Standard is that a specialized pharmacy residency program is structured to ensure the achievement of certain predetermined competencies. While the Standard requires a minimum one-year, full-time practice commitment or equivalent for the residency, there is no set way in which this time is to be assigned. Each of the Supplemental Standards and Learning Objectives for specialty residency training specifies those areas in which the resident's competence must be developed, and these should serve as the principal determinants by which programs are structured. The amount of time required to accom-

plish a minimum level of competence in each of these areas will vary from one resident to another. It is essential that the resident's academic accomplishments, prior experience, and personal professional career goals be taken into consideration in structuring each individual's program. (See section V.)

The accreditation program is conducted under the authority of the ASHP Board of Directors. The ASHP Regulations on Accreditation of Pharmacy Residencies[2] set forth the policies governing the accreditation program and describe the procedures to be followed in applying for accreditation of pharmacy residency programs.

Throughout this Standard, where the auxiliary verbs *shall* and *must* are used, an absolute requirement is implied. The words *should* and *may* denote a recommended guideline for compliance.

Part I—Qualifications of the Training Site

Principle I A

Specialized pharmacy residencies shall be conducted only in those practice settings where the governing bodies, personnel, and staff have committed to seek excellence in patient care, have sought and accepted outside appraisal, and have demonstrated substantial conformance with professionally developed and nationally applied practice and operational standards.

Requirements

1. A hospital that offers, or that participates in offering, a specialized pharmacy residency shall be accredited by the Joint Commission on Accreditation of Healthcare Organizations or the American Osteopathic Association.

2. Other practice settings that offer, or that participate in offering, specialized residency training shall have demonstrated substantial conformance with applicable professionally developed and nationally applied standards.

Interpretation. The most recent evaluation report, including specific evaluative comments regarding pharmacy services or other drug-related matters, will serve as evidence that this requirement has been met and shall be made available to the accreditation survey team.

Principle I B

Two or more practice sites, or a sponsoring organization working in cooperation with one or more practice sites, may jointly provide a specialized pharmacy residency.

Requirements

1. A specialized pharmacy residency program is depen-

dent on an environment in which all of the learning objectives prescribed in the Supplemental Standard can be met. It is appropriate for two or more practice sites, or a sponsoring organization (e.g., college of pharmacy) and one or more practice sites, to collaborate in conducting a specialized pharmacy residency program.

2. A college of pharmacy that participates in offering a specialized pharmacy residency shall be accredited by the American Council on Pharmaceutical Education.

Interpretation. Application for accreditation of a multisite specialty residency must be submitted in the name of the principal practice site (i.e., the practice site in which the majority of the residency program is centered). In the case of a sponsoring organization (e.g., college of pharmacy) that has one or more practice settings to provide for residency training, the application for accreditation must be completed by the sponsoring organization and the principal practice site.

Further qualifications for an accredited multisite residency program are set forth in parts II, III, and IV of this Standard.

Part II—Qualifications of the Residency Program Director and Preceptors

Principle II

Directors and preceptors of specialized residencies shall be individuals who maintain high professional ideals, who have distinguished themselves in practice, and who have the desire and the aptitude to teach.

Requirements

1. The director of pharmacy service in the practice site shall appoint a qualified member of his or her staff to serve as program director of the specialized pharmacy residency program.

Interpretation. The director of pharmacy service at the practice site has the ultimate responsibility for education and training of residents. Unless the director of pharmacy service is qualified according to requirements II-2 and II-3 below, he or she must appoint a program director from among those on the staff who are qualified. The program director must be accountable to the director of pharmacy service for the services he or she provides and for the conduct of the residency program. The residency program director is responsible for ensuring that the overall program goals and specific learning objectives are met, training schedules are maintained, appropriate preceptorship for each rotation or period of training is provided, and the resident evaluations based on the pre-established learning objectives are routinely conducted.

2. The program director shall have completed appropriate ASHP-accredited residency training or have equivalent experience, shall have earned the Doctor of Pharmacy or other appropriate advanced degree in pharmacy, and shall have two years of experience in the specialized area of pharmacy practice in which he or she serves as program director; alternatively, if lacking an advanced degree or postgraduate training,

he or she shall have had four years of experience in the specialized area of pharmacy practice in which he or she serves as program director.

Interpretation. Formal training in the area of specialization, such as postgraduate residency training or fellowship training, is allowable in meeting the years of experience requirement.

Any additional or more stringent requirements for the program director, as set forth in the Supplemental Standard, must be met.

3. The program director shall have demonstrated outstanding capabilities as a practitioner and as a teacher in the specialized area of pharmacy practice; further, he or she shall have made significant contributions to the development or improvement of the area of specialization in which he or she practices.

Interpretation. The program director serves as the resident's role model in the specialized area of pharmacy practice, as well as overall coordinator of the resident's education and training. Furthermore, the program director is expected to maintain ongoing responsibility and accountability for the provision of pharmaceutical care in the specialized area of training. It is critical, therefore, that the program director's skills as a practitioner and educator be exemplary. This may be characterized by the following:

- Having a progressive, documented record, demonstrating improvements in and contributions to the respective area of specialized pharmacy practice.
- Having received formal recognition by peers as a model practitioner.
- Holding appointments on the appropriate drug policy committees of the institution.
- Having demonstrated an ability to teach, including holding a faculty appointment in a college of pharmacy, college of medicine, or other college that awards a professional practice degree (baccalaureate or higher) in the health field. (An adjunct appointment or clinical appointment is acceptable.)
- Having demonstrated and documented evidence of the ability to direct and manage a pharmacy practice residency.
- Having a sustained record of contributing to the total body of knowledge in the specialized area of pharmacy practice through publications or formal presentations at professional meetings, to include publications in refereed national professional practice publications or scholarly papers at national conclaves.
- Regularly serving as a reviewer of contributed papers or manuscripts submitted for publication.

4. Multisite residency programs shall have one designated residency program director, whose appointment shall be agreed to in writing by each of the participating practice sites.

Interpretation. The residency program director for multisite residencies is the individual held accountable for the conduct and the quality of the residency program. If a department of pharmacy and college of pharmacy constitute the two organizations providing for residency training, then the director of pharmacy shall, in cooperation with the dean, delegate oversight for the program to a qualified individual within the pharmacy department or the college of pharmacy, provided that a clear line of accountability is established for the program between the director of pharmacy and this individual.

In the case of multisite, college-sponsored programs, the directors of pharmacy, in cooperation with the dean, must appoint a qualified individual to be program director.

5. The residency program director shall have considerable latitude in delegating preceptorial responsibilities for specific segments of the residency program to qualified pharmacy practitioners. The preceptors must have demonstrated outstanding strengths in the area of practice for which he or she serves as preceptor.

Interpretation. Each rotation or period of training must have a qualified pharmacist preceptor. Evaluation of a preceptor's qualifications shall be based on professional education and experience in the area of practice for which he or she shall serve as preceptor. All preceptors should have completed an ASHP-accredited residency and hold the Pharm.D. degree or have equivalent qualifications; further, all are expected to practice routinely in the area in which they serve as preceptor. The Standard does not preclude the use of physician preceptors in select elective "rotations"; however, a pharmacy practitioner must supervise the residency training experience as well as directly observe and provide evaluation of the resident's performance.

Part III—Selection and Qualifications of the Resident

Principle III

The applicant must be a highly motivated pharmacist having a sufficient foundation of broad skills and competence in pharmacy practice necessary for further professional development in a specialized area of pharmacy practice.

Requirements

1. The resident shall be a graduate of an accredited college of pharmacy and be licensed, or be eligible for licensure, in the state or jurisdiction in which the residency program is located. The resident should hold the Doctor of Pharmacy degree and should have completed an ASHP-accredited residency training program or have an equivalent level of prior experience in pharmacy practice.

Interpretation. The applicant must be a graduate of a college of pharmacy accredited by the American Council on Pharmaceutical Education or otherwise be eligible for licensure. The entering resident will be expected to have completed a comprehensive clerkship and externship program, such as is required in contemporary Doctor of Pharmacy curricula, or have had sufficient cumulative life experience to equal this entrance requirement.

A pharmacist who specializes in a focused area of pharmacy practice must have a sound foundation in the broader aspects of pharmacy services to relate to the goals and objectives set forth in each specialized supplemental standard. It is clear that an ASHP-accredited residency in pharmacy practice[3] provides the applicant with the level of

knowledge and skills needed to provide the fundamentals of pharmacy practice on which specialty training can be built. For that reason, a resident entering an ASHP-accredited specialized residency program should have completed an ASHP-accredited residency in pharmacy practice or have attained competencies similar to those expressed in the Draft Goals and Objectives for Residencies in Pharmacy Practice.[a] It is the program director's responsibility to assess applicants' baseline knowledge and skills and to ascertain that they qualify for admission.

Any additional or more stringent requirements for the resident, as set forth in the Supplemental Standard, must be met; further, nothing in this Standard and the Supplemental Standard shall prevent individual residency programs from setting more stringent entry-level requirements.

2. The residency program director shall establish a formal procedure for evaluating applicants' qualifications.

Interpretation. Typical admission criteria should include, but not be limited to, prior residency experience (including the evaluation of the resident's goals and objectives from previous residency training), academic transcripts, and submission of formal letters of recommendation from current and prior preceptors and faculty (including those individuals who provided residency and clerkship training), and from former employers. Personal interviews should be conducted. Residency applicants should be evaluated by all members of the staff who have major preceptorial responsibilities.

3. Final acceptance of the applicant shall be the responsibility of the director of pharmacy.

Interpretation. The director of pharmacy services is ultimately responsible for the pharmacy residency program. In the case of multisite residencies or those provided by a sponsoring organization and one or more practice sites, a mechanism shall be in place that permits the individuals who have responsibility for coordinating the residency programs to agree cooperatively upon selection of applicants.

Part IV—Residency Training Program and Pharmacy Service

Principle IV A

The training and education of residents in the provision of pharmaceutical care shall be of paramount importance in the overall structure and organization of a specialized pharmacy residency program.

Requirement

1. The pharmacy practice site shall conduct the residency in such a way as to ensure that any services the resident is required to provide complement, rather than compete with, the educational and experiential objectives of the program.

Interpretation. A specialized residency in pharmacy practice involves active participation by the resident in the provision of pharmaceutical care. This is best achieved when the resident is directly involved in making judgments regarding the specialized pharmaceutical care needs of patients.

Having responsibility adds understanding, confidence, and purpose and builds upon the resident's academic knowledge and professional background. A substantial portion of this participation must, of necessity, involve hands-on experience, since only through actual provision of care and involvement in decision-making processes can the resident be expected to gain an understanding of the knowledge, skills, and judgments required to carry out the specialized pharmaceutical care needs of patients. Through actual experience the resident learns how specialty practitioners provide pharmaceutical care and how their services are best coordinated with other disciplines involved with drug use throughout the practice site. Thus, the residency program should concentrate on developing the resident's ability to conceptualize, integrate, and transform accumulated experiences and knowledge into improved use of drugs in cooperation with the patient and other health care providers.

A residency is a full-time obligation; hence, the resident shall manage activities external to the residency so as not to interfere with the goals and objectives of the program as defined in this Standard.

Principle IV B

Specialized residency programs shall be predicated on the knowledge, attitudes, and skills required for contemporary pharmacy practice. The practice site offering the residency shall provide an exemplary training environment; further, the scope of pharmacy services at the site must be adequate to make possible the attainment of the residency program objectives set forth below.

Requirements

1. An accredited specialized pharmacy residency program shall develop the resident's competence in those areas set forth in the Learning Objectives that are specified in the Supplemental Standard for the specialized area in which the residency program is provided.

Interpretation. Using the Supplemental Standard and Learning Objectives, individualized learning objectives must be developed for each resident as required in section V and should specify the attitudes, skills, and knowledge the resident is expected to gain from each activity. These objectives then serve to guide the resident, as well as the program director and rotation preceptors responsible for the resident's experience, in the evaluation of achievement. The overall goals of the residency program must be in concert with the mission and needs of the pharmacy department.

2. The specialized area in which residency training is provided shall be an integral part of the health care organization's total program of pharmacy services, be organized in accordance with the principles of sound management under the direction of a legally qualified pharmacist, and have sufficient personnel and facilities for residency training. It shall comply with all applicable federal, state, and local laws, codes, statutes, and regulations governing pharmacy practice.

Interpretation. Any practice site that proposes to offer a pharmacy practice or specialty residency must offer a level of service sufficient in scope and quality to create an envi-

ronment throughout the site that is conducive to the support of such a program. The ASHP Statement on the Pharmacist's Clinical Role in Organized Health-Care Settings[4] and the ASHP Technical Assistance Bulletin on Assessment of Departmental Directions for Clinical Practice in Pharmacy[5] provide guidance in determining the extent to which pharmacy provides these services to inpatients. Moreover, in order to provide pharmaceutical care, pharmacists and residents must have access to patients' charts (or databases) and opportunity for chart notation. The document ASHP Guidelines for Obtaining Authorization for Documenting Pharmaceutical Care in Patient Medical Records[6] provides assistance in this area.

It is not acceptable to simulate residency experiences to substitute for nonexistent pharmacy services, nor is it acceptable to substitute academic courses for segments of the program that clearly require practice experience. The specialized pharmacy service area in which residency training is provided must comply with the provisions of part IV of the ASHP Accreditation Standard for Residency in Pharmacy Practice[3] that apply to the specialized area and any additional or more stringent requirements of the respective Supplemental Standard.

Essential aspects of administration and facilities needed in any practice site, and particularly one offering an ASHP-accredited residency, are outlined in the ASHP Guidelines: Minimum Standard for Pharmacies in Institutions.[7] Several key elements of management that the practice site must have in place include

*   A table of organization delineating the reporting lines of pharmacy service personnel, and corresponding written position descriptions.
*   A mission statement and strategic plan that include vision, values, and strategic goals and objectives that are clearly defined and documented. All staff members must be familiar with the intent and substance of these. As a department head in the institution, the pharmacy director is responsible for determining departmental objectives, with corresponding timetables, when appropriate, and these should be in accord with the established goals of the practice site.
*   Pertinent legal and regulatory requirements that must be met, and maintenance of documentation pertaining to compliance with such requirements.
*   Written policies and procedures for the pharmacy service, which must be kept current and supported with appropriate administrative mechanisms to ensure routine compliance.
*   Application of computer technology to pharmacy operations.

Additionally, a member of the pharmacy staff shall be a member of and actively participate in all committees of the medical staff or practice site (e.g., pharmacy and therapeutics committee, quality assurance committee, institutional review board) responsible for establishing policies concerning drugs, drug therapy, drug delivery devices, and any other drug-related matters pertaining to the specialized area of pharmacy practice.

3. There shall be an adequate number of pharmacists who practice regularly in the specialized area in which residents are being trained to ensure proper supervision and training of the residents.

Interpretation. The pharmacy service must have a sufficient complement and diversity of professional and technical staff to ensure that the department can provide the level of service required within the practice site and to which it is committed. While this Standard imposes no fixed ratio of full-time staff to residents, the number of well-qualified specialists on the staff must be adequate to provide supervision and guidance to the resident in each area of training outlined in the Supplemental Standard. One of these must serve as program director of the residency program. There is a fine line between the amount of preceptor supervision required during the resident's training and the degree of autonomy needed by the resident to provide direct patient care. Hence, pharmacy preceptors and the resident must work together closely to ensure that this fundamental element of the training program is met without compromising patient care through inadequate supervision.

Those who provide specialized pharmacy services must be accountable to the health care organization's pharmacy department head for those services.

All staff pharmacists shall be currently licensed to practice in one of the jurisdictions of the United States. Professional staff members, including the residents, should seek professional enrichment and must demonstrate their interest in maintaining competency. Ways in which these objectives may be met include, but are not limited to, the following: attending continuing-education programs, reading the professional literature, and participating in local, state, or national professional organizations.

The supportive-staff complement should be sufficient to handle all technical functions that can be appropriately assigned to them. The ASHP Technical Assistance Bulletin on Outcome Competencies and Training Guidelines for Institutional Pharmacy Technician Training Programs provides examples of functions that should be routinely delegated to technicians. It should be the goal of the department that all technical personnel have completed a formally organized training program.

4.   In the case of specialized residencies that involve more than one major training site (as described in principle I B of this Standard), the pharmacy service in each shall qualify under the provisions of this Standard.

Interpretation. The Society will apply the interpretive commentaries noted in requirements IV A-1 through IV B-4 above in reviewing the pharmacy service in any major training site. Sites used for periods of one month or less will not be considered major training sites. Such sites may account for no more than three months of the total residency program, and the involvement of any such site is subject to approval by the Society.

Further, nothing in this Standard shall exclude from consideration for accreditation those health care organizations that contract with outside vendors for pharmaceutical services (e.g., colleges of pharmacy and contract management firms), provided that the quality of the contracted services otherwise meets the intent of this Standard.

5.   The resident shall complete an appropriate project.

Interpretation. An investigation of some particular pharmacy issue must be completed as one of the requirements for the residency. This may be in the form of original research, a problem-solving exercise, or development, enhancement,

or evaluation of some aspect of pharmacy services. The residency director may require the resident to undertake one major project or several short-term projects.

Final reports, following an accepted manuscript style, shall be submitted by the resident prior to completion of the program, and the residency director shall require a formal presentation by the resident of obtained results.

All such projects shall be directed toward useful outcomes and should not merely be academic exercises for the sole purpose of satisfying this requirement.

Part V—Development of Individualized Learning Objectives

Principle V

The residency program shall be established from clearly defined and measurable outcome learning objectives.

Requirements

1.   A set of individualized learning objectives shall be documented for each resident at the beginning of the program. These resident objectives shall be developed using the learning objectives outlined in the respective ASHP Supplemental Standard to reflect the resident's entering knowledge, skills, and abilities.

Interpretation. Each incoming resident shall be evaluated to assess current knowledge, skills, and abilities. Based on this evaluation, the respective Supplemental Standard and Learning Objectives shall be modified to establish a set of individualized learning objectives for each resident. The Learning Objectives should stress outcomes rather than the process by which those outcomes are achieved and should serve to guide the residents, program director, and preceptors in the development of experiential learning and the assessment of its outcomes.

For residents who have not completed a prior ASHP-accredited residency or who have not had significant pharmacy practice experience, the program director must develop a process to assess the resident's competence in the four core areas of pharmacy practice (acute, ambulatory care, drug information and drug policy development, and practice management) specified in the ASHP Accreditation Standard for Residency in Pharmacy Practice.[3] Moreover, where appropriate to the setting, specific learning objectives must be added to the respective specialized set of required objectives to address any fundamental pharmacy practice deficiencies identified.

2.   An organized plan shall be developed and documented that defines the program structure and the types of learning experiences necessary to accomplish the individual resident's learning objectives established in requirement V-1.

Interpretation. The plan shall be developed by the residency program director and the preceptors, with input from the resident, as needed. The relative emphasis in specific areas of training should vary according to each resident's past experience and shall be guided by the resident's individualized learning objectives, as specified in principle V-1 above, not by the uniqueness of the site's services. Each plan shall be evaluated regularly and modified accordingly.

3. Each resident's activities shall be scheduled in advance and planned to make possible the attainment of the predetermined program goals and learning objectives.

Interpretation. The program director and preceptors, in cooperation with the resident, shall develop a training schedule that is based on the broad plan and is designed to achieve the predetermined goals and learning objectives for the residency program. The schedule shall be written in sufficient detail to give each resident a clear understanding of assignments and activities and must reflect the predetermined goals and learning objectives the program director expects each resident to achieve.

Part VI—Evaluation of Resident and Residency Program

Principle VI

The residency program must be evaluated to assess resident learning, preceptor performance, and the training environment.

Requirements

1. Continuous feedback to and communication with the resident shall be provided by the preceptor during each training segment, and a final evaluation, based on pre-established learning objectives, shall be conducted after every period of training.

Interpretation. Periodic evaluation throughout the course of the training segment is an essential means by which to provide residents with an assessment of ongoing performance. Therefore, both during and at the end of each period of training, the preceptor must evaluate the resident on the basis of pre-established learning objectives for that training segment. Strategies for assessing the accomplishment of each resident's objectives should be developed prior to each resident learning experience and communicated to the resident. In this way participants in the precepting/learning process will be fully informed of expectations and criteria used to measure success. All final evaluations must directly evaluate the learning objectives and be documented, reviewed with the resident by the preceptor, and signed by the resident and the program director. An assessment of the resident's communication skills (oral and written) and ability to interrelate with other health care professionals is required. When deficiencies are noted, appropriate remedial action must be taken.

2. The resident shall assess each period of training and corresponding preceptor.

Interpretation. The resident shall provide an overall assessment of the period of training and of precepting and mentoring techniques used by the preceptor responsible for the training segment; further, this shall be documented and reviewed by the resident with the program director and preceptor.

3. Each resident shall undertake periodic written self-evaluation; further, these evaluations shall be reviewed with the resident by the appropriate preceptor(s) and the residency program director.

Interpretation. Written self-evaluation reports shall be required of each resident by the residency program director and must be completed at least quarterly during the course of the training program. Each report shall be compared with the preceptor's evaluation of the resident to assist the resident, the preceptor, and the program director in identifying any unmet objectives that were established for the period of time covered by the report.

Part VII—Experimentation and Innovation

Principle VII

Experimentation and innovation in developing and implementing postgraduate residency training programs shall be encouraged.

Requirement

1. Experimental and innovative approaches to developing and implementing residency programs and alternative methods to meeting this Standard should be pursued; these activities must be adequately planned and coupled with an appropriate evaluation system.

Interpretation. The intent is to provide programs with an opportunity to explore new mechanisms to meet this Accreditation Standard while maintaining excellence in established program areas.

Particular areas of experimentation and innovation include, but are not limited to, structure and process of training segments, scheduling, program length, and affiliation with academic programs or differentiated practice sites. Program directors and preceptors desiring to explore program alternatives or methods that depart from current requirements in the Standard should provide assurances that quality in the residency program is not affected adversely; further, consultation with the ASHP Accreditation Services Division is strongly encouraged.

Part VIII—Certificate

Principle VIII

The pharmacy practice residency graduate's completion of the program shall be attested to by the accredited practice site(s).

Requirements

1. The practice site(s) and, if applicable, the sponsoring organization (e.g., college of pharmacy) shall recognize those pharmacists who have successfully completed the residency in a specialized area of pharmacy practice by awarding an appropriate certificate of residency.

Interpretation. It is the program director's prerogative and responsibility to award the certificate of residency. In accrediting a residency program, ASHP does not certify the individual resident. Reference may be made in the residency certificate to its ASHP-accredited status, in accordance with the provisions of the ASHP Regulations on Accreditation of Pharmacy Residencies.[2]

2. No certificate shall be issued to any individual who has failed to complete the practice site's prescribed program or to meet the intent of this Standard.

Interpretation. In issuing a certificate of residency to a pharmacist, the practice site attests that the individual has achieved the predetermined goals and objectives of the residency program in a specialized area of pharmacy practice. If the site knowingly issues an unearned certificate of residency, its accreditation by ASHP shall be subject to revocation.

References

1. American Society of Hospital Pharmacists. Definitions of pharmacy residencies and fellowships. *Am J Hosp Pharm.* 1987; 44:1141–4

2. American Society of Hospital Pharmacists. ASHP regulations on accreditation of pharmacy residencies. *Am J Hosp Pharm.* 1985; 42:2005–7.

3. American Society of Hospital Pharmacists. ASHP accreditation standard for residency in pharmacy practice (with emphasis on pharmaceutical care). *Am J Hosp Pharm.* 1992; 49:146–53.

4. American Society of Hospital Pharmacists. ASHP statement on the pharmacist's clinical role in organized health-care settings. *Am J Hosp Pharm.* 1989; 46: 2324–6.

5. American Society of Hospital Pharmacists. ASHP technical assistance bulletin on assessment of departmental directions for clinical practice in pharmacy. *Am J Hosp Pharm.* 1989; 46:339–41.

6. American Society of Hospital Pharmacists. ASHP guidelines for obtaining authorization for documenting pharmaceutical care in patient medical records. *Am J Hosp Pharm.* 1989; 46:338–9.

7. American Society of Hospital Pharmacists. ASHP guidelines: minimum standard for pharmacies in institutions. *Am J Hosp Pharm.* 1985; 42:372–5.

---

aDraft Goals and Objectives for Residencies in Pharmacy Practice, under review by the Commission on Credentialing.

Approved by the ASHP Board of Directors, April 27, 1994. Developed by the ASHP Commission on Credentialing. This revision of the Accreditation Standard takes effect April 27, 1995. Until that time, the current Standard, which was approved April 28, 1988, is in force.

The bibliographic citation for this document is as follows: American Society of Hospital Pharmacists. ASHP accreditation standard for specialized pharmacy residency training (with guide to interpretation). *Am J Hosp Pharm* 1994; 51:2034–41.

ASHP Supplemental Standard and Learning Objectives for Residency Training in Drug Information Practice

Preamble

Definition. A specialized residency in drug information practice is defined as an organized, directed postgraduate program of practical experience that centers on developing the competencies necessary to provide comprehensive drug information services in health care organizations.

Purpose and Philosophy. A specialized residency in drug information pharmacy practice must be organized and conducted to develop mastery of knowledge and an expert level of competency in this area of pharmacy, differentiated in scope, depth, and proficiency from the drug information activities of organized health care setting pharmacy practice residents. Objectives of such training shall include extensive experiences in providing comprehensive drug information services in an organization or several organizations, integrated with the organization's pharmaceutical care services, drug distribution systems, and the appropriate committees dealing with drug use.

Accreditation Authority. The ASHP Accreditation Standard for Specialized Pharmacy Residency Training,[1] taken together with this supplement, are the basic criteria used to evaluate drug information residency training programs in organizations applying for accreditation by the American Society of Hospital Pharmacists.

Qualifications of the Training Site. The training site must meet the requirements set forth in Part I of the ASHP Accreditation Standard for Specialized Pharmacy Residency Training. Facilities may include, but are not limited to, general hospitals, or health science centers, multihospital systems, health maintenance organizations, and pharmaceutical industries. A multisite residency program shall have one designated residency director, whose appointment shall be agreed to in writing by each of the participating practice sites.

Qualifications of the Pharmacy Service. Segments of residency training conducted as part of a pharmacy service in a health care organization must meet the requirements set forth in Part IV of the Accreditation Standard for Specialized Pharmacy Residency Training. The drug information service must have a least one pharmacist with an established practice in drug information. In addition, the pharmacy service must provide a comprehensive program of drug information services substantially more than that required in ASHP's Minimum Standard for Pharmacies in Institutions[2] The following specific requirements are established for the drug information service program.

1. *Physical facilities.* There shall be a defined area for the drug information center. Space shall be adequate to house the furniture, equipment, literature resources, and personnel of the drug information service.
2. *Resources.* There shall be a comprehensive drug information library with current primary, secondary, and tertiary sources. Adequate textbooks and periodicals

in appropriate pharmaceutical and biomedical subject areas shall be available in the drug information center or quickly accessible in another location. Computer-based resources, including indexing or abstracting services, shall be available in the drug information center. Reference texts shall be current and provide detailed information in at least the following areas: adverse effects, availability, chemistry, cost, dose, drugs of choice, drug administration, efficacy, formulations, incompatibilities, identification (foreign and American), indications, interactions, laws, mechanisms of action, nonprescription drugs, pathophysiology, pharmacokinetics, statistics, teratogenicity, and toxicology. The drug information center should be located near a medical library that, in turn, has access to a regional medical library.

3. *Staffing.* At least one full-time drug information specialist shall practice in the drug information center. Secretarial and clerical support shall be readily available to the drug information center staff.
4. *Availability of service.* The drug information center shall be open for service at least eight hours per day, Monday through Friday, with off-hours service capability through a paging system, answering service, or other mechanism.
5. *Scope of service.* The ASHP Accreditation Standard for Residency in Pharmacy Practice[3] sets forth the fundamental scope of pharmacy services that should be provided by health care organizations offering a residency program or segments of residency training.
6. *Review of quality.* There shall be an ongoing continuous quality improvement program to evaluate the activities of the pharmacy and drug information services.

Qualifications of the Program Director. The program director's qualifications shall meet the requirements set forth in Part II of the ASHP Accreditation Standard for Specialized Pharmacy Residency Training. The program director shall be proficient as a drug information specialist and shall demonstrate this through practice experience in his or her specialty. In addition, the program director shall maintain an active patient care involvement, through clinical consultations, other patient-oriented services provided through the drug information service, or routinely provided pharmaceutical care services.

Selection and Qualifications of the Resident. The resident must meet the requirements set forth in Part III of the ASHP Accreditation Standard for Specialized Pharmacy Residency Training.

Supplemental Goals and Objectives

Goals

1. Take personal responsibility for improving the pharmaceutical care of patients by advancing drug information practice.
2. Develop a plan to establish a drug information service

that includes requirements for physical space, personnel, budget, and equipment.

3. Design a continuous quality improvement plan for a drug information service.
4. Design a plan for the documentation of drug information services.
5. Design a drug information storage and retrieval system for the multi-user environment of a drug information center.
6. Develop and implement drug-use policies and procedures.
7. Employ advanced literature analysis skills in preparing drug information.
8. Contribute to the biomedical literature.
9. Communicate drug information clearly, orally and in writing.
10. Provide information support for investigational drug programs.
11. Ensure the quality of pharmacy and therapeutics committee decisions on drug use policy.
12. Develop strategies for improving an organized health care setting's adverse drug reaction program.
13. Develop strategies for improving an organized health care setting's drug use evaluation program.
14. Enhance health care professionals' skills in the retrieval, evaluation, and communication of drug information and the application of drug policy.
15. Understand the process that the department of pharmacy uses to meet accreditation requirements.
16. Conduct original experimental or descriptive research into drug information practice.
17. Manage the operation of a drug information center.
18. Integrate patient care skills with an advanced level of drug information skills to provide a higher level of direct patient care.
19. Maximize efficiency in performing drug information tasks through expert use of computer databases and electronic communications.
20. Publish newsletters providing pertinent drug use information for health care professionals in the organized health care setting.
21. Serve as a resource for the lay press in matters related to pharmacy practice and drug therapy.
22. Demonstrate ethical conduct in all activities related to drug information practice.

Objectives Associated with Goal Statement

The following are Terminal Objectives (TO) and Enabling Objectives (EO) associated with each goal statement.

Goal 1. Take personal responsibility for improving the pharmaceutical care of patients by advancing drug information practice.

TO 1.1 (Characterization) Lead the profession in improving the pharmaceutical care of patients by advancing drug information practice.

EO 1.1.1 (Synthesis) Write one's own philosophy of practice as a drug information specialist.

EO 1.1.2 (Characterization) Demonstrate an appreciation for one's professional obligation by contributing to the professional literature.

EO 1.1.3 (Characterization) Demonstrate appreciation for one's professional obligation by active participation in drug information specialty organizations.

EO 1.1.4 (Characterization) Use a systematic, ongoing process for self-assessment and to meet learning needs as required for excellence in drug information specialty practice.

Goal 2. Develop a plan to establish a drug information service that includes requirements for physical space, personnel, budget, and equipment.

TO 2.1 (Application) Use the principles of needs assessment to determine services to be offered by a proposed drug information service.

EO 2.1.1 (Comprehension) Discuss the components of a complete plan to establish a drug information service in a particular organized health care setting.

TO 2.2 (Evaluation) Appraise drug information resources relevant to the information needs of the organized health care setting.

EO 2.2.1 (Comprehension) Discuss the characteristics of published sources of information pertinent to drug information science.

EO 2.2.2 (Comprehension) Discuss the characteristics of online information resources pertinent to drug information science.

EO 2.2.3 (Comprehension) Discuss factors to consider when identifying the types of drug information resources required by a specific organized health care setting.

TO 2.3 (Synthesis) Devise a plan for accommodating the physical space needs of a proposed drug information service.

EO 2.3.1 (Comprehension) Describe criteria for effectively using space and for evaluating choice of location for a drug information service.

EO 2.3.2 (Comprehension) Discuss how the delivery of various drug information services may affect space and location requirements.

TO 2.4 (Synthesis) Formulate capital, personnel, operating, and revenue budgets for a proposed drug information service.

EO 2.4.1 (Synthesis) Formulate a drug information center capital budget.

EO 2.4.1.1 (Analysis) Identify items to include in the capital budget.

EO 2.4.1.2 (Application) Use a knowledge of the kinds of data required and appropriate resources to gather data to support the need for capital budget items, including equipment specifications and vendor options.

EO 2.4.1.3 (Evaluation) Determine specific capital budget items to submit for approval.

EO 2.4.1.4 (Application) Write a justification for items submitted for approval for the capital budget according to the institution's policies and procedures.

EO 2.4.2 (Synthesis) Formulate a drug information center personnel budget.

EO 2.4.2.1 (Analysis) Identify staffing requirements to include in the personnel budget.

EO 2.4.2.2 (Application) Use a knowledge of the kinds of data required and appropriate resources to gather data to support staffing requirements, including projected hours of staffing, salaries, overtime, differentials, turnover, workload analysis, and productivity records.

EO 2.4.2.3 (Synthesis) Formulate a budget plan that meets staffing needs.

EO 2.4.2.4 (Application) Write a justification for staffing resources submitted for approval for the personnel budget according to the institution's policies and procedures.

EO 2.4.3 (Synthesis) Formulate a drug information center operating budget.

EO 2.4.3.1 (Analysis) Identify items to include in the operating budget.

EO 2.4.3.2 (Application) Use a knowledge of the kinds of data required and appropriate resources to gather data to support the need for operating budget items, including fixed and variable expenses.

EO 2.4.3.3 (Evaluation) Determine operating budget accounts and funding levels to submit for approval.

EO 2.4.3.4 (Synthesis) Formulate a budget plan that secures needed operating budget accounts and funding levels.

EO 2.4.3.5 (Application) Write a justification for operating budget accounts and funding levels submitted for approval according to the institution's policies and procedures.

EO 2.4.4 (Comprehension) Discuss variables that would affect the revenue budget for a drug information center.

TO 2.5 (Comprehension) Discuss the tasks performed by personnel in a drug information center.

Goal 3. Design a continuous quality improvement (CQI) plan for a drug information service.

TO 3.1 (Synthesis) Formulate a CQI plan for a proposed drug information center.

EO 3.1.1 (Synthesis) Establish indicators, thresholds, and expected corrective actions.

EO 3.1.2 (Analysis) Determine the most appropriate person to perform each CQI activity.

Goal 4. Design a plan for the documentation of drug information services.

TO 4.1 (Synthesis) Formulate a plan to document the services of a proposed drug information service.

EO 4.1.1 (Comprehension) Discuss the elements of drug information services that should be documented.

EO 4.1.2 (Comprehension) Discuss systematic procedures for documenting drug information services.

Goal 5. Design a drug information storage and retrieval system [using electronic and/or manual processes] for the multi-user environment of a drug information center.

TO 5.1 (Synthesis) Design a drug information storage and retrieval system using electronic or manual processes, or both, for the multi-user environment of a drug information center.

EO 5.1.1 (Analysis) Determine what information in a drug information center is appropriate to store and retrieve.

EO 5.1.2 (Comprehension) Discuss characteristics of indexing options for storing and retrieving drug information and responding to drug information requests.

Goal 6. Develop and implement drug use policies and procedures.

TO 6.1 (Synthesis) Design policies and procedures that meet the needs of the organized health care setting.

EO 6.1.1 (Comprehension) Discuss the influence of organizational climate on the design and implementation of drug use policies and procedures.

EO 6.1.2 (Evaluation) Appraise current policies for congruence with the organized health care setting's mission, goals, and needs.

EO 6.1.3 (Synthesis) Formulate new or revised policies that are congruent with the organized health care setting's mission, goals, and needs.

EO 6.1.4 (Evaluation) Appraise current procedures for congruence with the organized health care setting's mission, goals, and needs.

EO 6.1.5 (Synthesis) Formulate new or revised procedures for congruence with the organized health care setting's mission, goals, and needs.

EO 6.1.6 (Evaluation) Appraise pharmaceutical manufacturer representative information for use in making drug use and drug use policy decisions.

EO 6.1.7 (Evaluation) Assess whether a pharmaceutical manufacturer's marketing and promotional activities are within the FDA regulatory guidelines.

EO 6.1.8 (Evaluation) Appraise current policies governing relations between the organized health care setting and the pharmaceutical industry to ensure that ethical practices are observed.

TO 6.2 (Synthesis) Formulate a plan that will implement a drug use policy.

EO 6.2.1 (Comprehension) Describe the key organizational players and entities in the implementation of a specific drug policy.

Goal 7. Employ advanced literature analysis skills in preparing drug information.

TO 7.1 (Synthesis) Prepare expert responses to complex drug information requests.

EO 7.1.1 (Comprehension) Discuss content and applicability of specialized sources of drug information.

EO 7.1.2 (Comprehension) Explain the application and interpretation of advanced statistical methods (e.g., meta-analysis, MANOVA).

EO 7.1.3 (Evaluation) Judge the adequacy of choice of quantitative or qualitative methods, or both, used to analyze data in a research study.

EO 7.1.4 (Evaluation) Assess the adequacy with which a research study's conclusions are supported by the study design and analysis of the data.

EO 7.1.5 (Analysis) Identify limitations to the generalizability of a specific research study.

EO 7.1.6 (Evaluation) Appraise drug information for the expertise and reputation of the source of information.

EO 7.1.7 (Evaluation) Determine instances in which a study conclusion is erroneously supported by a data display.

EO 7.1.8 (Comprehension) Discuss standards of care applicable to a specific drug information request.

EO 7.1.9 (Synthesis) In circumstances where there is no relevant information on which to base a response to a request for drug information, exercise clinical judgment to formulate a reasonable recommendation.

Goal 8. Contribute to the biomedical literature.

TO 8.1 (Synthesis) Write research articles, reviews, letters to the editor, or case reports that are suitable for publication.

EO 8.1.1 (Application) Use the "Uniform Requirements for Manuscripts Submitted to Biomedical Journals" in the preparation of research articles, reviews, letters to the editor, or case reports submitted for publication.

EO 8.1.2 (Application) Given a specific article, identify appropriate journals to which that article might be submitted for publication.

EO 8.1.3 (Evaluation) Given an identified topic related to pharmacy practice, appraise the publishability of an article on that topic.

EO 8.1.4 (Comprehension) Compare and contrast the reputations of biomedical journals.

EO 8.1.5 (Evaluation) Assess and edit others' articles prepared for publication.

Goal 9. Communicate drug information clearly, orally and in writing.

TO 9.1 (Synthesis) Organize all written and oral communication in a logical manner.

TO 9.2 (Synthesis) Design all communication at a level appropriate for the audience.

TO 9.3 (Synthesis) Construct each drug information communication using appropriate oral or written style, or both.

TO 9.4 (Synthesis) Design public presentations integrating advanced speaking skills while also meeting the needs of the group situation.

TO 9.5 (Synthesis) Formulate a listening strategy appropriate to each situation.

Goal 10. Provide information support for investigational drug programs.

TO 10.1 (Comprehension) Discuss the value of conducting investigational drug research studies.

TO 10.2 (Evaluation) Participate in determining the acceptability of research protocols for the organized health care setting.

EO 10.2.1 (Evaluation) Assess the adequacy of an investigational drug protocol's study design.

EO 10.2.2 (Comprehension) Discuss ethical and regulatory guidelines governing human research.

EO 10.2.3 (Comprehension) Discuss the financial implications of a research proposal for the organized health care setting.

EO 10.2.4 (Comprehension) Describe the overall process of human research approval.

EO 10.2.5 (Comprehension) Describe the functions and policies of the organized health care setting's investigational review board.

TO 10.3 (Evaluation) Participate in formulating investigational drug policy for the organized health care setting.

TO 10.4 (Application) Use an accepted system for storing and retrieving investigational drug protocols.

TO 10.5 (Application) Use an understanding of resources to identify a supplier for a given investigational drug.

Goal 11. Ensure the quality of pharmacy and therapeutics committee decisions on drug use policy.

TO 11.1 (Synthesis) Compile information for pharmacy and therapeutics committee decisions on drug use policy, based on an analysis of the committee's needs.

EO 11.1.1 (Comprehension) Discuss pertinent therapeutic issues for making drug use policy decisions.

EO 11.1.2 (Comprehension) Discuss ethical issues involved in making drug use policy decisions.

EO 11.1.3 (Comprehension) Discuss the contribution of organized health care setting statistics, a knowledge of key individuals and services, activity in the health care industry, and reimbursement issues that may affect drug use policy.

TO 11.2 (Evaluation) Determine proper drug use policy for recommendation to the P&T committee.

EO 11.2.1 (Comprehension) Describe the documentation required to support any drug use policy recommendation.

TO 11.3 (Synthesis) Design a communication strategy that will result in an informed evaluation of a drug use policy by the P&T committee.

EO 11.3.1 (Comprehension) Discuss factors to consider in developing a communication strategy that will result in an informed evaluation of a drug use policy by the P&T committee.

TO 11.4 (Synthesis) Design systematic follow-up that assesses the implementation and outcome of a drug use policy.

Goal 12. Develop strategies for improving an organized health care setting's adverse drug reaction program.

TO 12.1 (Synthesis) Formulate strategies for improvement of an organized health care setting's adverse drug reaction program.

EO 12.1.1 (Synthesis) Develop methods that identify trends that can lead to the prevention of adverse drug reactions.

EO 12.1.2 (Comprehension) Discuss the application of guidelines prepared by the Joint Commission on Accreditation of Healthcare Organizations and ASHP to the development and implementation of adverse drug reaction programs.

EO 12.1.3 (Comprehension) Discuss the application of various approaches to reversing adverse drug reaction trends.

TO 12.2 (Evaluation) Assess the impact on patient care of an organized health care setting's policy formulated to avert the occurrence of adverse drug reactions.

Goal 13. Develop strategies for improving an organized health care setting's drug use evaluation program.

TO 13.1 (Synthesis) Formulate strategies for improvement of an organized health care setting's drug use evaluation program.

EO 13.1.1 (Synthesis) Develop methods that identify trends in drug usage that should undergo study.

EO 13.1.2 (Comprehension) Discuss the application of guidelines prepared by the JCAHO, ASHP, and OBRA to the development and implementation of DUE programs.

TO 13.2 (Evaluation) Assess the impact on patient care of the drug use evaluation program.

Goal 14. Enhance health care professionals' skills in the retrieval, evaluation, and communication of drug information and the application of drug policy.

TO 14.1 (Synthesis) Design training for health care professionals in the retrieval, evaluation, and communication of drug information.

EO 14.1.1 (Comprehension) Explain skills in drug information of concern to health care professionals (drug literature evaluation, retrieval methods, use of resources).

TO 14.2 (Synthesis) Design training for health care professionals in the application of drug policy.

Goal 15. Understand the process that the department of pharmacy uses to meet accreditation and legal requirements.

TO 15.1 (Comprehension) Discuss strategies the department of pharmacy employs to comply with accreditation and legal requirements.

Goal 16. Conduct original experimental or descriptive research into drug information practice.

TO 16.1 (Synthesis) Conduct an experimental or descriptive research study of drug information practice that is suitable for publication.

 EO 16.1.1 (Evaluation) Determine a drug information topic suitable for study.

 EO 16.1.2 (Analysis) Identify resources required to conduct a specific research study

 EO 16.1.3 (Synthesis) Write a grant proposal for internal or external use that will secure the required resources for a specific research study.

 EO 16.1.4 (Comprehension) Discuss potential funding sources for a proposal for a specific research study.

 EO 16.1.5 (Application) Follow the plan set forth in the research proposal to conduct a research study.

Goal 17. Manage the operation of a drug information center.

TO 17.1 (Synthesis) Devise strategies for fiscally sound management of a drug information center.

TO 17.2 (Synthesis) Devise strategies for managing the human resources of a drug information center that result in an effective, efficient working environment.

 EO 17.2.1 (Comprehension) Describe the qualifications of personnel for a drug information center.

 EO 17.2.2 (Synthesis) Formulate recruitment strategies for a specific position in a drug information center.

 EO 17.2.3 (Synthesis) Develop an interviewing plan for the selection of potential employees.

 EO 17.2.4 (Synthesis) Design an employee evaluation system for a drug information center that is consistent with the organized health care setting's policies on human resource management.

 EO 17.2.5 (Application) Use the principles of progressive discipline to recommend disciplinary actions for drug information center employees.

 EO 17.2.6 (Synthesis) Design an orientation and training program for drug information center personnel that is consistent with the organized health care setting's human resources management policies.

TO 17.3 (Evaluation) Reassess the drug information needs of the organized health care setting on an ongoing basis.

TO 17.4 (Synthesis) Use information documented on services provided by the drug information center to generate reports that describe the center's productivity, quality, and patient outcomes.

TO 17.5 (Evaluation) Appraise a drug information center's continuous quality improvement program for effectiveness.

TO 17.6 (Synthesis) Design improvements in a drug information center's continuous quality improvement

program that will achieve the program's goals.

Goal 18. Integrate patient care skills with an advanced level of drug information skills for improving the pharmaceutical care of patients.

TO 18.1 (Synthesis) Consistently formulate solutions to a broad range of patient-specific drug information issues that maximize the achievement of pharmaceutical care outcomes.

TO 18.2 (Evaluation) Assess one's own practice for the successful integration of patient care and advanced drug information skills for improving direct patient care.

Goal 19. Maximize efficiency in performing drug information tasks through expert use of computer databases and electronic communications.

TO 19.1 (Evaluation) Appraise one's approach to performing drug information tasks for the most efficient use of computer technology.

 EO 19.1.1 (Evaluation) Determine the applicability of advanced computer technology such as networking and integrated software for performing drug information problem solving.

 EO 19.1.2 (Comprehension) Describe the characteristics of advanced sources of computerized drug information.

 EO 19.1.3 (Knowledge) State vendors of computerized drug information.

 EO 19.1.4 (Comprehension) Discuss emerging technology in information management.

Goal 20. Publish newsletters providing pertinent drug use information for health care professionals in the organized health care setting.

TO 20.1 (Synthesis) Create newsletters providing pertinent drug use information for health care professionals in the organized health care setting.

 EO 20.1.1 (Evaluation) Determine the appropriate format for a specific newsletter.

 EO 20.1.2 (Application) Use editing skills to edit material to fit a particular newsletter format.

 EO 20.1.3 (Application) Apply the principles of timeliness and inclusiveness in the circulation of a newsletter.

Goal 21. Serve as a resource for the lay press in matters related to pharmacy practice and drug therapy.

TO 21.1 (Synthesis) Formulate a considered response to inquiries from the lay press in matters related to pharmacy practice and drug therapy.

 EO 21.1.1 (Comprehension) Discuss the potential impact on the individual, the organized health care setting, and the public by responding to a specific inquiry from the lay press.

 EO 21.1.2 (Comprehension) Discuss the lack of control of the final disposition of information provided to the press.

 EO 21.1.3 (Synthesis) Construct a database in response to a lay press inquiry.

 EO 21.1.4 (Characterization) Give responses to interview questions that demonstrate public responsibility.

Goal 22. Demonstrate ethical conduct in all activities related to drug information practice.

TO 22.1 (Organization) Integrate consideration for ethics into each drug information response.

EO 22.1.1 (Application) Identify ethical issues in specific situations that involve the provision of drug information services.

EO 22.1.2 (Application) Identify the most appropriate party(ies) to make decisions regarding specific ethical issues with which the drug information specialist is confronted.

References

1. American Society of Hospital Pharmacists. ASHP accreditation standard for specialized pharmacy residency training. *Am J Hosp Pharm.* 1994; 51:2034–41.
2. American Society of Hospital Pharmacists. ASHP minimum standard for pharmacies in institutions. *Am J Hosp Pharm.* 1985; 42:372–5.
3. American Society of Hospital Pharmacists. ASHP accreditation standard for residency in pharmacy practice (with an emphasis on pharmaceutical care). *Am J Hosp Pharm.* 1992; 49:146–53.

Approved by the ASHP Board of Directors, April 27, 1994. Developed by a working group of ASHP drug information practitioners and the ASHP Commission on Credentialing. For currently existing programs, this revision of the accreditation standard takes effect April 27, 1995. Until that time, the current standard, which was approved September 24, 1982, is in force.

The bibliographic citation for this document is as follows: ASHP supplemental standard and learning objectives for residency training in drug information practice. In: Practice Standards of ASHP 1994–95. Hicks WE, ed. Bethesda, MD: American Society of Hospital Pharmacists; 1994.

ASHP Supplemental Standard and Learning Objectives for Residency Training in Geriatric Pharmacy Practice

Preamble

Definition. A residency in geriatric pharmacy practice is defined as a postgraduate program of organized training that meets the requirements set forth and approved by the American Society of Hospital Pharmacists. The "ASHP Accreditation Standard for Specialized Pharmacy Residency Training,"[1] together with this supplement, is the basic criteria used in evaluation of geriatric pharmacy residency training programs in institutions applying for accreditation by the American Society of Hospital Pharmacists.

A specialized residency in geriatric pharmacy practice should be organized and conducted to develop expert skills and competency in this area of pharmacy. Objectives of such training should include extensive experience in providing clinical pharmacy services to geriatric patients, as well as experience in the management of drug distribution systems in geriatric health-care facilities.

Qualifications of the Training Site. The parent facility for residency training in geriatric pharmacy practice shall be a long-term care facility or other organized health-care setting, including a hospital, which provides extensive geriatric services and which meets the requirements set forth in Standard I in the body of the "ASHP Accreditation Standard for Specialized Pharmacy Residency Training."[1] Ancillary facilities may be used as appropriate in pursuing the objectives for training outlined below.

The pharmacy practice setting in which the residency is based shall meet the requirements set forth in Standard II.[1] It shall have adequate facilities to carry out a broad scope of services.

Qualifications of the Preceptor. The area of specialization of the preceptor shall be geriatric pharmacy practice.

The following learning objectives shall be approved by the Commission on Credentialing following review annually by a committee appointed from the Special Interest Group on Geriatric Pharmacy Practice of the American Society of Hospital Pharmacists.

Learning Objectives

I. *General.* A resident who completes an accredited program in geriatric pharmacy practice shall be able to
   A. Identify the symptoms of a wide range of disease states commonly encountered in geriatric patients.
   B. Obtain a medication history and assess the patient's attitude toward compliance.
   C. Monitor drug therapy prospectively for potential drug-related problems (such as drug interactions) and recommend modifications in drug therapy, when appropriate, to circumvent these problems.
   D. Recommend, monitor, and assess pharma-

cotherapy for geriatric patients, taking into account those pathophysiologic factors that predispose the elderly to drug-related injury.
   E. Provide counseling on drug therapy for patients and families using appropriate communication principles.
   F. Participate in the education of students and professional staff members using appropriate teaching methods.
   G. Evaluate drug studies reported in the geriatric literature in terms of research design and validity of results.
   H. Communicate effectively with patients, staff, nurses, physicians, and professional peers.
   I. Evaluate an existing pharmacy service in a geriatric health-care facility in terms of federal and state regulations and ASHP minimum standards and propose any needed improvements.
   J. Apply drug audit criteria in evaluating the quality of drug therapy in a geriatric health-care facility.
   K. Demonstrate creativity by contribution to the practice of geriatric pharmacy and the science of gerontology.

II. *Specific.* In order to achieve these objectives, the resident must be able to speak with authority on the following subjects:
   A. *Demographics of aging.*
      1. Elderly population of the United States.
         a. Present.
         b. Predicted trends.
      2. Incidence of major disease states.
      3. Causes of death.
      4. Medication consumption patterns.
         a. Nonprescription.
         b. Prescription.
         c. Inpatient.
         d. Outpatient.
         e. Influencing factors.
   B. *Age-related alterations in physiology.*
      1. Sensory.
         a. Hearing.
         b. Vision.
         c. Touch.
         d. Taste.
      2. Physiologic.
         a. Weight.
         b. Fat/water ratio.
         c. Bone density.
      3. Renal.
         a. Renal physiology.
         b. Creatinine clearance.
      4. Hepatic.
         a. Hepatic physiology.
         b. Decreased hepatic function.
   C. *Common disease states in geriatrics.* For each disease state listed, the resident should be able to

discuss (1) clinical manifestations, (2) treatment, and (3) monitoring parameters.

1. Neurological disorders.
   a. Organic brain syndrome.
   b. Cerebrovascular accident (CVA).
   c. Seizure disorder secondary to CVA.
   d. Parkinson's disease.
2. Cardiovascular diseases.
   a. Arteriosclerotic heart disease.
   b. Hypertension.
   c. Congestive heart failure.
3. Musculoskeletal diseases.
   a. Osteoarthritis.
   b. Osteoporosis.
4. Gastrointestinal disorders.
   a. Constipation.
   b. Diarrhea.
5. Infections.
   a. Urinary tract infection.
   b. Upper respiratory infection.
   c. Skin.
6. Hematological diseases.
   a. Anemias (iron deficient, megaloblastic, blood loss, and chronic disease).
   b. Thrombosis and embolism.
7. Endocrine disorders.
   a. Diabetes mellitus.
   b. Hypothyroidism.
8. Decubitus ulcers.
9. Malignancies.

D. *Age-related pharmacokinetic alterations.*
1. Absorption.
   a. Gastric.
   b. Intestinal.
   c. Parenteral.
   d. Clinical significance.
2. Drug distribution.
   a. Volume of distribution.
   b. Fat/water ratio.
   c. Tissue permeability.
   d. Serum protein.
      i. Albumin.
      ii. Globulin.
   e. Clinical significance.
3. Drug clearance.
   a. Renal function.
   b. Hepatic function.
   c. Clinical significance.

E. *Age-related alterations of medication effect.*
1. General principles.
2. Alterations in response.
   a. Receptor sites.
   b. Idiosyncratic reactions.
   c. Decreased drug elimination.
3. Clinical implications.

F. *Social aspects of aging.*
1. Cultural.
2. Religious.
3. Ethnic.
4. Economic.

G. *Compliance to prescribed drug therapy of the elderly.*
1. Factors contributing to improper compliance.
   a. Memory loss.
   b. Sensory changes.

   c. Hearing disabilities.
   d. Learning disabilities.
2. Effect of safety closures on compliance.
3. Assessment of patient compliance and detection of improper compliance.
4. Compliance aids.
5. Pharmacist's role.

H. *Communication with the elderly.*
1. Age-related handicaps.
   a. Visual.
   b. Hearing.
   c. Mental.
2. Techniques.

I. *Medication education in the elderly.*
1. Need.
2. Techniques.
3. Resources.
4. Impact.

J. *Adverse reactions to medications in the elderly.*
1. Risk factors in the elderly.
2. Incidence.
3. Clinical manifestations.
4. Detection.
5. Management and prevention.
6. Pharmacist's role.

K. *Drug interactions in the elderly.*
1. General principles.
2. Drug–drug.
3. Drug–food.
4. Drug–alcohol.
5. Incidence.
   a. Outpatient.
   b. Inpatient.
6. Clinical significance.
7. Management and prevention.

L. *Drug abuse in the elderly.*
1. Alcohol.
2. Prescription drugs.
3. Nonprescription drugs.

M. *Considerations in terminal disease.*
1. Death and dying.
2. Hospice concept.
3. Drug therapy considerations.
   a. Analgesia.
   b. Long-term drug therapy.
   c. Marijuana.

N. *Considerations in chronic disease.*
1. Psychosocial aspects of chronic illness.
2. Long-term drug therapy.

O. *Use of unproven remedies by the elderly.*
1. "Fountain of youth" concept.
2. "Cures" for aging.
   a. Gerovital.
   b. Miscellaneous.

P. *Sexuality in the elderly.*
1. Sexual response patterns in the elderly.
2. Medication effect on sexuality.
   a. Gynecomastia.
   b. Impotence.
3. Treatment of sexual dysfunction.
   a. Androgenic hormones.
   b. Estrogenic hormones.
   c. Placebo.

Q. *Nutritional implications of aging.*
1. Nutritional requirements.

2. Nutritional patterns.
   a. Physical influence.
   b. Financial influence.
3. Food–drug interactions.

R. *Exercise programs for the elderly.*
   1. Exercise requirements.
   2. Exercise patterns.

S. *Health appliances and accessories used by the elderly.*
   1. Ostomy supplies.
   2. Canes.
   3. Walkers.
   4. Crutches.
   5. Miscellaneous.

T. *Implications of drug product selection for the elderly.*
   1. Explanation of generic medications.
   2. Pharmacist in drug product selection.
   3. How the elderly can save money with generic prescriptions.

U. *State and federal rules and regulations pertaining to the elderly.*
   1. Medicare and Medicaid conditions for participation.
      a. Skilled nursing facilities.
      b. Intermediate care facilities.
      c. Home health care.
   2. State laws and regulations.
      a. Skilled nursing facilities.
      b. Intermediate care facilities.
      c. Homes for the aged.
   3. National health insurance.
   4. Pharmacist's role in the development of regulations.

V. *Pharmacist's responsibility to the elderly.*
   1. Long-term care facilities.
      a. Skilled nursing facilities.
      b. Intermediate care facilities.
      c. Homes for the aged.
   2. Home health care.
   3. Community.
   4. Drug use review.
   5. Pharmaceutical services for the elderly.

Training

The resident's training schedule shall be directed toward the accomplishment of these objectives and shall include provisions for rotations or blocks of training in each of the following areas:

1. Inpatient care.
2. Ambulatory patient care.
3. Elective rotations (jointly agreed on by the resident and the preceptor).
4. Interdepartmental and extramural rotations wherever necessary to achieve the objectives.
5. Interdisciplinary continuing education activities such as attendance at clinical conferences, seminars, and grand rounds.

In addition, the schedule should make provision for the resident's participation in a clinical research project or for a self-directed investigation in an appropriate area. The preceptor should emphasize to the resident the need to report on research findings at professional meetings, and the preceptor should attempt to schedule the resident's participation in such forums to present this work.

When appropriate, the resident's training should be augmented with reading assignments and formal, didactic presentations by qualified health professionals.

Reference

1. American Society of Hospital Pharmacists. ASHP accreditation standard for specialized pharmacy residency training (with guide to interpretation). *Am J Hosp Pharm.* 1980; 37:1229–32.

Approved by the ASHP Board of Directors, September 24, 1982. The initial draft was based largely on work by William Simonson, Pharm.D., and Craig Caron, Pharm.D. Comments were sought from the SIG on Geriatric Pharmacy Practice, and the final document was approved by the Commission on Credentialing before submission to the Board of Directors.

The bibliographic citation for this document is as follows: American Society of Hospital Pharmacists. ASHP supplemental standard and learning objectives for residency training in geriatric pharmacy practice. *Am J Hosp Pharm.* 1982; 39:1972–4.

ASHP Accreditation Standard for Residency Training in Nuclear Pharmacy (with Guide to Interpretation)

Preamble

Definitions. A residency in nuclear pharmacy practice is defined as a postgraduate program of organized training that meets the requirements set forth and approved by the American Society of Hospital Pharmacists for training specialists in nuclear pharmacy practice.

The "Accreditation Standard for Residency Training in Nuclear Pharmacy" is the criterion used in evaluation of nuclear pharmacy residency training programs in institutions applying for accreditation by the American Society of Hospital Pharmacists. It is the Society's intent that one who completes an accredited residency in nuclear pharmacy practice will possess competencies that meet, and exceed to a considerable degree, those set forth in the "Nuclear Pharmacy Practice Standards."[1]

The interpretive narrative following each element of the Standard is intended to illustrate how the Standard will be interpreted by the accreditation site surveyors and the Society's Commission on Credentialing in evaluation of residency programs. The companion document to the Standard, the "ASHP Statement on Accreditation of Pharmacy Residencies,"[2] sets forth the policies governing the accreditation program and describes the procedures to be followed in applying for accreditation of pharmacy residency programs.

Objectives. The objectives for residency training in nuclear pharmacy are to ensure a continuing supply of well-qualified nuclear pharmacy specialists and to prepare practitioners for careers in this specialty who can (1) apply radiopharmaceutical theory in a practice or research-oriented setting with respect to both drug products and their clinical applications; (2) function effectively with nuclear medicine physicians, nuclear medicine technologists, radiation safety personnel, and other nuclear pharmacists; (3) apply the principles of radiation safety; (4) manage a nuclear pharmacy unit; and (5) contribute to the total knowledge in nuclear pharmacy and advance the level of nuclear pharmacy practice.

Application of the Standard. A fundamental principle of this Standard is that nuclear pharmacy residency programs are structured to ensure the achievement of certain predetermined competencies. While the Standard requires a minimum of 2000 hours training time for the residency, there is no set way in which this time is to be allotted. Standard V, below, specifies those areas in which the resident's competence must be developed, and these are the principal determinants by which programs are structured. Based on the resident's entering level of knowledge and skills, the training program may well vary in structure and in areas of emphasis for each resident.

Standard I. Qualifications of the Training Hospital

A. Nuclear pharmacy residency training programs shall be oriented to institutional practice and shall be based, in large part, in a hospital. The hospital shall be accredited by the Joint Commission on Accreditation of Hospitals or the American Osteopathic Association. Further, the hospital shall operate an organized nuclear medicine department and be licensed by the Environmental Protection Agency or the Nuclear Regulatory Commission and other appropriate agencies for all categories of radioactive byproduct materials used in humans.

B. Two or more institutions may join together to provide nuclear pharmacy residency training, provided that each institution meets the intent of this Standard.

C. Nuclear pharmacy residencies shall be conducted only in those institutions in which the educational benefits to the resident are considered of paramount importance in relation to the service benefits which the institution may obtain from the resident.

D. The institution must provide a wide range of nuclear medicine studies.

E. The institution shall be staffed with at least one board-certified nuclear medicine physician and one nuclear medicine technologist. Where two or more institutions are used as training sites, at least half of the participating institutions shall be staffed by at least one board-certified nuclear medicine physician and one board-certified nuclear medicine technologist.

Interpretation

I-A. Only those hospitals whose governing bodies, personnel, and professional staffs have collaborated to seek excellence, which have accepted outside appraisal, and which have demonstrated substantial conformance with professionally developed and nationally applied criteria should serve as training facilities for pharmacy residents. The standards of the Joint Commission on Accreditation of Hospitals[3] or the accreditation requirements of the American Osteopathic Association[4] will serve as the basic guides in evaluating the qualifications of the hospital.

Ancillary training sites may also be used in nuclear pharmacy training programs (e.g., centralized nuclear pharmacy facilities serving two or more medical centers), provided that such sites meet the requirements of Standard II of this document.

I-B. Application for accreditation of a multiple site nuclear pharmacy residency program must be submitted in the name of one corporate entity, which may be, for example, one of the participating institutions or an academic health science center to which one or more of the participating institutions belong.

I-C. A residency training program should provide experience in the technological aspects of nuclear pharmacy practice, in all aspects of radioactive drug use control in the hospital, in the clinical application of such drugs in the diagnosis and treatment of patients, and in the use of radionuclides as tracers in research. Participation by the resident in the activities of the nuclear pharmacy lends understanding, confidence, and purpose to his academically attained professional background. A significant portion of this participation must, of necessity, involve on-the-job training, since only through actual performance of some activities can the resident be expected to gain an appreciation and an understanding of the knowledge and skills required to carry out these activities. Through actual experience, the resident learns how these activities interrelate and are best coordinated with other activities and functions throughout the nuclear pharmacy unit and the nuclear medicine department.

The greater emphasis in residency training, however, should be concentrated on developing within the resident the ability to coordinate activities and conceptualize, integrate, and transform accumulated experiences and knowledge into improved nuclear pharmacy services. Furthermore, in order to guarantee that the educational benefits to the resident are of paramount importance when compared with any service benefits that may accrue to the institution, it shall be demonstrable that the nuclear pharmacy unit can capably carry out all of its service obligations in the absence of residents.

I-D. It is important that the nuclear pharmacy resident have a broad spectrum of experience in nuclear diagnostic and therapeutic studies. The training site must, therefore, provide experience in both routine and investigational nuclear medicine procedures involving various organ systems.

I-E. Since the nuclear pharmacist functions in an interdisciplinary environment, it is important that the nuclear pharmacy resident have regular professional contact with highly qualified specialists in related disciplines. Board certification in nuclear medicine, nuclear medicine science, and nuclear medicine technology implies special expertise in each of these respective areas.

Standard II. Qualifications of the Nuclear Pharmacy Service

A. The nuclear pharmacy service shall be organized in accordance with the principles of good management under the immediate supervision of a legally qualified pharmacist. It shall have sufficient staff, both professional and supportive, to carry out a broad scope of radiopharmaceutical services and shall comply (where applicable) with all federal, state, and local laws, codes, statutes, and regulations.

B. The nuclear pharmacy shall have physical facilities that are adequate to permit activities over a broad range of services including, but not limited to, the following professional and administrative areas:

1. Nuclear pharmacy administration.
2. Radiopharmaceutical distribution and inventory control.
3. Technology and quality control.
4. Radiotracer development and evaluation.
5. Radiopharmaceutical chemistry and tracer methodology.
6. Radiological health activities.
7. Clinical services.

It is necessary that a regular and continuing experience be provided in these activities, and it is not sufficient

to create artificial situations for residents to obtain this experience. If any of the designated activities or divisions of pharmaceutical practice are not available in the parent training site, arrangements shall be made with another nuclear pharmacy unit (or other facility acceptable to the American Society of Hospital Pharmacists) to provide the necessary experience.

C. The director of the nuclear pharmacy unit shall have the responsibility and the authority to carry out a broad scope of radiopharmaceutical services.

Interpretation

II-A. There should be an organizational chart for the nuclear pharmacy unit which illustrates the chain of authority and responsibility for personnel, depicts what functions the nuclear pharmacy service presumes to carry out, and shows the relationship between the nuclear pharmacy unit director, the director of the hospital pharmacy, and the director of nuclear medicine. Objectives should be clearly defined in written statements, and all staff members should be familiar with the intent and substance of the objectives, which should be in accord with the established objectives of the hospital pharmacy and the nuclear medicine department.

There should be written procedures for all routine transactions, functions, and operations in the nuclear pharmacy unit, and they should be kept current. Orientation of all new personnel should include a review of the scope and use of the policy and procedure manual. All personnel in the nuclear pharmacy unit should be thoroughly familiar with the procedures applicable to their respective areas of responsibility and should comply with them.

The professional personnel complement should be adequate to carry out the stated objectives for the nuclear pharmacy service. Professional staff members should be graduates of colleges of pharmacy accredited by the American Council on Pharmaceutical Education and should have received special postgraduate training or experience in nuclear pharmacy. They should be currently licensed to practice in the state in which the nuclear pharmacy unit operates. They should demonstrate their interest in maintaining professional competence by attending continuing education programs, reading the professional literature, and participating in their local, state, and national professional organizations.

II-B. A broad scope of services is essential to a well-rounded residency program. The ability of the hospital to provide an appropriate range of experiences for the nuclear pharmacy resident is determined in large part by the ability of the nuclear medicine department and the nuclear pharmacy service to provide well-operated, patient-oriented service programs in each of the specified areas of professional practice. It is not acceptable to synthesize training experiences to substitute for nonexistent service programs. Neither is it acceptable to substitute any academic college courses for experience in service programs, although didactic courses may be taken simultaneously with the experiential training. Required experience may be obtained in another nuclear pharmacy unit, but a written protocol for this training experience must be approved by the

American Society of Hospital Pharmacists. The Society reserves the right to request a survey of such sites.

Nuclear pharmacy administration. The functions performed in nuclear pharmacy administration include directing, organizing, staffing, planning, budgeting, controlling, coordinating, supervising, and reporting. Of primary importance is the existence of, and compliance with, formalized policies and procedures for administrative activities such as purchasing and inventory control, cost accounting, budgeting, personnel selection and management, policy and procedures development, handling correspondence, indexing and filing, control of regulated radiopharmaceuticals and supplies, interdepartmental and interinstitutional relationships, and periodic reporting to appropriate administrative agencies.

Radiopharmaceutical distribution and inventory control. The drug distribution system should provide for the preparation of radiopharmaceuticals on an around the clock basis. Twenty-four-hour staffing for the nuclear pharmacy (i.e., on-call services after normal working hours) is rapidly becoming a standard of practice.

The nuclear pharmacy should have an organized system of radiopharmaceutical and radioisotope inventory control. In addition, all nuclear pharmacists should be familiar with and comply with all institutional, local, county, state, and federal regulations concerning the transportation, packaging, labeling, and disposal of radioactive materials.

Technology and quality control. The primary purposes of these service activities are

1. To provide a product in a special dosage form, package size, or type when not commercially available.
2. To control the quality of all drugs manufactured, extemporaneously compounded, packaged, repackaged, or labeled within the nuclear pharmacy.
3. To monitor the performance of all staff members involved in product manipulation (e.g., aseptic technique).
4. To control the manufacture, storage, and distribution of investigational radiopharmaceuticals.
5. To perform comparative evaluation of the pharmaceutical quality of radiopharmaceutical products under consideration for eventual use by the nuclear pharmacy.
6. To provide assurance of radionuclidic, radiochemical, and pharmaceutical purity of all radiopharmaceuticals.

The pharmacy must have adequate personnel, space, and facilities to carry out these activities. When certain facilities (such as autoclaves) are not available, arrangements may be made with other departments to use theirs.

Radiotracer development and evaluation. The nuclear pharmacy unit must regularly participate in basic or clinical research projects related to the development of new or modified radiotracer drugs. It is important, therefore, that the staff be familiar with all aspects of new drug development, from the original concept of drug use to radiolabeling procedures and writing of IND applications. Further, the nuclear pharmacy unit must routinely coordinate clinical investiga-

tion procedures to determine the safety, sensitivity, specificity, accuracy, and predictive diagnostic values of the radioactive drugs involved in such studies. Associated with such procedures are the following: developing patient consent forms, securing approval from local human experimentation committees and radiation safety groups, planning of study protocols and data collection techniques, and contacting potential clinical investigators, among others. The nuclear pharmacy unit must also participate in postmarketing surveillance of new radiotracers.

Radiopharmaceutical chemistry and tracer methodology. In addition to services offered through provision of the usual daily radiopharmaceutical preparations and the technology and quality control activities applied to those functions, circumstances may exist where a more indepth evaluation of a radiopharmaceutical product may be necessary.

Additionally, a physician or researcher may require the formulation or synthesis of a special dosage form for administration to animals or patients. These services require highly specialized skills in radiopharmaceutical chemistry and tracer methodology. The primary activities related to this service area are

1. Preparation of "custom" radiochemical and radiopharmaceutical formulations, such as radioiodinated proteins and technetium labeling kits.
2. Determination of yields and purity of radiopharmaceutical products utilizing chromatographic methods or other separations and analytical techniques.
3. Calculation of the specific activity and specific concentration of radioactive solutions.
4. Performance of animal and human biodistribution tracer methodology studies on "custom" or pilot formulations for determination of pharmacologic and kinetic properties of these preparations, such as volumes of distribution, blood clearance rates, compartmental localization, and routes and rates of excretion from the body, as well as for calculation of radiation dosimetry.
5. Performance of animal and human biodistribution studies on commonly used radiopharmaceuticals to help identify causes for inappropriate distributions that may be seen clinically.
6. Evaluation of radionuclidic and radiochemical purity of precursors required for the manufacture of new radiopharmaceuticals.
7. Evaluation of sterility and pyrogenicity of radiopharmaceuticals after formulation (or in the investigation of a febrile patient reaction).
8. Evaluation of the shelf life of radiopharmaceutical products in storage (and after preparation) using radiochemical and biological tracer methodologies.

Radiological health activities. Since nuclear pharmacy personnel handle radioactive materials on a daily basis, policies must be developed and rigidly followed to insure their personal health and safety. Although in some environments it is the radiation safety officer who sets and enforces such policy, nuclear pharmacists should be responsible for supervision of ancillary personnel, visitors, and others in their purview. Professional attitudes are of paramount importance when considering radiation safety procedures. All nuclear pharmacy personnel should be thoroughly familiar with radiation protection policies, safety equipment, and all regulations (both internal and external) relating to this area. Posting and monitoring devices should be adequate to cover all possible circumstances involving storage, dispensing, quality control, or research functions. Appropriate procedures should be established for decontamination of personnel and equipment should spillage of radioactivity occur.

In some settings, nuclear pharmacists administer therapeutic agents such as radioactive iodine. In such cases, the pharmacist must observe all policies respecting his and the patient's safety.

Clinical services. Although most, if not all, of the service functions of the nuclear pharmacy have clinical components associated with them, clinical services are taken to be, for the purpose of this document, those functions identified in the following list:

1. Provision of oral and/or written consultations in such areas as unanticipated or illogical biodistribution of radiotracers, radiopharmaceutical formulation problems, interpretation of radiometrically determined drug serum levels, timely and appropriate radioactive drug use and administration, radiopharmaceutical kinetics, special patient preparation for nuclear medicine studies, and scheduling problems with nuclear medicine procedures and other diagnostic tests.

2. Monitoring the safety and efficacy of an individual patient's drug regimen using radiometric methods (e.g., early detection of doxorubicin cardiotoxicity via gated blood pool imaging and left ventricular ejection fraction determination).

3. Patient education and counseling on the use of radiopharmaceuticals in nuclear medicine procedures.

4. Initiation of and participation in clinical investigations in collaboration with appropriate staff members of affiliated hospitals and clinics (e.g., development of specialized radiometric techniques for evaluating pharmacologic effects and pharmacokinetics of drugs and investigation of new diagnostic radiopharmaceuticals).

5. Detection and reporting of adverse reactions to radiopharmaceuticals.

6. Conducting radiopharmaceutical use reviews (prospective and retrospective).

7. Participation in the education of medical, pharmacy, and nursing personnel.

8. Participation in management of medical diagnostic emergencies.

9. Preparation of patient individualized radiopharmaceuticals, and followup on the diagnostic accuracy and usefulness of these radiotracers.

10. Administration of therapeutic radiopharmaceuticals when this service is not precluded by specific local statutes.

11. The theoretical and practical use of radioassays in medicine.

In evaluating clinical service activities, the American Society of Hospital Pharmacists considers only those services performed by staff members and only those services that are continuously performed even in the absence of students and residents. Although it is not expected that every nuclear pharmacy in which a

residency program is conducted will necessarily be involved in each of the activities listed above, there must be a comprehensive program of clinical services. A nuclear pharmacy unit seeking to maintain an accredited residency program should provide for extensive patient contact and for strong and continuing interaction with the medical staff.

It is recognized that the degree of direct patient contact a nuclear pharmacist may have will vary from one practice site to another. In some instances, the nuclear pharmacist may serve as a consultant to the nuclear medicine physician who may, in turn, be a consultant to a primary care physician. Even so, it is often necessary for the nuclear pharmacist to make direct contact with the patient or primary care physician or both in order to complete certain consultation activities, e.g., to determine the reason for an alteration in radiopharmaceutical biodistribution or to determine the probability that a reported adverse reaction was caused by the administration of a radiopharmaceutical. Direct patient contact may also occur during drug history interviews taken prior to radiopharmaceutical administration, while explaining the procedures involved in a new radiotracer study when obtaining informed patient consent, in the process of monitoring patients' vital signs for the purpose of collecting data on the acute effects of investigational radiopharmaceuticals, and during the administration of therapeutic radiopharmaceuticals.

The provision of clinical services should be a stated objective of the nuclear pharmacy and should be addressed in the departmental policies and procedures, in position descriptions for the professional staff, and in the nuclear pharmacy director's management reports. Further, the director should have some system for evaluating the quality of clinical services provided by his staff.

II-C. Because of his overall responsibility for the residency program, the nuclear pharmacy director must have a wide latitude of freedom to coordinate and integrate the service and training functions. This is only possible if he has total responsibility and authority as administrative head to manage the nuclear pharmacy unit and coordinate its services and functions with those in the nuclear medicine department. Nothing in this Standard is designed to deny the authority of the physician to control his laboratory environment in cases where such facilities may be used in the nuclear pharmacy training program.

Standard III. Qualifications of the Residency Director and Preceptors

A. The director of the nuclear pharmacy service shall be the overall director of the residency training program and shall be subject to general administrative control and guidance by the director of pharmacy services, college dean, institutional director, or appropriate executive officer.

B. The residency director shall be a pharmacist, shall have completed a nuclear pharmacy residency accredited by the ASHP, and shall have had 2 years of administrative and clinical experience; or, if lacking a residency, shall have 5 years of experience in a nuclear pharmacy, a substantial part of which should have been of an administrative nature.

C. The residency director shall have demonstrated superior capabilities in the operation of a nuclear pharmacy service and shall have made significant contributions to the development or improvement of nuclear pharmacy practice.

D. The residency director shall have considerable latitude in delegating preceptorial responsibilities to the staff. Each individual designated as a preceptor must have demonstrated outstanding strengths in one or more areas of nuclear pharmacy practice. The residency director, however, is ultimately accountable for the overall quality of the residency training program.

E. There shall be at least one preceptor employed for each resident in the program.

F. The residency director shall be an active member of the American Society of Hospital Pharmacists. Other designated preceptors should also be members of the Society.

Interpretation

III-A. Nuclear pharmacy residency training programs that conform to the intent of this Accreditation Standard are designed to train nuclear pharmacy practitioners who are competent to provide a wide range of professional services, as well as administrative support and direction to others. Only the director of the nuclear pharmacy service is in a position to facilitate training in the total scope of operations of the unit. Further, the nuclear pharmacy director sets the overall tone of the training program. He does so by the personal philosophy he professes, by what he stands for, by the contributions he makes to his profession, and by his sense of values.

Since nuclear pharmacy residency programs may be based partly in sites other than hospitals (e.g., college of pharmacy or independent centralized facilities), they are subject to supervisory control by a broad range of administrators.

III-B. Administrative experience is interpreted to mean experience as a nuclear pharmacy head (director or manager) or as an assistant nuclear pharmacy head with responsibilities largely commensurate with those of the nuclear pharmacy director. Experience as a staff nuclear pharmacist with only partial or minimal supervisory responsibilities is not acceptable as administrative experience for purposes of meeting this requirement.

This section is not intended to be in conflict with, nor is it intended to preempt, nuclear pharmacy residency programs located in states where prior restrictions exist concerning the qualifications of the nuclear pharmacy director.

III-C. The following will be taken as evidence that the residency director meets the intent of this part of the Standard: publications in scientific and professional literature, attendance at and participation in continuing education programs, scholarly presentations to his peers, and interprofessional involvement with others in the nuclear medicine community.

III-D. Each preceptor should meet essentially the same qualifications as set forth in III-C.

III-E. The ratio of one preceptor to every resident is pre-scribed to assure that the requisite number of hours for supervision and tutorial time can be effectively met and to avoid exploitation of the resident.

Standard IV. Qualifications and Selection of the Applicant

A. The applicant should be a graduate of a school of pharmacy accredited by the American Council on Pharmaceutical Education.

B. The applicant should have a thorough grounding in patient-oriented (clinical) pharmacy services; further, the applicant should demonstrate some degree of knowledge and skills in nuclear pharmacy practice.

C. The applicant should be recommended by his college faculty, previous employers, or professional colleagues.

D. The applicant should be a member of the American Society of Hospital Pharmacists or, if not, he should become a member of the Society if accepted as a resident.

E. Final approval of the qualifications of the applicant and his acceptance shall be the responsibility of the nuclear pharmacy service director.

Interpretation

IV-A. It is permissible to admit graduates of pharmacy schools located outside the United States to accredited residency programs if other qualified residents are concurrently in training.

IV-B. Residency training in nuclear pharmacy practice is predicated on prior clerkship and externship training. For this reason, the entering resident will be expected to have completed a comprehensive clerkship and externship program, such as is required in contemporary doctor of pharmacy curricula, or have had sufficient cumulative life experience to equal this entrance requirement. Specifically, the resident should demonstrate a thorough familiarity with methods of patient workup, chart review, and other techniques which may be useful in assessing the ways in which different patients may respond to the administration of radiopharmaceutical agents. Prior work experience in nuclear pharmacy is also desirable.

It is the program director's responsibility to assess applicants' baseline knowledge and skills to ascertain that they qualify for admission.

IV-C. It is advisable also to conduct a personal interview with each qualified applicant before making final decisions.

IV-D. The resident has an obligation to his profession and himself to support his professional organizations. Membership and active participation in these organizations not only demonstrate a favorable attitude toward his profession but are most effective in broadening his career horizons by fostering a better understanding of the profession in society and the profession's obligations to the public it serves.

IV-E. Since residents become, in effect, members of the nuclear pharmacy staff, the director of the nuclear pharmacy service must have authority to accept or reject any applicant.

Standard V. Residency Training Program

A. Objectives for the residency program shall be set out in writing and shall be provided to each resident at the beginning of his program. The objectives shall relate both to the administrative and professional practice skills required in contemporary good nuclear pharmacy practice and shall describe the terminal competencies to be striven for in the residency program. Objectives for training in each of the following areas shall be included:

1. Nuclear pharmacy administration.
2. Radiopharmaceutical distribution and inventory control.
3. Technology and quality control.
4. Radiotracer development and evaluation.
5. Radiopharmaceutical chemistry and tracer methodology.
6. Radiological health activities.
7. Clinical services.
8. Educational experience and activities.
9. Research methodology.

B. Each resident's activities shall be scheduled in advance and shall be planned to make possible the attainment of the predetermined objectives. The overall schedule shall consist of a minimum of 2000 hours of training (residency-related) time, extending over a period of no less than 12 months.

C. Each resident shall maintain a record of his training activities which clearly delineates the scope and period of training. The residency director shall keep such records on file for review by the ASHP accreditation survey team.

D. Provision shall be made for formalized and regularly scheduled evaluation of the resident's achievement in terms of the objectives previously established.

Interpretation

V-A. The specific training activities and experiences in which the resident will participate (under each of the nine training areas listed) are subject to considerable variation because of the differences existing among facilities, training programs, residency directors, and residents. Furthermore, there are no clear lines of distinction among the nine major training areas with regard to the discrete activities that each encompasses. For the purpose of this Accreditation Standard, however, each of these areas is taken to include the specific training activities outlined below. The residency director should use these lists of activities as guidelines in developing training objectives for his program. The objectives should specify the attitudes, skills, and knowledge the resident should be expected to gain from each activity. These objectives then serve as guides for the residency director and other persons responsible for the resident's training in developing and supervising training experiences and in evaluating achievement.

Since this Accreditation Standard stresses outcomes more than the process by which those outcomes are achieved, the residency director should assess the entering resident's baseline knowledge and skills in each of the nine major areas of residency training as set forth above. This will eliminate unnecessary repetition of training which the resident may have previously received.

Once the residency director has satisfied himself that a resident has achieved the predetermined minimum level of competence in each of the areas, he may arrange for that resident to concentrate, during the time remaining in his program, on either administrative affairs, professional practice, or research methods. If an area of emphasis is to be pursued, an understanding on this point should be agreed on in advance by the residency director and the resident, and the predetermined objectives for training should identify the additional competencies to be achieved in the area of emphasis, above and beyond that expected of another resident whose program does not concentrate on that area.

Nuclear pharmacy administration. The objectives of the resident's training in nuclear pharmacy management are to orient him not only to the function and concepts of nuclear pharmacy management but also to the nuclear pharmacy director's philosophy of total service and to increase his knowledge, refine his skills, mold his attitudes, and develop his problem-solving abilities relating to personnel management, organization management, communications, and management of resources. The resident must learn to make judgments, set priorities, and assume responsibilities. The residency director must serve as the principal preceptor in this area of training.

The resident should receive orientation, instruction, and experience leading to competence in, but not restricted to, the following specific areas and activities:

1. Organization of the nuclear pharmacy.
2. Administrative and professional policies.
3. Development and maintenance of the policy and procedure manual.
4. Interdepartmental administrative activities (including orientation).
5. Hospital, college, or corporate staff meetings and administrative conferences (if appropriate).
6. Hospital committees (pharmacy and therapeutics committee, human use committee, safety committee, etc.).
7. Nuclear pharmacy staff meetings.
8. Intradepartmental communications.
9. Local, state, and federal laws and regulations (including Nuclear Regulatory Commission or its equivalent in agreement states, Radiation Safety, boards of pharmacy, Department of Transportation, and Environmental Protection Agency).
10. Personnel management and training.
11. Accounting and bookkeeping.
12. Departmental budgeting.
13. Contract services.
14. Departmental records and reports.
15. Office procedures (filing, handling correspondence, etc.).
16. Professional organization participation.
17. Safety practices (general and radiation safety).
18. Space and facilities planning.
19. Departmental quality assurance.
20. Evaluation of personnel dosimetry reports.
21. Completion and submission of documents re-

lated to licensure to local, state, and federal agencies.

Radiopharmaceutical distribution and inventory control. The objectives for the resident's training in this area are to develop his abilities in all aspects of drug use control in the nuclear pharmacy and to develop his philosophy about the responsibilities of the pharmacist in providing optimal radiopharmaceutical products for patient administration. The resident should receive orientation, instruction, and experience leading to competence in, but not restricted to, the following areas and activities:

1. Nuclear pharmacy service policies and procedures.
2. Standards, laws, and regulations.
3. Radiopharmaceutical product selection (in conjunction with other members of the nuclear medicine community).
4. Physicians' orders and their transmission (onto prescriptions, labels, etc.).
5. Containers and labeling.
6. Radiopharmaceutical literature.
7. Logistics of drug distribution/transportation.
8. Preparation of radiopharmaceuticals and labeling kits.
9. Ancillary supplies.
10. Investigational radiopharmaceuticals.
11. "After-hours" service.
12. Use of dose calibrators and other scintillation detection equipment.
13. Medication error reporting.
14. Electronic data processing applications.
15. Reporting of radiopharmaceutical problems relating to altered biodistribution.
16. Radiopharmaceutical recalls/obsolescence.
17. Radiopharmaceutical pricing and/or patient charges.
18. Radiopharmaceutical and supply procurement and inventory control.
19. Vehicle and equipment maintenance.
20. Nuclear pharmacy, transport vehicle, and packaging wipe tests and monitoring procedures.

Technology and quality control activities. The major objectives for the resident's training in this area are to enable him to procure or produce the highest quality radiopharmaceutical products and supplies for administration to patients, to protect the quality of these products until they are administered, and to protect the patient from receiving a mislabeled, misbranded, adulterated, or suboptimal drug. This area of training will develop or reinforce the resident's understanding of the physical, radiochemical, and compounding principles that influence dosage forms and govern their selection. The resident will also become familiar with factors affecting drug product stability (i.e., radiochemical purity) and the systems used to minimize compounding, packaging, and labeling errors.

Note: The pharmacist's undergraduate training in such areas as physical pharmacy, technology, pharmacology, medicinal chemistry, and biopharmaceutics may go a long way toward achieving those objectives stated above. The residency director should not overlook the need, however, to assess the resident's latent knowledge and skills in these areas and to schedule training activities as appropriate to complement the resident's baseline abilities. The director should obviously give considerable attention to the resident's ability to compound prescriptions for intravenous administration and other dosage forms requiring aseptic technique. The resident should receive orientation, instruction, and experience leading to competence in at least the following areas and activities:

1. Product formulation principles and theory.
2. Product procurement specifications.
3. Good manufacturing practices.
4. Use and operation of compounding, packaging, and radiolabeling procedures.
5. Packaging and labeling.
6. Storage and stability considerations.
7. Quality control procedures.
8. Records and reports.

Furthermore, the resident should receive orientation, instruction, and experience leading to competence in the following activities and areas relating specifically to sterile and/or radioactive products:

9. Principles and methods of sterilization.
10. Aseptic techniques and procedures.
11. Use and limitations of the laminar airflow hood.
12. Formulation, production, and quality control of injectables.
13. Radiochemical and radionuclidic purity testing, including use of scintillation detection equipment of these procedures.
14. Storage problems for sterile products.
15. Tonicity and pH adjustments and controls.
16. Radioactive/sterile syringe packaging.
17. Reconstitution of injectables.
18. Sterility and pyrogenicity testing.
19. Standards, laws, and regulations.
20. Space, equipment, and facilities planning.

Radiotracer development and evaluation. The objectives for training in this area are to familiarize the resident with preclinical and clinical drug trials. Residents will have an opportunity to be involved in actual investigational new drug research or data analysis or both. In addition, the resident will have some practice in completing application forms for drug development projects.

The resident's training should include, but not be limited to, the following areas:

1. Drug literature search/evaluation.
2. Design of preclinical/clinical trials.
3. Development of data collection forms.
4. Contacting clinicians for patient trials.
5. Design of patient consent forms.
6. Explanations of procedures to patients.
7. Analysis of data/scan results.
8. Writing of IND/NDA applications and revisions.
9. Calculation of sensitivity, specificity, accuracy, and predictive diagnostic values of nuclear medicine procedures.
10. Biodistribution studies.
11. Testing of radionuclidic and radiochemical purity, pyrogenicity, and sterility.
12. Acute, subacute, and chronic toxicity studies.
13. Calculating radiation dosimetry.

Radiopharmaceutical chemistry. The objectives for training in this area are to provide the resident with an understanding of the basic principles of radiochemistry as applied to the preparation and testing of radiopharmaceuticals. Included in this body of knowledge are the reactor and accelerator methods of production of radionuclides; the use of radionuclide generators, including their operation kinetics; the various methods of separation of isotopes; and the principles of chemistry that relate to the preparation of radiopharmaceuticals.

Since radiopharmaceuticals are used primarily for diagnostic purposes, it is essential that the resident understand the basic concepts of tracer methodology as they are applied to the clinical setting.

The resident should receive orientation, instruction, and experience leading to competence in, but not limited to, the following areas:

1. The radiochemistry of elements used in the production of radiopharmaceuticals.
2. The production of radionuclides.
3. Chromatography.
4. Radionuclide generators.
5. Radioactive decay equations.
6. Formulation of radiopharmaceutical products.
7. Chemistry of radiopharmaceutical production.

Radiological health activities. The objectives of training in this area are to instill in the resident the importance of radiological health concerns as they pertain to nuclear pharmacists and to provide a framework of training and experience that is adequate to satisfy state and federal licensing requirements.

The resident should receive orientation, instruction, and experience leading to competence in, but not limited to, the following areas:

1. Radiation biology, including factors affecting acute and delayed radiation injury, and the effects of radiation on cells (somatic and genetic).
2. Radiation safety precautions, including use of radiation monitoring equipment, methods for reduction of radiation exposure, wipe testing and surveying of packages, etc.
3. Rules and regulations concerning handling, transportation, and disposal of radioactive materials (i.e., Department of Transportation and Nuclear Regulatory Commission).
4. Radioactive decontamination procedures.
5. Radiation dosimetry.
6. Administration of therapeutic radiopharmaceuticals (safety aspects).
7. Considerations for special patient needs (e.g., in pediatric patients or pregnant patients).
8. Acceptable levels of radiation exposure for radiation workers.

Clinical services. The objectives for training in clinical services are to strengthen and reinforce the diagnostic and therapeutic knowledge that the resident should have brought to the residency as a result of prior education and training. It is expected that the resident will gain additional diagnostic and therapeutic knowledge and develop abilities in the clinical application of radioactive and nonradioactive drugs in patient management. Central to this area of the resident's training is the evaluation of radiotracer methodologies in relation to the special needs of individual patients.

The resident should receive orientation, instruction, and experience leading to competence in, but not limited to, the following areas and activities:

1. Patient medication histories.
2. Monitoring drug therapy using radiometric and nonradiometric methods.
3. Patient counseling and education.
4. Participation in management of medical emergencies, especially those requiring rapid diagnostic information.
5. Clinical trials with investigational radiopharmaceuticals.
6. Adverse drug reaction and drug problem identification/reporting.
7. Routine consultation with nuclear medicine personnel and primary care physicians.
8. Radiopharmaceutical use review.
9. Interdisciplinary educational activities.
10. "Troubleshooting" scans with altered biodistribution or biorouting of radiotracers due to iatrogenic causes, technical or drug formulation problems, or unanticipated pathophysiologic patient variability.
11. Interpretation of drug serum levels.
12. Predictive values from diagnostic tests, including radioassays.
13. Diagnostic test interferences and scheduling problems with nuclear medicine studies.
14. Administration of therapeutic radiopharmaceuticals.
15. Timeliness and appropriateness of nuclear medicine studies and other diagnostic modalities.
16. Radiopharmaceutical drug literature evaluation and utilization.
17. Use of radiotracer techniques to assist physicians and researchers.
18. Use of imaging devices and data acquisition and analysis equipment (computers) in diagnostic radiotracer studies.
19. Special patient preparation for nuclear medicine procedures.
20. Radiopharmaceutical kinetics.
21. Design and use of patient education materials (e.g., information about the nuclear medicine studies).

Educational experience and activities. The objectives of training in this area are to convey to the resident the attitude that it is his professional responsibility to maintain his competence through a planned program of self- and continuing education. An important corollary objective is for the resident to develop communication and teaching skills. The resident's training in this area should include, but not be limited to, the following:

1. Lecture and conference or case study topics presented by the residency director and other preceptors.
2. Review (on a continual basis) of current and past literature related to radiopharmacy practice.
3. Review of principles of education (e.g., learning objectives, lesson plans, and evaluation instruments).
4. Formal and informal presentations to various groups of students and professionals.
5. Conferences with residency director on a weekly basis for discussion and counsel (if more than one resident in program, a weekly group conference between the residency director and resi-

dents may be sufficient).

6. Attendance at and participation in seminars and continuing education programs on a local, state, regional, and national basis.

7. Development of a personal philosophy and strategy for lifelong continuing education.

Research methodology. The objectives of training in this area are to provide the resident with important basic skills to permit the design, implementation, and evaluation of research objectives that are not necessarily product or clinically oriented but that are oriented toward the gathering of experimental data by means other than those discussed above. This training shall include, but not be limited to, the following areas:

1. Statistics.
2. Liquid scintillation counting.
3. Autoradiography.
4. Tracer and indicator-dilution techniques.

V-B. The minimum total training hours and training period may be exceeded without limit but not reduced.

It is important that a schedule of activities for the residency training program be planned before the resident's arrival. The schedule should be written in sufficient detail to give the resident a clear understanding of each assignment and activity. The schedule must reflect the predetermined learning objectives and make possible their achievement. In fact, it may be desirable to integrate the learning objectives and the training schedule into one syllabus.

It is recognized that detailed planning of time schedules in advance is at best difficult and, frequently, almost impossible. The important aspect of this element of the Standard is not the existence of a detailed time (clock or calendar) schedule but rather that careful and conscientious planning goes into the development of the residency training program in advance of its initiation. The schedule may be thought of as the tool with which the objectives can be achieved and which aids in insuring that no objective is overlooked.

V-C. It is important that the resident maintain sufficient documentation of his training activities so that the residency director and other preceptor(s) can monitor his progress. Documentation for any given period of time (e.g., 1 month) should relate to the predetermined learning objectives for that period. Such records can thus serve as a basis for evaluation of the resident by his preceptors and for periodic self-examination by the resident.

V-D. The self-evaluation must relate to the resident's progress in achieving the preset learning objectives and should not be based solely on personality traits or other subjective criteria. When deficiencies are noted, appropriate remedial action must be taken. A written record of the periodic evaluation must be maintained and must be reviewed with the resident.

Standard VI. Certification

A. An appropriate certificate indicative of successful completion of the residency shall be awarded to the resident by the training institution on the recommendation of the nuclear pharmacy residency program director.

Interpretation

VI-A. Certification of completion of the nuclear pharmacy residency training program is the responsibility of the training institution. ASHP accredits only the training program—not the resident.

References

1. Nuclear pharmacy practice standards. Washington, DC: American Pharmaceutical Association; 1978.
2. American Society of Hospital Pharmacists. ASHP statement on accreditation of pharmacy residencies (with policies and procedures). *Am J Hosp Pharm.* 1980; 37:1221–3.
3. Accreditation manual for hospitals 1981. Chicago: Joint Commission on Accreditation of Hospitals; 1981.
4. Accreditation requirements of American Osteopathic Association. Chicago: American Osteopathic Association; 1981.

Approved by the ASHP Board of Directors, September 24–25, 1981. The initial draft was developed by William Hladik, M.S., and Allan Gobuty, Pharm.D. Comments were sought from the SIG on Nuclear Pharmacy, and the final document was approved by the Commission on Credentialing before submission to the Board of Directors.

The bibliographic citation for this document is as follows: American Society of Hospital Pharmacists. ASHP accreditation standard for residency training in nuclear pharmacy (with guide to interpretation). *Am J Hosp Pharm.* 1981; 38:1964–71.

ASHP Supplemental Standard and Learning Objectives for Residency Training in Nutritional Support Pharmacy Practice

Preamble

Definition. A residency in pharmacy practice nutritional support is defined as a postgraduate program of organized training that meets the requirements set forth and approved by the American Society of Hospital Pharmacists for training expert practitioners in this area of pharmacy. The "ASHP Accreditation Standard for Specialized Pharmacy Residency Training," together with this supplement, is the basic criteria used in evaluation of nutritional support pharmacy residency training programs in institutions applying for accreditation by the American Society of Hospital Pharmacists.

A specialty pharmacy residency in nutritional support services should be organized and conducted to develop expert skills and competency in providing clinical pharmacy services to patients receiving nutritional support, as well as experience in the management of a nutrition support service.

Qualifications of the Training Site. The parent facility for residency training in nutritional support pharmacy practice shall be a general hospital in which extensive nutritional support services are provided and which meets the requirements set forth in Standard I in the body of the "ASHP Accreditation Standard for Specialized Pharmacy Residency Training." Ancillary facilities (such as outpatient treatment units) may be used as appropriate in pursuing the objectives for training outlined below.

The pharmacy department in which the residency is based shall meet the requirements set forth in Standard II. It shall have adequate facilities to carry out a broad scope of services.

Qualifications of the Preceptor. The area of specialization of the preceptor shall be nutritional support practice. Additionally, the preceptor shall demonstrate proficiency as a clinical pharmacist.

The following learning objectives shall be approved by the Commission on Credentialing following review annually by a committee appointed from the Special Interest Group on Intravenous Therapy of the American Society of Hospital Pharmacists.

Learning Objectives

A resident who completes an accredited residency program in nutritional support pharmacy practice shall be able to

1. Conduct a patient interview, including drug history, and interpret the clinical significance, as related to nutrition, of the information obtained in the interview.
2. Perform a nutritional and metabolic assessment of the patient based on pertinent physical examination and laboratory variables.
3. Organize, evaluate, summarize, and communicate (either orally or in writing) the results of a nutritional assessment.
4. Identify the various types of nutritional disorders and the symptoms and pathophysiology associated with each.
5. Speak with authority on the utilization of substrates and the biochemistry of metabolism.
6. Develop an individualized nutritional regimen, including type of support (enteral or parenteral, or both), route of administration, formulation and selection of appropriate solutions, and rate of administration.
7. Monitor appropriate variables to assess patient progress.
8. Explain the therapeutic goals of a given nutrition support regimen and modifications of that regimen.
9. Recommend an appropriate nutritional regimen for a patient based on his or her unique clinical status and recommend appropriate modifications to an existing regimen.
10. Monitor drug therapy prospectively for potential drug–drug, drug–laboratory test, drug–nutrient, and drug–disease state interactions and recommend modifications in drug therapy, when appropriate, to avoid such interactions.
11. Discuss the effect of nutrition on drug therapy, including the effect of malnourishment on the pharmacokinetics of selected drugs.
12. Discuss how nutritional support, critical care management, and multiple drug therapy are interrelated.
13. Educate the patient or patient's family about the nutritional needs of the patient.
14. Conduct educational programs on nutrition support topics for students and professional staff members, using appropriate teaching methods.
15. Compound parenteral solutions, giving appropriate consideration to stability, sterility, compatibility, and accuracy.
16. Retrieve, evaluate, and communicate (orally and in writing) information from the biomedical literature relating to nutritional support.
17. Compare the various nutritional substrates and products available and state the rationale for the use of each.
18. Compare the features of various infusion devices used in the delivery of enteral and parenteral nutrition solutions.
19. Work effectively with other members of the nutritional support team (physicians, nurses, clinical dietitians, other pharmacists, and supportive personnel).
20. Outline an organizational structure for a nutritional support service and describe the roles and responsibilities of each member.
21. Participate in the ambulatory management of patients with nutritional problems and in the provision of home nutritional support.
22. Outline the historical development of nutritional support as a therapeutic modality and of nutritional support services.

In addition, the resident's competence in the following specific areas of nutritional support practice shall be developed:

A.   *Assessment*. The resident shall be able to

1.   Interview patients and evaluate the significance of changes in eating habits, weight loss, altered bowel habits, and any physical changes that may relate to nutritional status and support.

2.   Accurately obtain and evaluate anthropometric measurements.

3.   Identify laboratory variables used to assess visceral protein status and the significance and biological characteristics of the various visceral proteins.

4.   Evaluate the need for and results of laboratory tests for acid–base balance, serum electrolytes, vitamins, enzymes, and minerals.

5.   Identify any confirmed or suspected alterations in renal, hepatic, pancreatic, pulmonary, or cardiac function.

6.   Calculate basal energy expenditure and make reasonable estimates of daily caloric and protein requirements for enteral or parenteral support, or both.

7.   Identify feasible routes of administration for aggressive nutritional support, taking into account factors such as venous access, results of clotting studies, integrity of gastrointestinal tract, and mental status.

B.   *Nutritional Diagnosis*. The resident shall be able to

1.   Discuss primary nutritional diseases, including
   a.   Protein malnutrition.
   b.   Protein–calorie malnutrition.
   c.   Starvation and anorexia nervosa.
   d.   Obesity.
   e.   Vitamin and mineral deficiencies.
   f.   Others.

2.   Correlate and use data from interviews, physical assessment, and laboratory tests to categorize an individual's nutritional status.

3.   Identify drugs being taken that may
   a.   Interfere with laboratory tests used in nutritional assessment and diagnosis.
   b.   Complicate the patient's presentation, i.e., drugs causing diarrhea, constipation, etc.
   c.   Be pharmacokinetically altered by the pathophysiologic changes of malnutrition.
   d.   Potentially cause changes in acid–base or fluid–electrolyte balance.
   e.   Cause either an anabolic or catabolic response by tissues.

C.   *Nutritional Support Recommendations*. The resident shall be able to

1.   Recommend the most appropriate route of nutritional support (enteral or parenteral, or both) based on the appropriate patient data such as
   a.   Present nutritional status and calculated intake requirements.
   b.   Integrity of gastrointestinal tract, venous access sites, laboratory indices, and any fluid and electrolyte imbalances.
   c.   Patient's medical problems, plans, and prognosis.

2.   Discuss the various enteral products available with respect to
   a.   Indications and contraindications for use.
   b.   The composition and source of the protein, carbohydrates, and fat in the products.

c.   Electrolyte, vitamin, and mineral content.
d.   The caloric density of the various products.
e.   Stability, osmotic load, palatability, and viscosity.

3.   Discuss the parenteral nutritional products available with respect to
   a.   Indications and contraindications for use.
   b.   The composition and source of protein, carbohydrate, and fat in the products.
   c.   Electrolyte, vitamin, and mineral content.
   d.   The caloric density of the various products and solutions.
   e.   The proper route of administration of electrolyte, mineral, and vitamin preparations.

4.   Discuss the characteristics, indications, contraindications, and limitations in the use of
   a.   Protein-sparing nutrition.
   b.   Peripheral vein total parenteral nutrition.
   c.   Central vein total parenteral nutrition.
   d.   Cyclic central vein total parenteral nutrition.
   e.   Intravenous fat emulsions.
   f.   Nasogastric feedings.
   g.   Nasoduodenal feedings.
   h.   Gastrostomies.
   i.   Jejunostomies.

5.   Discuss the special considerations for the nutritional support of the renal failure patient, including
   a.   Alterations in the electrolytes to be administered.
   b.   Modification of trace mineral administration.
   c.   Modification of protein administration.
   d.   Concentration of parenteral nutrition fluids.
   e.   Alterations in drug elimination.
   f.   Acute versus chronic renal failure.
   g.   Effects of dialysis (hemodialysis and peritoneal dialysis) on nutritional needs.

6.   Discuss the special considerations for the nutritional support of the pancreatitic patient, including
   a.   Insulin administration.
   b.   Management of essential fatty acid deficiency and the use of intravenous fat emulsions and fat-containing diets.

7.   Discuss the special considerations for the nutritional support of the hepatic patient, including
   a.   Alterations in substrate utilization.
   b.   Modification of substrate administration.
   c.   Changes in drug metabolism.
   d.   Fluid and electrolyte management.

8.   Identify and communicate, orally or in writing, the therapeutic goals and endpoints of a given nutritional regimen for a patient.

D.   *Monitoring Nutritional Support*. The resident shall be able to

1.   Comment on the need for, and usefulness of, the following laboratory tests in monitoring patients on nutrition support regimens; comment on clinical significance of the results of each test:
   a.   Visceral protein levels such as transferrin and albumin.
   b.   Twenty-four-hour urine collections for

urea, creatinine, electrolytes, etc.

 c. Electrolyte, vitamin, and trace mineral determinations.

 d. Cholesterol, triglyceride, and free fatty acid levels.

 e. Blood urea nitrogen and ammonia levels.

 f. Serum and urinary glucose levels.

 g. Others specific to the particular institution.

2. Recommend appropriate changes in nutritional solutions or rate of administration, or both, based on pertinent laboratory data.

3. Make recommendations on the administration of insulin based on

 a. Past medical history.

 b. Blood glucose levels.

 c. Urinary sugar and acetone levels.

 d. Receiving of peritoneal or hemodialysis.

 e. Route of nutritional support.

4. Explain the rationale for gradually increasing or decreasing the rate of hyperalimentation

5. Discuss the importance of monitoring stool pH and frequency of stools in the patient receiving enteral support.

6. Compare and contrast the use of bolus and continuous enteral feedings in both the stomach and small bowel.

7. Develop a schedule for obtaining pertinent laboratory values and defend the rationale for that schedule (including the frequency for ordering the laboratory tests).

8. Accurately calculate a patient's intake of specific nutrients based on a daily intake and output record and a daily calorie count.

9. Describe commonly used techniques for determining clearance of intravenous fat emulsions.

10. Discuss the following manifestations of pathophysiology of malnutrition with respect to alterations in response to drug therapy:

 a. Hypoalbuminemia.

 b. Decreased enzymatic function.

 c. Decreased tissue perfusion.

 d. Decreased glomerular filtration.

 e. Edema.

 f. Decreased absorptive capacity of gastrointestinal tract.

 g. Loss of tissue mass and a decreased total cellular mass.

 h. Alterations in hormonal balance.

E. *Infusion Components and Systems.* The resident shall be able to

1. Discuss the indications for, limitations to, and characteristics of the following apparatus used in nutritional support:

 a. Pumps (various types).

 b. Controllers (various types).

 c. Subclavian central catheter.

 d. Permanent central venous catheters (e.g., Broviac and Hickman).

 e. Soft silicone rubber feeding tube.

 f. Gastrostomy and jejunostomy feeding tubes.

 g. Nasogastric tubes.

 h. Antecubital catheter.

 i. Final filtration devices.

 j. Solution formulators.

2. Discuss the following aspects of catheter care and dressing changes:

 a. Aseptic and dressing techniques.

 b. Relationship to complication rate.

F. *Ambulatory Care.* The resident shall be able to

1. Evaluate the appropriateness of home parenteral and enteral nutrition for a particular patient, taking into account

 a. Patient's medical condition and stability.

 b. Family support.

 c. Training of patient and family.

 d. Feasibility in scheduling routine laboratory monitoring.

 e. Provision of home supplies.

 f. Monitoring of home therapy.

 g. Reimbursement for services.

2. Propose appropriate treatment regimens for the ambulatory management of patients with nutritional problems, both for those treated in an ambulatory clinic environment and those receiving home care.

G. *Organizational Considerations of a Nutritional Support Service.* The resident shall be able to discuss the following considerations relating to the development and coordination of a nutritional support service:

1. Forming and organizing committees.

2. Identifying available resources within the institution.

3. Reporting structures.

4. Program justification.

5. Job descriptions.

6. Scope of services, including policies and procedures.

7. Mechanisms for intradepartmental and interdepartmental communication.

8. Reimbursement for services.

9. Educational and research responsibilities.

The resident's training schedule shall be directed toward the accomplishment of these objectives and shall provide the resident the opportunity to

1. Participate directly in the nutritional support of a wide range of patient populations, including internal medicine, surgical, and pediatric patients.

2. Participate in interdepartmental and extramural rotations wherever necessary to achieve the objectives outlined above.

3. Attend grand rounds, clinical conferences, seminars, and other interdisciplinary continuing education activities.

4. Make scholarly presentations on topics related to his area of expertise.

In addition, the schedule should make provision for the resident's participation in a clinical research project or for a self-directed investigation in an appropriate area. The preceptor should emphasize to the resident the need to report on research findings at professional meetings, and the preceptor should attempt to schedule the resident's participation in such forums to present this work.

When appropriate, the resident's training should be augmented with reading assignments and formal, didactic presentations by qualified health professionals.

Approved by the ASHP Board of Directors, September 24–25, 1981. The initial draft was developed by Timothy Vanderveen, Pharm.D., and Robert Parks, Pharm.D. Comments were sought from the SIG on Intravenous Therapy, and the final document was approved by the Commission on Credentialing before submission to the Board of Directors.

The bibliographic citation for this document is as follows: American Society of Hospital Pharmacists. ASHP supplemental standard and learning objectives for residency training in nutritional support pharmacy practice. *Am J Hosp Pharm*. 1981; 38:1971–3.

ASHP Supplemental Standard and Learning Objectives for Residency Training in Oncology Pharmacy Practice

Preamble

Definition. A specialized residency in oncology pharmacy practice is defined as an organized, directed postgraduate training program that centers on developing the competencies necessary to provide pharmaceutical care to cancer patients.

Purpose and Philosophy. The supplemental residency standard establishes criteria for the training and education of pharmacists in the fundamentals of exemplary contemporary pharmacy practice in organized health care systems dealing with cancer patients. An oncology pharmacy practice residency embraces the concept that oncology pharmacy practitioners must share in the responsibility and accountability for optimal drug therapy outcomes in cancer patients. Therefore, residencies in oncology pharmacy practice must provide residents with opportunities to function independently as practitioners through conceptualizing, integrating, and transforming accumulated experience and knowledge into improved drug therapy for cancer patients.

Accreditation Authority. The ASHP Accreditation Standard for Specialized Pharmacy Residency Training,[1] taken together with this supplement, are the basic criteria used to evaluate oncology pharmacy practice residency training programs in organizations applying for accreditation by the American Society of Hospital Pharmacists.

Qualifications of the Training Site. The training site must meet the requirements set forth in part I of the ASHP Accreditation Standard for Specialized Pharmacy Residency Training. Facilities that provide specialized residency training in oncology pharmacy practice shall be oncology treatment institutions or hospitals that provide comprehensive clinical and distributive oncology pharmacy services; these facilities should be involved in research endeavors in this field.

If needed, extramural experiences in other health care settings can be scheduled to augment the resident's training. Extramural experiences may be conducted either as full-time training activities (e.g., for a one-month block), or on a regularly scheduled part-time basis. If extramural experiences are scheduled for the purpose of pursuing one or more of the fundamental competencies outlined below, there must be a pharmacist preceptor who has defined responsibilities for monitoring the residents' progress and evaluating his or her accomplishments. The qualifications of the extramural experiences are subject to review and approval by the American Society of Hospital Pharmacists.

Qualifications of the Pharmacy Service. The pharmacy services must meet the requirements set forth in Part IV of the Accreditation Standard for Specialized Pharmacy Residency Training. The facility must have at least one pharmacist with an established practice in oncology clinical pharmacy. There should be an oncology pharmacy satellite that provides patient-specific services to cancer patients. In all circumstances, the pharmacy must show evidence that comprehensive clinical and distributive services care including adequate departmental administration, inpatient and outpatient drug inventory and control, ambulatory care oncology services, drug information resources, and an ongoing quality assurance program, are being provided to cancer patients.

Qualifications of the Program Director. The program director's qualifications shall meet the requirements set forth in Part II of the ASHP Accreditation Standard for Specialized Pharmacy Residency Training. The program director shall demonstrate proficiency as an oncology pharmacy practitioner and maintain an active patient-care involvement.

Selection and Qualifications of the Resident. In addition to meeting the requirements set forth in the ASHP Accreditation Standard for Specialized Pharmacy Residency Training, the resident must have previously completed an ASHP-accredited pharmacy practice residency or have had an equivalent level of prior experience in pharmacy practice.

Supplemental Goals and Objectives

Goals

1. Assume personal responsibility for improving pharmacy's care of oncology patients, including the prevention and treatment of disease.
2. Provide for the specialized needs of oncology patients while addressing the patient's total pharmaceutical care needs.
3. Design, recommend, and monitor patient-specific pharmacotherapy and immunotherapy for neoplastic and related diseases in cancer patients.
4. Counsel patients on proper drug use, drug interactions, and toxicities and, if pertinent, provide patient education on preparing anticancer and biologic agents.
5. Respond to requests for information about approved and investigational anticancer and biologic agents.
6. Prepare and present interdisciplinary educational activities on oncology pharmacy practice-related topics to health care professionals.
7. Participate on teams of health care professionals developing, implementing, monitoring, and analyzing research protocols for anticancer, biologic, or supportive-care therapy.
8. Develop and operate a system for preparing and distributing approved and investigational anticancer drugs.
9. Identify factors for measuring the quality of care provided by the oncology pharmacy service that can be used in a departmental continuous quality assurance program.
10. Communicate effectively with cancer patients, their caregivers, and oncology health care professionals.

Objectives Associated with Each Goal Statement. The following are Terminal Objectives (TO) and Enabling Objectives (EO) associated with each goal statement.

Goal 1. Assume personal responsibility for improving pharmacy's care of oncology patients, including the prevention and treatment of disease.

TO 1.1 (Characterization) Practice the delivery of pharmaceutical care to improve the outcome of oncology patients including the prevention and treatment of disease.

EO 1.1.1 (Synthesis) Write one's own philosophy of practice as an oncology pharmacy specialist.

Goal 2. Provide for the specialized needs of oncology patients while addressing the patient's total pharmaceutical care needs.

TO 2.1 (Synthesis) Generate patient care plans that reflect all aspects of the delivery of pharmaceutical care.

Goal 3. Design, recommend, and monitor patient-specific pharmacotherapy and immunotherapy for neoplastic and related diseases in cancer patients.

TO 3.1 (Synthesis) Create a patient database upon which to make pharmacologic therapeutic decisions for cancer patients.

EO 3.1.1 (Application) Use medical terminology and abbreviations particular to the discussion of cancer.

EO 3.1.2 (Comprehension) Discuss the epidemiology, etiology, presenting symptoms, pathophysiology, usual metastatic sites, associated diagnostic tests, treatments (pharmacotherapy, radiation therapy, and surgery), and prognosis of neoplastic diseases.

EO 3.1.3 (Comprehension) Discuss the etiology, presenting symptoms, pathophysiology, associated diagnostic tests, and treatments of cancer-related disorders.

EO 3.1.4 (Comprehension) Discuss the etiology, presenting symptoms, pathophysiology, associated diagnostic tests, and treatments of cancer-treatment related complications.

EO 3.1.5 (Comprehension) Discuss the clinical pharmacology; pharmacokinetics; pharmacodynamics; common doses, schedules, and administration techniques; and dose-related, dose-limiting, and cumulative toxicities of all FDA-approved cancer chemotherapeutic, hormonal, and biologic response-modifying agents.

EO 3.1.6 (Comprehension) Discuss the unique aspects of antineoplastic therapy related to drug resistance mechanisms, dose intensity, biochemical modulation, circadian drug delivery, radiation sensitizers, bone marrow transplantation conditioning regimens, and gene therapy.

EO 3.1.7 (Analysis) Discriminate organ system abnormalities that are cancer induced from those that are drug induced.

EO 3.1.8 (Synthesis) When interviewing to gather information for a patient database, modify interview strategies for patients and caregivers to accommodate their special emotional needs.

TO 3.2 (Synthesis) Formulate desired pharmacologic therapeutic outcomes for a cancer patient that reflect the integration of pertinent patient-specific data in relationship to disease-specific and drug-specific information.

(See **EO 3.1.2***)*
(See **EO 3.1.3***)*
(See **EO 3.1.4***)*
(See **EO 3.1.5***)*

TO 3.3 (Synthesis) Design a therapeutic regimen for a cancer patient with consideration for patient- and treatment-specific information and the organized health care setting's constraints.

(See **EO 3.1.2***)*
(See **EO 3.1.3***)*
(See **EO 3.1.4***)*
(See **EO 3.1.5***)*

EO 3.3.1 (Comprehension) Describe the physical, chemical, and economic considerations and potential complications of medication administration systems, including intravenous infusion pumps, ambulatory infusion pumps, intra-arterial pumps, central venous catheters, and enteral feeding systems.

EO 3.3.2 (Application) Use a knowledge of the special considerations of ambulatory care oncology patients when designing their pharmacotherapeutic plans.

TO 3.4 (Synthesis) Design a monitoring plan for a therapeutic regimen for a cancer patient that will determine achievement of desired pharmacologic therapeutic outcomes with consideration for patient- and treatment-specific information and the organized health care setting's specific constraints.

(See **EO 3.1.2***)*
(See **EO 3.1.3***)*
(See **EO 3.1.4***)*
(See **EO 3.1.5***)*

EO 3.4.1 (Comprehension) Discuss the use of radiologic exams, pathologic findings, and tumor markers to assess the effects of anticancer drug treatment.

TO 3.5 (Synthesis) Propose a therapeutic regimen and monitoring plan for the treatment of cancer, cancer-associated diseases, or treatment-related complications to a prescriber, a patient, or both.

TO 3.6 (Evaluation) Redesign a cancer patient's therapeutic regimen and monitoring plan based on an appraisal of the attainment of the specified pharmacologic therapeutic outcomes.

Goal 4. Counsel patients on proper drug use, drug interactions, and toxicities and, if pertinent, provide patient education on preparing anticancer and biologic agents.

TO 4.1 (Comprehension) Discuss with the preceptor proper drug use, drug interactions, toxicities, and remedial actions for toxicities associated with anticancer therapy.

TO 4.2 (Synthesis) Modify counseling strategies to accommodate the special emotional needs of the cancer patient.

TO 4.3 (Application) Instruct patients in the preparation and administration of anticancer and biologic agents according to sound educational practice for teaching complex kinesthetic and cognitive skills.

Goal 5. Respond to requests for information about approved and investigational anticancer and biologic agents.

TO 5.1 (Comprehension) Discuss the most likely reliable sources of information about approved and investigational anticancer and biologic agents.

TO 5.2 (Application) Use CANCERLIT, PDQ, and other literature sources specific to oncology pharmacy practice to retrieve drug information.

Goal 6. Prepare and present interdisciplinary educational activities on oncology pharmacy practice-related topics to health care professionals.

TO 6.1 (Evaluation) Appraise emerging issues in oncology pharmacy practice that would be suitable for interdisciplinary educational sessions.

TO 6.2 (Analysis) Discriminate aspects of oncology pharmacy practice within the practice setting that could be improved through interdisciplinary educational programs.

TO 6.3 (Analysis) Distinguish those aspects of a selected educational program topic that are pertinent for presentation to the selected audience.

TO 6.4 (Application) Use information sources relating to oncology pharmacy practice, such as abstracts, personal communications, and computer databases to prepare interdisciplinary educational presentations.

TO 6.5 (Evaluation) Appraise information for inclusion in an interdisciplinary educational presentation according to criteria unique to the oncology content area.

TO 6.6 (Synthesis) Design interdisciplinary educational programs on oncology pharmacy practice that reflect consideration of level of content and terminology suitable to the audience.

Goal 7. Participate on teams of health care professionals developing, implementing, monitoring, and analyzing research protocols for anticancer, biologic, or supportive-care therapy.

TO 7.1 (Comprehension) Describe the phases of the investigational drug development process and the objectives for each phase as it applies to approving anticancer and biologic compounds.

TO 7.2 (Comprehension) Discuss steps in the investigational protocol approval process.

TO 7.3 (Comprehension) Describe the purposes of standard sections of research protocols for anticancer, biologic, or supportive-care therapy.

TO 7.4 (Comprehension) Discuss factors that facilitate pharmacy participation in teams of health-care professionals developing, implementing, and monitoring research protocols for anticancer, biologic, or supportive care.

TO 7.5 (Synthesis) Create a pharmaceutical information section of a research protocol that includes all drugs used in the study.

TO 7.6 (Evaluation) Recommend modifications of the informed consent document related to the drug therapy used in an anticancer, biologic, or supportive-care study.

TO 7.7 (Analysis) Outline a plan for the drug administration aspects of a research protocol.

TO 7.8 (Application) Use the drug dose modifications section of a study to evaluate the appropriateness of a drug order involved in the study.

TO 7.9 (Comprehension) Describe proper procedures for reporting adverse reactions to investigational anticancer and biologic compounds.

Goal 8. Develop and operate a system for preparing and distributing approved and investigational anticancer drugs.

TO 8.1 (Comprehension) Discuss factors to consider when modifying a traditional pharmacy physical layout according to the special needs of operating an oncology pharmacy service.

TO 8.2 (Comprehension) Discuss specialized equipment needs required to operate an oncology pharmacy service.

TO 8.3 (Evaluation) Appraise a department's existing policies and procedures for preparation, distribution,

administration, and disposal of antineoplastic agents for conformance to guidelines for safe handling of antineoplastic agents.

TO 8.4 (Evaluation) Appraise a department's existing policies and procedures for securing and keeping records for investigational drugs.

TO 8.5 (Application) Secure investigational drugs according to guidelines specified for studies sponsored by the National Cancer Institute (NCI) or by industry. The category investigational drugs includes compassionate use, treatment IND, treatment referral center protocols, and Group C.

TO 8.6 (Application) Keep records of investigational drugs according to guidelines specified for NCI-sponsored or industry-sponsored drug studies.

TO 8.7 (Application) Prepare antineoplastic agents according to established guidelines.

Goal 9. Identify factors for measuring the quality of care provided by the oncology pharmacy service that can be used in a departmental continuous quality assurance program.

TO 9.1 (Analysis) Select outcomes of pharmaceutical care that would measure the quality of care provided by the oncology pharmacy service that can be used in a departmental continuous quality assurance program.

Goal 10. Communicate effectively with cancer patients, their caregivers, and oncology health care professionals.

TO 10.1 (Application) Use persuasive communication techniques.

TO 10.2 (Synthesis) Formulate communications that reflect sensitivity to the status, expertise, and emotional needs of the audience.

Core Experiences in Direct Patient Care

A residency in oncology pharmacy practice is dependent on the availability of a broad range of patient categories and professional practice experience. Therefore, it is expected that core experiences in direct patient care should occur in various patient care settings (i.e., acute care and ambulatory care settings), as appropriate.

1. Neoplastic diseases
   a. Breast cancer
   b. GI tract cancer
   c. Leukemias
   d. Lung cancer
   e. Lymphomas
   f. Prostate cancer
   g. Testicular cancer
   h. Central nervous system tumors
   i. Ovarian cancer
2. Disease-related or iatrogenic problems in the cancer patient
   a. Nausea and vomiting
   b. Infections in the immunocompromised host
   c. Acute and chronic pain
   d. Mucositis
   e. Nutrition support
   f. Extravasation
   g. Hypercalcemia of malignancy
   h. Malignant effusions
   i. Tumor compression syndromes (e.g., spinal cord compression)

    j. Syndrome of inappropriate secretion of antidiuretic hormone (SIADH)

3. Treatment procedures

    a. Bone marrow transplantation (autologous and allogeneic)

    b. Chemotherapy

    c. Radiation therapy

    d. Immunotherapy

    e. Surgery

4. Antineoplastic agents

    a. Drug resistance mechanisms

    b. Dose intensity

    c. Regional chemotherapy

    d. Biochemical modulation

    e. Circadian drug delivery

    f. Radiation sensitizers

    g. Bone marrow transplantation conditioning regimens

Reference

1. American Society of Hospital Pharmacists. ASHP accreditation standard for specialized pharmacy residency training. *Am J Hosp Pharm.* 1994; 51:2034–41.

Approved by the ASHP Board of Directors, April 27, 1994. Developed by a working group of ASHP oncology pharmacy practitioners and the ASHP Commission on Credentialing. For currently existing programs, this revision of the accreditation standard takes effect April 27, 1995. Until that time, the current standard, which was approved April 23, 1982, is in force.

The bibliographic citation for this document is as follows: ASHP supplemental standard and learning objectives for residency training in oncology pharmacy practice. In: Practice Standards of ASHP 1994–95. Hicks WE, ed. Bethesda, MD: American Society of Hospital Pharmacists; 1994.

ASHP Supplemental Standard and Learning Objectives for Residency Training in Pediatric Pharmacy Practice

Preamble

Definition. A specialized residency in pediatric pharmacy practice is defined as an organized, directed postgraduate program that centers on developing the competencies necessary to provide pharmaceutical care to pediatric patients.

Purpose and Philosophy. The supplemental residency standard establishes criteria for the training and education of pharmacists in the delivery of exemplary pharmaceutical care to pediatric patients. A pediatric pharmacy practice residency embraces the concept that pediatric pharmacy practitioners share in the responsibility and accountability for optimal outcomes in pediatric patients. Therefore, residencies in pediatric pharmacy practice must provide residents with the opportunities to function independently as practitioner through conceptualizing, integrating, and transforming accumulated experience and knowledge into improved drug therapy for pediatric patients.

Accreditation Authority. The ASHP Accreditation Standard for Specialized Pharmacy Residency Training, (1) taken together with this supplement, are the basic criteria used to evaluate pediatric pharmacy practice residency training programs applying for accreditation by the ASHP.

Qualifications of the Training Site. The training site must meet the requirements set forth in Part I of the "ASHP Accreditation Standard for Specialized Pharmacy Residency Training." (1) Facilities may include, but are not limited to, a tertiary care medical center, a freestanding pediatric hospital, or a general hospital that provides comprehensive clinical and distributive pediatric pharmacy services. Ancillary facilities may be used, as appropriate, in pursuing the objectives for training outlined below.

Qualifications of the Pharmacy Service. The pharmacy services must meet the requirements set forth in Part IV of the ASHP Accreditation Standard for Specialized Pharmacy Residency Training, (1) The facility must have at least one pharmacist with an established clinical practice in pediatrics. There should be a pediatric pharmacy satellite or similar facility that provides patient-specific services to pediatric patients. In all circumstances, the pharmacy department must show evidence that comprehensive clinical and distributive pharmacy services are being provided to pediatric patients.

Qualifications of the Program Director. The program director's qualifications shall meet the requirements set forth in Part II of the ASHP Accreditation Standard for Specialized Pharmacy Residency Training. (1) The program director shall demonstrate proficiency as a clinical pharmacist in the area of pediatric pharmacy services.

Selection and Qualifications of the Resident. In addition to meeting the requirements set forth in the ASHP Accreditation Standard for Specialized Pharmacy Residency Training, the resident *must* have previously completed an ASHP-Accredited Pharmacy Practice Residency or have had an equivalent level of prior experience in pharmacy practice.

Supplemental Goals and Objectives

Goals

1. Assume responsibility for developing a pharmacy practice philosophy that supports pharmaceutical care and pediatric pharmacy practice excellence.
2. Effectively communicate with children of varying ages.
3. Stay current with the pediatric drug therapy literature.
4. Deliver effective presentations to health care professionals and the public on topics related to pediatric pharmaceutical care.
5. Employ effective precepting skills in the training of pharmacy students and other health care professionals.
6. Maintain active involvement in local, state, and national pharmacy and pediatric organizations.
7. Design and execute a project involving pediatric pharmacy practice-related issues.
8. Conduct direct pediatric patient care activities using a consistent approach that reflects the philosophy of pharmaceutical care, and that is performed with the efficiency and depth of experience characteristic of an experienced pharmacist.
9. Design, recommend, implement, monitor, and evaluate patient-specific pharmacotherapy.
10. Anticipate potential fetal impact resulting from maternal exposure or genetic abnormalities.
11. Prepare medications in dosage and dosage forms suitable for pediatric patients.
12. Ensure that all forms of pediatric drugs, including parenterals, are administered using appropriate techniques.
13. Work effectively with multidisciplinary health care teams in the organized health-care setting.
14. Participate effectively in medical staff rounds of pediatric patients.
15. Provide medication-use education to caregivers or, when appropriate, to patients.
16. Ensure continuity of pharmaceutical care to and from the acute and ambulatory patient-care settings.
17. Document all pharmaceutical-care activities appropriately.
18. Participate in the management of pediatric medical emergency codes.
19. Assist in programs that center on disease prevention and wellness promotion.
20. Provide concise, applicable, and timely responses to requests for pediatric drug information from healthcare providers and patients.
21. Select a core library appropriate for a pediatric practice setting.
22. Maximize work efficiency through the use of computerized database retrieval systems retaining pediatric drug information.
23. Write newsletter articles that provide pertinent pediat-

ric drug-use information for health care professionals in the organized health-care setting.

24. Develop educational materials that assist the public in the understanding of drug-use issues or the management of their own drug therapy.

25. Utilize poison control information.

26. Conduct programs that center on pediatric poison and substance abuse prevention.

27. Participate in the formulary selection of drugs intended for pediatric use.

28. Participate in the ongoing modification of a health system's process for assessing, managing, preventing, and reporting medication errors.

29. Evaluate current organized health care setting policies and procedures for adequacy in meeting pediatric pharmacy needs.

30. Consult on the development or modification of selected policies for the selection and use of drugs intended for pediatric use in the organized health-care setting.

31. Assume responsibility for the organized health-care setting's ongoing adherence to its drug-use policies for drugs intended for pediatric use.

32. Conceptualize a comprehensive system of services to meet pediatric pharmacy needs.

33. Influence the organized health care setting's committees to achieve the goals of pediatric pharmacy practice.

Objectives Associated with Goal Statements. The following are Terminal Objectives (TO) and Enabling Objectives (EO) associated with each goal statement.

Goal 1. Assume responsibility for developing a pharmacy practice philosophy that supports pharmaceutical care and pediatric pharmacy practice excellence.

TO 1.1 (Organization) Prepare a statement of one's pharmacy practice philosophy that reflects pharmaceutical care and adherence to pediatric pharmacy practice excellence.

Goal 2. Effectively communicate with children of varying ages.

TO 2.1 (Synthesis) Modify communication strategies to communicate effectively with children of varying ages.

Goal 3. Stay current with the pediatric drug therapy literature.

TO 3.1 (Characterization) Adhere to a plan for staying current with the pediatric drug therapy literature.

Goal 4. Deliver effective presentations to health care professionals and the public on topics related to pediatric pharmaceutical care.

TO 4.1 (Synthesis) Design effective presentations for health care professionals and the public on topics related to pediatric pharmaceutical care.

TO 4.2 (Application) Use effective educational techniques to deliver presentations to health care professionals and the public on topics related to pediatric pharmaceutical care.

Goal 5. Employ effective precepting skills in the training of pharmacy students and other health care professionals.

TO 5.1 (Synthesis) Formulate precepting strategies to successfully facilitate the learning of pharmacy students and other health care professionals.

Goal 6. Maintain active involvement in local, state, and national pharmacy and pediatric organizations.

TO 6.1 (Organization) Demonstrate an acceptance of the importance of membership in pharmacy and pediatric organizations by being actively involved in local, state, and national associations.

Goal 7. Design and execute a project involving pediatric pharmacy practice-related issues.

TO 7.1 (Synthesis) Design and conduct a project whose focus is to evaluate or enhance the pharmaceutical care of pediatric patients.

EO 7.1.1 (Comprehension) Discuss the differences between conducting research on children and adults.

Goal 8. Conduct direct pediatric patient care activities using a consistent approach that reflects the philosophy of pharmaceutical care, and that is performed with the efficiency and depth of experience characteristic of an experienced pharmacist.

TO 8.1 (Synthesis) Devise efficient strategies for one's own direct patient-care activities that maximize the delivery of appropriate pharmaceutical care to each pediatric patient.

TO 8.2 (Synthesis) Formulate solutions to complex pediatric patient-care problems that maximize the achievement of pharmaceutical care outcomes.

Goal 9. Design, recommend, implement, monitor, and evaluate patient-specific pharmacotherapy.

TO P9.1 (Synthesis) Collect, generate, and organize all patient-specific information needed by the pharmacist to detect and resolve drug-related problems and to make appropriate drug therapy decisions.

EO P9.1.1 (Comprehension) Identify the types of information the pharmacist requires to detect and resolve drug-related problems and to make appropriate drug therapy decisions.

EO P9.1.2 (Comprehension) Discuss signs and symptoms, epidemiology, etiology, risk factors, pathogenesis, natural history of diseases, pathophysiology, and clinical course of diseases commonly encountered in the pediatric patients.

EO P9.1.3 (Comprehension) Discuss the mechanism of action, pharmacokinetics, pharmacodynamics, pharmacoeconomics, usual regimen (dose, schedule, form, route, and method of administration), indications, contraindications, interactions, adverse reactions, and therapeutics of drugs commonly used to treat pediatric patients.

EO P9.1.4 (Synthesis) Integrate effective communication techniques in interviews with patients, caregivers, health-care professionals, or others so that the patient-specific information needed by the pharmacist is collected.

EO P9.1.5 (Adaptation) When appropriate, measure patient vital signs and perform a screening physical assessment of the pediatric patient.

TO P9.2 (Evaluation) Appraise patients' current drug and non-drug therapy based on an integration of pathophysiologic, pharmacotherapeutic, pharmacokinetic, pharmacodynamic, economic, ethical, and legal considerations to as well as knowledge of the current literature and one's own practice experience to determine the presence of any of the following drug therapy problems:

1. drugs used with no medical indication
2. medical conditions for which there is no drug prescribed
3. drugs prescribed inappropriately for a particular medical condition
4. anything inappropriate in the current drug therapy regimen (dose, schedule, route of administration, method of administration)
5. presence of therapeutic duplication
6. prescription of drugs to which the patient is allergic
7. presence or potential for adverse drug events
8. presence of clinically significant drug–drug, drug–disease, drug–nutrient, or drug–laboratory test interactions
9. interference with medical therapy by social or recreational drug use
10. patient not receiving full benefit of prescribed drug therapy
11. treatment problems arising from financial impact of drug therapy on the patient
12. patient lack of understanding of their drug therapy

EO P9.2.1 (Evaluation) Prioritize patients' pharmacotherapy problems. Compile patient-specific information for the development of an individual pharmacotherapeutic plan for pediatric patients.

TO 9.3 (Evaluation) Appraise the appropriateness of pediatric patients' nutritional therapy.

EO 9.3.1 (Comprehension) Discuss pediatric growth and development.

EO 9.3.2 (Comprehension) Discuss nutritional needs of the pediatric patient in the different stages of growth and development.

EO 9.3.3 (Comprehension) Discuss the use of nutritional products to address the hydration, electrolyte, and nutritional requirements of the pediatric patient.

TO 9.4 (Evaluation) Using patient-specific information summarize pediatric patients' health-care needs.

EO 9.4.1 (Comprehension) Discuss social and environmental factors impacting the delivery of health care to pediatric patients.

EO 9.4.2 (Comprehension) Discuss the impact of pediatric patients' growth and development on changes in their health care needs.

TO 9.5 (Synthesis) Specify pharmacotherapeutic goals for a pediatric patient that integrate patient-specific data; age-specific, disease-specific, and drug-specific information; and ethical considerations.

EO 9.5.1 (Comprehension) Discuss those situations in which the interaction between age and disease alters the setting of pharmacotherapeutic goals for the pediatric patient

EO 9.5.2 (Comprehension) Discuss ethical considerations in setting pharmacotherapeutic goals for pediatric patients.

TO 9.6 (Synthesis) Design pharmacotherapeutic regimens, including modifications to existing drug therapy, that work to meet pediatric patients' pharmacotherapeutic goals.

TO 9.7 (Application) Recommend pharmacotherapeutic regimens to prescribers, caregivers, and, when appropriate, to pediatric patients in a way that is systematic, logical, and secures consensus from prescribers, caregivers and patients.

TO 9.8 (Synthesis) Design monitoring plans for pharmacotherapeutic regimens of pediatric patients that effectively evaluate achievement of the patient-specific pharmacotherapeutic goals.

EO 9.8.1 (Synthesis) Determine parameters to monitor that will measure achievement of pharmacotherapeutic goals for an approved pharmacotherapeutic regimen for pediatric patients (e.g., possible paradoxical effects).

EO 9.8.2 (Knowledge) Describe normal value ranges for parameters measured in pediatric patients.

EO 9.8.3 (Comprehension) Discuss the relationship between what are normal value ranges for parameters measured in pediatric patients and the influence of a disease state.

TO 9.9 (Evaluation) Interpret the relevance of each measured parameter in a monitoring plan for a pediatric patient when compared to the desired values.

TO 9.10 (Synthesis) Modify pediatric patients' pharmacotherapeutic regimens as necessary based on the evaluation of monitoring data.

Goal 10. Anticipate potential fetal impact resulting from maternal exposure or genetic abnormalities.

TO 10.1 (Comprehension) Discuss the relationship between maternal exposure and genetic abnormalities and neonatal outcomes.

TO 10.2 (Comprehension) Discuss interventions applied prior to delivery that can improve neonatal outcomes.

Goal 11. Prepare medications in dosage and dosage forms suitable for pediatric patients.

TO 11.1 (Synthesis) Modify the preparation of drug products to fit the needs of pediatric patients.

EO 11.1.1 (Evaluation) Determine when drug product preparation requires modification.

EO 11.l.2 (Evaluation) Appraise the drug literature for methods applicable to modifying drug preparation for pediatric patients.

Goal 12. Ensure that all forms of pediatric drugs, including parenterals, are administered using appropriate techniques.

TO 12.1 (Characterization) Assume responsibility for assuring that the recommended drug administration policy for pediatric patients is applied.

TO 12.2 (Synthesis) Write policies and procedures governing the appropriate administration of all forms of drugs, including parenterals, to pediatric patients.

Goal 13. Work effectively with multidisciplinary health care teams in the organized health-care setting.

TO 13.1 (Characterization) Propose membership on multidisciplinary teams affecting the pharmaceutical care of pediatric patients.

TO 13.2 (Synthesis) When participating on multidisciplinary teams, influence team decisions to reflect the principles of pediatric pharmaceutical care.

Goal 14. Participate effectively in medical staff rounds of pediatric patients.

TO 14.1 (Synthesis) Formulate appropriate responses to

drug therapy recommendation requests and drug policy questions occurring during medical staff rounds of pediatric patients.

EO 14.1.1 (Characterization) Demonstrate a commitment to maintaining a database of the pediatric literature to support participation in medical staff rounds.

EO 14.1.2 (Characterization) Demonstrate a commitment to maintaining current knowledge of the organized health-care setting's drug policies and procedures.

Goal 15. Provide medication-use education to caregivers or, when appropriate, to patients.

TO 15.1 (Synthesis) Design medication use education for caregivers or, when appropriate, for patients.

EO 15.1.1 (Comprehension) Describe factors to consider in evaluating the medication use educational needs of pediatric patients.

TO 15.2 (Application) Use effective patient education techniques to provide discharge counseling to caregivers and, when appropriate, pediatric patients, including information on drug therapy, adverse effects, compliance, appropriate use, handling, and drug administration.

Goal 16. Ensure continuity of pharmaceutical care to and from the acute and ambulatory patient-care settings.

TO P16.1 (Application) Use a systematic procedure to communicate pertinent pharmacotherapeutic information to and from the acute and ambulatory patient-care settings.

Goal 17. Document all pharmaceutical-care activities appropriately.

TO 17.1 (Organization) Integrate documentation into all pharmaceutical-care activities.

EO 17.1.1 (Comprehension) Explain the importance of documenting pharmaceutical-care activities.

EO 17.1.2 (Application) Follow institutional policies and procedures when documenting pharmaceutical-care activities.

EO 17.1.3 (Application) Report the results of ADRs to appropriate committees, product manufacturers, and the Food and Drug Administration (FDA).

EO 17.1.4 (Application) Report the outcome of a patient-specific corrective action plan to appropriate individuals or committees.

EO 17.1.5 (Application) When detecting a significant adverse drug event resulting from a drug product defect, report the event according to the health system's policies and procedures.

EO 17.1.6 (Application) Report the results of significant drug interactions to appropriate individuals and committees.

Goal 18. Participate in the management of pediatric medical emergency codes.

TO 18.1 (Synthesis) Formulate appropriate responses as the pharmacy team member in the management of pediatric emergency code situations.

EO 18.1.1 (Application) Follow established protocol procedures according to pediatric advanced life support (PALS) for emergency codes.

EO 18.1.2 (Synthesis) Devise appropriate drug therapy recommendations in pediatric emergency code situations.

EO 18.1.3 (Application) Calculate doses, prepare and dispense medications, as needed in a pediatric medical emergency code situation.

Goal 19. Assist in programs that center on disease prevention and wellness promotion.

TO 19.1 (Comprehension) Explain a program for health-care consumers that centers on disease prevention and wellness promotion.

Goal 20. Provide concise, applicable, and timely responses to requests for pediatric drug information from health-care providers and patients.

TO 20.1 Provide concise, applicable, and timely responses to requests for pediatric drug information from health-care providers and patients.

EO 20.1.1 (Comprehension) Discuss sources and the relative reliability of each source of pediatric drug information.

Goal 21. Select a core library appropriate for a pediatric practice setting.

TO 21.1 (Application) Use a knowledge of standard pediatric references to select a core library of primary, secondary, and tertiary references appropriate for a pediatric practice setting.

Goal 22. Maximize work efficiency through the use of computerized database retrieval systems retaining pediatric drug information.

TO 22.1 (Application) Demonstrate the use of varying computerized database retrieval systems that enhance one's ability to provide pediatric drug information (e.g., MicroMedex, Iowa System.)

Goal 23. Write newsletter articles that provide pertinent pediatric drug-use information for health care professionals in the organized health-care setting.

TO 23.1 (Application) Use a knowledge of the purpose of newsletters to write articles that provide pertinent pediatric drug use information for health-care professionals in the organized health-care setting.

EO 23.1.2 (Analysis) Identify topics for inclusion in a newsletter that meet the needs of the audience for information on pediatric pharmacy issues.

Goal 24. Develop educational materials that assist the public in the understanding of drug-use issues or the management of their own drug therapy.

TO 24.1 (Synthesis) Generate educational materials that assist the public in the understanding of drug-use issues or the management of an individual's drug therapy.

EO 24.1.1 (Comprehension) Explain consumer issues related to drug use or drug therapy management.

Goal 25. Utilize poison control information.

TO 25.1 (Application) Demonstrate correct usage of poison control information sources to efficiently respond to pediatric poisoning situations.

Goal 26. Conduct programs that center on pediatric poison and substance abuse prevention.

TO 26.1 (Application) Present programs that center on pediatric poison prevention or avoidance of substance abuse to children and adults.

Goal 27. Participate in the formulary selection of drugs intended for pediatric use.

TO 27.1 (Application) Use established concepts and principles to revise or implement an organized health-care setting's formulary selection of drugs intended for pediatric use.

EO 27.1.1 (Synthesis) Prepare pediatric-specific drug monographs that conform to acceptable guidelines (e.g., ASHP Technical Assistance Bulletins on Drug Formularies) for use by P&T committee members.

EO 27.1.2 (Evaluation) Make recommendations based on comparative reviews for formulary status of a new drug intended for pediatric use.

Goal 28. Participate in the ongoing modification of a health system's process for assessing, managing, preventing, and reporting medication errors.

TO 28.1 (Application) Use a knowledge of factors which affect the operation of an organized, integrated approach for minimizing medication errors to revise a health system's approach to handling medication errors.

EO 28.1.1 (Analysis) Use skill in continuous quality improvement (CQI) techniques such as brainstorming, flowcharting and cause-and-effect diagramming to identify possible causes of medication errors and their potential solutions.

EO 28.1.2 (Comprehension) Discuss methods for minimizing medication errors.

EO 28.1.3 (Comprehension) Discuss methods suitable for evaluating the effectiveness of a particular health system's process for minimizing medication errors.

Goal 29. Evaluate current organized health care setting policies and procedures for adequacy in meeting pediatric pharmacy needs.

TO 29.1 (Evaluation) Appraise current organized health care setting policies and procedures for adequacy in meeting pediatric pharmacy needs.

Goal 30. Consult on the development or modification of selected policies for the selection and use of drugs intended for pediatric use in the organized health-care setting.

TO 30.1 (Synthesis) Devise recommendations for the selection and use of drugs intended for pediatric use in the organized health-care setting.

Goal 31. Assume responsibility for the organized health-care setting's ongoing adherence to its drug-use policies for drugs intended for pediatric use.

TO 31.1 (Characterization) Demonstrate leadership in assuring the organized health care setting's adherence to its drug-use policies for drugs intended for pediatric use.

Goal 32. Conceptualize a comprehensive system of services to meet pediatric pharmacy needs.

TO 32.1 (Synthesis) Design a comprehensive system of services meeting pediatric pharmacy needs.

EO 32.1.1 (Comprehension) Discuss factors to be taken into consideration in meeting the unique pharmacy needs of pediatric patients.

Goal 33. Influence the organized health care setting's committees to achieve the goals of pediatric pharmacy practice.

TO 33.1 (Comprehension) Discuss the varying committee structures in different types of organized health care settings that may influence pediatric pharmacy practice.

TO 33.2 (Organization) Explain the importance of pharmacy participation on organized health care setting committees that influence pediatric pharmacy practice.

Reference

1. American Society of Hospital Pharmacists. ASHP Accreditation Standard for Specialized Pharmacy Residency Training. *Am J Hosp Pharm.* 1994; 51:2034–41.

Approved by the ASHP Board of Directors November 15, 1994. Developed by a working group of ASHP pediatric pharmacy practitioners and the ASHP Commission on Credentialing. For currently existing programs, this revision of the accreditation standard takes effect November 15, 1995. Until that time, the current standard, which was approved November 18, 1983, is in force.

The bibliographic citation for this document is as follows: ASHP supplemental standard and learning objectives for residency training in pediatric pharmacy practice. In: Practice Standards of ASHP 1995–96. Hicks, WE, ed. Bethesda, MD: American Society of Health-System Pharmacists; 1995.

ASHP Supplemental Standard and Learning Objectives for Residency Training in Adult Internal Medicine Pharmacy Practice

A specialized residency in internal medicine pharmacy practice is defined as a postgraduate program of organized education and training that meets the requirements set forth and approved by the American Society of Hospital Pharmacists. The "ASHP Accreditation Standard for Specialized Pharmacy Residency Training"[1] and this supplement describe the basic criteria used to evaluate internal medicine pharmacy residency training programs in institutions applying for accreditation by the American Society of Hospital Pharmacists.

A specialized residency in internal medicine pharmacy practice must be organized and conducted to develop a mastery of knowledge and an expert level of competency in this area, differentiating in scope, depth, and proficiency from skills expected of institutional pharmacy and general clinical pharmacy residents. Objectives of such training shall include extensive experiences in providing comprehensive clinical pharmacy services to inpatient adult internal medicine patients, as well as experience in the management of institutional drug distribution systems and the appropriate committees dealing with institutional drug use.

Qualifications of the Training Site

The parent facility for an accredited residency in internal medicine pharmacy practice shall meet the requirements set forth in Standard I in the body of the "ASHP Accreditation Standard for Specialized Pharmacy Residency Training."[1]

Qualifications of the Pharmacy Service

The pharmacy service in which an accredited internal medicine pharmacy practice residency is based must meet the requirements set forth in Standard II of the "ASHP Accreditation Standard for Specialized Pharmacy Residency Training."[1] In addition, the pharmacy department must provide a comprehensive program for inpatient pharmaceutical services, far surpassing that required in the "ASHP Minimum Standard for Pharmacies in Institutions."[2] The following specific requirements are established for the internal medicine pharmacy service program:

A. **Medical Records.** All patient-related records must be accessible to pharmacy personnel on a continuous basis.

B. **Drug Information Resources.** Each facility shall have a drug information center which maintains a centralized body of pharmaceutical and medical literature containing current primary, secondary, and tertiary literature sources. The drug information center should be located near a medical library which, in turn, has access to a regional medical library.

C. **Scope of Service.** Besides the fundamental scope of inpatient pharmaceutical services outlined in the "ASHP Minimum Standard for Pharmacies in Institutions,"[2] routine pharmaceutical services should also include the following:

1. Provision of patient-specific therapeutic and toxicologic information.
2. Patient monitoring for therapeutic and adverse effects of drug therapy.
3. Participation in ongoing drug use reviews, medical audits, and quality assurance.
4. Publication of therapeutics newsletters.
5. Experiential training and formal instruction of health professional students and residents.
6. Adverse drug reaction monitoring and reports.
7. Formal therapeutic and pharmacokinetic drug consultations.

The following pharmacy activities should also be provided where feasible: (1) formal nutritional support consultations and (2) participation in clinical drug investigations.

Qualifications of the Preceptor

Preceptors of accredited internal medicine pharmacy practice residencies must meet the requirements set forth in Standard III of the "ASHP Accreditation Standard for Specialized Pharmacy Residency Training."[1] The area of specialization of the preceptor shall be internal medicine pharmacy practice. Additionally, the preceptor shall demonstrate proficiency as a clinical pharmacist within this area of practice. The preceptor shall also maintain an active and consistent patient-care service responsibility, either through clinical consultations or other patient-oriented services.

Qualifications of the Applicant

In addition to meeting the requirements set forth in Standard IV of the "ASHP Accreditation Standard for Specialized Pharmacy Residency Training,"[1] the applicant should have completed formal academic instruction in the following subject areas or their equivalents: pathophysiology, pharmacokinetics, pharmacotherapeutics, communication techniques, drug literature evaluation, and drug study design.

Residency Training Program

The adult internal medicine pharmacy practice residency program shall be structured, organized, and administered in accordance with the requirements set forth in Standard V of the "ASHP Accreditation Standard for Specialized Pharmacy Residency Training."[1] (Note: The interpretation of this Standard shall be approved by the ASHP Commission on Credentialing following review annually by a committee appointed from the Special Interest Group on Adult Clinical Pharmacy Practice of the American Society of Hospital Pharmacists.)

A. **Learning Objectives.** A resident who completes an accredited residency program in internal medicine pharmacy practice shall be able to

1. Demonstrate professional responsibility, dedi-

cation, and maturity as well as the ability to communicate clearly, concisely, and effectively, both orally and in writing, in order to function as a productive member of a multidisciplinary health-care team.

2. Speak with authority on the pathology, pathophysiology, and pharmacotherapeutic and pharmacokinetic management of acute and chronic diseases commonly encountered in an inpatient internal medicine service.

3. Obtain and record patient medication histories which document previous drug therapy, drug interactions, drug-induced symptoms or diseases, noncompliance, drug misuse or abuse, and allergies or hypersensitivity reactions that may directly affect that patient's drug therapy treatment plan.

4. Use pertinent information gained from the patient and the medical record to
   a. Identify all patient problems that lend themselves to treatment with drugs or that may be caused by current drug therapy.
   b. Identify a rational goal of therapy for each problem.
   c. Ensure that each problem is being treated with drug(s) of choice for the patient and that (1) no other patient problem is adversely affected by the therapy and (2) no other patient problem alters the choice of therapy.
   d. Identify optimal variables for monitoring therapeutic outcomes, including adverse drug effects, and conduct the monitoring process.
   e. Recommend appropriate alterations in drug therapy when the goal is not reached or adverse effects occur.
   f. Screen for drug interactions and recommend appropriate changes in the drug regimen.
   g. Ensure that the patient complies with the therapeutic regimen.
   h. Evaluate any clinical change for possible drug cause.
   i. Refer pertinent drug and patient information to the appropriate health-care provider.

5. Write a formal drug therapy consult note, including recommendations on drug therapy treatment plans and therapeutic endpoints.

6. Counsel patients regarding appropriate procurement, use, and storage of therapeutic agents.

7. Contribute to the management of medical emergencies such as cardiac arrests and acute poisonings.

8. Develop, implement, and conduct quality-assurance programs to evaluate clinical pharmacy services.

9. Collaborate with the medical staff in developing, implementing, and conducting drug use review programs.

10. Conduct educational programs on the therapeutic aspects of patient care to health-care students and professional staff members, using appropriate teaching methods.

11. Assist in the administrative and clinical aspects of planning and implementing clinical pharmacy services, with emphasis on cost justification, documentation, and reimbursement of the clinical services as well as integration with distributive pharmacy functions.

12. Evaluate the delivery of pharmaceutical services and offer suggestions for improvement.

13. Work with the nursing staff to insure the safe, correct, and cost-efficient administration of drugs.

B. **Areas of Emphasis.** The resident's training program must occur in a multidisciplinary setting in which each member of the health-care team has a defined patient-care responsibility. It must be organized in a way that makes possible the attainment of the learning objectives. Exposure to a widely varied patient population is expected. The program shall be directed toward solving specific pharmacotherapeutic and pharmacokinetic problems of acute and chronic diseases that occur commonly in an inpatient adult medicine environment. These diseases should include, but not be limited to:

1. Infectious diseases.
   a. Respiratory tract infections.
   b. Tuberculosis.
   c. Endocarditis.
   d. Urinary tract infections.
   e. Sexually transmitted diseases.
   f. Meningitis.
   g. Joint and bone infections.
   h. Septic shock.
   i. Infections in immunocompromised hosts.
   j. Skin and soft tissue infections.

2. Cardiology.
   a. Arrhythmias.
   b. Congestive heart failure.
   c. Cardiogenic shock.
   d. Myocardial infarction.
   e. Hypertension.
   f. Angina.
   g. Thromboembolic disorders.

3. Gastroenterology.
   a. Management of nausea, vomiting, diarrhea, and constipation.
   b. Peptic ulcer disease.
   c. Hepatic diseases.
      i. Cirrhosis.
      ii. Hepatitis.
      iii. Drug induced.
   d. Inflammatory bowel disease.
   e. Pancreatitis.
   f. Esophageal reflux.

4. Renal.
   a. Drug induced.
   b. Acute renal failure.
   c. Chronic renal failure.
   d. Nephrotic syndrome.

5. Pulmonary.
   a. Asthma.
   b. Chronic obstructive pulmonary disease.
   c. Acute respiratory failure.

6. Rheumatology.
   a. Rheumatoid arthritis.
   b. Gout.
   c. Systemic lupus erythematosis.
   d. Degenerative joint disease.

7. Neurology.
   a. Pain control.
   b. Multiple sclerosis.
   c. Convulsive disorders.
   d. Parkinson's disease.
   e. Organic brain syndrome.
   f. Stroke.
   g. Myasthenia gravis.
8. Oncology/hematology.
   a. Anemias.
   b. Leukemias.
   c. Lymphomas.
   d. Solid tumors.
   e. Bleeding disorders.
9. Endocrinology.
   a. Diabetic ketoacidosis.
   b. Nonketoic hyperosmolar coma.
   c. Diabetes mellitus.
      i. Type I.
      ii. Type II.
   d. Hypothyroidism.
   e. Hyperthyroidism.
   f. Syndrome of inappropriate antidiuretic hormone.
   g. Diabetes insipidus.
   h. Metabolic bone disease.
   i. Adrenal disorders.
10. Nutritional/fluid and electrolytes.
    a. Total parenteral nutrition.
    b. Enteral nutrition.
    c. Dehydration.
    d. Acid–base disturbances.
    e. Fluid and electrolyte balance.

The program should also focus on drug literature analysis and associated communication skills.

C. **Extramural Experiences.** When appropriate, rotations or visitations to other health-care settings should be scheduled to augment the resident's training. Extramural rotations may be conducted either as full-time training activities (e.g., for a 1-month block) or on a regularly scheduled part-time basis. If extramural rotations are scheduled for the purpose of pursuing one or more of the fundamental objectives outlined above, there must be a pharmacist-preceptor who has defined responsibilities for monitoring the resident's progress and evaluating his accomplishments. A detailed set of objectives for extramural rotations must be prepared in advance. Extramural rotations must represent not more than 25% of the resident's experience. The qualifications of the extramural training site are subject to review and approval by the American Society of Hospital Pharmacists.

D. **Research Projects.** The residency training schedule shall make provision for the resident's participation in a directed or collaborative clinical research project. The purpose of such activities is to teach the application of the scientific method. The resident should submit a final report of the project, which should be of publishable quality.

References

1. American Society of Hospital Pharmacists. ASHP accreditation standard for specialized pharmacy residency training (with guide to interpretation). *Am J Hosp Pharm*. 1980; 37:1229–32.
2. American Society of Hospital Pharmacists. ASHP minimum standard for pharmacies in institutions. *Am J Hosp Pharm*. 1977; 34:1356–8.

Approved by the ASHP Board of Directors, April 26, 1984. Developed by the ASHP SIG on Adult Clinical Pharmacy Practice and approved by the ASHP Commission on Credentialing.

The bibliographic citation for this document is as follows: American Society of Hospital Pharmacists. ASHP supplemental standard and learning objectives for residency training in adult internal medicine pharmacy practice. *Am J Hosp Pharm*. 1984; 41:1383–5.

ASHP Supplemental Standard and Learning Objectives for Residency Training in Psychopharmacy Practice

Preamble

Definition. A specialized residency in psychopharmacy practice is defined as an organized, directed postgraduate program that centers on developing the competencies necessary to provide pharmaceutical care to psychiatric patients.

Purpose and Philosophy. The supplemental residency standard establishes criteria for the training and education of pharmacists in the delivery of exemplary pharmaceutical care to psychiatric patients. A psychopharmacy practice residency embraces the concept that psychopharmacy practitioners share in the responsibility and accountability for optimal drug therapy outcomes in psychiatric patients. Therefore, residencies in psychopharmacy practice must provide residents with the opportunities to function independently as practitioners through conceptualizing, integrating, and transforming accumulated experience and knowledge into improved drug therapy for psychiatric patients.

Accreditation Authority. The ASHP Accreditation Standard for Specialized Pharmacy Residency Training,[1] taken together with this supplement, are the basic criteria used to evaluate psychopharmacy pharmacy practice residency training programs applying for accreditation by the ASHP.

Qualifications of the Training Site. The training site must meet the requirements set forth in Part I of the ASHP Accreditation Standard for Specialized Pharmacy Residency Training. Facilities may include, but are not limited to, mental health institutions, or general hospitals or multihospital systems that provide extensive psychiatric services. Ancillary facilities such as outpatient treatment units may be used, as appropriate, in pursuing the objectives for training outlined in the goals and objectives.

Qualifications of the Pharmacy Service. If the residency is conducted as part of a pharmacy service in a health care organization, the pharmacy services must meet the requirements set forth in Part IV of the Accreditation Standard for Specialized Pharmacy Residency Training. The facility where the residency program is conducted must have at least one pharmacist with an established clinical practice in psychopharmacy.

Qualifications of the Program Director. The program director's qualifications shall meet the requirements set forth in Part II of the ASHP Accreditation Standard for Specialized Pharmacy Residency Training. The program director shall demonstrate proficiency as a clinical pharmacist in the area of psychopharmacy practice and shall be accessible for resident supervision. A multisite residency program shall have one designated residency program director whose appointment shall be agreed to in writing by each of the participating practice sites.

Selection and Qualifications of the Resident. The resident must meet the requirements set forth in the ASHP Accreditation Standard for Specialized Pharmacy Residency Training.

Supplemental Goals and Objectives

Goals

1. Conduct direct patient care activities for psychiatric patients, using a consistent approach that reflects the philosophy of pharmaceutical care and that is performed with efficiency and depth of experience characteristic of a psychiatric pharmacist.
2. Identify the appropriate roles of the pharmacist and others on the health care team in delivery of care to the psychiatric patient.
3. Identify psychiatric patients' health care needs.
4. Prepare patient-specific databases for patients that meet the pharmacist's needs for devising a patient care plan.
5. Provide input into the diagnostic process.
6. Appraise existing drug therapy of patients with mental disorders to determine the appropriateness of drug, dose, dosage regimen, route or method of administration, compliance, drug interactions, therapeutic duplications, therapeutic outcomes, and cost, and to avoid adverse drug reactions and other complications.
7. Participate in patients' psychotherapeutic treatment plans.
8. Specify treatment goals for psychiatric patients that consider patient-, disease-, and drug-specific information and ethical considerations.
9. Design pharmacotherapeutic regimens to achieve patient-specific treatment goals for psychiatric patients.
10. Recommend pharmacotherapeutic regimens to treatment teams and patients.
11. Design monitoring plans that effectively measure the achievement of treatment goals and take into account patient-specific factors.
12. Evaluate the outcomes of implementing psychiatric patients' pharmacotherapeutic regimens.
13. Ensure, whenever possible, continuity of pharmaceutical care of psychiatric patients to and from the institutional and noninstitutional patient care settings.
14. Provide individualized medication-use education to psychiatric patients and their caregivers, when applicable.
15. Document all pharmaceutical care activities appropriately.
16. Contribute to the psychiatric training of pharmacy students and other health care professionals and supportive personnel.
17. Deliver effective education on psychiatric topics to patients, the public, and health care professionals.
18. Design and execute a project or investigation in which application of the scientific method is demonstrated.
19. Select a core library appropriate for a psychiatric practice setting.
20. Stay current with psychiatric drug therapy literature.
21. Provide concise, applicable, and timely responses to requests for psychiatric drug information from health care providers and patients.
22. Provide inservice education on psychiatric pharmacy

topics to physicians, nurses, and other practitioners.

23. Deliver public awareness programs, when possible, that focus on the early recognition and treatment of mental disorders.

24. Participate in the ongoing revision of the drug formulary of an organized mental health care setting.

25. Participate in the development or modification of selected policies for the selection and use of drugs in the organized mental health care setting.

26. Participate in the ongoing modification of a drug-use evaluation (DUE) program in an organized mental health care setting.

27. Display compassion for patients.

28. Communicate clearly, orally and in writing.

29. Maximize work efficiency through the use of computers.

30. Recognize the importance of the history of psychopharmacy practice.

Core Goals

(Taken from Pharmacy Practice set of Model Goals and Objectives)

1. Take personal responsibility for improving the pharmaceutical care of patients.
2. Maintain a professional image.
3. Establish a commitment to life-long learning.
4. Maintain active involvement in local, state, and national pharmacy organizations.
5. Work to resolve practice problems efficiently.
6. Demonstrate ethical conduct in all activities related to pharmacy practice.
7. Maintain confidentiality of patient information.
8. Manage time effectively.
9. Work harmoniously on various committees in the organized mental health care setting.
10. Manage change effectively.
11. Model a practice management philosophy that supports pharmaceutical care and pharmacy practice excellence.
12. Evaluate current pharmacy services to determine if the services are meeting the health care needs of the patients.
13. Utilize systems used to document and report pharmacy patient care outcomes.
14. Judge each practice management issue for its relative importance to all other practice management issues and prioritize accordingly.
15. Contribute to the achievement of pharmacy goals through effective participation on an organization's committees.
16. Assist in ensuring departmental compliance with accreditation, legal, regulatory, and safety requirements (e.g., JCAHO requirements; ASHP standards, statements, and guidelines; state and federal laws regulating pharmacy practice; OSHA regulations).
17. Understand methods used to monitor and evaluate drug costs.
18. Participate in the management of the practice area's human resources.
19. Participate in the departmental quality improvement program.
20. Understand the appropriate relationship between the pharmacist and the pharmaceutical industry.

21. Assist in developing proposals for a new service.
22. Resolve conflicts through negotiation.
23. Work through the political and decision-making structure to accomplish one's practice area goals.
24. Participate in the pharmacy department's planning process.
25. Detect patterns in the occurrence of significant medication errors that signal the need to develop mechanisms to prevent their recurrence.
26. Manage the use of investigational drugs according to established protocols and the organized health care setting's policies and procedures.
27. Participate in the development and implementation of selected pharmacy department's policies and procedures.

Objectives Associated with Goal Statements. The following are Terminal Objectives (TO) and Enabling Objectives (EO) associated with each goal statement.

Goal 1. Conduct direct patient care activities for psychiatric patients, using a consistent approach that reflects the philosophy of pharmaceutical care and that is performed with efficiency and depth of experience characteristic of an experienced psychiatric pharmacist.

TO 1.1 (Synthesis) Devise efficient strategies for one's own direct patient care activities that maximize the delivery of appropriate pharmaceutical care to each psychiatric patient.

TO 1.2 (Synthesis) Formulate solutions to complex psychiatric patient care problems that maximize the achievement of pharmaceutical care outcomes.

Goal 2. Identify the appropriate roles of the pharmacist and others on the health care team in delivery of care to the psychiatric patient.

TO 2.1 (Synthesis) Devise a plan for managing psychiatric patients' health care needs that matches patients with appropriate members of the health care team.

EO 2.1.1 (Comprehension) Discuss the scope of psychopharmacy practice.

EO 2.1.2 (Comprehension) Discuss the multiple roles that a psychiatric pharmacist may fulfill.

EO 2.1.3 (Comprehension) Discuss the settings in which psychiatric pharmacists serve.

EO 2.1.4 (Comprehension) Discuss the interface of psychiatric pharmacy practice and psychiatry.

EO 2.1.5 (Comprehension) Discuss the roles of other members of a psychiatric patient treatment team.

EO 2.1.6 (Comprehension) Discuss the interrelationship of the pharmacist's patient care activities with those of other members of the psychiatric patient treatment team.

Goal 3. Identify psychiatric patients' health care needs.

TO 3.1 (Evaluation) Using a patient-specific database, summarize psychiatric patients' health care needs.

EO 3.1.1 (Comprehension) Describe psychosocial and environmental factors affecting the delivery of health care that should be considered when defining the health care needs of psychiatric patients.

Goal 4. Prepare patient-specific databases for patients that meet the pharmacist's needs for devising a patient care plan.

TO 4.1 (Synthesis) Generate patient-specific databases that meet the pharmacist's needs for making drug therapy recommendations for psychiatric patients.

EO 4.1.1 (Comprehension) Discuss the importance of including findings from a mental status examination, physical assessment, rating scale data, neurological assessment, psychosocial and rehabilitative evaluations, medicolegal documents, and compliance assessment when building a patient-specific database for a psychiatric patient.

EO 4.1.2 (Application) Use medical charts or records to identify information that may be pertinent to decisions on desired pharmacotherapeutic outcomes for psychiatric patients.

EO 4.1.2.1 (Application) Use standard medical terminology and abbreviations specific to mental health.

EO 4.1.2.2 (Application) Locate information required for a psychiatric patient-specific database that is contained in a mental status examination, physical assessment rating scales, neurobiologic assessments, psychosocial and rehabilitative evaluations, medicolegal documents, and compliance assessments.

EO 4.1.3 (Synthesis) Formulate an interview approach for patients, caregivers, family, health care professionals, or others that employs effective communication techniques to obtain information for a psychiatric patient's database.

EO 4.1.3.1 (Synthesis) When presented with a limited time frame, structure an interview that elicits maximum pertinent information from a patient who presents with functional or cognitive psychopathology.

EO 4.1.3.2 (Synthesis) When presented with a patient with an unknown history, formulate an interview strategy that will accommodate unknown patient characteristics.

EO 4.1.3.3 (Application) Use the principles of prevention and management of aggressive behavior, a basic understanding of the psychodynamics of human behavior, and the influence of the milieu and psychosocial stressors to formulate an interview approach for psychiatric patients.

EO 4.1.4 (Evaluation) Interpret observed patient behavior and interactions with others to collect data for a patient-specific database.

EO 4.1.5 (Synthesis) Devise strategies that maximize the reliability of results when administering standardized psychiatric and neurobiologic rating scales to patients.

EO 4.1.5.1 (Application) Use accepted procedures to administer and interpret standardized psychiatric rating scales and neurologic assessments.

EO 4.1.6 (Analysis) Determine the most likely reliable source of desired information to be gathered for a psychiatric patient's database.

EO 4.1.6.1 (Comprehension) Discuss factors that influence the reliability of sources of information of psychiatric patients.

EO 4.1.6.2 (Evaluation) Appraise the reliability of the psychiatric patient as a historian, including self-reports of compliance and medical or psychiatric history.

Goal 5. Provide input into the diagnostic process.

TO 5.1 (Evaluation) Integrate knowledge of the patient's target symptoms, longitudinal course, and other diagnostic techniques to assist in the formulation of a diagnosis.

EO 5.1.1 (Evaluation) Identify drug-responsive target symptoms for a psychiatric patient.

EO 5.1.1.1 (Comprehension) Discuss the concept of target symptoms.

EO 5.1.1.2 (Comprehension) Discuss the target symptom approach to the management of psychiatric patients.

EO 5.1.1.3 (Comprehension) Discuss the relative responsiveness of target symptoms to drug therapy.

EO 5.1.2 (Comprehension) Discuss the standardized categorization of mental disorders (e.g., the current edition of Diagnostic and Statistical Manual for Mental Disorders).

EO 5.1.3 (Comprehension) Discuss diagnostic criteria, including inherent controversies, for major mental disorders.

EO 5.1.4 (Comprehension) Discuss the relevance of neuroimaging studies, neurobiological laboratory findings, and other technologies in formulating a diagnosis.

Goal 6. Appraise existing drug therapy of patients with mental disorders to determine the appropriateness of drug, dose, dosage regimen and route or method of administration, compliance, drug interactions, therapeutic duplications, therapeutic outcomes, and cost, and to avoid adverse drug reactions and other complications.

TO 6.1 (Evaluation) Appraise existing drug therapy of patients with mental disorders using the patient-specific database and a benefit/risk analysis to determine the appropriateness of drug, dose, dosage regimen, route or method of administration, compliance, drug interactions, therapeutic duplications, therapeutic outcomes, and cost and to avoid adverse drug reactions and other complications.

EO 6.1.1 (Comprehension) Compare patient outcomes that are feasible in institutional versus noninstitutional settings.

EO 6.1.1.1 (Comprehension) Compare patient outcomes that are realistic for the acutely ill versus chronically ill patient and for the behaviorally stable versus unstable patient.

EO 6.1.2 (Comprehension) Discuss the conceptual framework, predisposing factors, age of onset, signs and symptoms, pathophysiology, clinical course, etiology, and treatment of diseases commonly encountered in the psychiatric setting.

EO 6.1.3 (Comprehension) Discuss the clinical application(s), method of administration, pharmacokinetics, pharmacology, therapeutic drug monitoring, and adverse effects and toxicity of CNS drugs.

EO 6.1.4 (Evaluation) Prioritize psychiatric patients' pharmacotherapy problems.

Goal 7. Participate in patients' psychotherapeutic treatment plans.

TO 7.1 (Application) Use psychotherapeutic and psychodynamic techniques to interact with psychiatric patients.

EO 7.1.1 (Comprehension) Discuss individual and group psychotherapeutic and psychodynamic techniques.

EO 7.1.2 (Comprehension) Discuss the factors to consider for using various individual and group psychotherapeutic and psychodynamic techniques.

Goal 8. Specify treatment goals for psychiatric patients that consider patient-, disease-, and drug-specific information and ethical considerations.

TO 8.1 (Synthesis) Specify treatment goals for psychiatric patients that integrate patient-specific, disease-specific, and drug-specific information, quality of life, and ethical considerations.

EO 8.1.1 (Application) Use skill in the performance of a quality-of-life assessment on a patient.

EO 8.1.2 (Comprehension) Compare and contrast the realistic limits of treatment outcomes in institutional versus noninstitutional settings.

EO 8.1.2.1 (Comprehension) Compare limits of treatment outcomes that are realistic for the acutely ill versus chronically ill and for the behaviorally stable versus unstable patient.

EO 8.1.3 (Comprehension) Discuss situations in which pharmacotherapy is secondary to overall patient treatment outcomes.

EO 8.1.3.1 (Comprehension) Discuss common forms of nondrug therapy used in the treatment of psychiatric and developmental disorders.

Goal 9. Design pharmacotherapeutic regimens to achieve patient-specific treatment goals for psychiatric patients.

TO 9.1 (Synthesis) Design or modify a psychiatric patient's pharmacotherapeutic regimen, using current drug knowledge, to meet treatment goals.

EO 9.1.1 (Comprehension) Discuss the use of psychoactive medications for non-FDA-approved indications.

Goal 10. Recommend pharmacotherapeutic regimens to treatment teams and patients.

TO 10.1 (Application) Recommend a pharmacotherapeutic regimen to the treatment team and patient in a way that is systematic and logical and secures consensus from the team and patient.

EO 10.1.1 (Comprehension) Discuss the process for the implementation and initiation of a patient-specific drug regimen.

EO 10.1.2 (Comprehension) Discuss various practice models that include pharmacist-initiated drug therapy orders.

Goal 11. Design monitoring plans that effectively measure the achievement of treatment goals, that prevent or minimize adverse reactions and drug interactions, and that take into account patient-specific factors.

TO 11.1 (Synthesis) Design monitoring plans for pharmacotherapeutic regimens that use a risk/benefit analysis that effectively evaluates achievement of the patient-specific treatment goals.

EO 11.1.1 (Evaluation) Select monitoring parameters for various patient populations, including but not limited to geriatrics, pediatrics, adolescents, chemically dependent patients, medically compromised patients, treatment-refractory populations, and patients with developmental disorders.

EO 11.1.1.1 (Comprehension) Discuss unique monitoring parameters specific for various patient populations, including but not limited to geriatrics, pediatrics, adolescents, chemically dependent patients, medically compromised patients, treatment-refractory populations, and patients with developmental disorders.

EO 11.1.2 (Evaluation) Select psychosocial factors pertinent for a particular psychiatric patient in the construction of a monitoring plan.

EO 11.1.2.1 (Comprehension) Discuss the psychosocial factors to be considered when constructing a monitoring plan for a psychiatric patient.

EO 11.1.3 (Evaluation) Describe the likelihood of a patient's compliance with a monitoring plan.

EO 11.1.3.1 (Comprehension) Discuss the importance of considering the psychiatric patient's health care beliefs when identifying issues of compliance.

EO 11.1.4 (Analysis) Identify sources of data for measuring the selected parameters.

EO 11.1.5 (Synthesis) Define a desirable value range for each selected parameter.

Goal 12. Evaluate the outcomes of implementing psychiatric patients' pharmacotherapeutic regimens.

TO 12.1 (Evaluation) Interpret the relevance of each measured parameter in a monitoring plan when compared with the desired values.

EO 12.1.1 (Comprehension) Discuss setting-specific policies and procedures, including laboratory tests, for monitoring drug therapy.

EO 12.1.2 (Comprehension) Describe factors that may contribute to unreliability of monitoring results (e.g., patient-specific factors, timing of monitoring tests, equipment errors, outpatient versus inpatient monitoring).

TO 12.2 (Synthesis) Modify a pharmacotherapeutic regimen as necessary, based on evaluation of objective and subjective findings.

Goal 13. Ensure, whenever possible, continuity of pharmaceutical care of psychiatric patients to and from the institutional and noninstitutional patient care settings.

TO 13.1 (Application) Use a systematic procedure to communicate pertinent pharmacotherapeutic information in patients' transition to and from institutional to noninstitutional patient care settings, whenever possible.

EO 13.1.1 (Comprehension) Discuss frameworks for the provision of psychiatric care and availability of patient-support systems.

Goal 14. Provide individualized medication-use education to psychiatric patients and their caregivers, when applicable.

TO 14.1 (Synthesis) Design individualized medication education for psychiatric patients and their caregivers, when applicable.

EO 14.1.1 (Analysis) Delineate information to include when providing medication education for psychiatric patients (e.g., side effects, indications, precautions).

EO 14.1.2 (Comprehension) Discuss the impact of the patient's mental status in defining the patient's medication education needs.

EO 14.1.3 (Comprehension) Discuss various psychotherapeutic techniques, including group therapy, that can be used to provide medication education.

TO 14.2 (Application) Use skill in individual and group techniques to provide effective medication education to a variety of psychiatric patients.

Goal 15. Document all pharmaceutical care activities appropriately.

TO 15.1 (Organization) Integrate documentation into all pharmaceutical care activities.

EO 15.1.1 (Application) Use site-specific format for recording the results of a psychopharmacy consultation.

EO 15.1.2 (Application) Use site-specific format for recording progress notes in the medical chart.

EO 15.1.3 (Application) Use site-specific format for recording patient findings (e.g., rating scales, mental status examinations).

Goal 16. Contribute to the psychiatric training of pharmacy students and other health care professionals and supportive personnel.

TO 16.1 (Application) Use sound educational techniques to teach psychiatric topics to pharmacy students, other health care professionals, and supportive personnel.

Goal 17. Deliver effective education on psychiatric topics to patients, the public, and health care professionals.

TO 17.1 (Application) Use effective educational techniques in all training and educational activities.

Goal 18. Design and execute a project or investigation in which application of the scientific method is demonstrated.

TO 18.1 (Synthesis) Design, alone or in conjunction with others, a project or investigation in which application of the scientific method is demonstrated.

EO 18.1.1 (Analysis) Identify potential issues that need to be studied.

EO 18.1.2 (Comprehension) Use a systematic procedure for performing a comprehensive literature search.

EO 18.1.3 (Synthesis) Generate questions to be answered by the project.

EO 18.1.4 (Synthesis) Design a project that will answer the questions identified.

TO 18.2 (Application) Execute a project or investigation, alone or in conjunction with others, in which application of the scientific method is demonstrated.

Goal 19. Select a core library appropriate for a psychiatric practice setting.

TO 19.1 (Application) Use a knowledge of standard references to select a core library of primary, secondary, and tertiary references appropriate for a psychiatric practice setting.

Goal 20. Stay current with psychiatric drug therapy literature.

TO 20.1 (Characterization) Adhere to a plan for staying current with psychiatric drug therapy literature.

Goal 21. Provide concise, applicable, and timely responses to requests for psychiatric drug information from health care providers and patients.

TO 21.1 (Evaluation) Determine from all available patient data and drug literature the appropriate information needed to respond to drug information requests.

TO 21.2 (Application) Use skill in drug literature evaluation to determine the quality of data gathered to respond to drug information requests.

TO 21.3 (Synthesis) Formulate responses to drug information requests based on analysis of the literature, patient-specific databases, or both.

TO 21.4 (Application) Prepare responses to drug information requests in the accepted format of the organized health care setting.

Goal 22. Provide inservice education on psychopharmacy topics to physicians, nurses, and other practitioners.

TO 22.1 (Synthesis) Design effective inservice education on psychopharmacy topics for physicians, nurses, and other practitioners on drug therapy issues.

Goal 23. Deliver public awareness programs, when possible, that focus on the early recognition, prevention, and treatment options of mental disorders.

TO 23.1 (Application) Use effective educational techniques to deliver public awareness programs, when possible, that focus on the early recognition, prevention, and treatment options of mental disorders.

Goal 24. Participate in the ongoing revision of the drug formulary of an organized mental health care setting.

TO 24.1 (Application) Use established concepts and principles to revise or implement the drug formulary of an organized mental health care setting.

Goal 25. Participate in the development or modification of selected policies for the selection and use of drugs in the organized mental health care setting.

TO 25.1 (Synthesis) Revise policies for the selection and use of drugs in the organized mental health care setting.

Goal 26. Participate in the ongoing modification of a drug-use evaluation (DUE) program in an organized mental health care setting.

TO 26.1 (Application) Use a knowledge of the factors that affect the design and implementation of an organized mental health care setting's drug-use evaluation (DUE) program to design a DUE.

Goal 27. Display compassion for patients.

TO 27.1 (Organization) Combine compassion with the delivery of pharmaceutical services.

EO 27.1.1 (Comprehension) Discuss the psychodynamics involved in displaying compassion and/or empathy toward psychiatric patients.

Goal 28. Communicate clearly, orally and in writing.

TO 28.1 (Synthesis) Organize all written or oral communication in a logical manner.

TO 28.2 (Application) Address all communication at the level appropriate for the audience.

TO 28.3 (Application) Use correct grammar, punctuation, spelling, style, and formatting conventions in the preparation of all written communications.

TO 28.4 (Complex Overt Response) Speak clearly and distinctly.

TO 28.5 (Application) Use public speaking skills to speak effectively in large and small group situations.

TO 28.6 (Application) Use listening skills consistently in the performance of job functions.

TO 28.7 (Application) Use a knowledge of the applicability of specific visual aids to enhance the effectiveness of communication.

TO 28.8 (Application) When appropriate, use persuasive communication techniques that maximize the possibility that the psychiatric patient will comply with the requested treatment plan.

TO 28.9 (Organization) Prepare all communications so that they reflect a positive image of pharmacy.

TO 28.10 (Application) Use effective strategies for communicating with patients who are non-English-speakers or who are impaired.

Goal 29. Maximize work efficiency through the use of computers.

TO 29.1 (Application) Demonstrate use of the computer in performing practice responsibilities.

EO 29.1.1 (Application) Use knowledge of medical information systems for psychiatric drug information to perform practice responsibilities.

Goal 30. Recognize the importance of the history of psychopharmacy practice.

TO 30.1 (Comprehension) Describe elements in the history of psychopharmacy practice that have contributed to the evolution of the practice.

EO 30.1.1 (Knowledge) State the history of psychopharmacy practice residency programs.

Core Goals and Objectives

(Taken from Pharmacy Practice set of Model Goals and Objectives)[a]

Goal 1. Take personal responsibility for improving the pharmaceutical care of patients.

TO 1.1 (Characterization) Prepare self to improve the pharmaceutical care of patients.

EO 1.1.1 (Characterization) Use a systematic, ongoing process to evaluate one's level of professional development and accomplish the learning needs required to provide excellent pharmaceutical care.

Goal 2. Maintain a professional image.

TO 2.1 (Application) Dress in attire that conveys a professional image.

TO 2.2 (Characterization) Consistently maintain personal self-control and professional decorum.

Goal 3. Establish a commitment to life-long learning.

TO 3.1 (Characterization) Use a systematic, on-going process to self-assess and meet learning needs.

Goal 4. Maintain active involvement in local, state, and national pharmacy organizations.

TO 4.1 (Application) Demonstrate an awareness for the importance of membership in pharmacy organizations by being actively involved in local, state, and national pharmacy associations.

Goal 5. Work to resolve practice problems efficiently.

TO 5.1 (Application) Demonstrate consistent use of a systematic approach to problem-solving.

TO 5.2 (Application) Use consensus building skills.

Goal 6. Demonstrate ethical conduct in all activities related to pharmacy practice.

TO 6.1 (Characterization) Act ethically in the conduct of all pharmacy practice activities.

Goal 7. Maintain confidentiality of patient information.

TO 7.1 (Application) Observe legal and ethical guidelines for safeguarding the confidentiality of patient information.

Goal 8. Manage time effectively.

TO 8.1 (Application) Use time management techniques to efficiently accomplish job responsibilities.

Goal 9. Work harmoniously on various committees in the organized mental health care setting.

TO 9.1 (Application) Use a knowledge of interpersonal skills to effectively manage working relationships.

Goal 10. Manage change effectively.

TO 10.1 (Application) Use a knowledge of the principles of change management to direct change to achieve departmental goals.

Goal 11. Model a practice management philosophy that supports pharmaceutical care and pharmacy practice excellence.

TO 11.1 (Characterization) Demonstrate leadership in fostering the philosophy of practice excellence in others.

Goal 12. Evaluate current pharmacy services to determine if the services are meeting the health care needs of the patients.

TO 12.1 (Evaluation) Appraise the organization's current pharmacy services for adequacy in meeting the health care needs of patients.

Goal 13. Utilize systems designed to document and report pharmacy patient care outcomes.

TO 13.1 (Comprehension) Describe the process of designing a system to report and document pharmacy patient care outcomes.

TO 13.2 (Application) Maintain an existing system that documents and reports pharmacy patient care outcomes.

Goal 14. Judge each practice management issue for its relative importance to all other practice management issues and prioritize accordingly.

TO 14.1 (Evaluation) Appraise practice management issues for their relative importance.

Goal 15. Contribute to the achievement of pharmacy goals through effective participation on an organization's committees.

TO 15.1 (Application) Use group participation skills when working on an organization's committees.

Goal 16. Assist in ensuring departmental compliance with accreditation, legal, regulatory, and safety requirements (e.g., JCAHO requirements; ASHP standards, statements, and guidelines; state and federal laws regulating pharmacy practice; OSHA regulations).

TO 16.1 (Comprehension) Discuss the effect upon practice area functions of accreditation, legal, regulatory, and safety requirements.

Goal 17. Understand methods used to monitor and evaluate drug costs.

TO 17.1 (Comprehension) Discuss the use of several methods used to monitor and evaluate drug costs.

Goal 18. Participate in the management of the practice area's human resources.

TO **18.1** (Comprehension) Describe recruitment strategies for a specific position.

TO **18.2** (Comprehension) Discuss the process used to interview and recommend practice area personnel for employment.

TO **18.3** (Comprehension) Describe the importance of orientation and training for practice area personnel.

TO **18.4** (Comprehension) Describe the components of a practice area employee evaluation system.

TO **18.5** (Comprehension) Discuss the principles and application of a progressive discipline process.

Goal 19. Participate in the departmental quality improvement program.

TO **19.1** (Application) Apply the guidelines of the department's quality improvement program to ensure quality improvement in assigned areas.

Goal 20. Understand the appropriate relationship between the pharmacist and the pharmaceutical industry.

TO **20.1** (Comprehension) Describe the role of the pharmacist in establishing policies for working with the pharmaceutical industry.

Goal 21. Assist in developing proposals for a new service.

TO **21.1** (Comprehension) Discuss the process for developing a proposal for a new service.

Goal 22. Resolve conflicts through negotiation.

TO **22.1** (Application) Use effective negotiation skills to resolve conflicts.

Goal 23. Work through the political and decision-making structure to accomplish one's practice area goals.

TO **23.1** (Application) Use knowledge of an organization's political and decision-making structure to influence accomplishing a practice area goal.

Goal 24. Participate in the pharmacy department's planning process.

TO **24.1** (Application) Participate in selected activities contributing to the development of the pharmacy department's objectives.

Goal 25. Detect patterns in the occurrence of significant medication errors that signal the need to develop mechanisms to prevent their recurrence.

TO **25.1** (Synthesis) Determine situations in which a medication error significantly impacts patient outcomes to justify the need to develop new mechanisms (e.g., additional polices and/or procedures) to prevent their recurrence.

Goal 26. Manage the use of investigational drugs according to established protocols, industry and governmental regulations, and the organized health care setting's policies and procedures.

TO **26.1** (Application) Manage the use of investigational drugs according to established protocols, industry and governmental regulations, and the organized health care setting's policies and procedures.

Goal 27. Participate in the development and implementation of selected pharmacy department's policies and procedures.

TO **27.1** (Application) Use standard management principles to develop selected policies and procedures that meet the needs of the pharmacy department.

Core Experiences in Direct Patient Care

For each of the following psychiatric, neurological, and developmental disorders, the resident should be able to describe pharmacotherapeutic treatments, their potential alternatives, and monitoring parameters for therapeutic effects and adverse reactions or toxicity:

1. Schizophrenia and other psychoses.
2. Mood disorders.
3. Anxiety disorders.
4. Sleep disorders.
5. Psychoactive substance-use disorders (including information on routes of administration of psychoactive substances and common street names).
6. Personality disorders.
7. Psychiatric disorders in the elderly.
8. Psychiatric disorders in children and adolescents.
9. Neurological disorders.
10. Developmental disorders.
11. Syndromes associated with aggression, hostility, and agitation.

The program coordinator should develop an experiential plan at the beginning of the program for each resident. The experiential component shall consist of the following required, selected, or elective learning experiences. The needs and interests of each resident and the attributes of the residency program should be utilized in the development of the experiential plan.

A. *Required Learning Experiences.* The resident's training shall include rotations or blocks of training in the following required areas:
   1. Adult inpatient psychiatry
   2. Outpatient clinic or day treatment center
B. *Selected Learning Experiences.* Two rotations from the following five areas shall be selected:
   1. Child and adolescent psychiatry
   2. Developmental disabilities
   3. Geriatric psychiatry
   4. Neurology
   5. Substance abuse treatment
C. *Elective Experiences.* Rotations in the following areas may be taken as electives:
   1. Administration
   2. Affective disorders
   3. Chronic or extended psychiatric care
   4. Consult and liaison psychiatry
   5. Eating disorders
   6. Emergency psychiatry
   7. Forensic psychiatry
   8. Intermediate psychiatric care
   9. Pregnancy and postpartum psychiatric disorders
   10. Psychopharmacology laboratory and pharmacokinetics
   11. Research
   12. Sleep disorders
   13. Other

Reference

1. American Society of Hospital Pharmacists. ASHP accreditation standard for specialized pharmacy residency training. *Am J Hosp Pharm* 1994; 51:2034–41.

ªDraft Goals and Objectives for Residencies in Pharmacy Practice, under review by the Commission on Credentialing.

Approved by the ASHP Board of Directors, April 27, 1994. Developed by a working group of ASHP psychopharmacy practitioners and the ASHP Commission on Credentialing. For currently existing programs, this revision of the accreditation standard takes effect April 27, 1995. Until that time, the current standard, which was approved March 20, 1980, is in force.

The bibliographic citation for this document is as follows: ASHP supplemental standard and learning objectives for residency training in psychopharmacy practice. In: Practice Standards of ASHP 1994–95. Hicks WE, ed. Bethesda, MD: American Society of Hospital Pharmacists; 1994.

ASHP Supplemental Standard and Learning Objectives for Residency Training in Hospital Pharmacy Administration

Introduction

Definition. A specialized residency in hospital pharmacy administration is defined as an organized, directed, postgraduate program of practical experience in hospital pharmacy administration.

Accreditation Authority. The "ASHP Accreditation Standard for Specialized Pharmacy Residency Training,"[1] together with this Supplemental Standard, sets forth the basic criteria to be used in the evaluation of such programs in hospitals applying for accreditation by the American Society of Hospital Pharmacists. Other elements of accreditation authority are specified in the "ASHP Accreditation Standard for Specialized Pharmacy Residency Training."

Application of the Standard. The manner in which this Supplemental Standard will be interpreted is specified in the "ASHP Accreditation Standard for Specialized Pharmacy Residency Training."

Part I—Qualifications of the Training Site

The training site must meet the requirements set forth in Part I of the "ASHP Accreditation Standard for Specialized Pharmacy Training."

Part II—Qualifications of the Pharmacy Service

A specialized residency in hospital pharmacy administration is predicated in large part on the service programs provided by the pharmacy department, since the resident must learn to manage these programs. It is essential that a broad scope of pharmacy services be provided by the hospital conducting such a residency program. Therefore, in addition to meeting the service requirements set forth in Part II of the "ASHP Accreditation Standard for Specialized Pharmacy Residency Training," *all areas* of the pharmacy service program also must comply with the provisions of Part II of the "ASHP Accreditation Standard for Hospital Pharmacy Residency Training."[2]

Further, the total number of residents must not exceed a level where close preceptorship by the department head is compromised.

Part III—Qualifications of the Program Director

Hospital pharmacy residency training programs are designed to train institutional pharmacy practitioners who have the competency to provide a wide range of professional services and to provide administrative support and direction to others. The only appropriate director of such a program, therefore, is the director of the pharmacy department in which the residency is based. It is this individual who sets the tone of the program through personal philosophy, personal beliefs, contributions to the profession, and sense of values.

In addition to meeting the requirements set forth in Part III of the "ASHP Accreditation Standard for Specialized Pharmacy Residency Training," the residency director shall have completed a hospital pharmacy residency accredited by ASHP (or obtained an equivalent level of practical experience) and shall have had at least 5 years of management experience at the assistant director level (or equivalent) or higher in a pharmacy meeting the requirements of the "ASHP Guidelines: Minimum Standard for Pharmacies in Institutions,"[3] 2 years of which shall have been as director.

Part IV—Selection and Qualifications of the Resident

In addition to meeting the requirements set forth in the "ASHP Accreditation Standard for Specialized Pharmacy Residency Training," the resident must have previously completed an ASHP-accredited hospital or clinical pharmacy residency training program or had an equivalent level of prior experience in hospital pharmacy practice.

This requirement does not preclude from consideration for accreditation those 2-year residency programs that accept residents who have not previously completed a hospital pharmacy or clinical pharmacy residency, provided that (1) the total number of hours of residency training time over the 2 years is at least 4000, (2) the first 2000 hours meet the requirements of the "ASHP Accreditation Standard for Hospital Pharmacy Residency Training,"[2] and (3) the remaining 2000 hours are devoted solely to the objectives for training set forth in Part V below.

Part V—Residency Training Program

Principle VA

The specialized residency training program shall be organized in accordance with sound educational principles.

A specialized residency program in hospital pharmacy administration must comply with the requirements set forth in Principle VA of the "ASHP Accreditation Standard for Specialized Pharmacy Residency Training."

Principle VB

The residency training program shall be predicated on the knowledge, attitudes, skills, and abilities required in contemporary hospital pharmacy management and administration.

Requirement

The training program shall provide for practical experiences in all functions of hospital pharmacy management and administration and for development of the knowledge and skills associated with those functions.

Interpretation. In addition to the requirements set forth in Principle VB of the "ASHP Accreditation Standard for Specialized Pharmacy Residency Training," a specialized residency program in hospital pharmacy administration must ensure that, through a combination of didactic training and experience, the resident shall achieve a level of competence consistent with the goals and objectives noted herein for such a program.

The primary teaching environment for the residency is the pharmacy department. It is thus critical that the resident first and foremost become thoroughly familiar with the structure, organization, governance, operations, policies, procedures, staff, history, plans, mission, strategies, and philosophy of the department and the hospital. This can be achieved by various mechanisms, which must be clearly delineated at the beginning of the resident's training. These training methodologies can consist of a combination of, but not limited to, the following: review of documents, discussions, lectures, conferences, site visits, scheduled rotations, attendance at meetings, interviews, and special projects. It is expected that the resident will also gain a working understanding of most institutional health-care environments. For example, a residency program conducted in a nonprofit hospital must also include adequate emphasis on issues of structure, organization, and philosophy in for-profit institutions. Similarly, programs conducted in specialized hospitals must make provisions to ensure that the resident has a thorough understanding and familiarity with other types of institutional pharmacy operations.

The program must, as a minimum, prepare the resident for practice at the management level in a wide variety of health-care settings. In addition to an academically well prepared and highly motivated resident, this requires a training program that helps the resident develop a sound philosophy of practice, maturity, creativity, judgment, and problem-solving skills. This level of skill and maturity can be achieved only in a program that emphasizes a high degree of direct involvement by the resident in the management of the department under the individual supervision of qualified preceptors and the director. The program must be designed to reduce the level of supervision and scrutiny gradually as the resident's skills and knowledge increase.

Learning Objectives

At the completion of the residency, the resident shall be able to

Human Resource Management

A. Analyze and develop manpower needs and develop a program to recruit, screen, interview, hire, orient, and train new employees.

B. Develop departmental guidelines to evaluate objectively performance appraisals, performance objectives, and disciplinary action.

C. Develop an employee incentive and retention program.

D. Implement an employee development program.

E. Make salary determinations and position classifications for new and promoted personnel based on a thorough understanding of the institution's wage and salary determination policy.

Financial Planning and Monitoring

A. Prepare a departmental capital, operational, revenue, and personnel budget, including but not limited to the following:

1. Current and forthcoming fiscal year's expenses by line item.

2. Supporting data and program justification using established productivity measurements.

3. Financial statements and related management reports.

4. Salary and nonsalary requirements for new or expanded programs and services.

5. Capital budget based on the best interest of the hospital, its patients, and the department.

6. Appropriate fee schedule for delineated services of the department.

Cost Accounting and Productivity

A. Maintain and analyze a manpower planning and productivity reporting program.

B. Identify and calculate costs of various pharmaceutical products and services.

C. Perform cost–benefit analysis of new pharmacy programs to be implemented and evaluate existing programs or services.

D. Develop and implement various cost-containment programs (i.e., target drug programs).

E. Investigate and prepare reports explaining and justifying variances in the monthly operating expense budget, using monthly and year-to-date figures.

Purchasing and Inventory Control

A. Develop and implement a purchasing program, including but not limited to the following:

1. A competitive bidding program.

2. A prime vendor or direct purchase agreement that would be advantageous to the department and the hospital.

B. Develop a system of drug purchasing, inventory, and management.

C. Develop a system of controlled substance distribution, purchasing, and inventory.

D. Develop a system of recordkeeping and documentation for all pharmaceutical purchases (i.e., audit trail).

E. Develop a quality-assurance (QA) program for pharmaceutical purchases, inventory management, and controlled substance distribution.

F. Evaluate alternative purchasing arrangements such as group purchasing.

Departmental Operations

A. Develop departmental policies and procedures and devise a plan for their implementation.

B. Develop new clinical and drug information service programs, including setting measurable goals and priorities for the provision of clinical and drug information services, cost justification of potential services, developing and implementing changes in physician prescribing habits, ensuring staff competence, and quality assurance.

C. Implement a quality-assurance program for the department that is integrated with the institution's quality-assurance program.

D. Develop or implement, or both, departmental safety and security programs.

E.   Develop and assess departmental goals and objectives consistent with the hospital's goals and objectives.

F.   Develop and implement a disaster preparedness program for the department.

G.   Develop a formulary control system, including but not limited to the following:
  1. Guidelines for drug use evaluation in the hospital.
  2. A program to handle nonformulary drug requests.
  3. A method of tracking nonformulary drug use in the hospital.
  4. A program (such as restricted drug categories) to influence prescribing behavior.

H.   Prepare the department for a Joint Commission on Accreditation of Healthcare Organizations (JCAHO) survey and effectively respond to any deficiencies cited.

I.   Evaluate the department's need for automated systems and implement those systems appropriately.

J.   Analyze the need for, develop, and implement diversified pharmaceutical services.

K.   Develop plan(s) to market new pharmacy program(s) within the institution.

Areas of Emphasis

The resident shall receive orientation, instruction, and experience leading to competence in, but not limited to, the following aspects of hospital pharmacy management and administration:[a]

A.   Hospital organization—corporate structure of hospitals (for-profit and not-for-profit), subsidiary corporations (e.g., home health-care facilities and emergency centers), multihospital systems, and managed care systems, including responsibilities of professional department heads in the hospital and organizational structure.

B.   Mission statements of the hospital and the pharmacy department and how these interrelate.

C.   Planning (developing a plan for achieving the department's mission)—goals and objectives, needs assessment, priorities, cost analysis, timetables, and assessing new markets for pharmacy services.

D.   Organization of the pharmacy service and its interrelationships with hospital administration, medical staff, nursing staff, and other departments.

E.   Human resource management:
  1. Federal, state, and local laws and/or policies as they pertain to personnel management.
  2. Hiring practices, recruitment, interviewing, and selection and orientation of professional and nonprofessional employees.
  3. Job descriptions, performance objectives, performance appraisals, and interviews for professional and nonprofessional staff.
  4. Employee morale and motivation.
  5. Collective bargaining and impact on employee–employer relationships.
  6. Various management approaches (e.g., participative and delegatory management styles) and the effectiveness of each.
  7. Staff training and development and continuing education programs.
  8. Determination of manpower needs and work schedule preparation. The resident should have ample opportunity to apply these skills through specific supervisory assignments (e.g., filling in during the absence of administrative or supervisory personnel).

F.   Managing financial resources:
  1. Determining departmental expenses and revenues.
  2. Policies and procedures for payment and other forms of reimbursement.
  3. Financial statements and related management reports.
  4. Budgeting—forecasting, preparing, controlling, and analyzing revenue and expense budgets.
  5. Cost–benefit analysis and cost-containment programs.
  6. Financial analysis of purchasing contracts.
  7. Pricing products and services.
  8. Forecasts for future needs (multilayer plan).

  The resident should have experience in maintaining the department's monthly financial statistics ledger and reports, designing and completing a financial audit, and participating in the budget preparation process and the total system of financial management.

G.   Purchasing and inventory management:
  1. Methods of maximizing competition in purchasing.
  2. Direct versus wholesale purchasing.
  3. Methods and criteria for evaluating multiple source drugs and vendor bid responses.
  4. Pharmacy purchasing procedures for ordering, executing purchase orders, and stat procurements, including the purchasing of controlled drugs and tax-free alcohol.
  5. Procedures for receiving drugs in terms of accuracy and security.
  6. Appropriate methods of defining the privileges and responsibilities of manufacturers' representatives within the hospital.
  7. Systems of inventory control used in pharmacy practice, including methods of setting inventory goals and achieving higher turnover rates and methods of handling return merchandise and drug recalls.
  8. Physical and perpetual inventory systems.
  9. Considerations of inhouse packaging, repackaging, and manufacturing.
  10. Considerations in the design of storage facilities for drugs.

  The resident should have experience in developing departmental purchasing strategies (group contracts and bids), buying for the department (e.g., filling in during the absence of the departmental buyer), and conducting the annual departmental physical inventory.

H.   Physical resources management:
  1. Efficient and productive use of space and facilities.
  2. Maintenance of existing facilities to comply with environmental safety standards.
  3. Planning for new facilities and evaluation and selection of equipment and supplies.
  4. Security considerations and systems.

I.   Departmental operations:

1. Laws, regulations, and standards affecting hospital pharmacy practice.
2. Policy and procedure manual—purposes, organization, and maintenance.
3. The formulary system—how it works, role of the pharmacy and therapeutics committee, and legal considerations in selection of therapeutic alternatives.
4. Administrative considerations of drug distribution and control systems—the department's goal (endpoint) for the drug distribution and control program, overall system design, special personnel considerations (e.g., use and supervision of technicians), special handling procedures (e.g., for controlled substances, intravenous solutions, investigational drugs, and cytotoxic agents), computer applications, quality assurance, patient safety, personnel safety, and security measures.
5. Administrative considerations of clinical and drug information service programs—departmental goals in these areas, setting priorities for the provision of clinical and drug information services, cost justification of potential services, computer applications, ensuring staff competence, and quality assurance.
6. Information management—applications of word processors and computers to pharmacy operations, including preparation of various management reports, formulary maintenance, inventory management, drug distribution applications, patient drug therapy monitoring, drug use review activities, and database services, among others.
7. Intradepartmental communications.
8. Quality-assurance programs, including those related to product quality.
9. Departmental safety and security.

J. The training program shall also provide for development of the resident's knowledge and skills in the following areas:
1. Communication—the resident should have assignments aimed at developing oral and written communication skills.
2. Problem solving and decisionmaking.
3. Methods used to evaluate health-care systems such as cost–benefit analysis and cost-effectiveness studies.
4. Leadership training.
5. Professional ethics.
6. Concept development.

Part VI—Certification

The residency graduate's competence shall be attested to by the health-care organization in accordance with Part VI of the "ASHP Accreditation Standard for Specialized Pharmacy Residency Training."

References

1. American Society of Hospital Pharmacists. ASHP accreditation standard for specialized pharmacy residency training. *Am J Hosp Pharm.* 1980; 37:1229–32.
2. American Society of Hospital Pharmacists. ASHP accreditation standard for hospital pharmacy residency training. *Am J Hosp Pharm.* 1985; 42:2008–18.
3. American Society of Hospital Pharmacists. ASHP guidelines: minimum standard for pharmacies in institutions. *Am J Hosp Pharm.* 1985; 42:372–5.

[a]At the discretion of the director, residents who through previous education and training can demonstrate a thorough knowledge of a specific area may not be required to complete that aspect of the curriculum.

Approved by the ASHP Board of Directors, April 28, 1988. Developed by the ASHP Commission on Credentialing. Supersedes the "ASHP Accreditation Standard for Advanced Residency in Hospital Pharmacy Administration," which was approved November 20–21, 1985. This revision of the Accreditation Standard takes effect immediately.

The bibliographic citation for this document is as follows: American Society of Hospital Pharmacists. ASHP supplemental standard and learning objectives for residency training in hospital pharmacy administration. *Am J Hosp Pharm.* 1988; 45:1930–3.

ASHP Supplemental Standard and Learning Objectives for Residency Training in Clinical Pharmacokinetics Practice

Introduction

Definition. A specialized residency in clinical pharmacokinetics practice is defined as an organized, directed, postgraduate program of practical experience in clinical pharmacokinetics practice.

Accreditation Authority. The "ASHP Accreditation Standard for Specialized Residency Training,"[1] together with this Supplemental Standard, sets forth the basic criteria used in evaluation of clinical pharmacokinetics residency training programs in health-care organizations applying for accreditation by the American Society of Hospital Pharmacists. Other elements of accreditation authority are specified in the "ASHP Accreditation Standard for Specialized Pharmacy Residency Training."

Application of the Standard. A specialized residency in clinical pharmacokinetics practice should be organized and conducted to develop expert skills and competency in this area of pharmacy practice. The manner in which this Supplemental Standard will be interpreted is specified in the "ASHP Accreditation Standard for Specialized Pharmacy Residency Training."

Part I—Qualifications of the Training Site

The training site must meet the requirements set forth in Part I of the "ASHP Accreditation Standard for Specialized Pharmacy Residency Training." Ancillary facilities (such as outpatient treatment units) may be used as appropriate in pursuing the objectives for training outlined below.

Part II—Qualifications of the Pharmacy Service

The pharmacy program in which the residency is based must meet the service requirements set forth in Part II of the "ASHP Accreditation Standard for Specialized Pharmacy Residency Training." An established clinical pharmacokinetics service must be an integral part of the department's overall pharmacy service program.

Part III—Qualifications of the Program Coordinator

The program coordinator's qualifications shall meet the requirements set forth in Part III of the "ASHP Accreditation Standard for Specialized Pharmacy Residency Training."

Part IV—Selection and Qualifications of the Resident

Selection and qualifications of the resident shall meet the requirements set forth in Part IV of the "ASHP Accreditation Standard for Specialized Pharmacy Residency Training."

Part V—Residency Training Program

Principle VA

The specialized residency training program shall be organized in accordance with sound educational principles.

A specialized residency program in clinical pharmacokinetics practice must comply with the requirements set forth in Principle VA of the "ASHP Accreditation Standard for Specialized Pharmacy Residency Training."

Principle VB

The residency training program shall be predicated on the knowledge, attitudes, skills, and abilities required in contemporary clinical pharmacokinetics practice.

Requirement

The training program shall provide for experiential training in clinical pharmacokinetics practice and for development of the knowledge and skills associated with those functions.

Interpretation. In addition to the requirements set forth in Principle VB of the "ASHP Accreditation Standard for Specialized Pharmacy Residency Training," a specialized residency program in clinical pharmacokinetics practice must ensure that, through a combination of didactic training and experience, the resident shall achieve a level of competence consistent with the goals and objectives noted herein for such a program. Advanced study in pharmacokinetic and pharmacodynamic principles, both theoretical and applied, should be strongly encouraged.

The resident's training shall include rotations or blocks of training in each of the following areas:

1. Wide variety of pediatric and adult inpatient and outpatient service areas (e.g., critical care units, medicine, surgery, and hemodialysis unit).
2. Elective rotations (jointly agreed on by the resident and the preceptor).
3. Clinical laboratory (or laboratories) performing drug analyses.
4. Interdepartmental and extramural rotations as needed to achieve the stated objectives.
5. Interdisciplinary continuing education activities such as participation at grand rounds, clinical conferences, and seminars.

I. *Learning Objectives*

At the completion of the residency, the resident shall be able to

1. Conduct a patient interview and interpret the results of the interview.

2. Conduct a pharmacokinetic and pharmacodynamic assessment of patients receiving drugs that have a narrow therapeutic index (relatively little difference between toxic and effective concentrations) or marked variability in their disposition.

3. Define the monitoring parameters to include drug concentrations as well as therapeutic endpoints for the safe and efficacious use of each drug used in a patient.

4. Devise an initial dosage regimen and monitoring strategy using pharmacokinetic principles and methods for drugs with a narrow therapeutic range or marked variability in their disposition.

5. Assess and monitor the clinical pharmacokinetics of drugs with a narrow therapeutic range or marked variability in their disposition, evaluate patient-specific pharmacokinetic parameter(s), and recommend modifications in drug therapy based on the changes in the patient's condition that alter drug pharmacokinetics.

6. Integrate pharmacodynamics and pharmacokinetics with the pathophysiology of a patient's disease(s).

7. Monitor patients for drug dose–concentration and concentration–effect responses.

8. Monitor drug therapy prospectively for potential drug–drug, drug–laboratory test, drug–diet, drug–disease state, and drug–condition interactions and recommend modifications in drug therapy, when appropriate, to minimize such interactions.

9. Monitor patients for adverse drug reactions and toxic responses using pharmacokinetic principles and measured drug concentrations.

10. Recommend appropriate revisions in drug therapy using pharmacokinetic principles when appropriate (e.g., any untoward drug effect has been detected, desired drug concentration not achieved, or therapeutic endpoint not achieved).

11. Take a medication history, assess the patient's attitude toward compliance, and evaluate the influence of these factors on measured drug concentrations and observed pharmacologic effects.

12. Provide patient counseling on the appropriate drug use.

13. Provide informal and formal education services on pharmacokinetic and pharmacodynamic principles to students and professional staff members using appropriate teaching methods.

14. Serve on the health-care team providing primary or consultative care through the applications of clinical pharmacokinetic principles to individual patients receiving drugs with a narrow therapeutic index.

15. Prospectively formulate and recommend individualized drug dosage regimens based on the pharmacokinetic principles of the drug, the purpose of the medication, concurrent diseases and drug therapy, and the patient's clinical database.

16. Demonstrate competency in devising individualized dosage regimens using pharmacokinetic models and various support systems (e.g., handheld calculators, microcomputers, or mainframe computers).

17. Recommend the adjustment of dosage regimens in response to drug concentrations or other biochemical or clinical markers.

18. Recommend appropriate blood sampling times and analytical methodologies for individualizing patient drug therapy.

19. Describe the clinical manifestations of the potential toxicities associated with a patient's medication, assess the cause of the toxicity using pharmacokinetic and pharmacodynamic principles, and recommend the appropriate course of action.

20. Develop and conduct a protocol to characterize the pharmacokinetics of a drug in the clinical setting.

21. Evaluate drug studies reported in the biopharmaceutic and pharmacokinetic literature in terms of research design, validity of results, and clinical applications.

22. Communicate effectively with patients, staff, nurses, physicians, and professional peers.

23. Plan, implement, and evaluate the administrative and clinical aspects of clinical pharmacokinetic services in a given practice site.

24. Demonstrate creativity by contribution to the literature and practice of clinical pharmacy and to the science of clinical pharmacokinetics.

25. Apply pharmacokinetic and pharmacodynamic principles to therapeutic agents for which serum concentrations are not routinely monitored.

II. *Areas of Emphasis*

The resident shall receive orientation, instruction, and experience leading to competence in, but not limited to, the following aspects of clinical pharmacokinetics practice:

A. ***Communication and Assessment Skills.*** The resident shall be able to

1. Define the demographic and biochemical characteristics for a patient that are required to formulate a pharmacokinetic assessment.

2. Define selected drug- and patient-specific information (i.e., disease status and concurrent therapy) required to perform a pharmacokinetic assessment.

3. Interpret clinical laboratory data, including drug concentrations, required to formulate a pharmacokinetic assessment.

4. Define all pharmacokinetic terms and principles used in pharmacokinetic assessments.

5. List appropriate target concentrations and drug effects expected to be observed in a patient.

6. Demonstrate effective written and oral communication skills with physicians, nurses, and other health-care practitioners.

B. ***Pharmacokinetics.*** The resident shall be able to describe the following for each drug listed in section C below:

1. The application of linear mathematic models (one- and two-compartment) to patient-specific dosage regimen calculations using the concepts of biologic half-life, apparent volume of distribution, and clearance.

2. The application of nonlinear or Michaelis–Menten kinetic models to patient-specific dosage regimen calculations using the concepts of V_{max} and K_m.

3. The applications of Bayesian principles or population pharmacokinetics and analyses in clinical pharmacokinetic assessments.

4. Drug absorption using the concepts of rate constants, lag time, t_{max}, C_{max}, and moment theory.

5. Processes controlling gastrointestinal absorption of drugs administered as liquids: mechanisms, sites, and the role of gastrointestinal motility and transit rate.

6. Gastrointestinal absorption of solid dosage forms: dissolution kinetics and the roles of particle size, salt or crystal form, dosage formulation, and physiological parameters (i.e., gastrointestinal pH and role of gastrointestinal enzymes).

7. Assessment of bioavailability and bioequivalence of drug products, including a critical examination of data necessary to make a rational drug product selection.

8. First-pass metabolism, including the roles of hepatic or gut wall metabolism, the effect on pharmacokinetic parameters and drug concentrations, and representative examples.

9. First-pass metabolism and Michaelis–Menten kinetics, including the applicability of these combinations to the comparison of sustained release preparations with controlled-release oral preparations.

10. Biopharmaceutics of diverse dosage forms (e.g., oral, controlled-release, injectable, ophthalmic, topical, rectal, inhalation, and newly developed dosage forms).

11. Drug distribution processes, including the roles of protein binding, organ perfusion rates, muscle mass, and weight.

12. Pharmacokinetics of drug elimination processes, including the physiological and physical–chemical considerations pertaining to renal excretion, biliary excretion, and hepatic biotransformation.

13. Pharmacodynamics (concentration–effect relationships) of clinical responses and adverse effects.

14. The effects of the following diseases on the pharmacokinetics of each drug listed in section C below: renal, hepatic, malabsorption, diseases affecting systemic hemodynamics and organ blood flow (i.e., congestive heart failure and myocardial infarction), thyroid and other endocrine disorders, and diseases affecting distribution and protein concentrations.

15. The pharmacokinetic and pharmacodynamic basis of drug interactions: mechanisms (i.e., induction, competitive inhibition, and noncompetitive inhibition) and representative examples.

16. The concepts of autoinduction with changes in pharmacokinetic parameters (i.e., clearance, elimination rate constants, and half-life) and drug concentrations as the liver enzymes become maximally induced at a particular dose for a particular drug.

17. Genetic and environmental sources for intersubject variation in pharmacokinetic parameters.

18. Age-dependent processes and changes in drug pharmacokinetics: placental transfer; pharmacokinetics in the neonate; breast milk transfer; and the infant, child, adolescent, and geriatric patient.

19. Influence of hemodialysis, peritoneal dialysis, hemoperfusion, adsorbents (gastric dialysis), and emetics on drug pharmacokinetics.

20. The statistical approaches, pharmacokinetic models, and methods of application to patient-specific databases for computerized and noncomputerized dosing algorithms used in clinical pharmacokinetics practice.

21. A plan for the initiation, implementation, and evaluation of a clinical pharmacokinetics pharmacy practice in existing health-care institutions.

C. **Clinical Application of Pharmacokinetics.** The resident shall be able to complete the following for the majority of drugs listed at the end of this section:

1. Discuss the pharmacology and mechanism of action.

2. Describe the therapeutic indications.

3. Describe the pharmacokinetics (see section B above).

4. List the therapeutic range of drug concentrations.

5. List the clinical indications for measuring drug concentrations.

6. Discuss the relationship of drug concentration, efficacy, and toxicity.

7. Describe the time course and adverse effects relative to therapeutic effects.

8. Describe the appropriate dosing regimens, dose ranges, relative efficacy, and adverse effects.

9. Discuss the advantages and disadvantages of various dosing methods (i.e., guidelines, nomograms, and pharmacokinetics) available.

10. Identify those patients who are likely to derive maximal benefit from clinical pharmacokinetic pharmacy practice.

11. Calculate a dosage regimen based on pharmacokinetic principles and patient characteristics before obtaining drug concentrations.

12. Recommend the appropriate specimen sample collection (i.e., time and number of samples) to ensure optimal use of the drug concentration that is measured.

13. Calculate an optimal dosage regimen for an individual patient using available drug concentrations with the appropriate pharmacokinetic method.

14. Recommend subsequent dosage regimens, laboratory monitoring, and drug concentration monitoring based on patient response, pharmacokinetic principles, and drug concentrations.

15. Effectively communicate (orally and in written form) all pharmacokinetic recommendations with professional staff and patients.

16. Assess the effectiveness of dosage individualization on the care of the patient.

17. Document cost–benefit and risk–benefit of clinical pharmacokinetics pharmacy practice.

18. Educate pharmacists, physicians, nurses, and other clinical practitioners on pharmacokinetic principles to improve drug safety and efficacy.

Drugs for which pharmacokinetic parameters exist include:

Amikacin	Methotrexate
Amiodarone	Mexiletine
Amitriptyline	Netilmicin
Carbamazepine	Nortriptyline
Chloramphenicol	Phenobarbital
Cyclosporine	Phenytoin
Desipramine	Primidone
Digitoxin	Procainamide
Digoxin	Propranolol
Disopyramide	Quinidine
Ethosuximide	Salicylates
Flecainide	Theophylline
Gentamicin	Tobramycin
Heparin	Tocainide
Imipramine	Valproic acid
Lidocaine	Vancomycin
Lithium	Warfarin

D. *Analysis of Drug Concentrations.* For each drug listed in section C above, the resident shall be able to
1. List the commonly available assay procedures.
2. Describe the theory, methodology, and relative cost of the following assay procedures: microbiological, gas chromatography, gas chromatography–mass spectrometry, high performance liquid chromatography, radioimmunoassay, homogeneous enzyme immunoassay, and fluorescence polarization immunoassay.
3. Describe the specificity, sensitivity, and comparative performance of each of the analytical techniques listed in 2 above.
4. Formulate properly timed specimen collection strategies as related to the assay performance for appropriate drug analysis and pharmacokinetic evaluation.

5. Discuss the influence of diseases and protein binding on drug concentration analysis.
6. List the indications for determining unbound drug concentrations.
7. Outline the steps involved in specimen collection and sample storage (including labeling and record-keeping) before analysis of drug concentrations.

Part VI—Certification

The residency graduate's competence shall be attested to by the health-care organization in accordance with Part VI of the "ASHP Accreditation Standard for Specialized Pharmacy Residency Training."

Reference

1. American Society of Hospital Pharmacists. ASHP accreditation standard for specialized pharmacy residency training. *Am J Hosp Pharm.* 1980; 37:1229–32.

Approved by the ASHP Board of Directors, April 28, 1988. Developed by the ASHP Commission on Credentialing in conjunction with the SIG on Clinical Pharmacokinetics Practice.

The bibliographic citation for this document is as follows: American Society of Hospital Pharmacists. ASHP supplemental standard and learning objectives for residency training in clinical pharmocokinetics practice. *Am J Hosp Pharm.* 1988; 45:1934–7.

ASHP Supplemental Standard and Learning Objectives for Residency Training in Critical Care Pharmacy Practice

Introduction

Definition. A specialized residency in critical care pharmacy practice is defined as an organized, directed postgraduate program of practical experience in providing clinical pharmacy services to critically ill patients.

Accreditation Authority. The "ASHP Accreditation Standard for Specialized Pharmacy Residency Training,"[1] together with this Supplemental Standard, sets forth the primary criteria used to evaluate critical care pharmacy residency training programs in health care organizations applying for accreditation by the American Society of Hospital Pharmacists. Other elements of accreditation authority are specified in the "ASHP Accreditation Standard for Specialized Pharmacy Residency Training."

Objectives. Specialized residency training in critical care pharmacy practice should be directed toward developing expert knowledge and skills in this specialty of pharmacy practice. The specialized residency in critical care pharmacy practice must meet the objectives set forth in the "ASHP Accreditation Standard for Specialized Pharmacy Residency Training."

Application of the Standard. A specialized residency in critical care pharmacy practice should be organized and conducted to develop expert skills and competencies in this area of pharmacy practice. The manner in which this Supplemental Standard will be interpreted is specified in the "ASHP Accreditation Standard for Specialized Pharmacy Residency Training."

Part I—Qualifications of the Training Site

The training site must meet the requirements set forth in Part I of the "ASHP Accreditation Standard for Specialized Pharmacy Residency Training." Ancillary facilities may be used as appropriate in pursuing the objectives for training outlined below. The facility that provides specialized residency training in critical care pharmacy shall be either a tertiary care center, a level-1 trauma center, or a general hospital that provides comprehensive clinical and distributive critical care pharmacy services.

Part II—Qualifications of the Pharmacy Service

The pharmacy program in which the residency is based must meet the service requirements set forth in Part II of the "ASHP Accreditation Standard for Specialized Pharmacy Residency Training." The facility must have at least one pharmacist with an established clinical practice in critical care. There should be a critical care pharmacy satellite that provides patient-specific services to critical care patients. In all circumstances, the pharmacy department must show evidence that comprehensive clinical and distributive pharmacy services are being provided to critically ill patients.

Part III—Qualifications of the Program Coordinator

The program coordinator's qualifications shall meet the requirements set forth in Part III of the "ASHP Accreditation Standard for Specialized Pharmacy Residency Training." The program coordinator shall demonstrate proficiency as a clinical pharmacist in the area of critical care pharmacy services.

Part IV—Selection and Qualifications of the Resident

In addition to meeting the requirements set forth in the "ASHP Accreditation Standard for Specialized Pharmacy Residency Training," the resident *must* have previously completed an ASHP-accredited hospital or clinical pharmacy residency training program or have had an equivalent level of prior experience in hospital pharmacy practice.

Part V—Residency Training Program

Principle VA

The specialized residency training program shall be organized in accordance with sound educational principles.

A specialized residency program in critical care pharmacy practice must comply with the requirements set forth in Principle VA of the "ASHP Accreditation Standard for Specialized Pharmacy Residency Training."

Principle VB

The residency training program shall be predicated on the knowledge, attitudes, skills, and abilities required to conduct a critical care pharmacy practice.

Requirement

The training program shall provide for experiential training in critical care pharmacy practice and for development of the knowledge and skills needed to provide comprehensive clinical pharmacy services to critically ill patients.

Interpretation. In addition to the requirements set forth in Principle VB of the "ASHP Accreditation Standard for Specialized Pharmacy Residency Training," a specialized residency program in critical care pharmacy practice must ensure that, through a combination of didactic training and clinical experience, the resident shall achieve a level of competence consistent with the goals and objectives noted herein for such a program. Advanced study in pathophysiologic and pharmacotherapeutic principles, both theoretical and applied, should be strongly encouraged. The resident's involvement in applied research in critical care pharmacotherapy should be encouraged.

I. *Learning Objectives*

A resident who completes an accredited program in critical care pharmacy practice shall be able to

1. Organize and operate a critical care pharmacy service, including physical accommodations, reference sources, computer applications, professional and supportive personnel, budgeting, relationships with other health-care departments, patient flow, assumed or designated responsibilities, and documentation of services.
2. Implement a modern drug distribution system (unit dose, intravenous admixtures, and patient profiles) in a critical care unit.
3. Administer drugs to critical care patients by using proper technique.
4. Discuss the pathophysiology of commonly encountered acute medical problems (see areas of emphasis) with physicians and other health-care providers.
5. Monitor the progression of diseases or effects of therapy by using clinical symptoms, laboratory data, information generated by hemodynamic monitoring techniques, and other relevant data.
6. Discuss the use of mechanical ventilators in critically ill patients and describe the potential adverse effects of mechanical ventilation and its effects on the pharmacokinetics of drugs in these patients.
7. Discuss the implications of intra-aortic balloon counterpulsation devices, intracranial pressure monitoring devices, pulmonary artery catheters, biventricular or monoventricular assist devices, and dialysis equipment on the pharmacotherapy of critically ill patients.
8. Identify how multiorgan system failure alters the therapeutic response to many drugs commonly administered to critically ill patients.
9. Anticipate therapeutic dilemmas and formulate appropriate alternatives.
10. Develop therapeutic priorities in managing the acute and chronic problems of the patient.
11. Prevent, detect, and manage adverse drug reactions and drug interactions in critically ill patients.
12. Apply pharmacokinetic and pharmacodynamic principles to the critically ill patient and recommend serum drug concentration sampling times to achieve cost-effective drug monitoring.
13. Determine the need for fluid and electrolyte therapy and recommend appropriate diluents and admixture concentrations to meet patient-specific needs.
14. Demonstrate competency in determining the nutritional requirements of critically ill patients and ensure the delivery of adequate nutrition.
15. Demonstrate competency in monitoring drug therapy, fluid and electrolyte therapy, and nutritional support in critically ill patients.
16. Integrate the pharmacologic needs of the patient with the other aspects of patient-care delivery by the critical care team.
17. Balance efficacy data with information on drug cost and other formulary considerations when recommending therapeutic alternatives.
18. Demonstrate skills in writing progress notes and consultations in such areas as drug therapy selection, pharmacokinetics, nutritional support, toxicology, and therapeutic monitoring.
19. Participate as an effective member of the cardiopulmonary resuscitation team and participate in the management of other emergency situations that require pharmacologic intervention. Certification in advanced cardiac life support is required. The resident should be involved in cardiopulmonary resuscitation. Dispensing medications, recording drugs and events during resuscitation, providing drug information during resuscitation, or teaching resuscitation pharmacology to other clinicians shall constitute active involvement in cardiopulmonary resuscitation.
20. Work with the nursing staff to ensure the safe, accurate, and correct administration of drugs.
21. State advantages and disadvantages of parenteral and nonparenteral drug delivery in the critical care setting and discuss drug delivery devices and equipment.
22. State common physical and chemical drug incompatibilities and prevent their occurrence in critically ill patients.
23. State the potential vesicating nature of intravenous drug preparations commonly used in critically ill patients and recommend appropriate management.
24. Participate in interdisciplinary continuing education activities (e.g., grand rounds, research seminars, clinical conferences, and inservice programs).
25. Demonstrate knowledge of infection control principles.
26. Develop protocols for drug administration in critically ill patients in cooperation with the medical and nursing staff.
27. Evaluate the critical care literature and apply new information to the care of patients.
28. Present formal and informal lectures on critical care therapeutic topics to pharmacists, physicians, medical students, nurses, and other health-care providers.
29. Serve as a preceptor and role model for baccalaureate pharmacy students and/or doctor of pharmacy candidates during their critical care rotations.
30. Identify areas of research involving the use of drugs, drug delivery devices, or drug monitoring in critically ill patients.
31. Participate in ongoing research involving the use of drugs, drug delivery devices, or drug monitoring techniques in critically ill patients.
32. Prepare and publish original research, case reports, and critical reviews of the literature in refereed journals.

II. *Areas of Emphasis*

The advanced resident should participate in the care of a variety of patients in specialized critical care units such as coronary care, medical intensive care, general surgery intensive care, neurosurgical/neurotrauma intensive care, thoracic intensive care, burn intensive care, shock/trauma, pulmonary intensive care, emergency medicine, and neonatal/pediatric intensive care. Experience in a coronary care unit, a medical intensive care unit (ICU), and a surgical ICU is mandatory. If the training site does not subdivide its critical care units, the resident must still have direct patient-care experience with medical and surgical intensive care patients during the majority of the specialized residency training program. Elective rotations (jointly agreed on by the resident and the preceptor) in subspecialties with direct application to critical care pharmacy practice (e.g., nutrition support, nephrology, infectious disease, neurology, cardiology, and pulmonary medicine) should be encouraged.

Didactic discussions, reading assignments, case presentations, written assignments, and direct patient-care experience will allow the resident to understand and appreciate the implications of drug therapy on the following areas of emphasis:

A. Hemodynamic and physiologic monitoring.
  1. Cardiovascular and pulmonary physiology and pathophysiology.
  2. Pulmonary artery catheterization.
  3. Hemodynamic and oxygen delivery profiles.
  4. Noninvasive monitoring parameters.
  5. Physiologic scoring indices (e.g., APACHE II Score, Glasgow Coma Scale, and Champion Trauma Score).
B. Shock and related problems.
  1. Cardiogenic shock.
  2. Septic shock.
  3. Hypovolemic or hemorrhagic shock.
  4. Anaphylactic shock.
  5. Neurogenic (spinal) shock.
  6. Multiple organ system failure.
  7. Management of heat stroke.
  8. Management of hypothermia.
  9. Metabolic response to shock/trauma and potential effects on drug kinetics.
C. Pulmonary.
  1. Arterial blood gas analysis (invasive and non-invasive).
  2. Pulmonary function studies.
  3. Principles of mechanical ventilation.
  4. Oxygen therapy.
  5. Adult respiratory distress syndrome.
  6. Acute ventilatory failure.
  7. Aspiration pneumonia.
  8. Status asthmaticus.
  9. Pulmonary embolism.
  10. Pneumothorax and hemothorax.
  11. Theophylline pharmacokinetics.
  12. Drug-induced lung disease.
  13. Inhalation therapy.
D. Intravenous therapy.
  1. Nutrition support in patients with liver disease, renal disease, pulmonary disease, septic shock, surgery, or trauma.
  2. Fluid and electrolyte therapy.
  3. Colloid and crystalloid fluid replacement.
  4. Isotonicity principles.
  5. Physical and chemical drug incompatibilities.
  6. Intravenous access.
E. Cardiovascular.
  1. Cardiopulmonary resuscitation.
  2. Arrhythmias.
  3. Cardiogenic pulmonary edema and congestive heart failure.
  4. Acute myocardial infarction and thrombolytic therapy.
  5. Hypertensive emergencies.
  6. Use of vasoactive and inotropic drugs.
  7. Use of intra-aortic balloon counterpulsation and ventricular assist devices.
  8. Unstable angina.
  9. Effect of cardiovascular diseases on drug kinetics.
  10. Interpretation of common electrocardiogram ab-

normalities seen in acute situations.
  11. Principles of electrophysiologic testing.
  12. Percutaneous transluminal coronary angioplasty.
  13. Valvular surgery and valvuloplasty.
  14. Coronary artery surgery.
  15. Cardiac transplantation.
  16. Myocardial contusion.
F. Renal.
  1. Dialysis, ultrafiltration, and hemoperfusion.
  2. Acute renal failure.
  3. Chronic renal failure.
  4. Acid–base balance.
  5. Drug dosing in renal failure.
  6. Effects of dialysis on drug kinetics.
  7. Renal transplantation.
  8. Fluid and electrolyte disorders.
  9. Diabetes insipidus.
  10. Syndrome of inappropriate antidiuretic hormone.
  11. Rhabdomyolysis.
G. Neurology
  1. Status epilepticus.
  2. Cerebral edema and intracranial hypertension.
  3. Head trauma.
  4. Cerebral resuscitation.
  5. Peripheral neurologic problems.
  6. Anticonvulsant pharmacokinetics.
  7. Myasthenia gravis.
  8. Cerebrovascular accidents.
  9. Coma—metabolic, anoxic, traumatic, and infectious.
H. Gastrointestinal.
  1. Stress ulceration.
  2. Bleeding varices.
  3. Acute upper and lower gastrointestinal bleeding.
  4. Enteral nutrition.
  5. Pancreatitis.
I. Hepatic.
  1. Liver failure.
  2. Hepatorenal syndrome.
  3. Portal hypertension and portal systemic encephalopathy.
  4. Hepatitis.
  5. Effects of reduced liver blood flow and diminished hepatocellular function on drug clearance.
  6. Liver transplantation.
J. Burns.
  1. Fluid resuscitation.
  2. Topical and systemic antibiotics.
  3. Smoke inhalation.
  4. Effects of burns on drug kinetics.
  5. Infection control and treatment.
K. Endocrine.
  1. Acute adrenal insufficiency.
  2. Diabetic ketoacidosis and nonketotic coma.
  3. Thyroid storm and ICU hypothyroid states.
  4. Pheochromocytoma.
  5. Hyperparathyroid states.
  6. Hypoglycemia.
L. Hematology.
  1. Blood component therapy.
  2. Bleeding disorders in the ICU.
  3. Fibrinolytics and anticoagulants.
  4. Fibrinolytic and anticoagulant antidotes.
  5. Disseminated intravascular coagulopathy.
  6. Drug-induced blood dyscrasias.

M. Infectious diseases.
1. Meningitis/encephalitis.
2. Nosocomial infection.
3. Antibiotic prophylaxis.
4. Antibiotic pharmacokinetics in the critically ill patient.
5. Intra-abdominal abscess.
6. Infections in the immunocompromised host.
7. Infection control.
8. Pneumonia and bronchitis.
9. Endocarditis.
10. Acquired immunodeficiency syndrome.
11. Sepsis.
12. Wound infection.

N. Pediatrics (optional).
1. Hyperbilirubinemia.
2. Reye's syndrome.
3. Neonatal respiratory distress syndrome.
4. Premature apnea.
5. Meconium aspiration.
6. Exchange transfusion.
7. Neonatal and pediatric pharmacokinetics.
8. Pediatric infections.

O. Psychiatry.
1. ICU psychosis.
2. Drug-induced psychosis.
3. Neuroleptic malignant syndrome.
4. Management of the combative patient.
5. Use of anxiolytics, antidepressants, and neuro-leptics.
6. Substance abuse and alcohol withdrawal syndromes.

P. Analgesia and anesthesia.
1. Acute and chronic pain management.
2. Hemodynamic and respiratory effects of analgesics.
3. Patient-controlled analgesia.
4. Opioid tolerance, withdrawal, and addiction.
5. Use of neuromuscular blocking drugs.
6. Malignant hyperthermia.

Q. Drug overdose.
1. Management of acute ingestion of drugs and household poisonings.
2. Pharmacokinetic considerations in drug overdose.
3. Extracorporeal methods for drug removal.

III. *Research Project*

A residency project in adult or pediatric critical care or emergency medicine is encouraged. The purposes of the residency project are to teach the application of the scientific method and to provide experience in conducting clinical research.

IV. *Extramural Experiences*

When appropriate, rotations in or visits to other health-care settings and attendance at professional meetings should be scheduled to augment the resident's training. Extramural rotations may be conducted either as full-time training activities (e.g., for a 1-month block) or on a regularly scheduled part-time basis. If extramural rotations are scheduled for the purpose of pursuing one or more of the fundamental learning objectives outlined above, there must be a pharmacist–preceptor who has defined responsibilities for monitoring the resident's progress and evaluating his or her accomplishments. A detailed set of objectives for extramural rotations must be prepared in advance. Extramural rotations must represent not more than 25% of the resident's experience. The qualifications of the extramural training site are subject to review and approval by ASHP.

Part VI—Certification

Principle VI

The residency graduate's competence shall be attested to by the health-care organization in accordance with Part VI of the "ASHP Accreditation Standard for Specialized Pharmacy Residency Training."

Reference

1. American Society of Hospital Pharmacists. ASHP accreditation standard for specialized pharmacy residency training. *Am J Hosp Pharm*. 1988; 45:1924–30.

Approved by the ASHP Board of Directors, November 15–16, 1989. Developed by the ASHP Commission on Credentialing in conjunction with the Specialty Practice Group on Critical Care Pharmacy Practice.

The bibliographic citation for this document is as follows: American Society of Hospital Pharmacists. ASHP supplemental standard and learning objectives for residency training in critical care pharmacy practice. *Am J Hosp Pharm*. 1990; 47:609–12.

ASHP Supplemental Standard and Learning Objectives for Residency Training in Primary Care Pharmacy Practice

Introduction

Definition. A specialized residency in primary care pharmacy practice is defined as an organized, directed, postgraduate program of practical experience in providing clinical pharmacy services to ambulatory patients.

Accreditation Authority. The "ASHP Accreditation Standard for Specialized Pharmacy Residency Training,"[1] together with this Supplemental Standard, sets forth the primary criteria used to evaluate primary care pharmacy residency training programs in health-care organizations applying for accreditation by the American Society of Hospital Pharmacists. Other elements of accreditation authority are specified in the "ASHP Accreditation Standard for Specialized Pharmacy Residency Training."[1]

Objectives. Specialized residency training in primary care pharmacy practice should be directed toward developing expert knowledge and skills in this specialty of pharmacy practice. The specialized residency in primary care pharmacy practice must meet the objectives set forth in the "ASHP Accreditation Standard for Specialized Pharmacy Residency Training."[1]

Application of the Standard. A specialized residency in primary care pharmacy practice should be organized and conducted to develop expert skills and competencies in this area of pharmacy practice. The manner in which this Supplemental Standard will be interpreted is specified in the "ASHP Accreditation Standard for Specialized Pharmacy Residency Training."[1]

Part I—Qualifications of the Training Site

The training site must meet the requirements set forth in Part I of the "ASHP Accreditation Standard for Specialized Pharmacy Residency Training."[1] Facilities may include, but are not limited to, institutional primary care settings, satellite clinics, and noninstitutional ambulatory health-care systems, including group medical practices and health maintenance organizations.

Part II—Qualifications of the Pharmacy Service

The pharmacy program in which the residency is based must meet the service requirements set forth in Part II of the "ASHP Accreditation Standard for Specialized Pharmacy Residency Training."[1] The facility must have at least one pharmacist with an established clinical practice in primary care. In addition, the pharmacy service must provide a comprehensive program of primary care services, substantially more than that required in the "ASHP Guidelines: Minimum Standard for Ambulatory Care Pharmaceutical Services."[2] The following specific requirements are established for the ambulatory care service program:

1. *Medical Records.* All patient-related records must be accessible before, during, and after the provision of clinical pharmacy services.
2. *Drug Information Resources.* Each facility shall maintain a centralized body of pharmaceutical and medical literature containing current primary, secondary, and tertiary literature sources.
3. *Scope of Service.* The "ASHP Statement on the Provision of Pharmaceutical Services in Ambulatory Care Settings"[3] sets forth the fundamental scope of services that should be provided by such a program. Provision of nonprescription drugs and health-related devices and appliances is included within the intent of this requirement.
4. *Preceptors Serving as Independent Proprietors.* In those instances where the preceptor may also serve as sole proprietor of an independent (noninstitutional) ambulatory care setting, particular attention should be focused on section II-B of the "ASHP Accreditation Standard for Specialized Pharmacy Residency Training."[1] Administrative and business concerns of the preceptor in such a setting should not be allowed to detract from the objectives of the residency program.
5. *Review of Quality.* There shall be an ongoing quality-assurance program to evaluate the pharmacy services being provided.

Part III—Qualifications of the Program Coordinator

The program coordinator's qualifications shall meet the requirements set forth in Part III of the "ASHP Accreditation Standard for Specialized Pharmacy Residency Training."[1] The program coordinator shall demonstrate proficiency as a clinical pharmacist in the area of primary care pharmacy services. Further, the program coordinator should be a member of the Specialty Practice Group on Primary Care.

Part IV—Selection and Qualifications of the Resident

The resident must meet the requirements set forth in the "ASHP Accreditation Standard for Specialized Pharmacy Residency Training."[1]

Part V—Residency Training Program

Principle VA

The specialized residency training program shall be organized in accordance with sound educational principles.

A specialized residency program in primary care pharmacy practice must comply with the requirements set forth in Principle VA of the "ASHP Accreditation Standard for

Specialized Pharmacy Residency Training."[1]

Principle VB

The residency training program shall be predicated on the knowledge, attitudes, skills, and abilities required to conduct a primary care pharmacy practice.

Requirement

The training program shall provide for experiential training in primary care pharmacy practice and for development of the knowledge and skills needed to provide comprehensive clinical pharmacy services to ambulatory patients.

Interpretation. In addition to the requirements set forth in Principle VB of the "ASHP Accreditation Standard for Specialized Pharmacy Residency Training,"[1] a specialized residency program in primary care pharmacy practice must ensure that, through a combination of didactic training and clinical experience, the resident will achieve a level of competence consistent with the goals and objectives noted herein for such a program. Advanced study in pathophysiology, chronic disease management and prevention, physical assessment, communication techniques, and drug literature evaluation may be necessary. The resident's involvement in applied research in primary care pharmacotherapy should be encouraged.

I.   **Learning Objectives.** A resident who completes an accredited program in primary care pharmacy practice shall be able to

    A.   Serve on a health-care team providing primary or consultative care.

    B.   Conduct a patient interview and interpret the results of the interview.

    C.   Take a medication history, assess the patient's attitude toward compliance, evaluate the influence of these factors on therapeutic response, and initiate strategies to correct noncompliant behavior.

    D.   Effectively counsel patients on drug use.

    E.   List and explain the monitoring parameters and therapeutic endpoints for the safe and efficacious use of each drug used in a patient.

    F.   Prospectively monitor drug therapy for potential drug–drug, drug–laboratory test, drug–diet, drug–disease, and drug–condition interactions and recommend modifications in drug therapy, when appropriate, to minimize such interactions.

    G.   Use interviews, physical assessment skills, and interpretation of laboratory test results to monitor therapy for adverse and therapeutic effects.

    H.   Prospectively formulate individualized drug regimens based on the purpose of the medication(s), concurrent disease(s) and drug therapies, pharmacokinetic parameters of the drug(s), cost effectiveness, and the patient's clinical condition.

    I.   Describe the clinical manifestations of potential toxicities associated with a patient's medication, assess the significance of the toxicity, and recommend an appropriate course of action.

    J.   Develop and conduct drug and drug-related (e.g., medication administration devices) research, including formal clinical drug investigations.

    K.   Evaluate drug studies in the literature in terms of research methodology, validity of results, and clinical applicability.

    L.   Communicate effectively with patients, physicians, nurses, other health professionals, and peers.

    M.   Develop criteria for safe and effective drug use and coordinate drug use evaluation as described by the Joint Commission on Accreditation of Healthcare Organizations.

    N.   Identify factors for measuring the quality of care provided by the pharmacy service that could be used in the development of a departmental quality-assurance program.

    O.   Explain the organization and operation of the outpatient pharmacy department. This could include physical accommodations, reference sources, computer applications, professional and supportive personnel, budgeting, relationships with other health-care departments, assumed or designated responsibilities, and documentation of services.

    P.   Develop computer skills to assist in the conduct of professional activities.

II.   *Areas of Emphasis.* The resident shall receive orientation, instruction, and experience in primary care patient management. This training must occur in a multidisciplinary setting in which each member of the health-care team has a defined patient-care responsibility. Whenever possible, this training should be provided directly in the patient-care environment. When this is not possible, training may be provided through required readings or in didactic lectures. This training should include, but not be limited to, the following aspects of primary care pharmacy practice:

    A.   *Communication and assessment skills.* The resident shall be able to

       1.   Take a complete and thorough drug history including current medications (prescription, nonprescription, and illicit drugs), significant prior medications, response to prior drug therapy, drug allergies and adverse effects, alcohol consumption, and smoking status.

       2.   Review the patient's medical records to gather information relevant to a patient's drug therapy including disease states, concurrent therapies, and response to prior therapy and then use the information gathered in formulating a treatment plan.

       3.   Interpret laboratory data relating to therapeutic response.

       4.   Determine monitoring parameters and therapeutic endpoints for the treatment prescribed.

       5.   Demonstrate effective written and oral communication skills with physicians, nurses, and other health-care practitioners. Documentation of written skills should be in the form of written progress notes or formal consultations in the patient's chart and interdepartmental memoranda.

Whenever possible, residents should be taught skills that will allow them to function as independent practitioners in the management of chronic diseases. To develop these skills, residents need additional training in pharmacy-managed clinics, after which they should be able to

1. Take a complete and accurate history of the primary medical problem and other medical illnesses that may have an impact on the disease state treated.
2. Apply the physical assessment skills necessary to manage a patient's treatment effectively.
3. Assess the acuteness and severity of reported symptoms and act on this assessment by reassuring the patient, initiating or adjusting medication when appropriate, or referring the patient to another health-care practitioner or clinic.

B. *Chronic disease management.* Residents shall gain experience in providing services to a wide variety of patients with common chronic disease states. Training shall provide the resident with the experience necessary to identify disease status, determine appropriate drug therapy, and assist in determining and monitoring therapeutic endpoints and evaluating laboratory and clinical data necessary for patient followup. Based on the clinical data available, the resident shall be able to formulate treatment plans for patients in a variety of ambulatory care settings, including home health care. The disease states may include, but not be limited to, the following:

1. Diabetes mellitus.
2. Hypertension.
3. Seizure disorders.
4. Parkinsonism.
5. Rheumatoid arthritis.
6. Tuberculosis.
7. Chronic obstructive pulmonary disease.
8. Asthma.
9. Angina pectoris.
10. Congestive heart failure.
11. Thromboembolic disorders.
12. Neoplastic disease.
13. Renal failure and renal transplantation.
14. Peptic ulcer disease.
15. Ulcerative colitis.
16. Thyroid disorders.
17. Gout.
18. Anemias.
19. Glaucoma.
20. Intractable pain and chronic pain syndromes (e.g., depression, osteoarthritis, irritable bowel syndrome, and gastroesophageal reflux disease).
21. Psychiatric disorders.
22. Lipid disorders.

C. *Acute care triage.* Residents shall be familiar with common acute diseases in primary care practice. They shall be able to identify symptoms, judge the acuteness and severity of the medical problem, and define appropriate actions to follow in helping to resolve the problem. Specific disease states may include, but not be limited to, the following:

1. Upper respiratory infections.
2. Headaches.
3. Diarrhea.
4. Otitis media.
5. Allergic dermatitis.
6. Acne.
7. Local fungal infections.
8. Allergic rhinitis.
9. Viral gastroenteritis.
10. Streptococcal pharyngitis.
11. Parasitic infections.
12. Sexually transmitted diseases.
13. Urinary tract infections.
14. Constipation.

D. *Preventive care.* Residents should be knowledgeable about measures for preventing illness. These measures may include, but are not limited to, the following areas:

1. Nutrition.
2. Hygiene.
3. Exercise programs.
4. Alcohol and drug abuse rehabilitation.
5. Smoking cessation program.
6. Weight reduction program.
7. Stress reduction program.
8. Immunizations.
9. Dietary management of diabetes, hyperlipidemia, and hypertension.
10. Diagnostic test materials.

E. *Self-care.* Residents should be familiar with commonly used nonprescription medications and understand how they relate to the patient's other therapy. They should also identify the potential drug–drug and drug–disease state interactions of nonprescription medications.

F. *Emergency care.* Residents shall be familiar with basic principles of emergency care. They shall be trained in basic cardiopulmonary resuscitation techniques.

G. *Family planning.* Residents should be familiar with family planning and perinatal care. Topics that should be included are:

1. Contraception.
2. Pregnancy testing.
3. Teratogenicity.
4. Sexually transmitted diseases.

H. *Therapy modification for special patient groups.* Residents shall be familiar with patient characteristics that may require therapeutic modifications and know how to make such modifications. These include

1. Renal failure.
2. Liver failure.
3. Breastfeeding.
4. Geriatric patients.
5. Pediatric patients.

I. *Devices.* Residents should have an understanding of the appropriate use of medical devices to assist in the management of patient illnesses. These may include, but are not limited to

1. Nutrition delivery systems.
2. Drug delivery systems.
3. Prosthetic devices.
4. Home health-care supplies (e.g., nebulizers,

monitoring devices, and diagnostic test kits).

5. Ostomy supplies.
6. Oxygen systems.
7. Surgical appliances.
8. Durable medical equipment.

J. *Drug literature analysis.* The training program shall develop the resident's ability to appraise critically the medical and pharmaceutical literature. An attempt should be made to develop the resident's learning habits so that learning becomes a lifelong pursuit. This may be accomplished through discussions of assigned reading, development of "journal clubs," or sharing papers for review.

K. *Development of new clinical services.* When possible, residents should be involved in the development of new clinical services at the residency training site, from early planning stages to final implementation. When this is not possible, detailed guidance shall be provided to the residents to familiarize them with what is needed to establish a clinical practice in a variety of ambulatory care settings, including home health care. The goal of this area is to make it possible for residents to develop new clinical practice sites on completion of their training.

L. *Personal computer skills.* Training in the use of common personal computer programs should be a part of the residency training. These may include word processing, database management, spreadsheet, graphics, pharmacokinetic, communications, and statistical analysis programs. The programs taught should be those that will enhance the resident's professional skills.

Part VI—Certification

Principle VI

The residency graduate's competence shall be attested to by the health-care organization in accordance with Part VI of the "ASHP Accreditation Standard for Specialized Pharmacy Residency Training."[1]

References

1. American Society of Hospital Pharmacists. ASHP accreditation standard for specialized pharmacy residency training. *Am J Hosp Pharm.* 1988; 45:1924–30.
2. American Society of Hospital Pharmacists. ASHP guidelines: minimum standard for ambulatory-care pharmaceutical services. *Am J Hosp Pharm.* 1982; 39:316.
3. American Society of Hospital Pharmacists. ASHP statement on the provision of pharmaceutical services in ambulatory care settings. *Am J Hosp Pharm.* 1980; 37:1095.

Approved by the ASHP Board of Directors, April 26, 1990. Developed by the ASHP Commission on Credentialing in cooperation with the Specialty Practice Group on Primary Care.

The bibliographic citation for this document is as follows: American Society of Hospital Pharmacists. ASHP supplemental standard and learning objectives for residency training in primary care pharmacy practice. *Am J Hosp Pharm.* 1990; 47:1851–4.

ASHP Supplemental Standard and Learning Objectives for Residency Training in Pharmacotherapy Practice

Preamble

Definition. A specialized residency in pharmacotherapy practice is defined as an organized, directed postgraduate program that centers on developing a mastery of knowledge and an expert level of competency in pharmacotherapy. Pharmacotherapy specialists ensure the safe, appropriate, and economical use of drugs in patients through the application of specialized skills, knowledge, and functions in patient care. Among their specialized functions are to collect and interpret data to design, recommend, implement, monitor, and modify patient-specific pharmacotherapy; interpret, generate, and disseminate drug therapy knowledge; and design, recommend, implement, monitor, and modify system-specific policies and procedures in collaboration with other professionals to optimize health care. A specialized residency in pharmacotherapy should be a minimum of 12 months in length and is designed to build on those competencies developed by a Residency in Pharmacy Practice.

Purpose and Philosophy. The supplemental residency standard establishes criteria for the training and education of pharmacists to deliver exemplary pharmacotherapy to patients. A pharmacotherapy practice residency embraces the concept that pharmacotherapy practitioners share in the responsibility and accountability for optimal drug therapy outcomes. Therefore, residencies in pharmacotherapy practice must provide residents with opportunities to function independently as practitioners by conceptualizing and integrating accumulated experience and knowledge and transforming it into improved drug therapy for patients.

Accreditation Authority. The ASHP Accreditation Standard for Specialized Pharmacy Residency Training,[1] together with this supplement, provides the basic criteria used to evaluate pharmacotherapy practice residency programs applying for accreditation by ASHP. Where a difference in criteria exists between these two documents, those contained in this supplement shall prevail.

Qualifications of the Training Site. The training site must meet the requirements set forth in Part I of the ASHP Accreditation Standard for Specialized Pharmacy Residency Training. Facilities may include, but are not limited to, tertiary care medical centers, ambulatory care settings, general hospitals, or other health systems that provide extensive patient care services where pharmacotherapists function as professionals on the health care team and have been delegated responsibility for ensuring the safe, appropriate, and economical use of drugs.

Qualifications of the Pharmacy Service. When the residency is conducted as part of a pharmacy in a health system, the pharmacy services must meet the requirements set forth in Part IV of the Accreditation Standard for Specialized Pharmacy Residency Training, including the provision of comprehensive clinical pharmacy services. The residency program must provide the following training components:

- Availability of comprehensive pharmacotherapy experiences in patients with acute and chronic diseases from a variety of patient populations (e.g., internal medicine, surgery, pediatrics, psychiatry, geriatrics).
- Active participation as a professional on the health care team.
- Conduct of patient medication interviews and counseling.
- Interpretation and application of pharmacokinetic data and principles to patient care.
- Participation in the creation and dissemination of new knowledge in pharmacotherapy.
- Provision of patient- and population-specific drug information to health professionals and patients.
- Participation in drug-use evaluations, medical disease audits, and quality assurance assessments, as well as service on appropriate institutional committees.

Qualifications of the Program Director. The program director's qualifications shall meet the requirements set forth in Part II of the ASHP Accreditation Standard for Specialized Pharmacy Residency Training. The program director must be a clinical pharmacist with demonstrated expertise in pharmacotherapy practice, as exemplified by (a) specialty residency training followed by a minimum of three years of practice experience or equivalent (i.e., five years of practice experience), (b) board certification in pharmacotherapy, and (c) maintenance of an active patient care service responsibility. The program director should participate in professional pharmacy associations appropriate to his or her area of practice. Other pharmacist preceptors must be able to demonstrate pharmacotherapy expertise in the area for which they serve as preceptors.

Selection and Qualifications of the Resident. The resident must meet the requirements set forth in the ASHP Accreditation Standard for Specialized Pharmacy Residency Training. The pharmacotherapy residency program is designed to train highly committed pharmacists to provide exceptional pharmacy services in their area of practice. It is not intended to provide general pharmacy practice competencies but to build on such experiences to create a pharmacotherapy specialist. To this end, residency candidates must have (a) earned a Doctor of Pharmacy degree from an ACPE-accredited school or college of pharmacy (or equivalent) and (b) previously completed an ASHP-accredited pharmacy practice residency (or be able to demonstrate equivalent clinical practice experience to the satisfaction of the program director). The resident should participate in professional pharmacy associations appropriate to his or her area of practice.

Pharmacotherapy Goals

Practice Foundation Skills

Goals

S1. Take personal responsibility for improving the pharmacotherapy provided to patients.

S2. Demonstrate ethical conduct in all pharmacotherapy activities.
S3. Establish a commitment to lifelong learning.
S4. Maintain active involvement in local, state, national, and international pharmacy organizations.
S5. Communicate clearly orally and in writing.
S6. Solve practice problems efficiently.
S7. Work harmoniously with others in the health system.
S8. Display compassion for patients.
S9. Maintain confidentiality of patient information.
S10. Contribute to the training of pharmacy students and other health care professionals and support personnel.
S11. Arrange and store information in an organized manner.

Direct Patient Care

Provide quality patient care by using a pharmacy practice methodology

Goals

P1. Conduct those aspects of direct patient care activities undertaken by the pharmacotherapist in the acute care and ambulatory care settings using a consistent approach that reflects the philosophy of pharmaceutical care and that is performed with the efficiency and depth of experience characteristic of an experienced pharmacotherapist.
P2. Design, recommend, implement, monitor, and evaluate patient-specific pharmacotherapy.
P3. Provide drug- and nondrug-use education to patients.
P4. Ensure continuity of pharmaceutical care to and from acute care and ambulatory care settings.
P5. Document all pharmacotherapy activities appropriately.

Provide quality patient care through participation in medical systems

P6. Participate effectively in medical staff rounds.
P7. Present programs that center on disease prevention and wellness promotion.

Interpret, Generate, and Disseminate Knowledge in Pharmacotherapy

Provide drug information and medication-use education

Goals

I1. Provide concise, applicable, comprehensive, and timely responses to requests for drug information from patients, the public, and health care providers.
I2. Prepare and disseminate drug information.
I3. Coordinate inservice education of physicians, nurses, and other clinical practitioners.

Participate in developing and evaluating drug-use policies

I4. Provide pharmacotherapy expertise in the development of the health system's drug-use, patient care, and research-related policies.
I5. Assume responsibility for the health system's ongoing adherence to its drug-use policies.
I6. Generate and disseminate new knowledge in pharmacotherapy (e.g., review article, case report or series, original research).

Practice Management

Develop personal practice management skills

Goals

M1. Model a practice that supports pharmacotherapy practice research and education excellence.
M2. Understand the process for establishing a pharmacotherapy specialty residency in one's own health system.
M3. Work effectively within the political and decision-making structure to accomplish one's practice area goals.
M4. Prioritize job responsibilities.

Manage integrated pharmaceutical care services

M5. Evaluate current pharmacy services to determine if the services are meeting the health care needs of the patients.

Objectives

Terminal objectives (TO) and enabling objectives (EO) associated with the goals are listed.

Practice Foundation Skills

Goal S1. Take personal responsibility for improving the pharmacotherapy provided to patients.
TO S1.1 (Characterization) Prepare self to improve the pharmacotherapy provided to patients.

Goal S2. Demonstrate ethical conduct in all pharmacotherapy activities.
TO S2.1 (Characterization) Act ethically in the conduct of all pharmacotherapy activities.

Goal S3. Establish a commitment to lifelong learning.
TO S3.1 (Characterization) Use a systematic, ongoing process to self-assess and meet learning needs.

Goal S4. Maintain active involvement in local, state, national, and international pharmacy organizations.
TO S4.1 (Characterization) Practice commitment to achieving the advancement of pharmacotherapy by being actively involved in professional associations at the local, state, and national levels.

Goal S5. Communicate clearly orally and in writing.
TO S5.1 (Synthesis) Organize all written or oral communication in a logical manner.
TO S5.2 (Application) Address all communication at the level appropriate for the audience.
TO S5.3 (Application) Use correct grammar, punctuation, spelling, style, and formatting conventions in the preparation of all written communications.
TO S5.4 (Complex overt response) Speak clearly and distinctly.
TO S5.5 (Application) Use public speaking skills to speak effectively in large and small group situations.
TO S5.6 (Application) Use listening skills consistently in the performance of job functions.
TO S5.7 (Application) Use a knowledge of the applicability of specific visual aids to enhance the effectiveness of communications.

TO S5.8 (Application) When appropriate, use persuasive communication techniques effectively.

TO S5.9 (Organization) Prepare all communications so that they reflect a positive image of pharmacy.

TO S5.10 (Application) Use effective strategies for communicating with patients who are non-English speakers or who are impaired (e.g., blind, deaf, cognitively impaired, illiterate).

Goal S6. Solve practice problems efficiently.

TO S6.1 (Application) Demonstrate consistent use of a systematic approach to problem solving.

TO S6.2 (Application) Use consensus-building skills.

Goal S7. Work harmoniously with others in the health system.

TO S7.1 (Application) Use a knowledge of interpersonal skills to effectively manage working relationships.

Goal S8. Display compassion for patients.

TO S8.1 (Organization) Combine compassion with the provision of pharmacotherapy.

Goal S9. Maintain confidentiality of patient information.

TO S9.1 (Application) Observe legal and ethical guidelines for safeguarding the confidentiality of patient information.

Goal S10. Contribute to the training of pharmacy students and other health care professionals and support personnel.

TO S10.1 (Application) Use sound educational techniques to teach pharmacy students, other health care professionals, and support personnel.

Goal S11. Arrange and store information in an organized manner.

TO S11.1 (Characterization) Adhere to an efficient system for organizing and storing information related to one's practice.

Direct Patient Care

Provide quality patient care by using a pharmacy practice methodology

Goal P1. Conduct those aspects of direct patient care activities undertaken by the pharmacotherapist in the acute care and ambulatory care settings using a consistent approach that reflects the philosophy of pharmaceutical care and that is performed with the efficiency and depth of experience characteristic of an experienced pharmacotherapist.

TO P1.1 (Synthesis) Devise efficient strategies appropriate for the practice of pharmacotherapy that maximize the delivery of pharmaceutical care to each patient within a limited time frame.

TO P1.2 (Synthesis) For the broad range of complex patient care problems encountered by the pharmacotherapist, consistently formulate solutions that maximize the achievement of pharmaceutical care outcomes.

Goal P2. Design, recommend, implement, monitor, and evaluate patient-specific pharmacotherapy. (When provided as part of the practice of pharmaceutical care, this goal always involves a series of integrated, interrelated steps. To facilitate teaching and assessment, these five steps are detailed below as separate but related goal areas.)

Goal P2A. Build the information base needed to design a drug therapy regimen.

TO P2A.1 (Synthesis) Collect, generate, and organize all patient-specific information needed by the pharmacotherapist to detect and resolve drug-related problems and to make appropriate drug therapy decisions.

EO P2A.1.1 (Comprehension) Identify the types of information the pharmacotherapist requires to detect and resolve drug-related problems and to make appropriate drug therapy decisions.

EO P2A.1.2 (Comprehension) Discuss the signs and symptoms, epidemiology, etiology, risk factors, pathogenesis, natural history, pathophysiology, and clinical course of the diseases specified in the appendix.

EO P2A.1.2.1 (Comprehension) Discuss the relationship to each other of the major anatomical landmarks of the body.

EO P2A.1.2.1.1 (Knowledge) Identify all the major anatomical landmarks of the body.

EO P2A.1.2.2 (Comprehension) Describe the normal functioning of the body's major organ systems and their interrelationship.

EO P2A.1.3 (Comprehension) Discuss the mechanism of action, pharmacokinetics, pharmacodynamics, pharmacoeconomics, usual regimen (dosage, schedule, form, route, and method of administration), indications, contraindications, interactions, adverse reactions, and therapeutics of all drugs applicable to the diseases listed in the appendix.

EO P2A.1.4 (Comprehension) Discuss various forms of drug and nondrug therapy, including lifestyle modification and the use of devices for disease prevention and treatment, for all diseases listed in the appendix.

EO P2A.1.5 (Synthesis) Integrate effective communication techniques in interviews with patients, caregivers, health care professionals, or others so that the patient-specific information needed by the pharmacotherapist is collected.

EO P2A.1.6 (Adaptation) When appropriate, measure patients' vital signs and use appropriate physical assessment skills to screen the cardiovascular, pulmonary, dermatologic, and neurologic systems.

TO P2A.2 (Evaluation) Appraise patients' current drug and nondrug therapy on the basis of an integration of pathophysiologic, pharmacotherapeutic, pharmacokinetic, pharmacodynamic, economic, ethical, and legal considerations; knowledge of the current literature; and one's own practice experience to determine the presence of any of the following drug therapy problems:

1. Drugs used with no medical indication.
2. Medical conditions for which there is no drug prescribed.
3. Drugs prescribed inappropriately for a particular medical condition.
4. Anything inappropriate in the current drug therapy regimen (dosage, schedule, route of administration, method of administration).
5. Presence of therapeutic duplication.
6. Prescription of drugs to which the patient is allergic.
7. Presence or potential for adverse drug events.
8. Presence of clinically significant drug–drug, drug–disease, drug–nutrient, or drug–laboratory test interactions.
9. Interference with medical therapy by social or recreational drug use.

10. Patient not receiving full benefit of prescribed drug therapy.

11. Treatment problems arising from financial impact of drug therapy on the patient.

12. Patients' lack of understanding of drug therapy.

EO P2A.2.1 (Evaluation) Prioritize patients' pharmacotherapy problems.

Goal P2B. Design pharmacotherapeutic regimens.

TO P2B.1 (Evaluation) Using an organized collection of patient-specific information, summarize patients' health care needs.

TO P2B.2 (Synthesis) Specify drug and nondrug therapy goals for patients that integrate pathophysiologic, pharmacotherapeutic, pharmacokinetic, pharmacodynamic, economic, ethical, and legal concerns; knowledge of current literature; and one's own practice experience with patient–specific and quality-of-life considerations.

TO P2B.3 (Synthesis) Design pharmacotherapeutic regimens, including modification of existing drug and nondrug therapy, that meet the goals established for patients and integrate pathophysiologic, pharmacotherapeutic, pharmacokinetic, pharmacodynamic, economic, ethical, and legal concerns; knowledge of current literature; and one's own practice experience with patient-specific and quality-of-life considerations.

TO P2B.4 (Application) In a systematic, logical, and consensus-seeking manner, recommend a pharmacotherapeutic regimen to prescribers and patients.

TO P2B.5 (Evaluation) When appropriate, initiate or modify drug therapy orders according to the health system's policy.

Goal P2C. Design monitoring plans for pharmacotherapeutic regimens.

TO P2C.1 (Synthesis) Design monitoring plans for pharmacotherapeutic regimens that effectively evaluate achievement of the patient-specific drug and nondrug therapy goals and that integrate pathophysiologic, pharmacotherapeutic, pharmacokinetic, pharmacodynamic, economic, ethical, and legal concerns; knowledge of current literature; and one's own practice experience with patient-specific and quality-of-life considerations.

EO P2C.1.1 (Comprehension) Discuss parameters to monitor that will measure achievement of drug and nondrug goals for a pharmacotherapeutic regimen for the diseases listed in the appendix.

EO P2C.1.2 (Comprehension) Discuss the frequency and criticality of monitoring parameter measurements.

TO P2C.2 (Application) When appropriate, order laboratory tests required by a monitoring plan according to the health system's policies and procedures.

Goal P2D. Redesign pharmacotherapeutic regimens and corresponding monitoring plans.

TO P2D.1 (Evaluation) Interpret the meaning of monitoring data by integrating normal and abnormal patient-specific data with one's practice experience.

TO P2D.2 (Synthesis) Modify a pharmacotherapeutic regimen as necessary, on the basis of evaluation of monitoring data, integrating pathophysiologic, pharmacotherapeutic, pharmacokinetic, pharmacodynamic, economic, ethical, and legal concerns; knowledge of current literature; and one's own practice experience with patient-specific and quality-of-life considerations.

Goal P3. Provide drug- and nondrug-use education to patients.

TO P3.1 (Synthesis) Design patient education regarding drug use and lifestyle modification, by using knowledge of current biomedical literature and one's own practice experience.

Goal P4. Ensure continuity of pharmaceutical care to and from acute care and ambulatory patient care settings.

TO P4.1 (Application) Use a systematic procedure to communicate pertinent pharmacotherapeutic information to and from acute care and ambulatory care settings.

Goal P5. Document all pharmacotherapy activities appropriately.

TO P5.1 (Organization) Integrate documentation into all pharmacotherapy activities.

EO P5.1.1 (Comprehension) Explain the importance of documenting pharmacotherapy activities.

EO P5.1.2 (Application) Follow institutional policies and procedures when documenting pharmacotherapy activities.

EO P5.1.3 (Application) Report the results of adverse drug reactions to appropriate committees, product manufacturers, and the Food and Drug Administration.

EO P5.1.4 (Application) Report the outcome of a patient-specific corrective action plan to appropriate individuals or committees.

EO P5.1.5 (Application) When detecting a significant adverse drug event resulting from a drug product defect, report the event according to the health system's policies and procedures.

EO P5.1.6 (Application) Report the results of significant drug interactions to appropriate individuals and committees.

Provide quality patient care through participation in medical systems

Goal P6. Participate effectively in medical staff rounds.

TO P6.1 (Synthesis) Provide comprehensive and authoritative information during medical staff rounds, using a style that ensures acceptance of the information and recommendations presented.

EO P6.1.1 (Analysis) Determine situations in which the pharmacist should be assertive in providing information.

Goal P7. Present programs that center on disease prevention and wellness promotion.

TO P7.1 (Synthesis) Design programs for the general public that center on disease prevention and wellness promotion.

Interpret, Generate, and Disseminate Knowledge in Pharmacotherapy

Provide drug information and medication-use education

Goal I1. Provide concise, applicable, comprehensive, and timely responses to requests for drug information from patients, the public, and health care providers.

TO I1.1 (Analysis) Discriminate between the requesters' statements of need and the actual drug information needs by asking for appropriate additional information.

TO I1.2 (Synthesis) Formulate a systematic, efficient, and thorough procedure for retrieving drug information, including the use of a National Library of Medicine search.

EO I1.2.1 (Comprehension) Discuss the strengths and weaknesses of manual and electronic methods of retrieving biomedical literature.

EO I1.2.2 (Knowledge) State sources of information for the pathophysiologic, pharmacotherapeutic, pharmacokinetic, pharmacodynamic, therapeutic, economic, ethical, and legal concerns of diseases listed in the appendix.

TO I1.3 (Evaluation) Determine from all relevant data and biomedical literature the appropriate information to evaluate to respond to a drug information request.

TO I1.4 (Evaluation) Appraise drug literature to determine the quality of data gathered to respond to drug information requests.

EO I1.4.1 (Analysis) Assess the potential for bias of the author or preparer of all forms of drug information.

EO I1.4.2 (Evaluation) Appraise study methodology to determine whether or not a study's methodology is adequate to support its conclusions.

EO I1.4.2.1 (Evaluation) Determine that the endpoint established for a study is appropriate.

EO I1.4.2.1.1 (Comprehension) Discuss methods used to test study endpoint (e.g., pulmonary function studies).

EO I1.4.2.2 (Comprehension) Discuss the effects on study outcomes of various methods of patient selection (e.g., volunteers, patients, or patients with different disease severity).

EO I1.4.2.3 (Comprehension) Discuss the effects on study outcomes of various methods of blinding (e.g., double-blind, single-blind, open research designs).

EO I1.4.2.4 (Comprehension) Discuss the effects on study outcomes of various methods of drug assay and quality assurance procedures (e.g., high-performance liquid chromatography, assay coefficient of variation).

EO I1.4.2.5 (Comprehension) Discuss the effects on study outcomes of various methods of data analysis (e.g., pharmacokinetics, pharmacoeconomics, and pharmacodynamics).

EO I1.4.2.6 (Comprehension) Discuss the effects on study outcomes of various statistical methods used for data analysis (e.g., t test, analysis of variance).

EO I1.4.2.7 (Application) Determine if a study finding is or is not clinically significant.

EO I1.4.2.8 (Comprehension) Discuss the strengths and limitations of different study designs.

TO I1.5 (Evaluation) Determine that a study's conclusions are supported by the study results.

EO I1.5.1 (Comprehension) Discuss how data from a study can be applied to expanded patient populations.

TO I1.6 (Synthesis) Formulate responses to drug information requests on the basis of analysis of the literature and one's own practice experience.

TO I1.7 (Evaluation) Assess the effectiveness of drug information recommendations.

Goal I2. Prepare and disseminate drug information.

TO I2.1 (Synthesis) Edit or author a newsletter providing pertinent pharmacotherapeutic information that meets the needs and interests of the reader.

EO I2.1.1 (Application) Use editing skills to revise newsletter articles for publication.

TO I2.2 (Synthesis) Write timely and authoritative consultations and notes according to the health system's policies and procedures.

EO I2.2.1 (Comprehension) Discuss the content and format of formal consultations.

EO I2.2.2 (Comprehension) Discuss the content and format of a progress note.

TO I2.3 (Evaluation) Determine the adequacy of a drug monograph for submission to the health system's pharmacy and therapeutics committee.

Goal I3. Coordinate inservice education of physicians, nurses, and other clinical practitioners.

TO I3.1 (Evaluation) Determine inservice education needs of the health system's physicians, nurses, and other practitioners on drug therapy issues.

TO I3.2 (Synthesis) Devise an overall strategy for meeting the inservice education needs of the health system's physicians, nurses, and other practitioners on drug therapy issues.

Participate in developing and evaluating drug-use policies

Goal I4. Provide pharmacotherapy expertise in the development of the health system's drug-use, patient care, and research-related policies.

TO I4.1 (Comprehension) Discuss the role of the pharmacotherapist in the establishment of a health system's formulary.

TO I4.2 (Synthesis) Establish and review criteria by which a specific drug or drug category selection can be continually updated.

TO I4.3 (Synthesis) Design drug-use evaluations as needed to resolve drug therapy problems.

TO I4.4 (Synthesis) Provide authoritative pharmacotherapeutic guidance to a team developing a collaborative treatment algorithm (e.g., critical pathways such as diabetic ketoacidosis, total hip arthroplasty).

EO I4.4.1 (Comprehension) Discuss the principles guiding the structure of a critical pathway.

TO I4.5 (Synthesis) Provide authoritative pharmacotherapeutic guidance to a health system research committee (e.g., institutional review board, human rights, research and development, animal care).

Goal I5. Assume responsibility for the health system's ongoing adherence to its drug-use policies.

TO I5.1 (Characterization) Demonstrate leadership in ensuring the health system's adherence to its drug-use policies.

Goal I6. Generate and disseminate new knowledge in pharmacotherapy (e.g., review article, case report or series, original research).

TO I6.1 (Comprehension) Discuss sources of and procedures for securing funding of investigations of pharmacotherapy-related issues.

TO I6.2 (Synthesis) Design investigations of pharmacotherapy-related issues that use the scientific method.

EO I6.2.1 (Comprehension) Discuss the application of the scientific method to the design of investigations.

EO I6.2.2 (Comprehension) Discuss the application of regulatory requirements for coordinating research in humans or animals to the design of investigations.

EO I6.2.3 (Evaluation) Defend the selection of a design methodology for an investigation (pharmacokinetics, pharmacoepidemiology, pharmacoeconomics, pharmacodynamics, pharmacotherapeutics, toxicology, analytical methodology, drug-use evaluation, pharmacometrics, survey, or psychosocial aspects of the use of drugs by society).

EO I6.2.4 (Comprehension) Discuss the use of various analytical methodologies (e.g., assay, protein-binding test) in the design of investigations.

EO I6.2.5 (Evaluation) Defend the choice of a particular statistical method for analyzing data in an investigation.

TO I6.3 (Application) Execute an investigation of a pharmacotherapy-related issue according to the specified design.

EO I6.3.1 (Comprehension) Explain methods for the management of data collected in an investigation.

TO I6.4 (Evaluation) Analyze data collected in an investigation of a pharmacotherapy-related issue to draw appropriate conclusions.

EO I6.4.1 (Comprehension) Discuss the relationship between the results of an investigation and conclusions that may be drawn from it.

TO I6.5 (Synthesis) Prepare a manuscript describing an investigation of a pharmacotherapy-related issue that is suitable for submission to a particular peer-reviewed publication.

EO I6.5.1 (Comprehension) Explain the uniform requirements for manuscripts submitted to biomedical journals, developed by the International Committee of Medical Journal Editors.

EO I6.5.2 (Application) Use a knowledge of where to locate publication policies and procedures to secure information needed to prepare a manuscript for publication.

Practice Management

Develop personal practice management skills

Goal M1. Model a practice that supports pharmacotherapy practice research and education excellence.

TO M1.1 (Characterization) Demonstrate leadership in fostering excellence in pharmacotherapy in others.

Goal M2. Understand the process for establishing a pharmacotherapy specialty residency in one's own health system.

TO M2.1 (Comprehension) Describe the process and resources needed to establish a pharmacotherapy specialty residency in a particular health system.

Goal M3. Work effectively within the political and decision-making structure to accomplish one's practice area goals.

TO M3.1 (Synthesis) Formulate effective strategies for influencing the health system's political and decision-making structure to accomplish a pharmacotherapy practice goal.

Goal M4. Prioritize job responsibilities.

TO M4.1 (Evaluation) Appraise each job responsibility for its relative importance to all job responsibilities and prioritize accordingly.

Manage integrated pharmaceutical care services

Goal M5. Evaluate current pharmacy services to determine if the services are meeting the health care needs of the patients.

TO M5.1 (Evaluation) Determine if pharmacotherapy services met the desired patient care outcomes for the past year.

Appendix—Diseases Covered in Residency Goals and Objectives

Bone and Joint
Required
- Bone and joint infections
- Rheumatoid arthritis
- Degenerative joint disease
- Osteoporosis
- Gout

Elective
- Osteomalacia
- Seronegative spondyloarthropathies

Cardiovascular
Required
- Hypertension
- Congestive heart failure
- Arrhythmias
- Ischemic heart disease
- Acute myocardial infarction
- Thromboembolic disorders
- Hyperlipidemias
- Stroke
- Cardiopulmonary resuscitation
- Hypertensive crisis/urgencies/emergencies
- Endocarditis
- Peripheral vascular disease
- Cor pulmonale

Elective
- Congenital heart disease
- Valvular heart disease
- Primary pulmonary hypertension
- Aortic stenosis

Dermatologic
Required
- Skin and soft tissue infections
- Acne
- Fungal infections
- Eczema
- Drug rashes
- Urticaria

Elective
- Burns
- Skin cancer
- Psoriasis
- Pressure sores

Endocrine and Exocrine
Required
- Diabetes mellitus
- Breast cancer/testicular cancer
- Thyroid disorders
- Osteoporosis

Elective

Diabetes insipidus
Tumors of the endocrine system
Adrenal disorders
Female endocrine disorders

Eye, Ear, Nose, and Throat
Required
Otitis
Glaucoma
Pharyngitis
Ophthalmic infections
Sinusitis
Elective
Head and neck cancer
Epiglottitis

Fluid and Electrolytes/Metabolic
Required
Parenteral and enteral nutrition
Fluid and electrolytes
Phosphate/magnesium/calcium
Acid–base

Gastrointestinal
Required
Gastroesophageal motility disorders
Nausea/vomiting
Peptic ulcer disease
Stress ulcer disease/upper gastrointestinal hemorrhage
Cirrhosis/hepatitis
Pancreatitis
Inflammatory bowel disease
Intra-abdominal infections
Elective
Zollinger-Ellison syndrome
Malabsorption syndrome
Lower gastrointestinal bleeding
Gastrointestinal cancers
Gastroesophageal reflux disease
Cholelithiasis
Gastrointestinal infections

Genitourinary
Required
Urinary tract infections
Sexually transmitted diseases
Prostatitis/prostatic hypertrophy
Contraception
Elective
Enuresis/urinary incontinence
Reproductive disorders
Prostate cancer
Tumors of the ureter/bladder
Sexual dysfunction/impotence

Hematologic
Required
Anemias
Clotting factor disorders
Disseminated intravascular coagulation
Sickle cell disease
Elective
Acute and chronic leukemia
Porphyria
G6PD deficiency

Thrombotic thrombocytopenic purpura

Immunologic
Required
Acquired immunodeficiency syndrome
Anaphylaxis
Allergic rhinitis
Immunodeficiency diseases
Stevens-Johnson syndrome
Elective
Lymphomas
Kawasaki disease
Angioedema
Polymyositis
Scleroderma
Sjögren's syndrome
Organ transplantation

Neurologic
Required
Epilepsy/status epilepticus
Pain management
Central nervous system hemorrhage
Central nervous system infections
Headache/migraine
Peripheral neuropathy
Elective
Tremors
Neuromuscular diseases/myasthenia gravis
Parkinson's disease
Head trauma

Psychiatric
Required
Drug or alcohol overdose
Anxiety disorders
Depressive disorders
Dementia
Delirium
Elective
Substance-induced organic mental disorders
Schizophrenia
Bipolar disorders
Organic mental syndromes
Disorders evident in infancy and childhood
Sleep disorders

Renal
Required
Acute and chronic renal failure
Upper urinary tract infections
Acid–base disorders
Dialysis
Elective
Kidney tumors
Congenital renal disease
Nephrolithiasis
Glomerulonephritis

Respiratory
Required
Asthma
Chronic obstructive pulmonary disease/emphysema
Pneumonia
Adult respiratory distress syndrome

Acute respiratory failure
Tuberculosis
Lung cancer
Elective
Cystic fibrosis
Apnea of prematurity
Bronchopulmonary dysplasia
Neonatal respiratory distress syndrome
Sleep apnea
Fat embolism syndrome

Multisystem Diseases
Required
Sepsis/shock
Antimicrobial prophylaxis
Systemic fungal infections
Toxicology
Vaccines, toxoids, immunobiologicals, and
diagnostics
Elective
Trauma/surgery
Parasitic disease
Inborn errors of metabolism
Nutritional deficiency

Reference

1. American Society of Hospital Pharmacists. ASHP
    Accreditation Standard for Specialized Pharmacy Resi-
    dency Training (with Guide to Interpretation). *Am J
    Hosp Pharm.* 1994; 51:2034–41.

Approved by the ASHP Board of Directors, September 22, 1995.
Approved by the ACCP Board of Regents, November 11, 1995.
(Note: The Preamble to the document approved by the ACCP Board
of Regents included modifications that were not contained in the
document approved by the ASHP Board in September. On November 18, 1995, the ASHP Board of Directors reviewed and approved
the modified Preamble.)

Developed jointly by the ASHP Commission on Credentialing and
the American College of Clinical Pharmacy.

The bibliographic citation for this document is as follows:
American Society of Health-System Pharmacists. ASHP supplemental standard and learning objectives for residency training
in pharmacotherapy practice. *Am J Health-Syst. Pharm.* 1996;
53:59–66.

ASHP Supplemental Standard and Learning Objectives for Residency Training in Infectious Diseases Pharmacy Practice

Preamble

Definition. A specialized residency in infectious diseases pharmacy practice is defined as an organized, directed postgraduate program that centers on developing the competencies necessary to provide pharmaceutical care to patients with infectious diseases.

Purpose and Philosophy. The supplemental residency standard establishes criteria for the training and education of pharmacists in the delivery of exemplary pharmaceutical care to patients with infectious diseases. An infectious diseases pharmacy practice residency embraces the concept that infectious diseases pharmacy practitioners share in the responsibility and accountability for optimal drug therapy outcomes. Therefore, residencies in infectious diseases pharmacy practice must provide residents with opportunities to function independently as practitioners through conceptualizing, integrating, and transforming accumulated experience and knowledge into improved drug therapy for patients.

Accreditation Authority. The ASHP Accreditation Standard for Specialized Pharmacy Residency Training[1], taken together with this supplement, provides the basic criteria used to evaluate infectious diseases pharmacy practice residency training programs applying for accreditation by ASHP.

Qualifications of the Training Site. The training site must meet the requirements set forth in Part I of the ASHP Accreditation Standard for Specialized Pharmacy Residency Training. Facilities may include, but are not limited to, tertiary care medical centers, general hospitals, or other health systems that provide extensive infectious disease services. Ancillary facilities such as outpatient treatment units may be used, as appropriate, in pursuing the objectives for training outlined in the goals and objectives.

Qualifications of the Pharmacy Service. When the residency is conducted as part of a pharmacy service in a health system, the pharmacy services must meet the requirements set forth in Part IV of the Accreditation Standard for Specialized Pharmacy Residency Training. The facility where the residency program is conducted must have at least one pharmacist with an established clinical practice in infectious diseases pharmacy.

Qualifications of the Program Director. The program director's qualifications shall meet the requirements set forth in Part II of the ASHP Accreditation Standard for Specialized Pharmacy Residency Training. The program director shall demonstrate proficiency as a clinical pharmacist in the area of infectious diseases pharmacy practice and shall be accessible for resident supervision. A multisite residency program shall have one designated residency program director whose appointment shall be agreed to in writing by each of the participating practice sites.

Selection and Qualifications of the Resident. The resident must meet the requirements set forth in the ASHP Accreditation Standard for Specialized Pharmacy Residency Training.

Infectious Disease Goals

Practice Foundation Skills

Goals

S1: Take personal responsibility for improving the pharmaceutical care of patients.

S2: Solve practice problems efficiently.

S3: Appreciate the need to adapt pharmaceutical care for the culturally diverse.

S4: Maintain active involvement in local, state, and national professional organizations that support infectious diseases pharmacy practice.

S5: Contribute to the training of pharmacy students and other health care professionals and support personnel.

S6: Design and execute investigations of infectious diseases-related issues.

S7: Understand the process of establishing an infectious diseases pharmacy practice specialty residency program.

S8: Understand how to evaluate the potential for an employment opportunity to meet professional and personal goals.

S9: Adhere to an interdisciplinary approach to antimicrobial management.

Direct Patient Care

Provide quality patient care by using a pharmacy practice methodology

Goals

P1: Conduct direct patient care activities using a consistent approach that reflects the philosophy of pharmaceutical care and that is performed with the efficiency and depth of experience characteristic of an experienced infectious diseases pharmacy specialist.

P2: Design, recommend, monitor, and evaluate patient-specific infectious diseases pharmacotherapy. (When provided as part of the practice of pharmaceutical care, the design, recommendation, monitoring, and evaluation of patient-specific pharmacotherapy is always a series of integrated, interrelated steps. These five steps are detailed below as separate but related goal areas to facilitate teaching and assessment.)

P2A: Build the information base needed to design an anti-infective[a] regimen.

P2B: Design pharmacotherapeutic regimens.

P2C: Design monitoring plans for anti-infective regimens.

P2D: Recommend anti-infective regimens and corresponding monitoring plans.

P2E: Redesign anti-infective regimens and corresponding monitoring plans based on evaluation of monitoring data.

P3: Provide education on anti-infective use to patients and caregivers.

P4: Ensure continuity of pharmaceutical care across health care settings.

P5: Document all pharmaceutical care activities appropriately.

Provide quality patient care through participation in medical systems

P6: Participate effectively in patient care rounds.

P7: Design programs that center on prevention of infectious diseases.

Drug Information and Drug Policy Development

Provide drug information and medication-use education

Goals

I1: Provide concise, applicable, and timely responses to requests for information from health care providers and patients relative to infectious diseases and anti-infective use.

I2: Select a core library, including computerized databases, appropriate for an infectious diseases pharmacy practice setting.

I3: Prepare and disseminate written information on anti-infective therapy.

I4: Prepare and verbally disseminate information on anti-infective therapy.

I5: Participate in the ongoing revision of the anti-infectives section of a health system's drug formulary.

I6: Participate in the development or modification of treatment protocols for infectious diseases.

I7: Participate in the development or modification of identified policies for the selection and use of anti-infectives.

I8: Participate in the development, implementation, and evaluation of the health system's drug-use evaluation (DUE) program.

Practice Management

Develop practice management skills

Goals

M1: Model a practice management philosophy that supports pharmaceutical care and pharmacy practice excellence.

M2: Work through the political and decision-making structure to accomplish one's practice area goals.

M3: Contribute to the achievement of pharmacy goals through effective participation on an organization's committees.

M4: Evaluate current pharmacy services to determine whether the services are meeting the needs of patients with infectious diseases.

M5: Participate in the development of proposals for new infectious diseases pharmacy services.

M6: Contribute to the achievement of health system goals for patient care using drug cost, outcome, and pharmacoeconomic information.

M7: Participate in the management of the practice area's human resources.

M8: Assist the health system in achieving compliance with accreditation, legal, regulatory, and safety requirements related to the use anti-infective agents (e.g., JCAHO requirements; ASHP standards, state and federal laws regulating pharmacy practice; OSHA regulations).

M9: Participate in the health system's quality improvement program.

M10: Conduct relations with the pharmaceutical industry in an ethical manner.

M11: Manage the use of investigational anti-infective agents according to established protocols and the health system's policies and procedures.

Objectives

Terminal objectives (TO) and enabling objectives (EO) associated with the goals are listed.

Practice Foundation Skills

Goal S1. Take personal responsibility for improving the pharmaceutical care of patients.

> **TO S1.1** (Characterization) Prepare self to improve the pharmaceutical care of patients with infectious diseases.
>
> > **EO S1.1.1** (Synthesis) Write one's own philosophy of practice as an infectious diseases specialist.
> >
> > **EO S1.1.2** (Characterization) Use a systematic, ongoing process to evaluate one's level of professional development and accomplish the learning needs required to provide pharmaceutical care.
>
> **TO S1.2** (Characterization) Demonstrate leadership in ensuring the health system's adherence to its drug-use and infection control policies.
>
> **TO S1.3** (Characterization) Display initiative in identifying and resolving pharmacy-related patient care problems.

Goal S2. Solve practice problems efficiently.

> **TO S2.1** (Synthesis) Devise efficient strategies for solving practice problems encountered by the infectious diseases pharmacist.

Goal S3. Appreciate the need to adapt pharmaceutical care for the culturally diverse.

> **TO S3.1** (Comprehension) Discuss the need to adapt the pharmaceutical care plan for patients of diverse cultural backgrounds.

Goal S4. Maintain active involvement in local, state, and national professional organizations that support infectious disease pharmacy practice.

> **TO S4.1** (Valuing) Demonstrate an awareness of the importance of membership in pharmacy organizations that support infectious diseases pharmacy practice by being actively involved in local, state, and national professional associations.

Goal S5. Contribute to the training of pharmacy students and other health care professionals and support personnel.

TO S5.1 (Application) Use sound educational techniques in teaching infectious diseases pharmacotherapy principles and practices to pharmacy students, other health care professionals, and support personnel.

Goal S6. Design and execute investigations of infectious diseases-related issues.

TO S6.1 (Synthesis) Design investigations of infectious diseases-related issues.

EO S6.1.1 (Analysis) Identify issues that need to be studied.

EO S6.1.2 (Synthesis) Generate questions to be answered by an investigation.

EO S6.1.3 (Synthesis) Design a study that will answer the questions identified.

TO S6.2 (Application) Execute an investigation of infectious diseases-related issues that follows an established design. (This is not intended to be an extensive study or a research project but an investigation that is appropriate for residency training.)

EO S6.2.1 (Application) Use a systematic procedure to collect data.

EO S6.2.2 (Analysis) Draw valid conclusions through evaluation of the data.

EO S6.2.3 (Application) Report the results of an investigation into infectious diseases-related issues in the appropriate media.

EO S6.2.4 (Application) Write a report of the results of an investigation in a format suitable for publication.

Goal S7. Understand the process of establishing an infectious diseases pharmacy practice specialty residency program.

TO S7.1 (Comprehension) Discuss the steps involved in establishing a pharmacy practice residency program at a particular site.

Goal S8. Understand how to evaluate the potential for an employment opportunity to meet professional and personal goals.

TO S8.1 (Comprehension) Discuss a process for evaluating the potential of an employment opportunity for meeting one's professional and personal goals.

Goal S9. Adhere to an interdisciplinary approach to antimicrobial management.

TO S9.1 (Characterization) Consistently practice using an interdisciplinary approach to antimicrobial management.

Direct Patient Care

Provide quality patient care by using a pharmacy practice methodology

Goal P1. Conduct direct patient care activities using a consistent approach that reflects the philosophy of pharmaceutical care and is performed with the efficiency and depth of experience characteristic of an infectious diseases pharmacy specialist.

TO P1.1 (Organization) Demonstrate commitment to the responsibility for patients having an infection by consistently delivering their pharmaceutical care while maximizing safety precautions.

TO P1.2 (Synthesis) Devise efficient strategies for one's own direct patient care activities that maximize the delivery of appropriate pharmaceutical care to each patient within a limited time frame.

TO P1.3 (Synthesis) Formulate solutions to complex infectious diseases patient care problems that maximize the achievement of desired pharmaceutical care outcomes.

Goal P2. Design, recommend, monitor, and evaluate patient-specific infectious diseases pharmacotherapy. (When provided as part of the practice of pharmaceutical care, the design, recommendation, monitoring, and evaluation of patient-specific pharmacotherapy is always a series of integrated, interrelated steps. These five steps are detailed below as separate, but related goal areas to facilitate teaching and assessment.)

Goal P2A. Build the information base needed to design an anti-infective regimen.

TO P2A.1 (Synthesis) Collect and organize all patient-specific information needed by the infectious diseases specialist to detect and resolve anti-infective-related problems and to make appropriate drug therapy recommendations.

EO P2A.1.1 (Comprehension) Identify the types of information the infectious diseases specialist requires to detect and resolve anti-infective-related problems and to make appropriate drug therapy recommendations.

EO P2A.1.2 (Comprehension) Discuss signs and symptoms, epidemiology, risk factors, pathogenesis, pathophysiology, natural history of disease, clinical course, etiology, and treatment of those infectious diseases listed in Appendix B.

EO P2A.1.3 (Comprehension) Discuss the mechanism of action, pharmacokinetics, pharmacodynamics, usual regimen (dose, schedule, form, route, and method of administration), indications, contraindications, interactions, adverse reactions, relative efficacies, and pharmacoeconomics of anti-infectives.

TO P2A.2 (Analysis) Determine the presence of any of the following problems or concerns in the patient's current drug therapy:

1. Drugs used with no medical indication.
2. Medical conditions for which there is no drug prescribed.
3. Drugs prescribed inappropriately for a particular medical condition.
4. Anything inappropriate in the current drug therapy regimen (dose, schedule, route of administration, method of administration).
5. Presence of therapeutic duplication.
6. Drugs to which the patient is allergic.
7. Presence or potential for adverse drug events.
8. Presence of clinically significant drug–drug, drug–disease, drug–nutrient, or drug–laboratory test interactions.
9. Interference with medical therapy by social or recreational drug use.
10. Patient not receiving full benefit of prescribed drug therapy.
11. Treatment problems arising from financial impact of drug therapy on the patient.
12. Patient lack of understanding of his or her drug therapy.

EO P2A.2.1 (Comprehension) Discuss factors affecting patient compliance with prescribed anti-infective regimens.

EO P2A.2.2 (Comprehension) Discuss factors to consider when comparing the benefits and risks of an alternative anti-infective therapy.

EO P2A.2.3 (Comprehension) Discuss factors to consider when trying to determine the likelihood that a reaction is occurring because of an anti-infective.

EO P2A.2.4 (Comprehension) Discuss acceptable approaches to the therapeutic management of an adverse reaction to an anti-infective.

EO P2A.2.5 (Evaluation) Prioritize patients' pharmacotherapy problems.

Goal P2B. Design pharmacotherapeutic regimens.

TO P2B.1 (Synthesis) Using an organized collection of patient-specific information, summarize patients' health care needs.

TO P2B.2 (Synthesis) Specify pharmacotherapeutic goals for a patient that integrate patient-specific data, disease-specific and drug-specific information, and economic, ethical, and quality-of-life considerations.

TO P2B.3 (Synthesis) Design an anti-infective regimen, including modifications to existing therapy, that meets the pharmacotherapeutic goals established for a patient.

EO P2B.3.1 (Comprehension) Discuss additional concerns with compliance, cost, and route of administration when making decisions on anti-infective regimens for patients in various health care settings.

Goal P2C. Design monitoring plans for anti-infective regimens.

TO P2C.1 (Synthesis) Design monitoring plans for anti-infective regimens that effectively evaluate achievement of the patient-specific pharmacotherapeutic goals.

EO P2C.1.1 (Synthesis) Determine parameters to monitor that will measure achievement of pharmacotherapeutic goals for an anti-infective regimen.

EO P2C.1.1.1 (Knowledge) State specific monitoring parameters for anti-infective regimens for diseases and anti-infectives listed in Appendix A.

EO P2C.1.2 (Analysis) Identify the most reliable sources of data for measuring the selected parameters.

EO P2C.1.3 (Synthesis) Define a desirable value range for each selected parameter taking into account patient-specific information.

Goal P2D. Recommend anti-infective regimens and corresponding monitoring plans.

TO P2D.1 (Application) Recommend an anti-infective regimen and corresponding monitoring plan to prescribers and patients in a way that is systematic and logical and secures consensus from the prescriber and patient.

Goal P2E. Redesign anti-infective regimens and corresponding monitoring plans based on evaluation of monitoring data.

TO P2E.1 (Analysis) Interpret the meaning of each parameter measurement in a collection of monitoring data by comparing it to the desired value.

EO P2E.1.1 (Comprehension) Explain factors that may contribute to the unreliability of monitoring results (e.g., patient-specific factors, timing of monitoring tests, equipment errors, outpatient versus inpatient monitoring).

TO P2E.2 (Synthesis) Modify a plan as necessary based on evaluation of monitoring data.

EO P2E.2.1 (Synthesis) Appropriately modify anti-infective therapy once monitoring data is obtained.

Goal P3. Provide education on anti-infective use to patients and caregivers.

TO P3.1 (Synthesis) Design education on anti-infective use for patients and caregivers that effectively meets their needs.

Goal P4. Ensure continuity of pharmaceutical care across health care settings.

TO P4.1 (Application) Use a systematic procedure to communicate pertinent pharmacotherapeutic information across health care settings.

Goal P5. Document all pharmaceutical care activities appropriately.

TO P5.1 (Organization) Integrate documentation into all pharmaceutical care activities.

Provide quality patient care through participation in medical systems

Goal P6. Participate effectively in patient care rounds.

TO P6.1 (Synthesis) Formulate appropriate responses to anti-infective drug therapy requests and drug policy questions occurring during patient care rounds.

EO P6.1.1 (Characterization) Demonstrate a commitment to maintaining a database to support participation in patient care rounds.

EO P6.1.2 (Characterization) Demonstrate a commitment to maintaining current knowledge of the organized health care setting's anti-infective policies and procedures.

Goal P7. Participate effectively on infection control committees.

TO P7.1 (Organization) Demonstrate commitment to the responsibility for the prevention of spread of diseases by providing leadership on infection control committees.

TO P7.2 (Synthesis) Revise policies for infection control and disease prevention.

Goal P8. Design programs that center on prevention of infectious diseases.

TO P8.1 (Synthesis) Design programs aimed at preventing the transmission of infectious diseases.

TO P8.2 (Synthesis) Formulate an immunization program for targeted patient populations.

Drug Information and Drug Policy Development

Provide drug information and medication-use education

Goal I1. Provide concise, applicable, and timely responses to requests for information from health care providers and patients relative to infectious diseases and anti-infective use.

TO I1.1 (Synthesis) Formulate a systematic, efficient, and thorough procedure for retrieving information on infectious diseases and anti-infective use.

EO I1.1.1 (Analysis) Identify the most relevant sources of information regarding infectious diseases and anti-infective agents, including sources of unpublished data.

TO I1.2 (Evaluation) Appraise the infectious disease literature to determine the quality of data gathered to respond to drug information requests.

EO I1.2.1 (Evaluation) Appraise adequacy of study methodology to support the study's conclusions.

EO I1.2.1.1 (Evaluation) Determine whether the endpoint established for a study is appropriate.

EO I1.2.1.1.1 (Comprehension) Discuss methods used to test study endpoint (e.g., microbiological procedures).

EO I1.2.1.2 (Comprehension) Discuss the effects on study outcomes of various methods of patient selection (e.g., volunteers, patients, or patients with different disease severity).

EO I1.2.1.3 (Comprehension) Discuss the effects on study outcomes of various methods of blinding (e.g., double-blind, single-blind, or open research designs).

EO I1.2.1.4 (Comprehension) Discuss the effects on study outcomes of various methods of drug assay and quality assurance procedures (e.g., HPLC, assay CV).

EO I1.2.1.5 (Comprehension) Discuss the effects on study outcomes of various methods of data analysis (e.g., pharmacokinetics, pharmacoeconomics, and pharmacodynamics).

EO I1.2.1.6 (Comprehension) Discuss the effects on study outcomes of various statistical methods used for data analysis (e.g., *t* test, ANOVA).

EO I1.2.1.7 (Application) Determine if a study is or is not clinically significant.

EO I1.2.1.8 (Comprehension) Discuss the strengths and limitations of different study designs.

EO I1.2.2 (Analysis) Determine that a study's conclusions are supported by the study results.

EO I1.2.3 (Application) Use published guidelines to help evaluate the results of a pharmacoeconomic publication.

EO I1.2.4 (Comprehension) Discuss how data from a study can be applied to expanded patient populations.

TO I1.3 (Synthesis) Formulate responses to drug information requests in oral or written format as appropriate to the request.

TO I1.4 (Evaluation) Assess the effectiveness of drug information recommendations.

Goal I2. Select a core library, including computerized databases, appropriate for an infectious diseases pharmacy practice setting.

TO I2.1 (Application) Use a knowledge of standard references and databases to select a core library of primary, secondary, and tertiary references appropriate for an infectious diseases pharmacy practice setting.

Goal I3. Prepare and disseminate written information on anti-infective therapy.

TO I3.1 (Synthesis) Edit and author a newsletter providing pertinent anti-infective therapy information that meets the needs and interests of the reader.

EO I3.1.1 (Application) Use editing and writing skills to revise newsletter articles for publication.

TO I3.2 (Synthesis) Write timely and authoritative consults and notes according to the health system's policies and procedures.

TO I3.3 (Evaluation) Determine the adequacy of an anti-infective drug monograph for submission to the health system's Pharmacy & Therapeutics (P&T) committee.

TO I3.4 (Synthesis) Write authoritative manuscripts, suitable for publication, that address issues in anti-infective therapy.

TO I3.5 (Synthesis) Generate educational materials that assist the public in the understanding of drug-use issues or the management of an individual's drug therapy.

Goal I4. Prepare and disseminate oral information on anti-infective therapy.

TO I4.1 (Characterization) Speak with confidence and authority when presenting information on anti-infective therapy to health care personnel and the public.

TO I4.2 (Synthesis) Design effective educational programs for pharmacists, physicians, nurses, and other practitioners on anti-infective therapy issues (e.g., inservice, lecture, seminar).

TO I4.3 (Application) Use effective educational techniques to present programs for pharmacists, physicians, nurses, and other practitioners on anti-infective therapy issues (e.g., inservice, lecture, seminar).

Participate in developing and evaluating drug-use policies

Goal I5. Participate in the ongoing revision of the anti-infectives section of a health system's drug formulary.

TO I5.1 (Application) Use established concepts and principles to revise the anti-infective section of a health system's drug formulary, if applicable.

EO I5.1.1 (Comprehension) Explain the purpose and organization of an anti-infective subcommittee of the P&T committee.

EO I5.1.2 (Application) Use a knowledge of relevant factors to estimate the impact of cost information on specific decisions of the P&T committee.

EO I5.1.3 (Analysis) Make recommendations for formulary status of a new anti-infective based on comparative reviews.

EO I5.1.4 (Analysis) Make recommendations for drug class decisions based on comparative reviews.

EO I5.1.5 (Analysis) Make recommendations on formulary status based on periodic review of non-formulary anti-infective use.

EO I5.1.6 (Application) Use a knowledge of relevant factors to estimate the impact of cost information on specific decisions of the P&T committee.

EO I5.1.7 (Comprehension) Discuss the contribution of pharmacoeconomic data to formulary decisions and drug marketing strategies.

Goal I6. Participate in the development or modification of treatment protocols for infectious diseases.

TO I6.1 (Synthesis) Contribute the pharmacy perspective to an interdisciplinary team developing treatment protocols using anti-infectives.

Goal I7. Participate in the development or modification of identified policies for the selection and use of anti-infectives.

TO I7.1 (Synthesis) Revise policies for the selection and use of anti-infectives.

Goal I8. Participate in the development, implementation, and evaluation of the health system's drug-use evaluation (DUE) program.

TO I8.1 (Synthesis) Design an anti-infective DUE that fits the health system's goals and mission statement.

EO I8.1.1 (Analysis) Identify appropriate topics for an anti-infective DUE in a specific health system.

TO I8.2 (Application) Conduct a DUE using accepted methodology.

TO I8.3 (Evaluation) Appraise the results of a DUE.

Practice Management

Develop personal practice management skills

Goal M1. Model a practice management philosophy that supports pharmaceutical care and pharmacy practice excellence.

TO M1.1 (Characterization) Demonstrate leadership in fostering the philosophy of practice excellence in others.

TO M1.2 (Characterization) Demonstrate leadership in promoting interdisciplinary team management.

Goal M2. Work through the political and decision-making structure to accomplish one's practice area goals.

TO M2.1 (Application) Use knowledge of an organization's political and decision-making structure to influence the accomplishment of a practice area goal.

EO M2.1.1 (Analysis) Identify individuals in the formal and informal organizational structure who are key decision-makers or who have significant influence on the decision-making process.

Goal M3. Contribute to the achievement of pharmacy goals through effective participation on an organization's committees.

TO M3.1 (Application) Use group participation skills when working on an organization's committees.

EO M3.1.1 (Comprehension) Discuss the specific site needs of various types of group meetings.

EO M3.1.2 (Analysis) Determine what information resulting from committee meetings should be supplied to various individuals or groups.

Manage integrated pharmaceutical care services

Goal M4. Evaluate current pharmacy services to determine whether the services are meeting the needs of patients with infectious diseases.

TO M4.1 (Evaluation) Appraise the organization's current pharmacy services for adequacy in meeting the needs of infectious diseases patients.

Goal M5. Participate in the development of proposals for new infectious diseases pharmacy services.

TO M5.1 (Synthesis) Design the pharmacy contribution to a proposal for a new service that involves the use of anti-infectives.

Goal M6. Contribute to the achievement of health system goals for patient care using drug cost, outcome, and pharmacoeconomic information.

TO M6.1 (Evaluation) Appraise anti-infective costs using conventional methodology.

TO M6.2 (Synthesis) Modify clinical practice based on outcome findings.

EO M6.2.1 (Evaluation) Assess patient outcomes for specific infectious diseases.

TO M6.3 (Synthesis) Modify clinical practice based on pharmacoeconomic data.

EO M6.3.1 (Synthesis) Design a pharmacoeconomic evaluation of anti-infective therapy for selected diseases.

EO M6.3.1.1 (Comprehension) Discuss the components of a pharmacoeconomic analysis.

EO M6.3.1.2 (Comprehension) Discuss the methodologies employed in the evaluation of pharmacoeconomic data.

Goal M7. Participate in the management of the practice area's human resources.

TO M7.1 (Synthesis) Write a job description for an infectious diseases pharmacist that matches with department needs and the health system's policies and procedures.

TO M7.2 (Synthesis) Formulate appropriate interview strategies for job candidates.

TO M7.3 (Comprehension) Explain the components of an employee evaluation system.

TO M7.4 (Comprehension) Discuss the principles and application of a progressive discipline process.

Goal M8. Assist the health system in achieving compliance with accreditation, legal, regulatory, and safety requirements related to the use anti-infective agents (e.g., JCAHO requirements; ASHP standards, statements, and guidelines; state and federal laws regulating pharmacy practice; OSHA regulations).

TO M8.1 (Evaluation) Determine appropriate activities and documentation to meet accreditation, legal, regulatory, and safety requirements in the area of infectious diseases.

Goal M9. Participate in the health system's quality improvement program.

TO M9.1 (Synthesis) Contribute to the development of guidelines to ensure quality improvement in the treatment of infectious diseases.

Goal M10. Conduct relations with the pharmaceutical industry in an ethical manner.

TO M10.1 (Synthesis) Formulate ethically appropriate strategies for one's contacts with the pharmaceutical industry.

Goal M11. Manage the use of investigational anti-infective agents according to established protocols and the health system's policies and procedures.

TO M11.1 (Application) Manage the use of anti-infective agents according to established protocols and the health system's policies and procedures.

Appendix A

The program director should develop an experiential plan at the beginning of the program for each resident. The experiential component shall consist of the following required and elective learning experiences. The needs and interest of each resident and the attributes of the residency program should be utilized in the development of the experiential plan.

A. ***Required Learning Experiences.*** The resident's training shall provide learning experiences that encompass multidisciplinary and independent pharmacy patient care. Therefore, training should be varied and of sufficient depth to prepare an independent pharmacy practitioner focused on diseases and antibiotic management. Required areas of training shall include the following:
1. Foundations of microbiology laboratory assessments, parameters and values.
2. Infectious disease consult service serving adult and pediatric patients.
3. Ambulatory care infectious diseases clinic.
4. Antimicrobial-use surveillance programs.

B. ***Elective Experiences.*** Learning experiences in the following areas may be taken as electives:
1. Medical intensive care.
2. Inpatient surgery service.
3. Inpatient medical service.
4. Medical oncology service.
5. Inpatient AIDS service.
6. Ambulatory care AIDS clinic.
7. Drug information center.
8. Solid organ or bone marrow transplantation services.
9. Limited basic or clinical research.
10. Pharmaceutical industry.
11. Infection control.
12. Pharmacoeconomics/health economics.

Appendix B

Through a broad range of practice experiences, the resident in infectious diseases pharmacy practice should develop an extensive knowledge base in the area of infectious diseases pharmacy practice. The following represents areas of content that should be incorporated into the residency curriculum.

A. ***General Content Areas***
1. Microbial virulence factors.
2. Host defense mechanisms.
3. Epidemiology of infectious diseases.
4. Medical microbiology laboratory assessments, parameters and values.

B. ***Principles of Anti-Infective Therapy***
1. General pharmacodynamics of anti-infectives.
   a. Mechanisms of anti-infective action.
   b. Mechanisms of anti-infective resistance.
   c. Mechanisms of post-antibiotic effect and bactericidal activity.
   d. Principles of synergy and antagonism.
2. Comparative pharmacology of anti-infectives.
   a. Antibacterials.
   b. Antifungals.
   c. Antivirals.
   d. Antiparasitics.
   e. Immunomodulators.
3. Therapeutic use of anti-infectives.
   a. Immunizations.
   b. Empiric use of anti-infectives.
   c. Prophylactic use of anti-infectives.
   d. Combination anti-infective therapies.
   e. Desensitization.
   f. Anti-infective-induced illness.
   g. Appropriate discontinuation of anti-infectives.

C. ***Therapeutics of Major Clinical Syndromes***
1. Upper-respiratory-tract infections.
2. Lower-respiratory-tract infections.
3. Urinary-tract infections.
4. Sepsis.
5. Intra-abdominal infections.
6. Cardiovascular infections.
7. Central nervous system infections.
8. Skin and soft-tissue infections.
9. Gastrointestinal infections.
10. Bone and joint infections.
11. Sexually transmitted diseases.
12. Infections of reproductive organs.
13. Ophthalmologic infections.
14. Viral hepatitis.
15. Human immunodeficiency virus (HIV) infection and AIDS (including opportunistic infections).
16. Special problems and miscellaneous syndromes.
    a. Nosocomial infections.
    b. Infections in the compromised host.
    c. Peri-operative infections.
    d. Burn injury.
    e. Bite injury.
    f. Zoonoses (e.g., rabies).
17. Tuberculosis and other mycobacterial infections.

Reference

1. American Society of Hospital Pharmacists. ASHP Accreditation Standard for Specialized Pharmacy Residency Training (with Guide to Interpretation). *American Journal of Hospital Pharmacists.* 1994; 51: 2034–41.

---

[a]Anti-infective: This term includes antibacterials, antifungals, antivirals, antiparasitics, vaccines, and biological response modifiers employed in the management of infectious diseases.

Approved by the ASHP Board of Directors, November 18, 1995. Developed by a working group of infectious diseases pharmacy practitioners representing ASHP, the Society of Infectious Disease Pharmacists (SIDP), and the ASHP Commission on Credentialing.

The bibliographic citation for this document is as follows: ASHP supplemental standard and learning objectives for residency training in infectious diseases pharmacy practice. In: *Practice Standards of ASHP 1996–97.* Deffenbaugh J, ed. Bethesda, MD: American Society of Health-System Pharmacists; 1996.

ASHP Technician Training Program Accreditation Regulations and Standards

ASHP Regulations on Accreditation of Hospital Pharmacy Technician Training Programs

Preamble

Hospital pharmacists have long recognized the need for a corps of technically trained supportive personnel in the field of hospital pharmacy. This need arises from the fact that the practice of hospital pharmacy encompasses a complex set of tasks, some of which require the knowledge and judgment of a pharmacist but many others of which do not. Without the benefit of a technically trained adjunctive work force, hospital pharmacists would be compelled to devote much of their own time and energies to the performance of technical tasks rather than to those patient-care pursuits for which they have been trained.

ASHP supports the effective use of qualified technicians in all institutional pharmacy settings; further, the Society recognizes an obligation to promulgate standards for the training of such personnel. To ensure a continuing supply of well-qualified technicians for hospital pharmacy practice, an accreditation program is conducted by the Society.

Objectives

The objectives of the accreditation program are (1) to upgrade and standardize the formal training that hospital pharmacy technicians receive; (2) to guide, assist, and recognize those hospitals and academic institutions that wish to support the profession by operating such programs; (3) to provide criteria for the prospective technician trainee in the selection of a program by identifying those institutions conducting accredited pharmacy technician training programs; and (4) to provide hospitals and related health agencies a basis for determining the level of competency of pharmacy technicians by identifying those technicians who have successfully completed accredited technician training programs.

Authority

The program for accreditation of hospital pharmacy technician training programs is conducted by the authority of the Board of Directors of ASHP under the direction of the Commission on Credentialing. All matters of policy relating to the accreditation program considered by the Commission on Credentialing shall be submitted for approval to the Board of Directors of the Society. The Commission on Credentialing shall review and evaluate applications and survey reports submitted and shall be specifically delegated by the Board of Directors to take final action on all applications for accreditation, in accordance with the policies and procedures set forth herein. The minutes of all transactions of the Commission on Credentialing shall be submitted to the Board of Directors for its review.

Policies

The following policies apply to the technician training accreditation program:

1. ***Initial Evaluation of Training Program.***

   a. The accreditation program shall be conducted as a service of ASHP to institutions voluntarily requesting evaluation of their programs.

   b. To be eligible for accreditation, a program must have been in operation for one full training cycle and have at least one graduate. (If accreditation is granted, it shall be retroactive to the date on which a valid and complete application, including all requested supporting documents, is received by the Society's Director of Accreditation Services.)

   c. Program evaluation shall be by site survey for which an appropriate fee, established by the Board of Directors, shall be assessed to the institution.

   d. Programs shall be reviewed by hospital pharmacists or hospital pharmacy educators appointed by the Society's Director of Accreditation Services.

2. ***Certificate of Accreditation.***

   a. A certificate of accreditation will be issued by the Society's Board of Directors to those institutions for whom accreditation is approved; however, the certificate remains the property of ASHP and shall be returned to the Society at any time accreditation is withdrawn.

   b. Any reference by an institution to accreditation by the Society in certificates, catalogs, bulletins, communications, or other forms of publicity shall state only the following: "(Name of Institution) is accredited for pharmacy technician training by the American Society of Hospital Pharmacists."

3. ***Continuing Evaluation of Accredited Programs.***

   a. The Society regards evaluation of accredited technician training programs as a continuous process; accordingly, the Commission on Credentialing shall request program directors of accredited programs to submit periodic written status reports to assist the Commission in evaluating the continued conformance of individual programs to the Accreditation Standard. Written reports shall be required from program directors at least every 2 years.

   b. Accredited training programs shall be reexamined by site visit at least every 4 years.

   c. Any major change in the organization of a program will be considered justification for immediate reevaluation.

   d. A survey fee, as established by the ASHP Board of Directors, shall be assessed to the institution for reaccreditation site visits.

4. ***Withdrawal of Accreditation.***

   a. Accreditation of a pharmacy technician training program may be withdrawn by the Society for any of the reasons stated below.

      (1) Accredited programs that no longer meet the requirements of the Society's "Accreditation Standard for Pharmacy Technician

Training Programs" shall have accreditation withdrawn.

(2) Accredited programs without a technician trainee for 2 consecutive years shall have accreditation withdrawn.

(3) Accreditation shall be withdrawn if the program director is replaced by another individual whose qualifications do not meet the requirements of the Accreditation Standard.

b. The institution shall submit a new application and undergo reevaluation to regain accreditation.

c. Accreditation shall not be withdrawn without first notifying the institution of the specific reasons why its program does not meet the Society's "Accreditation Standard for Pharmacy Technician Training Programs." In such instances, the institution shall be granted an appropriate specified period of time to correct deficiencies.

d. The institution shall have the right to appeal the decision of the Commission on Credentialing.

Accreditation Procedures

1. *Application for Accreditation.*

a. Application forms may be requested from the American Society of Hospital Pharmacists, Director of Accreditation Services, 7272 Wisconsin Avenue, Bethesda, MD 20814. These forms should be filled out in duplicate. One copy of the application should be signed by the chief executive officer of the institution seeking accreditation and the director of the technician training program and submitted, along with the supporting documents specified in the application instructions, to the Society's Director of Accreditation Services. The duplicate copy should be retained for the applicant's files.

b. The Director of Accreditation Services will acknowledge receipt of the application and review it to make a preliminary judgment about the applicant's conformance to the basic requirements of the Accreditation Standard. If the Director feels that the program fails to meet the criteria of the Accreditation Standard in some fundamental way, he will notify the signatories of the application accordingly and advise against scheduling a site visit until the problems have been corrected. The applicant is not bound, however, to accept the Director's advice to delay the accreditation application.

2. *Site Visit.*

a. At a mutually convenient time, the Society will send a survey team to review the training program. Instructions for preparation for the site visit (list of documents to be made available to the team, suggested itinerary, etc.) will be sent to the program director well in advance. Normally, the site visit is conducted in 1 working day by a team of two people.

b. In the case of a program conducted by an academic institution, arrangements must be made by the institution for the survey team to conduct an onsite review of the practical training sites.

3. *Survey Report.*

a. At the end of the survey, the survey team will complete a report, consisting of a checklist and written comment, that will be reviewed with the program director and chief executive officer (or his representative). A copy of the report will be given to the institution. The original will be sent by the team to the Society's Director of Accreditation Services.

b. The institution will be given 30 days in which to respond to the survey report. Response should be in writing and sent to the Director of Accreditation Services.

c. The institution's accreditation application file, including the surveyors' report, plus any written comments received from the institution, will be reviewed by the Commission on Credentialing at its next meeting. The Commission will resolve any factual issues at that time.

d. Notice of action taken by the Commission will be sent to the chief executive officer of the institution and the technician program director, along with a list of any deficiencies that the Commission considered in arriving at its decision and recommendations for overcoming those deficiencies. The report will indicate that the Commission has acted either (1) to accredit or reaccredit the program for a period not to exceed 2 years or (2) to withhold or withdraw accreditation.

4. *Appeal of Commission Decision.*

a. *Notification of intent to appeal.* In the event that the Commission shall fail to accredit or reaccredit fully a program, the institution's chief executive officer may appeal the decision of the Commission to an appeal board on the grounds that the decision of the Commission was arbitrary, prejudiced, biased, capricious, or based on incorrect application of the Standards to the institution. The chief executive officer must notify the Director of Accreditation Services, in writing by registered or certified mail within 10 days after receipt of the Commission's decision, of the institution's intent to appeal. The institution must state clearly on what grounds the appeal is being made. The institution shall then have an additional 30 days in which to prepare for its presentation to an appeal board.

b. *Appeal board.* On receipt of an appeal notice, the Director of Accreditation Services shall proceed to constitute an ad hoc appeal board. The appeal board shall consist of one member of the Society's Board of Directors, who shall be appointed by the President of ASHP and who shall serve as chairman, and two directors of accredited pharmacy technician training programs, neither of whom is a member of the Commission on Credentialing, one to be named by the appellant and one by the chairman of the Commission. In addition, a hospital administrator shall be appointed by the President of the Society to serve in a nonvoting, ex officio capacity on the appeal board. The Director of Accreditation Services shall serve as secretary of the appeal board. As soon as appointments to the appeal board have been made, the Director of Accreditation Services shall immediately forward to all appeal board members copies of all written documentation considered by the Commission in rendering its decision.

c. *Hearing.* The appeal board shall have convened in not less than 30 days nor more than 60 days from the date of receipt of an appeal notice by the Director of Accreditation Services. The Director of Accreditation Services shall notify appellants and appeal board members, at least 30 days in advance, of the date, time, and place of the hearing. The institution filing the appeal may be represented at the hearing by one or more appropriate officials and shall be given the opportunity at such hearing to present written, or written and oral, evidence and argument tending to refute or overcome the findings and decision of the Commission on Credentialing. The Director of Accreditation Services shall represent the Commission at the hearing.

The appeal board shall advise the appellant of the board's decision, in writing by registered or certified mail, within 10 days of the date of the hearing. The decision of the appeal board is final and binding on both the appellant and ASHP.

d. *Appeal board expenses.* The appellant shall be responsible for all expenses incurred by its own representatives at the appeal board hearing and shall pay all reasonable travel, living, and incidental expenses incurred by its appointee to the appeal board. Expenses incurred by the other board members and the Director of Accreditation Services shall be borne by ASHP.

Approved by the ASHP Board of Directors, April 23–24, 1987. Developed by the ASHP Commission on Credentialing. Supersedes the previous regulations approved November 20–21, 1985. The current revision reflects a change in policy with respect to the cycle of site visits; previously, such visits were required "at least every 2 years," whereas the policy now is for onsite inspections "at least every 4 years" supplemented by written reports from the training program at least every 2 years.

The bibliographic citation for this document is as follows: American Society of Hospital Pharmacists. ASHP regulations on accreditation of hospital pharmacy technician training programs. *Am J Hosp Pharm.* 1987; 44:2741–3.

ASHP Accreditation Standard for Pharmacy Technician Training Programs

Part I—Administrative Responsibility for the Training Program

A. Pharmacy technician training programs may be conducted by either health-care or academic institutions. These institutions must be accredited, when applicable, by the appropriate agency and shall be responsible for ensuring that the following requirements have been met:

1. The trainee's practical experience is obtained in qualified training site(s) that meet the requirements set forth in Parts II and III.

2. The program director shall meet the requirements set forth in Part IV.

B. When requested, the health-care or academic institution shall provide the trainee applicant with information concerning the purpose of the training program, prospects for employment, and realistic salary expectations.

C. A program director shall be named whose authority and responsibilities are commensurate with those of other allied health, technical, or vocational training programs offered by the institution. This individual shall have appropriate authority to direct all aspects of training. The director need not be a pharmacist; however, there must be a sufficient complement of pharmacists on the faculty to meet all instructional objectives.

D. An advisory committee comprising a broad-based group of pharmacists, faculty, and pharmacy technicians must be established and have specific authority for the following:

1. Determining that the curriculum makes possible the attainment of all learning objectives set forth in Part VI.

2. Approving practice training sites.

3. Validating admission criteria.

4. Validating criteria for successful completion of the program.

E. Nothing in this Standard shall prevent individual training programs from establishing more stringent requirements than those specified herein. Further, in instances where more stringent requirements have been established or adopted by state law, regulation, or governmental agency, those requirements will take precedence for the purposes of accreditation by ASHP of programs within the corresponding state or jurisdiction.

Part II—Qualifications of the Training Site

A. A health-care facility that offers, or participates in offering, a technician training program shall be accredited by the Joint Commission on Accreditation of Healthcare Organizations or the American Osteopathic Association.

B. Other practice sites (e.g., community pharmacies) that participate in technician training shall have demonstrated substantial conformance with applicable professionally developed and nationally applied practice standards.

C. All practice sites shall comply (where applicable) with all federal, state, and local laws, codes, statutes, regulations, and licensing requirements.

D. Technician training sites shall conduct the practice component of the program in such a way as to ensure that any services the technician trainee is required to provide complement, rather than compete with, the educational and experiential objectives of the program.

Part III—Qualifications of the Pharmacy Service

A. All pharmacies involved in technician training shall be organized in accordance with the principles of good management under the direction of a legally qualified pharmacist and with sufficient appropriate personnel to provide a broad scope of pharmaceutical services to all patients served.

B. The training site(s) used for experiential training shall have adequate facilities to carry out services that meet, when applicable, the intent of the "ASHP Guidelines: Minimum Standard for Pharmacies in Institutions"[1] or the "ASHP Guidelines on Pharmaceutical Services for Ambulatory Patients."[2] It is necessary that practice experience be part of regular, ongoing services; hence, it is not sufficient to create "artificial situations" in which trainees can obtain this experience.

C. Pharmacies involved in technician training must be neat and orderly and must project a highly professional image.

Part IV—Qualifications of the Program Director and Preceptors

A. The technician training program shall be subject to similar general administrative control and guidance employed by the institution for other allied health-care training programs. If the program is conducted by an academic institution, the program director must ensure that pharmacists or designees oversee and guide all experiential training of the pharmacy technician trainees at the practice site.

B. The program director is encouraged to be a member of a national pharmacy organization and the corresponding state affiliate. All other program faculty and preceptors should also hold active membership in these organizations.

C. The program director shall have considerable latitude in delegating preceptorial responsibilities for the technician training program to others on staff. Each individual designated as an instructor must have demonstrated competence in one or more related areas of pharmacy practice and possess an ability to teach. The program director, or designee, is ultimately accountable for the overall quality of the trainee's practical experience.

D. Persons who supervise experiential training must meet the following qualifications:

1. The hospital pharmacy director, or designee, shall supervise experiential hospital pharmacy training. This individual shall have had at least 5 years' experience in a pharmacy that meets the requirements of the "ASHP Guidelines: Minimum Standard for Pharmacies in Institutions."[1]

2. All experiential training that occurs outside the hospital setting must be coordinated by a pharmacist or designee with sufficient knowledge and skills to provide a sound educational experience. Further, this individual must have demonstrated sufficient contribution and commitment to pharmacy practice and patient care.

Part V—Qualifications and Selection of the Applicant

A. The applicant must be a high school graduate or possess a high school equivalency certificate.

B. Final approval of the qualifications of the applicant for acceptance as a trainee shall be the responsibility of the director of the technician training program.

Part VI—Technician Training Program

A. The technician training program must include didactic, laboratory, and practice components structured to allow trainees to achieve the program objectives. Objectives for the technician training program shall be in writing and shall be provided to each trainee at the beginning of the program. The objectives shall relate to the technical skills required in contemporary pharmacy practice and shall describe the terminal competencies to be striven for in the training program.[a] The training program shall be based on the following objectives:

1. The technician should demonstrate appropriate knowledge and understanding of pharmacy's role in the health-care industry, including quality improvement processes that may be used to monitor pharmacy's ability to fulfill its responsibilities within a given health-care system.

2. The technician should have a thorough knowledge and understanding of the duties and responsibilities of pharmacy technicians, including standards of ethics governing pharmacy practice.

3. The technician should have a working knowledge of the pharmaceutical and medical terms, abbreviations, and symbols commonly used in the prescribing, dispensing, administering, and charting of medications in the institution.

4. The technician should have a working knowledge of the general chemical and physical properties of drugs handled in the manufacturing and packaging operations used in the delivery of pharmaceutical services.

5. The technician should be able to perform the arithmetical calculations required for the usual dosage determinations and solution preparation.

6. The technician should be able to perform the essential functions relating to drug purchasing and inventory control.

7. The technician should demonstrate a working knowledge of drug dosages, routes of administration, and mechanical, automatic, or robotic drug delivery systems.

8. The technician should have a working knowledge of the procedures and operations relating to the manufacturing, packaging, and labeling of drug products.

9. The technician should have a working knowledge of the procedures and operations relating to aseptic compounding and parenteral admixture operations.

10. The technician should exhibit the ability to perform the usual technician functions associated with contemporary drug distribution systems.

11. The technician should be able to perform the manipulative and recordkeeping functions associated with the dispensing of prescriptions for ambulatory patients, including the completion of universal insurance claim forms when necessary.

B. Appropriate laboratory exercises, including computerized application of recordkeeping and drug distribution systems, shall be used to reinforce classroom instruction before onsite experiential training commences.

C. All instructors and trainees must be thoroughly familiar with the requirements of this Standard.

D. Each trainee's activities shall be scheduled in advance and shall be planned to enable the trainee to attain the predetermined objectives. The training schedule shall consist of a minimum of 600 hours of training (contact) time, extending over a period of 15 weeks or longer.

E. A broad plan for each student shall be developed and documented at the beginning of the program.

F. Records of training activities that clearly delineate the scope and period of training shall be maintained. The program director shall keep these records on file.

G. The program director shall arrange for formalized and regularly scheduled evaluation of the trainee's achievement in terms of the objectives previously established.

Part VII—Experimentation and Innovation

A. Experimental and innovative approaches to developing and implementing pharmacy technician training programs and alternative methods for meeting this Standard shall be encouraged.

B. These experimental and innovative activities must be adequately planned and coupled with an appropriate evaluation system.

Part VIII—Certificate

A. The accredited program shall recognize those pharmacy technicians who have completed successfully the pharmacy technician training program by awarding an appropriate certificate or diploma.

B. No certificate shall be issued to any individual who has failed to complete the prescribed program or to meet the intent of this Standard.

References

1. American Society of Hospital Pharmacists. ASHP guidelines: minimum standard for pharmacies in insti-

tutions. *Am J Hosp Pharm.* 1985; 42:372–5.
2. American Society of Hospital Pharmacists. ASHP guidelines on pharmaceutical services for ambulatory patients. *Am J Hosp Pharm.* 1991; 48:311–5.

---

[a]The "ASHP Technical Assistance Bulletin on Outcome Competencies and Training Guidelines for Institutional Pharmacy Technician Training Programs" (*Am J Hosp Pharm.* 1982; 39:317–20) is recommended as a guide.

Approved by the ASHP Board of Directors, September 25, 1992. Developed by the ASHP Commission on Credentialing. Supersedes the previous versions approved on April 23, 1982, and revised November 17–18, 1983, and November 20–21, 1985.

The bibliographic citation for this document is as follows: American Society of Hospital Pharmacists. ASHP accreditation standard for pharmacy technician training programs. *Am J Hosp Pharm.* 1993; 50:124–6.

ASHP-Endorsed Documents

Code of Ethics for Pharmacists

Preamble

Pharmacists are health professionals who assist individuals in making the best use of medications. This Code, prepared and supported by pharmacists, is intended to state publicly the principles that form the fundamental basis of the roles and responsibilities of pharmacists. These principles, based on moral obligations and virtues, are established to guide pharmacists in relationships with patients, health professionals, and society.

Principles

I.   *A pharmacist respects the covenantal relationship between the patient and pharmacist.*

Interpretation: Considering the patient–pharmacist relationship as a covenant means that a pharmacist has moral obligations in response to the gift of trust received from society. In return for this gift, a pharmacist promises to help individuals achieve optimum benefit from their medications, to be committed to their welfare, and to maintain their trust.

II. *A pharmacist promotes the good of every patient in a caring, compassionate, and confidential manner.*

Interpretation: A pharmacist places concern for the well-being of the patient at the center of professional practice. In doing so, a pharmacist considers needs stated by the patient as well as those defined by health science. A pharmacist is dedicated to protecting the dignity of the patient. With a caring attitude and a compassionate spirit, a pharmacist focuses on serving the patient in a private and confidential manner.

III. *A pharmacist respects the autonomy and dignity of each patient.*

Interpretation: A pharmacist promotes the right of self-determination and recognizes individual self-worth by encouraging patients to participate in decisions about their health. A pharmacist communicates with patients in terms that are understandable. In all cases, a pharmacist respects personal and cultural differences among patients.

IV. *A pharmacist acts with honesty and integrity in professional relationships.*

Interpretation: A pharmacist has a duty to tell the truth and to act with conviction of conscience. A pharmacist avoids discriminatory practices, behavior or work conditions that impair professional judgment, and actions that compromise dedication to the best interests of patients.

V.   *A pharmacist maintains professional competence.*

Interpretation: A pharmacist has a duty to maintain knowledge and abilities as new medications, devices, and technologies become available and as health information advances.

VI. *A pharmacist respects the values and abilities of colleagues and other health professionals.*

Interpretation: When appropriate, a pharmacist asks for the consultation of colleagues or other health professionals or refers the patient. A pharmacist acknowledges that colleagues and other health professionals may differ in the beliefs and values they apply to the care of the patient.

VII. *A pharmacist serves individual, community, and societal needs.*

Interpretation: The primary obligation of a pharmacist is to individual patients. However, the obligations of a pharmacist may at times extend beyond the individual to the community and society. In these situations, the pharmacist recognizes the responsibilities that accompany these obligations and acts accordingly.

VIII.*A pharmacist seeks justice in the distribution of health resources.*

Interpretation: When health resources are allocated, a pharmacist is fair and equitable, balancing the needs of patients and society.

Endorsed by the American Society of Health-System Pharmacists House of Delegates on June 3, 1996. Proceedings of the 47th annual session of the ASHP House of Delegates. *Am J Health-Syst Pharm.* 1996; 53:1805. ASHP Reports.

White Paper on Pharmacy Technicians
Recommendations of Pharmacy Practitioner Organizations on the Functions, Training, and Regulation of Technicians

Introduction

Pharmacy technicians will have a growing role as pharmacists depend on them to facilitate expansion of the profession's scope of practice.

Most pharmacists probably agree with the above statement about pharmacy technicians, although many may have questions about how the profession should nurture the development of this component of the pharmacy work force. These questions involve issues related to the functions, training, and regulation of technicians.

This white paper expresses the views of the endorsing organizations on these matters and is offered for the information and guidance of all elements of the profession, including pharmacy practice managers, supervising pharmacists, pharmacy technicians, technician educators, and state boards of pharmacy.

Definitions

In the interest of good communications and sound decision-making, it is important to use terms such as *pharmacy technician*, *registration*, *licensure*, and *certification* carefully and consistently. The following authoritative definitions are used for purposes of this paper and are advocated for use throughout pharmacy:

Pharmacy Technician: An individual working in a pharmacy who, under the supervision of a licensed pharmacist, assists in pharmacy activities that do not require the professional judgment of the pharmacist.[1]

Licensure: The process by which an agency of government grants permission to an individual to engage in a given occupation upon finding that the applicant has attained the minimal degree of competency necessary to ensure that the public health, safety, and welfare will be reasonably well protected.[2] Within pharmacy, pharmacists are licensed by state boards of pharmacy.

Registration: The process of making a list or being enrolled in an existing list.[3] Within pharmacy, some state boards have elected to register technicians who work under the supervision of licensed pharmacists.

Certification: The process by which a nongovernmental agency or association grants recognition to an individual who has met certain predetermined qualifications specified by that agency or association.[2] Within pharmacy, technicians may voluntarily choose to become certified through an examination process administered by the Pharmacy Technician Certification Board.

When an examination is used in a credentialing process such as certification or licensure, the examination must meet rigorous psychometric and legal standards for the sake of fairness to credentialing candidates and for protection of the credentialing body.

Reasons for the Growing Role of Pharmacy Technicians

There is widespread acceptance among practicing pharmacists today that their primary mission is to help people make the best use of medications. Pharmacists want to practice their profession in a way that permits them to take personal responsibility for facilitating the achievement of predefined outcomes from medication-related care that improve a patient's quality of life. The profession is in the process, on many fronts, of re-engineering practice along the lines of this practice model, which is called pharmaceutical care or pharmacist care.

A key element in the profession's strategy for achieving pharmaceutical care is for the pharmacist to delegate routine functions to well-qualified, appropriately supervised pharmacy technicians. This will help permit pharmacists to free up time to focus on the medication-related problems of the patients they serve. Pharmacy's commitment to pharmaceutical care has significant societal implications; for ambulatory patients in the United States, the cost to the health care system of medication-related problems is approximately $77 billion annually.[4]

Coinciding with the pharmacist's desire to transform the mission of practice are a number of factors that have led pharmacy managers to reassess how traditional pharmaceutical services are provided. Key among these factors is mandatory pharmacist counseling of ambulatory patients. Other relevant developments include a sharp erosion of margins on prescription dispensing services and cost containment in all sectors of health care delivery. Partly in response to all these factors, more pharmacy practice managers are interested in employing technicians to assist the pharmacist.

Current Status of Pharmacy Technicians

Although pharmacists have used various types of supportive personnel in their practices for decades, the occupation of "pharmacy technician" is still in the process of becoming defined consistently throughout the profession. Progress is being made (although some would say it is sluggish) in reaching consensus on questions such as the knowledge, skills, and abilities required of technicians; functions of technicians; training requirements; appropriate level of supervision; and recognition by regulatory bodies.

Number of Pharmacy Technicians. There is no definitive information on the number of pharmacy technicians in the United States. A recent survey estimated that approximately 47,000 pharmacy technicians work in hospitals.[5] There are approximately 53,000 community pharmacies in the country; if, on average, 1.5 technicians are employed per pharmacy, there would be about 80,000 technicians in this sector of practice. Technicians also assist pharmacists in settings such as long-term-care facilities, mail service pharmacies, and home care organizations. An estimate of 150,000 pharmacy technicians in total seems reasonable.

Knowledge, Skills, and Abilities of Technicians. The 1991–1994 Scope of Pharmacy Practice Project conducted a national task analysis of technicians in all states and in a wide array of practice settings. The results of that project[6] are the best available data on the functions pharmacy technicians perform and on the knowledge they need in order to perform those functions. These findings have been the basis for the new voluntary national certification program for technicians and the model curriculum for pharmacy technicians that is under development (see below). Further, the results should be used by pharmacy more broadly to help establish a professionwide plan for the development of the occupation of pharmacy technician.

Among the findings of the Scope project were the following data on how pharmacy technicians, on average, divide their time:

1. Pharmacy technicians spend more than 26% of their time on collecting, organizing, and evaluating information in the process of assisting pharmacists in serving patients.
2. Pharmacy technicians devote more than 21% of their time developing and managing medication distribution and control systems; about half of this time is in the specific area of preparing, dispensing, distributing, and administering medications.
3. Pharmacy technicians spend less than 7% of their time providing drug information and education.

Functions of Technicians. The nature of the work that technicians perform in pharmacy practice varies widely; this is true for the following reasons:

1. The training and, hence, qualifications, of technicians vary widely.
2. The beliefs and values that pharmacists have with respect to the use of technicians vary widely.
3. State pharmacy practice laws vary in what pharmacists are allowed to delegate to technicians.
4. State pharmacy practice laws limit, to differing degrees, the ratio of technicians to pharmacists.

Technician Training. The training that current technicians have received is quite variable. In hospitals, one third of pharmacy technicians have received formal training, and the balance have been trained informally on the job.[5] In community pharmacy practice, most technicians have on-the-job training only.

There are at least 90 formal technician training programs nationwide, many of them at community colleges or technical schools.[7] There is a national accreditation service for pharmacy technician training programs; 44 programs are accredited.[8] The standards for national accreditation call for a minimum of 600 hours of training (contact) time, extending over a period of 15 weeks or longer.[9]

A consortium of national pharmacy organizations is currently developing a model curriculum for technician training. This work is based on the results of the Scope of Pharmacy Practice Project. Those developing the model curriculum hope that it will, over time, stimulate a higher level of standardization in the training of technicians. The groups involved in the initial steps of this project are the American Society of Health-System Pharmacists, the American Association of Colleges of Pharmacy, the American Association of Pharmacy Technicians, the American Pharmaceutical Association, and the Pharmacy Technician Educators Council.

Effect of Technology on Future Demand for Technicians. In counterbalance to the professional practice imperatives in pharmacy, the advancement of drug product distribution technology may serve to reduce future demand for pharmacy technicians. While this is a plausible development, its magnitude is difficult to predict. Nevertheless, it seems likely that there will be a sizable demand for pharmacy technicians for some time to come, although the functions that technicians perform and the knowledge and skills they need will change as practice technology evolves.

State Board of Pharmacy Regulation. The role of state boards of pharmacy is to protect the health and safety of the public in its interface with pharmacy services. State boards establish minimum standards for practicing pharmacists and license those who meet the qualifications. State boards also establish minimum standards for pharmacy facilities and license those that comply. Pharmacist and pharmacy licenses may be revoked if the state board has evidence that the public is at risk as a result, for example, of failure to comply with legal requirements. Through their firm control over who may practice as a pharmacist, state boards extend their reach to the work of nonlicensed personnel who work under the pharmacist's supervision.

State boards of pharmacy currently deal with technicians in a variety of ways.[a] Some do not acknowledge the existence of technicians; some limit the type of pharmacies that are permitted to employ technicians; many establish technician-to-pharmacist ratios; some have training requirements for technicians; and some register technicians. Because of the growing importance of technicians in pharmacy practice, many state boards of pharmacy are reassessing their stance with respect to this component of the pharmacy work force.

Some state boards of pharmacy have concluded that the registration of pharmacy technicians allows them to safeguard the public by tracking the technician work force and preventing individuals with documented problems (such as substance abuse or drug-product diversion) from serving as pharmacy technicians. State boards sometimes call their registration process "licensure" even though it is more akin to registration and does not meet the standard definition of licensure that is noted in the Definitions section of this paper. An important distinction is that licensure is a public sanction to engage in an occupation and is based on an objective determination (such as through a written examination) that the individual is qualified to do so. In the case of a health occupation, state licensure is designed to protect the public health.

Pharmacy Technician Certification. A voluntary national certification program for pharmacy technicians was launched in 1995 by the Pharmacy Technician Certification Board (PTCB), an independent testing agency established by the American Pharmaceutical Association, the American Society of Health-System Pharmacists, the Illinois Council of Health-System Pharmacists, and the Michigan Pharmacists Association. The two state organizations involved in this partnership had previously conducted separate certification programs that were franchised to other states. Approximately 8500 technicians had been certified by the Illinois and Michigan programs; most of them are expected to transfer their certification to the national program.

The examination developed by PTCB was based on the results of the Scope of Pharmacy Practice Project as supplemented by the expertise of the PTCB Certification Council and the PTCB Pharmacy Technician Resource Panel. These two bodies within PTCB consist of pharmacists, pharmacy technicians, and pharmacy technician educators who are very familiar with the functions of pharmacy technicians in all practice settings. PTCB exam development was guided by the standards of the National Commission for Certifying Agencies, the American Psychological Association, and the U.S. Equal Employment Opportunity Commission. The exam was given at more than 100 sites throughout the United States on three occasions in 1995. The 7900 technicians who applied to take the exam came from all areas of pharmacy practice.

The pharmacy technician certification exam measures mastery of knowledge; it does not test competence, and it does not supplant the need for licensed-pharmacist control over pharmacy operations. For employers, the certification program offers evidence that a certified individual possesses knowledge that has been shown to be important in the work of technicians; that evidence can aid hiring and promotion decisions. For technicians, the program offers an opportunity to gain recognition for having command of knowledge that is central to their work.[10,11]

Pharmacy Manpower Issues. The Pew Health Professions Commission recently released a report that urged reductions in the number of physicians, nurses, and pharmacists by 10–25% for the purpose of meeting the needs of an "emerging new health system."[12] For pharmacy, the report encouraged the profession to concentrate on clinical pharmacy (pharmaceutical care) and system management and to work with other health care providers. The use of pharmacy technicians will allow pharmacists to meet the challenges outlined by the Pew commission while fulfilling pharmacists' legally mandated role of overseeing the safe distribution of prescription medications.

Quality Assurance in Pharmacy Practice. Under the current system of regulating pharmacy practice in the United States, the pharmacist–pharmacy technician relationship depends on the licensed pharmacist retaining responsibility for the functions that the pharmacy technician performs. This is appropriate and in the public's best interest. Any compromise in this arrangement would set the stage for competing occupations in the distribution of medications, which would be confusing and wasteful. Pharmacists have a responsibility to ensure that the technicians they employ are well trained and appropriately supervised, and that they work under the guidance of clear policies and procedures that are based on the principles of continuous quality improvement. It is appropriate for state boards of pharmacy to review the written policies and procedures that govern the use of technicians in a licensed pharmacy.

Recommendations

1. ***Registration versus Licensure.*** In states where the board of pharmacy wishes to exercise some direct oversight of technicians, a system of registration should be used; state boards should not license pharmacy technicians. The state board of pharmacy should continue to hold licensed pharmacists accountable for the

quality of pharmacy service that is provided under their charge. If a registry of technicians is available, pharmacists should consult it in evaluating potential employment of individuals as pharmacy technicians.

2. ***Innovation in the Use of Pharmacy Technicians.*** The profession of pharmacy should actively stimulate innovation in the use of pharmacy technicians in ways that enhance the value of pharmacy's contributions to health care; among the elements of this effort should be the following:
   a. Foster widespread and thorough understanding of the principle that licensed pharmacists are accountable for the work that pharmacy technicians perform under their supervision.
   b. Reassess mandated arbitrary ratios of technicians to pharmacists and mandated arbitrary limitations on technician functions, based on the premise that these matters are for the supervising pharmacist to decide.
   c. Foster understanding of the value of certification of pharmacy technicians.
   d. Provide educational programs on improving the quality assurance methods that pharmacists apply to the work of technicians.

3. ***Pharmacy Technician Training.*** The profession of pharmacy should begin to plan for the promulgation of uniform national standards for pharmacy technician training. This process will evolve over time, just as standards for pharmacist education have evolved. Recognition among pharmacists of the need for uniform standards for technician training will grow as the perceived value of technicians in pharmacy practice continues to increase.

4. ***Scope of Pharmacy Practice.*** The profession of pharmacy should maintain current information on the scope of practice of pharmacists and pharmacy technicians. In order to maintain contemporary programs for the licensure of pharmacists and the certification of technicians, it is essential that up-to-date and accurate information be collected on the dimensions of their practices.

Conclusion

In this time of upheaval in health care, it is vital for pharmacy to position itself as a health profession that is closely aligned with important needs of patients. That is why such strong support has been given throughout the profession to the modern mission of the pharmacist, namely, helping people make the best use of medications. It will be difficult for the profession to fully achieve this mission without the use of well-qualified, appropriately supervised pharmacy technicians.

Although there is a compelling need for pharmacists to expand the purview of their professional practice, there is also a need for pharmacists to maintain control over all aspects of drug product handling in the patient care arena, including dispensing and compounding. No other discipline is as well qualified to ensure public safety in this important aspect of health care. Further, the economic foundation of community pharmacy practice is still tied to prescription dispensing.

At this point in history, the imperatives facing pharmacy with respect to pharmacy technicians are twofold: Maintain pharmacist accountability for the work of pharmacy technicians and foster innovation in the use of technicians under the supervision of pharmacists. These imperatives will be met by state board of pharmacy *licensure of pharmacists* and, where deemed appropriate, *registration of technicians*. The public will be well served by this approach.

References

1. Pharmacy Technician Certification Board. 1995 candidate handbook—national pharmacy technician certification examination. Washington, DC: Pharmacy Technician Certification Board; 1995:15.
2. Credentialing health manpower. Washington, DC: U.S. Department of Health, Education and Welfare, 1977 Jul; DHEW publication no. (OS)77-50057.
3. Black's law dictionary. 5th ed. St. Paul: West; 1979.
4. Johnson JA, Bootman JL. Drug-related morbidity and mortality: a cost-of-illness model. *Arch Intern Med.* 1995; 155:1949–56.
5. Santell JP. ASHP national survey of hospital-based pharmaceutical services—1994. *Am J Health-Syst Pharm.* 1995; 52:1179–98.
6. Summary of the final report of the Scope of Pharmacy Practice Project. *Am J Hosp Pharm.* 1994; 51:2179–82.
7. Pharmacy technician education and training—1995 directory. Cincinnati: Harvey Whitney Books; 1995.
8. Pharmacy technician program directory—1995. Bethesda, MD: American Society of Health-System Pharmacists; 1995.
9. American Society of Hospital Pharmacists. ASHP accreditation standard for pharmacy technician training programs. *Am J Hosp Pharm.* 1993; 50:124–6.
10. Zellmer WA. Pharmacy technicians, part 1: national certification. *Am J Health-Syst Pharm.* 1995; 52:918.
11. Smith JE. The national voluntary certification program for pharmacy technicians. *Am J Health-Syst Pharm.* 1995; 52: 2026–9.
12. Pew Health Professions Commission. Critical challenges: revitalizing the health professions for the twenty-first century. San Francisco: UCSF Center for Health Professions; 1995.

---

[a]Data on the status of technicians and nonpharmacist personnel in the 50 states, the District of Columbia, and Puerto Rico, published in the National Association of Boards of Pharmacy 1995–96 *Survey of Pharmacy Law*, can be obtained from the ASHP Professional Practice and Scientific Affairs Division.

Endorsed by the ASHP Board of Directors in March 1996 and by the American Pharmaceutical Association Board of Trustees in April 1996. This document is also being published in the *Journal of the American Pharmaceutical Association*.

The bibliographic citation for this document is as follows: American Society of Health-System Pharmacists. White paper on pharmacy technicians. *Am J Health-Syst Pharm.* 1996; 53:1991–4.

Index

━━━ A

Administration
  ambulatory care, 54
  correctional facilities, 86
  pharmacokinetic services, 14
  pharmacy services, hospital, acute care, 35
Adverse drug reactions, 3, 58, 107
  pediatrics, 84
  reporting, 59, 79, 107
Affiliated chapters, collective bargaining, 7
After-hours pharmacy
  service, 36, 68, 107
Ambulatory care, pharmacy services, 54
  drug distribution system, 55
  facilities and equipment, 54
  patient counseling, 55
  patient education, 55
  pediatrics, 84
  pharmaceutical care, 55
American Council on Pharmaceutical Education, 9
Anesthesiology and surgery, pharmacy services, 159
Angiotensin-converting-enzyme inhibitors, 208
Anticoagulant therapy, 194
Anti-infective agents
  dosage schedules, 223, 253
  nonsurgical prophylaxis, 251
    rational drug therapy, 11
  surgical prophylaxis, 221
Antimicrobial prophylaxis, 221, 251
Antimicrobial resistance, 199, 202
  surveillance program, 199
Antineoplastic agents (See Hazardous drugs)
Aseptic technique, 12, 174
Automated dispensing device, 27

━━━ B

Bacterial infections, anti-infective agents, 251, 221
Beyond-use date, 185 (See also Expiration dates)
Biological safety cabinets
  certification, 141
  classification, 140, 151
  decontamination, 142
Bring-in medications, 38, 68, 107

━━━ C

Catheters
  patency, 197
  saline flushing, 197
Certification, biological safety cabinets, 141
Charting by exception, 27
Charts (See Medical records)
Clinical care plans
  definition, 96
  development process, 98
  home health care, 77
  multidisciplinary, 26
  pharmacy and therapeutics committee, 97
Clinical fellowships, 276
Clinical pharmacy services, 155
  compensation, 13, 49
  reimbursement, 13, 49
Clinical practice guidelines
  antimicrobial prophylaxis in surgery, 221
  heart failure, 208
  insulin-dependent diabetes mellitus, 205
  multidrug-resistant tuberculosis, 202
  pneumococcal resistance, 199
Clinical research, 15
Code of Ethics, 378
Collective bargaining, 7
Compassionate use medications, 45
Compensation (See also Reimbursement)
  clinical pharmacy services, 13, 49
  pharmaceutical care, 25
  third-party, 13, 49
Competitive bidding, 31, 103, 153
Compounding
  nonsterile products, 182, 187
  ophthalmic preparations, 169
  sterile products, 171
Comprehensive Drug Abuse Prevention and Control
  Act of 1970, 113
Computerization, drug control, 109
Conflicts of interest, 61
Continuing education, 9
  home health care, 79
  industry-funded, 61
Controlled substances, 113
  dispensing, 118
  diversion, 118
  labeling, 119
  methadone, 122
  order forms, 116
  partial filling, 119
  pilferage, 121
  records and inventory, 115
  refills, 119

registration, 114
security, 120
surgery and anesthesiology, 162
storage, 120
transfers, 117
waste disposal, 117
Correctional facilities, 86
Cost-containment, drug product, 153
Counseling, patient (*See* Patient counseling)
Critical pathway (*See* Clinical care plans)
Cytotoxics (*See* Hazardous drugs)

D

Decontamination, biological safety cabinets, 142
Department-focused functions, 26
Directly observed therapy, 202
Discounts, drug product, 31
Disinfectants, 11
Dispensing
controlled substances, 118
investigational drugs, 47
nonpharmacists, 56
Diversion, controlled substances, 121
Documentation
home health care, 78
immunization, 166
medication information requests, 94
non-sterile products, 185
patient counseling, 34
patient education, 34
pharmaceutical care, 43, 91
research, 41
Dosage schedules, anti-infective agents, 223, 251
Drug, definition (FDA), 19
Drug administration, 106
hazardous drugs, 146
Drug administration device, 19
definition, 17
problems, 17
Drug delivery system, definition, 17
Drug distribution system, 19
ambulatory care, 55
correctional facilities, 87
home health care, 78
hospitals, 37
investigational drugs, 47
unit-dose, 10, 104, 124
Drug information, 36 (*See also* Medication information)
correctional facilities, 88
pediatrics, 84
Drug misadventuring, 58, 66, 108
Drug product
cost-containment, 153

discounts, 31
evaluation, 134
pilferage, 154
recalls, 109
returns, 31
selection, 3, 63, 134
waste, 154
Drug therapy monitoring, 77, 92
pediatrics, 84
Drug use control, 19, 37, 108
investigational drugs, 46
Drug use evaluation (*See* Medication-use evaluation)
Drug use review (*See* Medication-use evaluation)

E

Economic status, pharmacists, 7
Education
continuing, 9
infection control, 12
Emergency medications, 107
Employment (*See* Personnel, pharmacy)
End-product evaluation, sterile products, 175
Equipment (*See* Facilities and equipment)
Ethics, 61, 378
Expiration dates, 111, 117, 175, 185 (*See also* Beyond-use date)

F

Facilities and equipment
ambulatory care, 54
hospital, 38
nonsterile products, 182
sterile products, 173
Fellowships, clinical
definition, 276
guidelines, 276
Food and Drug Administration
MedWatch, 60
Formulary, 3, 63, 134, 155, 165
content and organization, 126
definition, 5
Formulary system, 3, 62, 126, 134, 155, 165
correctional facilities, 88
definition, 5

G

Generic equivalence, 5
Generic substitution, 64
Gloves, permeability, 143
Glycemic control, 205

H

Hazardous drugs (*See* Antineoplastic agents, Cytotoxics)
administration, 146
handling, 136
reproductive risks, 136, 137, 139
spill kits, 148
waste disposal, 109, 148
Health care reform, 25
Heparin, 197
Home health care, 76

I

Immunization, 165
Industry, pharmaceutical, 61, 81
Infection control programs, 11
Information
management, 157
medication, 93
patient-specific, 90
Informed consent, 45
Infusion devices, 77, 197
Institutional review board, 45
Insulin-dependent diabetes mellitus, 205
International Normalized Ratio, 194
International Sensitivity Index, 194
Interviews (*See* Personnel, pharmacy)
Inventory control, 153
controlled substances, 116
investigational drugs, 47
Investigational drugs, 45
Investigator
clinical studies, 45
research, 42

L

Labeling
controlled substances, 119
hazardous drugs, 145
nonsterile products, 186
sterile products, 175
unit-dose, 111, 124
unlabeled use, 20
Laminar-airflow hoods, 173
Laws
Comprehensive Drug Abuse Prevention
and Control Act of 1970, 113
National Childhood Vaccine Injury Act of 1986, 166
Omnibus Budget Reconciliation Act of 1990, 32
Poison Prevention Packaging Act of 1970, 106
Safe Medical Devices Act of 1990, 17

M

Medical records (charts), 43, 55
home health care, 76
Medication errors, 66, 108
classification, 72
pediatrics, 84
reporting, 73
Medication information (*See also* Drug information)
Activities, 93
Requests, 93
Resources, 94
Medication-use evaluation, 3, 51, 62, 108 (*See* Drug
use evaluation, Drug use review)
pediatrics, 84
MedWatch, 60
Methadone, 122
treatment programs, 123
Mission
ASHP, 2
pharmacist, 3

N

Narcotic treatment program, 123
National Childhood Vaccine Injury Act of 1986, 166
National Commission on Correctional Health Care, 86
Night cabinets (*See* After-hours pharmacy service)
Nondistributive services (*See* Clinical pharmacy
services; Pharmaceutical care)
Nonformulary drugs, 63
Nonsterile products
compounding, 182, 187
documentation, 185
expiration dates, 185
labeling, 186
packaging, 186
records, 185
stability, 185
storage, 184
Nosocomial infections, 11

O

Omnibus Budget Reconciliation Act of 1990, 32
Ophthalmic preparations, compounding, 169
Outcomes, pharmaceutical care, 22

P

Packaging
nonsterile products, 186
unit-dose, 111, 124
Patient counseling, 16, 32

ambulatory care, 55
home health care, 77
immunization, 166
Patient education, 16, 32
ambulatory care, 55
home health care, 77
immunization, 166
infection control, 12
pediatrics, 84
Patient-focused care, 26
Peripheral indwelling intermittent infusion devices, 197
Personnel, pharmacy, 33, 189
background verification, 190
interviews, 189
job offer, 190
management, 156
position description, 189
recruitment, 189
retention, 191
Pharmaceutical care
ambulatory care, 55
definition, 22
documentation, 43, 91
health care reform, 25
health care system, 25
home health care, 76
hospital, 35
outcomes, 22
patient counseling, 32
patient education, 32
patient-focused care, 26
standardized method, 90
Pharmaceutical manufacturer, selecting, 30
Pharmacokinetic services, 14
pediatrics, 84
Pharmacy and therapeutics committee, 3, 5, 62, 126, 134, 155
Pharmacy services
after-hours, 107
ambulatory care, 54
clinical, 49, 155
correctional facilities, 86
drug information, 36
home health care, 76
hospitals, 35
medication information, 91
minimum standards, 35
patient counseling, 16, 32
patient education, 16, 32
pediatrics, 83
pharmacokinetic, 14, 84
surgery and anesthesiology, 159
Pharmacy technician
accreditation regulations, 370
certification, 380
definitions, 129, 379
training, 129, 373, 379
Pilferage
controlled substances, 121
drug products, 154
Pneumococcal resistance, 199
Poison Prevention Packaging Act of 1970, 106
Policy and procedure manual, 102
Position description (See Personnel, pharmacy)
Procurement, drug products, 31
Productivity, 156
Professional relations, industry, pharmaceutical, 61
Promotional activities, 61, 81
Prothrombin time, 194
Purchasing, 102, 153

Q

Quality assurance (quality control)
sterile products, 171
Quality of life, 23

R

Rational drug therapy, anti-infective agents, 11
Recalls, drug, 109
Records, 103
controlled substances, 115
immunization, 166
investigational drugs, 46
nonsterile products, 185
Recruitment (See Personnel, pharmacy)
Re-engineering, 26
Registration, controlled substances, 114
Reimbursement (See also Compensation)
clinical pharmacy services, 13, 49
immunization, 167
pharmaceutical care, 25
unlabeled uses, 21
Reporting
adverse drug reaction, 59, 79, 107
drug administration device problem, 17
medication error, 73, 108
(drug) product problem, 109
research, 41
Representatives, pharmaceutical (vendor, industry, sales), 81, 107
Reproductive risks, hazardous drugs, 136, 137, 139
Research, 15, 39, 61
correctional facilities, 89
documentation, 41
investigator, 42

methods, 41
reporting, 41
Residencies
   accreditation regulations, 277
   adult internal medicine pharmacy practice, 326
   clinical fellowship, 273
   clinical pharmacokinetics practice, 341
   critical care pharmacy practice, 345
   definition, 274
   drug information practice, 295
   geriatric pharmacy practice, 301
   hospital pharmacy administration, 337
   infectious disease pharmacy practice, 361
   nuclear pharmacy, 304
   nutritional support pharmacy practice, 313
   oncology pharmacy practice, 317
   pediatric pharmacy practice, 321
   pharmacotherapy practice, 353
   pharmacy practice, 280
   primary care pharmacy practice, 349
   psychopharmacy practice, 329
   specialized pharmacy, 288
Respirators, hazardous drug, 142
Retention (See Personnel, pharmacy)
Risk level classification, sterile products, 171

S

Safe Medical Devices Act of 1990, 17
Sales representatives (See Representatives, pharmaceutical)
Samples, 38, 82, 107
Single unit package, definition, 111
Sodium chloride injection, 197
Spill kits, 148
Stability, nonsterile products, 185
Sterile products
   compounding, 171
   end-product evaluation, 175
   expiration dates, 175
   facilities and equipment, 173
   labeling, 175
   ophthalmic preparations, 169
   quality assurance, 171
   risk level classification, 171
   storage, 173
Sterilization, 11
Storage
   controlled substances, 120
   investigational drugs, 47
   nonsterile products, 184
   sterile products, 173
Supplier, selecting, 30
Support personnel (See also Pharmacy technician)

definition, 129
Surgery and anesthesiology
   controlled substances, 162
   pharmacy services, 159
Surgery, anti-infective agents, 221
Stop orders, 104

T

Technicians (See Pharmacy technician)
Therapeutic equivalence, 5, 64
Therapeutic interchange, 64
Therapeutic purpose, 37
Third-party payment systems, 13, 47
Toxicity, environmental, hazardous drugs, 109, 136
Training
   nonsterile products compounding, 184
   pharmacy technicians, 129, 370
   sterile products compounding, 173
Treatment guidelines, 63
Treatment IND, 45

U

Unapproved use (See Unlabeled use)
Unit-dose, 124
   drug distribution system, 10
   package, definition, 111
Unlabeled use, definition, 20
   reimbursement, 21

V

Vaccination, pneumococcal, 200
Vendors' representatives (See Representatives, pharmaceutical)

W

Warfarin, 194
Waste, drug product, 154
Waste disposal
   controlled substances, 117
   hazardous drugs, 109, 148
Work redesign, 26

ASHP POLICIES
1982–97

**American Society of
Health-System Pharmacists™**

7272 Wisconsin Avenue
Bethesda, Maryland 20814
(301) 657-3000

Contents

Introduction 391

Policies

      1997 Policies 392

      1996 Policies 393

      1995 Policies 394

      1994 Policies 394

      1993 Policies 395

      1992 Policies 396

      1991 Policies 396

      1990 Policies 398

      1989 Policies 399

      1988 Policies 400

      1987 Policies 401

      1986 Policies 403

      1985 Policies 403

      1984 Policies 405

      1983 Policies 407

      1982 Policies 409

Index 411

Introduction

ASHP Policies 1982–97 is a catalog of professional policy positions adopted by the ASHP House of Delegates (HOD), organized from the most current year, 1997, back to those adopted fifteen years earlier, 1982. The foundations for ASHP's policies are its Mission Statement and its purposes as stated in the ASHP Charter. The American Society of Health-System Pharmacists (ASHP) is the professional association for pharmacists in health systems helping people make the best use of medications. Current membership is 30,000.

The mission of ASHP is to represent its members and to provide leadership that will enable pharmacists in organized health-care settings to (1) extend pharmaceutical care focused on achieving positive patient outcomes through drug therapy; (2) provide services that foster the efficacy, safety, and cost-effectiveness of drug use; (3) contribute to programs and services that emphasize the health needs of the public and the prevention of disease; and (4) promote pharmacy as an essential component of the health care team.

The purposes of ASHP, as stated in the ASHP Charter, are as follows:

1. To advance public health by promoting the professional interests of pharmacists practicing in hospitals and other organized health-care settings through:
   a. Fostering pharmaceutical services aimed at drug-use control and rational drug therapy.
   b. Developing professional standards for pharmaceutical services.
   c. Fostering an adequate supply of well-trained, competent pharmacists and associated personnel.
   d. Developing and conducting programs for maintaining and improving the competence of pharmacists and associated personnel.
   e. Disseminating information about pharmaceutical services and rational drug use.
   f. Improving communication among pharmacists, other members of the health-care industry, and the public.
   g. Promoting research in the health and pharmaceutical sciences and in pharmaceutical services.
   h. Promoting the economic welfare of pharmacists and associated personnel.
2. To foster rational drug use in society such as through advocating appropriate public policies toward that end.

3. To pursue any other lawful activity that may be authorized by ASHP's Board of Directors.

Each policy in this catalog is identified by a four-digit number; the first two digits show the year that the policy was approved by the HOD, and the third and fourth digits are sequencing numbers. Background information on any policy can be found in that year's August issue of the *American Journal of Health-System Pharmacy* under "Proceedings of the Annual Session of the ASHP House of Delegates." The "Source" for each policy indicates how the policy was introduced to the HOD, e.g., in a report of a council, through the Chairman of the Board, or as a resolution.

During 1996–1997, the policy-recommending bodies of ASHP, at the direction of the Board of Directors, began a sunset review of the existing ASHP policies. Some bodies implemented processes to review policies, whereas others proceeded to recommend that certain policies be continued, revised, or discontinued. Recommendations for revisions or discontinuations were presented to the 1997 ASHP HOD for action. The content of the ASHP Policies of 1982–97 reflects the HOD's actions.

ASHP Policies are published annually in a separate document and, starting in 1997–98, also within the *Practice Standards of ASHP*. *Practice Standards* includes ASHP Statements (declarations and explanations of basic philosophy or principles, approved by the Board of Directors and the House of Delegates), ASHP Guidelines (general advice on implementation of pharmacy practice programs, approved by the Board of Directors), ASHP Technical Assistance Bulletins (specific, detailed advice on pharmacy programs or functions as developed by an ASHP staff division in consultation with experts, approved by the Board of Directors), ASHP Therapeutic Guidelines (thorough, systematically developed advice for health-care professionals on appropriate use of medications for specific clinical circumstances), ASHP Therapeutic Position Statements (concise statements that respond to specific therapeutic issues of concern to health care consumers and pharmacists, as developed through the guidance of the ASHP Commission on Therapeutics, approved by the Board of Directors), and ASHP Residency Accreditation Regulations and Standards (requirements for ASHP-accredited postgraduate residency and technician training programs).

Policies

1997 Policies

9701
DIRECT-TO-CONSUMER ADVERTISING OF PHARMACEUTICALS
Source: Council on Legal and Public Affairs and the Board of Directors

To support direct-to-consumer advertising that is educational in nature about prescription drug therapies for certain medical conditions and appropriately includes pharmacists as a source of information; further,

To oppose direct-to-consumer advertising of specific prescription drug products; further,

To support the development of legislation or regulation that would require nonprescription drug advertising to state prominently the benefits and risks associated with product use that should be discussed with the consumer's pharmacist or physician.

9702
DRUG SAMPLES
Source: Council on Legal and Public Affairs

To oppose drug sampling or similar drug marketing programs that (1) do not provide the elements of pharmaceutical care, (2) result in poor drug control, allowing patients to receive improperly labeled and packaged, deteriorated, outdated, and unrecorded drugs, (3) provide access to prescription drugs by unauthorized, untrained personnel, (4) may encourage inappropriate prescribing habits, or (5) may increase the cost of treatment for all patients.

9703
MANUFACTURER-SPONSORED PATIENT-ASSISTANCE PROGRAMS
Source: Council on Legal and Public Affairs

To encourage pharmaceutical manufacturers to (1) extend their patient assistance programs to serve the needs of both uninsured and underinsured patients, (2) enhance access to and availability of such programs, and (3) incorporate the elements of pharmaceutical care into these programs.

9704
PHARMACY TECHNICIANS
Source: Council on Legal and Public Affairs

To support registration by state boards of pharmacy and voluntary certification for technical personnel in pharmacy consistent with recommendations contained in the ASHP–APhA White Paper on Pharmacy Technicians (*Am J Health-Syst Pharm.* 1996; 53:1793–6); further,

To oppose state licensure of pharmacy technical personnel because the state boards should hold pharmacists accountable for the quality of pharmacy service that is provided under their charge.

(*Note:* Certification is the process by which a nongovernmental agency or association grants recognition to an individual who has met certain predetermined qualifications specified by that agency or association.

Licensure is the process by which an agency of government grants permission to an individual to engage in a given occupation upon a finding that the applicant has attained the minimal degree of competency necessary to ensure that the public health, safety, and welfare will be reasonably well protected.

Registration is the process of making a list or being enrolled in an existing list.)

(*Note:* This policy supersedes ASHP Policy 9302).

9705
PHARMACIST EDUCATION OF CONSUMERS
Source: Council on Legal and Public Affairs and the Board of Directors

To encourage pharmaceutical manufacturers to utilize pharmacists as the preferred mechanism to educate consumers about drug therapies, particularly new and emerging therapies.

9706
TWENTY-FOUR-HOUR ACCESS TO PHARMACISTS
Source: Council on Professional Affairs

To support the principle that all patients should have 24-hour access to a pharmacist responsible for their care.

9707
PEDIATRIC DOSAGE FORMS
Source: Council on Professional Affairs

To support efforts that stimulate development of pediatric dosage forms of drug products.

9708
EXPRESSION OF THERAPEUTIC PURPOSE OF PRESCRIBING
Source: Council on Professional Affairs

To support the routine expression by prescribers of the condition being treated or the therapeutic purpose of medication with or in every prescription and medication order.

9709
REPORTING MEDICATION ERRORS AND ADVERSE DRUG REACTIONS
Source: Council on Professional Affairs

To encourage pharmacists to exert leadership in establishing a nonthreatening, confidential atmosphere in their work places to encourage pharmacy staff and others to report actual and suspected medication errors and adverse drug reactions in a timely manner.

9710
IMAGE OF AND OPPORTUNITIES FOR HEALTH-SYSTEM PHARMACISTS
Source: Council on Educational Affairs

To develop and implement a public relations plan promoting the professional image of health-system pharmacists to the general public, other health-care professionals, and, especially, health-system decision-makers; further,

To provide ASHP informational and recruitment materials identifying career opportunities for pharmacists practicing in organized health-care settings.

1996 Policies

9601
STANDARDIZATION OF DRUG MEDICATION FORMULARY SYSTEMS
Source: Council on Administrative Affairs

To support the concept of a standardized medication formulary system among components of integrated health systems when standardization leads to improved patient outcomes; further,

To include in the formulary-standardization process the direct involvement of the health system's physicians, pharmacists, and other appropriate health care professionals.

9602
ELECTRONIC INFORMATION SYSTEMS
Source: Council on Administrative Affairs

To advocate the use of electronic information systems, with appropriate security controls, that enable the sharing of patient-specific data among the components of an integrated health system; further,

To strongly encourage health-system administrators, regulatory bodies, and other appropriate groups to provide pharmacists full access to patient-specific clinical data within an integrated system.

9603
ASHP STATEMENT ON SUPPORTIVE PERSONNEL
Source: Council on Educational Affairs

To discontinue the October 1970 ASHP Statement on Supportive Personnel in Hospital Pharmacy; further,

To delete ASHP policies 8218, 8313, 8602, 8604, and 8714.

9606
FDA REFORM
Source: Council on Legal and Public Affairs

To support continued definition of the Food and Drug Administration's public health mission in terms of product approval, labeling approval, manufacturing oversight, and marketing oversight, while deferring to state regulation and professional self-regulation on matters related to the use of drugs, biologics, and medical devices; further,

To support the allocation of sufficient federal resources to allow the FDA to meet its defined public health mission; further,

To support management reforms at the FDA that allow timely and cost-effective approval of drugs, biologics, and medical devices, without compromising the agency's vital mandate of ensuring that new products are safe and effective and that all products and manufacturers meet minimum quality standards; further,

To support the appointment of practicing pharmacists to FDA advisory committees as one mechanism of ensuring that decisions made by the agency incorporate the unique knowledge of the profession of pharmacy for the further benefit of the patient.

9607
CODE OF ETHICS
Source: Council on Legal and Public Affairs

To endorse the Code of Ethics for Pharmacists.

9608
USE OF COLOR TO IDENTIFY DRUG PRODUCTS
Source: Council on Professional Affairs

To support the reading of drug product labels as the most important means of identifying drug products; further,

To oppose reliance on color by health professionals and other to identify drug products; and further,

To oppose actions by manufacturers of drug products and others to promulgate reliance on color to identify drug products.

9609
HUMAN FACTORS CONCEPTS
Source: Council on Professional Affairs

To encourage pharmacists to apply human factors concepts (human errors related to inadequate systems or environment) in the prevention, analysis, and reporting of medication errors; further,

To encourage research (in conjunction with other groups, as appropriate) to identify human factors causes of medication errors and opportunities for their prevention.

9611
ASHP STATEMENT ON THE PHARMACIST'S CLINICAL ROLE IN ORGANIZED HEALTH-CARE SETTINGS
Source: Council on Professional Affairs

To discontinue the ASHP Statement on the Pharmacist's Clinical Role in Organized Health-Care Settings, dated June 5, 1989.

9613
THE EXPANDED ROLE OF PHARMACY TECHNICIANS
Source: House of Delegates Resolution

That ASHP study the potential for greater technician involvement in the organization, such as by appointing a technician member to an ASHP council and by creating a technician seat in the ASHP House of Delegates.

9614
DUES AUTHORITY
Source: Chairman of the Board of Directors

To delegate to the Board of Directors the authority to adjust annually the ASHP membership dues rate for the purpose of covering increased costs of existing membership services for a period of the next five years, 1997–2001; further,

To limit any increases in dues by the Board of Directors, under this authorization, to the annual percentage increase in the Consumer Price Index for all Urban Consumers.

1995 Policies

9501
DRUG FORMULARY SYSTEM MANAGEMENT
Source: Council on Administrative Affairs

To support the concept that management of a drug formulary system must be based first and foremost on clinical principles and must include the active and direct involvement of physicians, pharmacists, and other appropriate health care professionals.

9502
ASHP CONTINUING-EDUCATION ACTIVITIES AND NONTRADITIONAL PHARM.D. PROGRAMS
Source: Council on Administrative Affairs

To develop ASHP continuing-education activities and materials, in both meeting and nonmeeting formats, to address the competencies identified by the American Association of Colleges of Pharmacy (AACP) Center for the Advancement of Pharmaceutical Education Advisory Panel on Educational Outcomes and the ASHP Model for Pharmacy Practice Residency Learning Demonstration Project; further

To use the work of the AACP Center for the Advancement of Pharmaceutical Education and the ASHP model for Pharmacy Practice Residency Learning Demonstration Project to develop continuing-education activities that could be either approved for college credit or potentially accepted as evidence of competency for applicants to nontraditional Pharm.D. programs.

This policy was reviewed in 1996 by the Council on Educational Affairs and by the Board of Directors and was found to still be appropriate.

9503
MODEL CONTINUING EDUCATION REGULATIONS
Source: Council on Educational Affairs

To pursue with the National Association of Boards of Pharmacy the inclusion of model continuing-education regulations as part of the new model regulations for pharmacy practice.

9504
ASHP STATEMENT ON THE PHARMACIST'S RESPONSIBILITY FOR DISTRIBUTION AND CONTROL OF DRUG PRODUCTS
Source: Council on Professional Affairs

To approve the ASHP Statement on the Pharmacist's Responsibility for Distribution and Control of Drug Products. (*Note:* this Statement supersedes a document of the same title dated June 1, 1992.)

9505
ASHP STATEMENT ON THE ROLE OF THE PHARMACIST IN PATIENT-FOCUSED CARE
Source: Council on Professional Affairs

To approve the ASHP Statement on the Role of the Pharmacist in Patient-Focused Care. (*Note:* This document will be published in the August 15, 1995, issue of *AJHP.*)

9506
TIME OF THE ASHP MIDYEAR CLINICAL MEETING
Source: House of Delegates Resolution

Motion: ASHP should study the time of the ASHP Midyear Clinical Meeting, consider other possible times, discuss meeting scheduling and planning with other organizations, and investigate the economic and practical feasibility of moving the ASHP Midyear Meeting to another time of the year in the future. A report of this should be presented to the 1996 House of Delegates.

1994 Policies

9401
PATIENT-FOCUSED CARE
Source: Council on Administrative Affairs

To support the concept of patient-focused care when it (a) is planned and implemented with pharmacists' involvement; (b) fosters the provision of pharmaceutical care; and (c) is motivated by a goal of improved patient care.

9402
ELECTRONIC ENTRY OF MEDICATION ORDERS
Source: Council on Administrative Affairs

To support, as the preferred method of prescribing, direct electronic entry of medication orders by the prescriber, with provisions for the pharmacist to review the order's appropriateness.

9403
MULTIDISCIPLINARY ACTION PLANS FOR PATIENT CARE (CARE MAPS)
Source: Council on Administrative Affairs

To support pharmacists as integral participants in the development of multidisciplinary action plans for patient care (care MAPs).

9404
PHARMACIST PRESCRIBING

Source: Council on Legal and Public Affairs

To pursue the development of legislative and regulatory provisions that allow for prescribing by the pharmacist as a component of pharmaceutical care.

9406
PATIENT'S RIGHT TO CHOOSE

Source: Council on Legal and Public Affairs

To support the right of the patient to choose and to give instructions regarding his or her health care.

9407
PRIMARY AND PREVENTIVE CARE

Source: Council on Professional Affairs

To support primary and preventive care roles for pharmacists in the provision of pharmaceutical care; further,

To collaborate with physician, nursing, and health-system administrator groups in pursuit of these goals.

This policy was reviewed in 1996 by the Council on Professional Affairs and by the Board of Directors and was found to still be appropriate.

9409
NABP MODEL PHARMACY PRACTICE ACT LANGUAGE ON THE RESPONSIBILITY OF THE PHARMACIST FOR OVERALL MEDICATION DISTRIBUTION SYSTEMS

Source: House of Delegates Resolution

ASHP should work with the National Association of Boards of Pharmacy to clarify language in the Model Pharmacy Practice Act concerning the responsibility of the pharmacist for the overall medication distribution system and to eliminate specific task requirements, allowing practitioners to focus on improving drug therapy through formulation of a therapeutic plan and detection, prevention, and resolution of medication-related problems.

9410
PRESCRIBING AUTHORITY FOR PHARMACISTS

Source: House of Delegates Resolution

That ASHP actively support state societies in the development and use of state-level prescribing authority for pharmacists.

9411
NAME CHANGE

Source: Chairman of the Board of Directors

To change the name of the "American Society of Hospital Pharmacists, Inc. (ASHP)" to the "American Society of Health-System Pharmacists, Inc. (ASHP)", effective January 1, 1995; further,

To amend the ASHP Charter, Article Second, by deleting "Hospital" and substituting "Health-System"; further,

To amend and restate the ASHP Bylaws, Article 1.1, to conform to the amended ASHP Charter; further,

To declare that this Charter amendment is "advisable," and direct that the Charter amendment be submitted to the House of Delegates and the membership for consideration.

(*Note:* The ASHP membership approved this action by mail ballot, September 1994.)

1993 Policies

9303
HEALTH-CARE REFORM

Source: Council on Legal and Public Affairs

To endorse the document "Principles for Including Medications and Pharmaceutical Care in Health Care Systems."

9304
ASHP STATEMENT ON PHARMACEUTICAL CARE

Source: Council on Professional Affairs

To approve the "ASHP Statement on Pharmaceutical Care."

(*Definition:* The mission of the pharmacist is to provide pharmaceutical care. Pharmaceutical care is the direct, responsible provision of medication-related care for the purpose of achieving definite outcomes that improve a patient's quality of life.)

9306
ASHP STATEMENT ON THE PHARMACIST'S ROLE WITH RESPECT TO DRUG DELIVERY SYSTEMS AND ADMINISTRATION DEVICES

Source: Council on Professional Affairs

To approve the "ASHP Statement on the Pharmacist's Role with Respect to Drug Delivery Systems and Administration Devices."

9307
DRUG DISTRIBUTION SYSTEMS IN ORGANIZED HEALTH-CARE SYSTEMS

Source: House of Delegates Resolution

To support the utilization of accurate methods of dispensing of medication that can free the pharmacist to focus on direct patient care.

This policy was reviewed in 1996 by the Council on Professional Affairs and by the Board of Directors and was found to still be appropriate.

9308
REIMBURSEMENT STATUS FOR CLINICAL PHARMACY SERVICES

Source: House of Delegates Resolution

To support the necessary processes to establish standards for clinical pharmacy documentation and to foster a direct relationship with third-party payers that facilitates a reimbursement status.

9309
EXPIRATION DATING OF PHARMACEUTICAL PRODUCTS

Source: House of Delegates Resolution

To support and actively promote the maximal extension of expiration dates of pharmaceutical products as a means of reducing health-care costs and to recommend that pharmaceutical manufacturers review their procedures to accomplish this end.

This policy was reviewed in 1996 by the Council on Professional Affairs and by the Board of Directors and was found to still be appropriate.

9310
RECOGNITION OF ONCOLOGY PHARMACY PRACTICE AS A SPECIALTY
Source: Chairman of the Board of Directors

To endorse a petition to the Board of Pharmaceutical Specialties (BPS) requesting recognition of oncology pharmacy practice as a specialty.

1992 Policies

9201
HUMAN IMMUNODEFICIENCY VIRUS (HIV) POSITIVE EMPLOYEES
Source: Council on Administrative Affairs

To adopt the position that mandatory routine testing of health-care workers for infection with the human immunodeficiency virus is unnecessary; further,

To support the use of universal precautions for infection control.

9202
NEEDLE-FREE DRUG PREPARATION AND ADMINISTRATION SYSTEMS
Source: Council on Administrative Affairs

To encourage manufacturers' efforts to create cost-effective drug preparation and drug administration systems that do not require needles.

9204
ELECTRONIC COMMUNICATION OF MEDICAL INFORMATION
Source: Council on Legal and Public Affairs

To support the use of electronic devices to transmit medical information, including prescriptions and drug orders, among practitioners and patients; further,

To encourage state policymakers to address the issues surrounding the conveyance of medical information, including prescriptions and drug orders, by electronic means.

9205
AUTOMATED SYSTEMS
Source: Council on Legal and Public Affairs

To support the use of current and emerging technology in the advancement of pharmaceutical care; further,

To encourage a review and evaluation of the state and federal legal and regulatory status of new technologies as they apply to pharmacy practice.

9206
MEDICATION-ERROR REPORTING
Source: Council on Professional Affairs

To support the concept of a multidisciplinary reporting system for medication errors that is (a) designed to collect data to identify preventable serious errors and opportunities for drug use improvement and (b) designed to maintain confidentiality; further,

To review and evaluate pilot medication error reporting efforts in order to study their effectiveness and the utility of the data they produce.

9207
AVERSIVE FLAVORING
Source: Council on Professional Affairs

To endorse the March 24, 1991, resolution of the American Association of Poison Control Centers concerning the addition of aversive flavoring to potentially toxic products.

9208
ASHP STATEMENT ON THE USE OF MEDICATIONS FOR UNLABELED USES
Source: Council on Professional Affairs

To approve the "ASHP Statement on the Use of Medications for Unlabeled Uses."

9209
ASHP STATEMENT ON THE PHARMACY AND THERAPEUTICS COMMITTEE
Source: Council on Professional Affairs

To approve the "ASHP Statement on the Pharmacy and Therapeutics Committee."

9211
TAMPER-EVIDENT PACKAGING ON TOPICAL PRODUCTS
Source: House of Delegates Resolution

ASHP should support the standardization and requirement of tamper-evident packaging on all topical products, including all dermatologicals and nonprescription products.

This policy was reviewed in 1996 by the Council on Professional Affairs and by the Board of Directors and was found to still be appropriate.

1991 Policies

9101
DECLARATION OF INTENT BY THE AMERICAN COUNCIL ON PHARMACEUTICAL EDUCATION
Source: Council on Educational Affairs

To reaffirm the official policy of ASHP to support the Doctor of Pharmacy degree as the single entry-level degree for professional pharmacy practice; further,

To strongly encourage the development of viable and widely available external and nontraditional Doctor of Pharmacy degree programs; further,

To be an active participant in the American Council on Pharmaceutical Education (ACPE) process for the revision of accreditation standards for entry-level education in pharmacy; further,

To provide the ACPE with appropriate documents and background materials in order to demonstrate the ASHP position and support for ACPE's intent on this important issue; further,

To actively investigate the long-range impact that the single entry-level degree will have on residency education, availability of experiential training sites, graduate education, and continuing education programs.

9103
DRUG TESTING
Source: Council on Legal and Public Affairs

To recognize the use of pre-employment drug testing or drug testing for cause during employment based on defined criteria and with appropriate validation procedures; further,

To support employer-sponsored drug programs that include a policy and process that promote the recovery of impaired individuals.

9104
CLOSED DISTRIBUTION SYSTEMS
Source: Council on Legal and Public Affairs

To reiterate support for the current system of drug distribution in which prescribers and pharmacists exercise their professional responsibilities on behalf of patients; further,

To acknowledge that there may be limited circumstances in which constraints on the traditional drug distribution mechanism may be appropriate if the following principles are met:

1. The requirements are based upon scientific evidence fully disclosed and evaluated by physicians, pharmacists, and others;
2. There is scientific consensus that the requirements are necessary and represent the least restrictive means to achieve safe and effective patient care;
3. The cost of the product and any associated product or services are identified for purposes of reimbursement, mechanisms are provided to compensate providers for special services, and duplicate costs are avoided;
4. All requirements are stated in functional, objective terms so that any provider who meets the criteria may participate in the care of patients; and,
5. The requirements do not interfere with professional practice of pharmacists, physicians, and others.

9105
DRUG PRICING
Source: Council on Legal and Public Affairs

To support the principle of prudent purchase of pharmaceutical products and related supplies by public and private entities using appropriate professional practices to achieve that end; further,

To encourage government support of existing local professional activities already practiced in organized health-care settings that are methods to promote quality and cost-effective pharmaceutical care for patients.

(*Note:* These methods include, without limitation, concepts such as drug-use review, formulary systems, pharmacy and therapeutics committees, and patient counseling.)

9106
MEDICAL DEVICES
Source: Council on Legal and Public Affairs

To support public and private initiatives to clarify and define the relationship among drugs, devices, and new technologies in order to promote safety and effectiveness as well as better delivery of patient care.

9107
COMPOUNDING VERSUS MANUFACTURING
Source: Council on Legal and Public Affairs

To support the principle that compounding, when done to meet anticipatory patient needs, is part of the practice of pharmacy and is not manufacturing; further,

To reaffirm the need for ASHP to develop pharmacy practice standards related to anticipatory compounding in organized health-care settings; further,

To foster educational efforts relating to pharmacy compounding in organized health-care settings.

9108
EMPLOYEE TESTING
Source: Council on Legal and Public Affairs

To oppose the use of truth-verification testing such as polygraphs as routine employment practices because of the possible interference with the rights of individuals; further,

To recognize the limited use of such testing during employment where such testing may protect the rights of individuals against false witness.

9110
PHARMACEUTICAL WASTE
Source: Council on Professional Affairs

To encourage hospital pharmacy departments to recycle waste materials; further,

To encourage pharmaceutical manufacturers to explore how they may assist pharmacy departments in their waste-recycling efforts; further,

To encourage pharmaceutical manufacturers to streamline packaging of drug products to reduce waste materials.

This policy was reviewed in 1996 by the Council on Professional Affairs and by the Board of Directors and was found to still be appropriate.

9111
ASHP STATEMENT ON PHARMACEUTICAL RESEARCH IN ORGANIZED HEALTH-CARE SETTINGS
Source: Council on Professional Affairs

To approve the "ASHP Statement on Pharmaceutical Research in Organized Health-Care Settings."

9112
DRUG ADMINISTRATION
Source: Council on Professional Affairs

To encourage pharmacists to pursue means to ensure the integrity of the drug delivery process, including drug administration; further,

To encourage education and training of pharmacists as preparation for participation in all aspects of the medication administration process.

9113
PHARMACISTS' ROLE IN IMMUNIZATION
Source: Council on Professional Affairs

To affirm that pharmacists have a public health and individual–patient responsibility in immunization; further,

To encourage pharmacists to seek opportunities for involvement in immunization programs.

9114
ASHP STATEMENT ON THE PHARMACIST'S ROLE IN PATIENT-EDUCATION PROGRAMS
Source: Council on Professional Affairs

To approve the "ASHP Statement on the Pharmacist's Role in Patient-Education Programs."

9116
ASHP STATEMENT ON THE PROVISION OF PHARMACEUTICAL SERVICES IN AMBULATORY CARE SETTINGS
Source: Council on Professional Affairs

To discontinue the "ASHP Statement on the Provision of Pharmaceutical Services in Ambulatory Care Settings."

9118
STATEMENT OF PRINCIPLE FOR PHARMACISTS' RELATIONSHIP WITH INDUSTRY
Source: House of Delegates Resolution

That ASHP take the initiative to formulate a statement of principle defining the professional standards of conduct for the pharmacist's working relationship with the pharmaceutical industry.

9119
STANDARDIZED PROTOCOL FOR WORKLOAD DATA COLLECTION AND REPORTING BY SOFTWARE VENDORS
Source: House of Delegates Resolution

To recommend that ASHP, through the Special Projects Division or by any other means deemed appropriate by the Board of Directors, work with hospital pharmacy computer systems software vendors to establish a forum for discussion regarding future needs for information technology.

Further, that ASHP (1) support the adoption and use of a standardized protocol for collecting and reporting workload data from pharmacy computer software programs and (2) encourage its members to help with the adoption of the uniform workload standards by discussing the standards at their system user group meetings.

9120
ALCOHOL AND PROFESSIONAL RESPONSIBILITIES OF PHARMACISTS
Source: House of Delegates New Business

That alcohol is a drug and should be used with the respect and concern afforded to any drug;

That pharmacists should extend their professional obligations and responsibilities to alcohol use by individuals and themselves;

That pharmacists have an obligation to ensure that, if consumed, alcohol is used only responsibly;

That pharmacists, by example in their personal conduct, should foster awareness of the nature of alcohol and responsible use of alcohol by those who choose to use alcohol; and

That ASHP and its members continue to support and foster impaired-pharmacist programs as a means of providing opportunities for such individuals to rehabilitate themselves.

9121
LIMITED AUTHORITY TO ADJUST THE DUES RATE
Source: Chairman of the Board of Directors

To delegate to the Board of Directors for a five-year period (covering the dues rate for calendar years 1992 through 1996) the authority to adjust annually the ASHP membership dues rate for the purpose of covering increased costs of existing membership services; further,

To limit any increases in dues to the annual percentage increase in the *Consumer Price Index for All Urban Consumers*.

9122
RECOGNITION OF PSYCHOPHARMACY PRACTICE AS A SPECIALTY
Source: Chairman of the Board of Directors

To endorse a petition to the Board of Pharmaceutical Specialties (BPS) requesting recognition of psychopharmacy practice as a specialty.

1990 Policies

9001
REIMBURSEMENT FOR UNLABELED USES OF FDA-APPROVED DRUG PRODUCTS
Source: Council on Administrative Affairs

To support third-party reimbursement for FDA-approved drug products appropriately prescribed for unlabeled uses; further,

To seek endorsement of this payment policy by other professional organizations.

9002
ASHP STATEMENT ON CONTINUING EDUCATION
Source: Council on Educational Affairs

To approve the revised "ASHP Statement on Continuing Education."

9003
DRUG PRODUCT PRICES
Source: Council on Legal and Public Affairs

To support existing laws and legitimate practices that allow organized health-care settings to purchase drug products and related supplies at prices that minimize health-care costs.

9004
HOME INTRAVENOUS THERAPY
Source: Council on Legal and Public Affairs

To support the implementation of a home intravenous therapy benefit under federal and private medical plans, along with an appropriate level of reimbursement for the pharmaceutical services, supplies, and equipment associated with this type of health care.

9005
GENERIC DRUG PRODUCTS
Source: Council on Legal and Public Affairs

To encourage pharmacists in organized health-care settings to assume a greater leadership role in legislative and other arenas relating to drug product selection and evaluation.

9006
NONDISCRIMINATORY PHARMACEUTICAL CARE
Source: Council on Professional Affairs

To adopt the following positions in regard to nondiscriminatory pharmaceutical care:

* All patients have the right to privacy, respect, confidentiality, and high-quality pharmaceutical care.
* No patient should be refused pharmaceutical care or denied these rights based solely on diagnosis.
* Pharmacists must always act in the best interest of individual patients while not placing society as a whole at risk.

This policy was reviewed in 1996 by the Council on Professional Affairs and by the Board of Directors and was found to still be appropriate.

9007
DRUG NAMES, LABELING, AND PACKAGING
Source: Council on Professional Affairs

To urge drug manufacturers and FDA to involve practicing pharmacists, nurses, and physicians in decisions about drug names, labeling, and packaging; further,

To inform pharmacists, and others as appropriate, about specific drug names, labeling, and packaging that have documented association with medication errors.

9008
STANDARDIZED PROTOCOL FOR INFORMATION EXCHANGE BETWEEN HOSPITALS
Source: House of Delegates Resolution

To support the adoption and use of a standardized protocol to facilitate information exchange within and between hospital data processing systems.

9009
STUDENT MEMBERSHIP DUES
Source: House of Delegates Resolution

To recommend a rollback in the student membership dues rate to the pre-January 1, 1990 level.

9010
GENERIC PHARMACEUTICAL TESTING
Source: House of Delegates Resolution

To support and foster legislative and regulatory initiatives designed to improve and restore public and professional confidence in the drug approval and regulatory process in which all relevant data are subject to public scrutiny.

9011
DRUG NOMENCLATURE
Source: House of Delegates Resolution

To work with the FDA, USP, and pharmaceutical industry to assure that drug products are named in a manner that clearly and without confusion permits identification of ingredients' strengths and changes.

1989 Policies

8901
PRACTITIONERS' DOCUMENTATION OF PHARMACEUTICAL SERVICES
Source: Council on Administrative Affairs

To incorporate into existing ASHP practice standards language that encourages documentation of pharmaceutical services and discusses the impact that such services have on patient outcomes.

8902
ORGANIZATIONAL RESIZING OF THE DEPARTMENT OF PHARMACY
Source: Council on Administrative Affairs

To advocate the implementation of a productivity-monitoring system in each department of pharmacy that would include a component analyzing the productivity changes and their impact on patient outcome indicators; further,

To continue communication with external consulting firms that are evaluating departments of pharmacy on the value of pharmaceutical services and on the use of accurate data to assess productivity and staffing levels in the department; further,

To promote the value of PharmaTrend to external consulting firms and to encourage an evaluation of the feasibility of expanding the types of measurements and indicators for clinical services contained in PharmaTrend.

8903
POLITICAL ACTION COMMITTEE (PAC)
Source: Council on Legal and Public Affairs

To establish a PAC to assist ASHP in its federal legislative efforts.

8904

ASHP STATEMENT ON THE PHARMACIST'S ROLE: DRUG DELIVERY SYSTEMS AND ADMINISTRATION DEVICES

Source: Council on Professional Affairs

To approve the "ASHP Statement on the Pharmacist's Role with Respect to Drug Delivery Systems and Administration Devices."

8905

ASHP STATEMENT ON THE PHARMACIST'S ROLE IN CLINICAL PHARMACOKINETIC SERVICES

Source: Council on Professional Affairs

To approve the "ASHP Statement on the Pharmacist's Role in Clinical Pharmacokinetic Services."

8906

ASHP STATEMENT ON THE PHARMACIST'S CLINICAL ROLE IN ORGANIZED HEALTH-CARE SETTINGS

Source: Council on Professional Affairs

To approve the "ASHP Statement on the Pharmacist's Clinical Role in Organized Health-Care Settings."

8907

ASHP STATEMENT ON UNIT DOSE DRUG DISTRIBUTION

Source: Council on Professional Affairs

To approve the "ASHP Statement on Unit Dose Drug Distribution."

8908

ALCOHOL ABUSE IN SOCIETY

Source: Council on Professional Affairs

To join with other interested organizations, as opportunities arise, in statements of concern regarding the health risks associated with alcohol as a potential substance of abuse.

1988 Policies

8801

PHARMACISTS IN MANAGED-CARE SETTINGS

Source: Council on Administrative Affairs

To assume a leadership role as a membership organization in meeting the unique needs of pharmacists practicing in managed-care settings (e.g., health maintenance organizations, preferred provider organizations, and independent practice associations).

8802

EDUCATIONAL PROGRAM RESOURCES FOR AFFILIATED STATE CHAPTERS

Source: Council on Educational Affairs

To identify potential educational program resources and support mechanisms that would assist ASHP-affiliated state chapters to plan, organize, and implement statewide continuing education programs; further,

To investigate the availability of ASHP resources for assisting affiliated state chapters in meeting their educational programming and support mechanism needs.

This policy was reviewed in 1996 by the Council on Educational Affairs and by the Board of Directors and was found to still be appropriate.

8804

EMPLOYEE DRUG TESTING

Source: Council on Legal and Public Affairs

To oppose the use of truth-verification testing (such as polygraphs and body tissue/fluid analyses) and all forms of integrity testing as routine employment practices because of the possible interference with the rights of individuals; further,

To recognize the limited use of such testing during employment in exceptional situations where such testing may protect the rights of individuals against false witness.

(*Note*: House of Delegates' approval of this recommendation would amend the following policy adopted by the House of Delegates in June 1986:

To oppose the use of truth-verification testing (such as polygraphs) and integrity testing as a routine employment practice because of the possible interference with the rights of individuals; further,

To recognize the limited use of such testing during employment in those exceptional situations where such testing may protect the rights of individuals against false witness.)

8805

PAIN MANAGEMENT EDUCATION

Source: Council on Legal and Public Affairs

To work with other national health-care organizations in educating health professionals about the proper administration of pain management therapy; further,

To increase the Society's efforts in offering educational programs addressing the issue of pain management therapy.

8806

ASHP STATEMENT ON THE PHARMACIST'S CLINICAL ROLE IN ORGANIZED HEALTH-CARE SETTINGS

Source: Council on Professional Affairs

To approve the "ASHP Statement on the Pharmacist's Clinical Role in Organized Health-Care Settings."

8807

TOBACCO AND TOBACCO PRODUCTS

Source: Council on Professional Affairs

To discourage the use and distribution of tobacco and tobacco products in and by pharmacies; further,

To seek, within the bounds of public law and policy, to eliminate the use and distribution of tobacco and tobacco products in meeting rooms and corridors at ASHP-sponsored continuing education events; further,

To join with other interested organizations in statements and expressions of opposition to the use of tobacco and tobacco products.

This policy was reviewed in 1996 by the Council on Professional Affairs and by the Board of Directors and was found to still be appropriate.

8808
HUMAN IMMUNODEFICIENCY VIRUS INFECTIONS
Source: Council on Professional Affairs

To seek input in the decisions of government and other organizations to express the concerns of pharmacists with regard to the handling of drugs and drug-related devices for the treatment and prevention of human immunodeficiency virus (HIV) infections; further,

To continue to inform pharmacists about drug and drug-related developments in the treatment of HIV infections.

This policy was reviewed in 1996 by the Council on Professional Affairs and by the Board of Directors and was found to still be appropriate.

8809
COUNCIL ON THERAPEUTICS
Source: SIG Cabinet

To create a new council or other body to be concerned with issues related to rational drug use in society; further,

To establish, within its purview, the development of drug therapy consensus documents; further,

To encourage the creation of this new council or other body as soon as possible.

8810
PROMOTION OF PHARMACISTS' PROFESSIONAL IMAGE
Source: House of Delegates Resolution

To develop a formalized public relations campaign to promote the professional image of pharmacists practicing in organized health-care settings.

8811
MECHANISM FOR PERIODIC REEXAMINATION OF ASHP'S ORGANIZATIONAL STRUCTURE AND GOVERNING PROCESS
Source: House of Delegates Resolution

To ask the Chairman of the House to develop a mechanism for establishing periodically a self-review task force to reexamine the organizational structure and governing processes of ASHP.

8812
RECOGNITION OF NUTRITIONAL SUPPORT PHARMACY PRACTICE AS A SPECIALTY
Source: Chairman of the Board of Directors

To endorse the petition to the Board of Pharmaceutical Specialties requesting recognition of nutritional support pharmacy practice as a specialty.

8814
CLINICAL PHARMACY AND ITS RELATIONSHIP TO THE INSTITUTION
Source: Chairman of the Board of Directors

To discontinue the document "ASHP and AHA Statement on Clinical Pharmacy and Its Relationship to the Institution."

1987 Policies

8701
PHARMACISTS' ROLE IN DRUG PROCUREMENT PROCESS
Source: Council on Administrative Affairs

To continue developing communication links with larger group purchasing arrangements and multi-institutional alliances in order to define the key points in the drug distribution system where pharmacists have maximum impact on the selection and acquisition of cost-effective products and services; further,

To encourage the Joint Commission on Accreditation of Hospitals (JCAH) to reemphasize the pharmacist's role in controlling the drug procurement process (as stated in JCAH Standard III for Pharmaceutical Services) in its accreditation surveys.

8702
PHARMACEUTICAL SERVICES IN ALTERNATIVE DELIVERY SITES
Source: Council on Administrative Affairs

To reemphasize existing ASHP policy regarding the pharmacy's responsibility in the procurement, distribution, and control of all drug products used within the health-care system.

(*Note*: Existing policy is found in "ASHP Guidelines: Minimum Standard for Pharmacies in Institutions" and "ASHP Statement on the Provision of Pharmaceutical Services in Ambulatory Care Settings.")

8703
STANDARD COMPUTER FORMATTING
Source: Council on Administrative Affairs

To support the technology and application of electronic data interchange in institutional pharmacies and to evaluate the implementation and benefits of this technology for pharmacy departments; further,

To encourage pharmaceutical wholesalers to use a standard coding format for electronic data interchange that is consistent with the needs of pharmacy departments in organized health-care settings; further,

To advocate the development of both formal and informal liaisons with other interested health-care associations to ensure that the interests of pharmacy are fully represented in the implementation of electronic data interchange technology.

8704
NATIONAL MANPOWER DATA SYSTEM
Source: Council on Educational Affairs

To endorse the development and implementation of a national pharmacy manpower data system; further,

To consider committing the appropriate resources to support a data system after reviewing the goals and objectives of the project.

This policy was reviewed in 1996 by the Council on Educational Affairs and by the Board of Directors and was found to still be appropriate.

8705
ASSESSMENT SURVEY OF CONTINUING EDUCATION NEEDS
Source: Council on Educational Affairs

To develop and implement an ongoing continuing education needs assessment survey that will assist in planning, organizing, and administering future educational programs.

This policy was reviewed in 1996 by the Council on Educational Affairs and by the Board of Directors and was found to still be appropriate.

8706
STAFF DEVELOPMENT PROGRAMS AND RESOURCES
Source: Council on Educational Affairs

To encourage pharmacy directors to support staff development programs in an effort to improve the quality of work life; further,

To assist pharmacy directors with staff development initiatives by providing a variety of educational programs, services, and resource materials.

This policy was reviewed in 1996 by the Council on Educational Affairs and by the Board of Directors and was found to still be appropriate.

8707
VACCINE AVAILABILITY
Source: Council on Legal and Public Affairs

To support federal efforts intended to ensure the continued availability and affordability of vaccines and other drug products in a manner that maintains their highest possible quality and provides adequate incentives for ongoing research, development, and distribution.

8708
THERAPEUTIC INTERCHANGE
Source: Council on Legal and Public Affairs

To support the concept of therapeutic interchange of various drug products by pharmacists under arrangements where pharmacists and authorized prescribers interrelate on the behalf of patient care.

8709
CODES ON SOLID DOSAGE FORMS OF PRESCRIPTION DRUG PRODUCTS
Source: Council on Legal and Public Affairs

To support efforts requiring manufacturers of solid dosage form prescription drug products to imprint a readily identifiable code indicating the manufacturer of the drug product and the product's ingredients; further,

To make information on transition of the codes readily available.

8710
DISCONTINUANCE OF "ASHP STATEMENT OF GOALS FOR INSTITUTIONAL PHARMACY"
Source: Council on Professional Affairs

To discontinue the "ASHP Statement of Goals for Institutional Pharmacy."

8711
CLINICAL INVESTIGATION OF DRUGS USED IN ELDERLY AND PEDIATRIC PATIENTS
Source: House of Delegates Resolution

To support clinical trial, patient-inclusion criteria that do not preclude trials of therapeutic agents in elderly and pediatric patients; and to support inclusion of appropriate surveillance mechanisms in such clinical trials to monitor informed consent and to prevent abuse of elderly and pediatric participants.

This policy was reviewed in 1996 by the Council on Professional Affairs and by the Board of Directors and was found to still be appropriate.

8712
THE PHARMACEUTICAL INDUSTRY AND DESIGN OF INVESTIGATIONAL STUDIES IN INSTITUTIONS
Source: House of Delegates Resolution

To develop a recommended procedural model for the pharmaceutical industry and other sponsors of clinical studies to use in the promotion, development, and implementation of investigational drug studies in institutions; and to educate the pharmaceutical industry and other sponsors of clinical studies in the key aspects of pharmacy involvement in investigational drug studies and the importance of adherence to this recommended model.

8713
DRUG ABUSE
Source: Chairman of the Board of Directors

To direct increased educational efforts with regard to drug abuse toward appropriate health-care personnel.

8715
RESIDENCY PROGRAMS
Source: Chairman of the Board of Directors

To encourage residency program directors to seek accreditation when applicable accreditation standards and processes exist as a means toward ensuring and conveying program quality.

This policy was reviewed in 1996 by the Council on Educational Affairs and by the Board of Directors and was found to still be appropriate.

1986 Policies

8605
GRADUATE MEDICAL EDUCATION
Source: Council on Legal and Public Affairs

To support legislation that ensures funding for hospital pharmacy residency programs consistent with the needs of the profession; further,

To oppose legislation involving reimbursement levels for graduate medical education that adversely affects pharmacy residencies at a rate disproportionate to other residency programs.

8607
PHARMACY CRIME
Source: Council on Legal and Public Affairs

To urge government officials to enforce fully the pharmacy crime laws in accord with statutory requirements.

8609
COUNTERFEITING
Source: Council on Legal and Public Affairs

To encourage FDA to take the steps necessary to ensure that all drug products entering the country be thoroughly inspected to establish that they have not been adulterated or misbranded; further,

To urge Congress to provide adequate funding or authority to impose user fees to accomplish this objective.

8610
PHARMACY TECHNICIANS
Source: Council on Legal and Public Affairs

To work toward the removal of legislative and regulatory barriers preventing pharmacists from delegating certain technical activities to other trained personnel.

8611
"DESIGNER DRUGS"
Source: Council on Legal and Public Affairs

To support efforts to limit the use of "designer drugs" and to minimize their risks.

8612
INTERNATIONAL SYSTEM OF UNITS
Source: Council on Professional Affairs

To not advocate, at this time, adoption of the International System of Units (SI units) as the exclusive labeling for drug dosages and concentrations; further,

To urge labelers to include: (1) units of mass, volume, or percentage concentrations and (2) moles or millimoles in labeling until the health professions and the public can be educated and be comfortable with use of SI units in prescribing and labeling drug products.

This policy was reviewed in 1996 by the Council on Professional Affairs and by the Board of Directors and was found to still be appropriate.

8613
ELIMINATION OF APOTHECARY SYSTEM
Source: Council on Professional Affairs

To recommend to all health professions and to the Pharmaceutical Manufacturers Association (PMA) that the apothecary system be eliminated in referring to dosage quantities and strengths.

This policy was reviewed in 1996 by the Council on Professional Affairs and by the Board of Directors and was found to still be appropriate.

8614
MEDICATION ERRORS AND RISK MANAGEMENT
Source: Council on Professional Affairs

To urge that pharmacists be included in hospitals' risk-management processes; further,

To emphasize the subject of medication errors in ASHP's publications and educational programs.

8616
INVESTIGATIONAL USE OF DRUGS
Source: Council on Professional Affairs

To reaffirm and publicize existing ASHP policy concerning the pharmacist's responsibilities for the control of the investigational use of drugs; further,

To urge pharmacists to develop formal liaison relationships between institutional review boards and pharmacy and therapeutics committees.

8619
NONTRADITIONAL PHARMACY PRACTICE SETTINGS
Source: Council on Professional Affairs

To give appropriate emphasis to pharmacy practice settings outside the hospital in future revisions of ASHP Statements, Guidelines, and Technical Assistance Bulletins.

8620
STATEMENT ON THE PHARMACIST'S ROLE IN INFECTION CONTROL
Source: Council on Professional Affairs

To approve the "ASHP Statement on the Pharmacist's Role in Infection Control."

1985 Policies

8501
MARKETING OF SERVICES
Source: Council on Administrative Affairs

To encourage hospital administrators and pharmacists to analyze the appropriateness of potential expanded services (e.g., home health-care and ambulatory care centers) in relation to a hospital's mission statement and to identify services that meet a hospital's needs; further,

To encourage hospital administrators and pharmacists to consult their hospital's legal staff on the ethics and implications associated with marketing specific auxiliary pharmaceutical services.

8502
IMPAIRED PHARMACISTS
Source: Council on Administrative Affairs

To recommend that hospitals actively address the issue of the impaired pharmacist.

8503
USE OF BAR CODES IN HOSPITAL PHARMACY
Source: Council on Administrative Affairs

To support the application of bar code technology in hospital pharmacies and to evaluate the improvements in this technology and the benefits that bar coding may offer to a hospital pharmacy department; further,

To encourage the appointment of an ASHP representative to the American Hospital Association (AHA)/Health Industry Bar Code Council Task Force on Implementation of the Health Industry Bar Code Standard; further,

To advocate the development of both formal and informal liaisons with AHA and the Health Industry Bar Code Council on the implementation of the bar code standard.

8504
STATEMENT ON THIRD-PARTY COMPENSATION FOR CLINICAL SERVICES BY PHARMACISTS
Source: Council on Administrative Affairs

To approve the "ASHP Statement on Third-Party Compensation for Clinical Services by Pharmacists."

8505
RELATIONSHIP BETWEEN PRACTICE SITES AND EDUCATIONAL INSTITUTIONS
Source: Council on Educational Affairs

To reaffirm ASHP's commitment to practitioner input in undergraduate education and to restate the importance of the institutional environment as a site for undergraduate training; further,

To continue discussions with the American Association of Colleges of Pharmacy (AACP) on defining and developing appropriate methods of organizational relationships between hospitals and colleges of pharmacy that permit a balance of patient care and service, as well as educational and research objectives of both institutions in a mutually beneficial manner; further,

To include the administrative interests of both the hospital and the college in defining these organizational relationships to assure compatibility of institutional (e.g., hospital or university) and departmental (e.g., pharmacy department and department in the college) objectives; further,

To develop jointly with AACP model contracts, agreements, and memoranda of understanding for use by hospitals and schools; further,

To develop jointly with AACP appropriate support materials to assist pharmacists in developing cost analyses and other materials required to justify active participation of a hospital in undergraduate pharmacy education.

8506
INTERNSHIP, EXTERNSHIP, AND CLERKSHIP
Source: Council on Educational Affairs

To endorse the recommendation of the APhA Task Force on Pharmacy Education and the statement in the proposed American Council on Pharmaceutical Education Accreditation Standard that states: "The curriculum should contain an externship and a clerkship of such quality and quantity to serve in lieu of the internship requirement."

This policy was reviewed in 1996 by the Council on Educational Affairs and by the Board of Directors and was found to still be appropriate.

8507
CAREER COUNSELING
Source: Council on Educational Affairs

To urge colleges of pharmacy to develop career counseling programs to make students aware of postgraduate career options, including residency training and career paths in various types of practice; further,

To urge that career counseling occur in a structured manner early in the curriculum and be continued throughout the curriculum; further,

To urge practitioners in various organized health-care settings to make themselves available to colleges of pharmacy for participation in both structured and unstructured career counseling.

This policy was reviewed in 1996 by the Council on Educational Affairs and by the Board of Directors and was found to still be appropriate.

8508
EXTERNAL DEGREE PROGRAMS AND INITIATIVES FOR HELPING PRACTITIONERS UPGRADE SKILLS
Source: Council on Educational Affairs

To encourage the broadest possible consortial approach to developing viable and widely available external degree programs within the shortest possible time; further,

To urge schools of pharmacy to develop flexible mechanisms that permit full-time practitioners to participate in courses in the contemporary curriculum and to urge directors of pharmacy to encourage staff participation in part-time academic work and to develop appropriate and flexible work hours to permit full-time staff to become part-time students; further,

To urge educational consortia, colleges of pharmacy, and other organizations to evaluate options in addition to a formal external degree program that can assist practitioners in upgrading their skills and to encourage these groups to develop a curricular approach to continuing education aimed at improving practice competence; further,

To urge these groups to develop measurable performance criteria for competence.

This policy was reviewed in 1996 by the Council on Educational Affairs and by the Board of Directors and was found to still be appropriate.

8510
ORGAN TRANSPLANT LEGISLATION
Source: Council on Legal and Public Affairs

To support the coverage of outpatient drugs, specifically immunosuppressive drugs, and related professional services of pharmacists needed by organ transplant patients if organ transplantation is paid for through public or private health insurance plans.

8511
PHARMACIST DISPENSING OF CERTAIN DRUGS
Source: Council on Legal and Public Affairs

To support improvement of availability, accessibility, and cost-effectiveness of health care through appropriate changes in applicable federal statutes and regulations to authorize pharmacists to dispense certain drug products directly to patients (after appropriate professional consultation) without a prescription; further,

To base such support on the following principles:

1. The profession is willing and able to make appropriate therapeutic decisions.
2. The drug products involved are appropriate for pharmacists' professional judgment based on the medical conditions to be treated, potential adverse effects (as indicated in approved labeling), and epidemiological factors.
3. Appropriate regulatory requirements exist for data collection for postmarketing surveillance and adverse drug reaction reporting.

8512
FDA REVIEW OF DRUG PRODUCTS FOR SAFETY AND EFFICACY
Source: Council on Legal and Public Affairs

To seek appropriate statutory, regulatory, and policy changes to assure that all drug products marketed in a new dosage form, or marketed for a new indication or new route of administration, be evaluated to determine safety and efficacy for the intended use as set forth in the products' labeling.

8514
NATIONAL DRUG CODE
Source: Council on Legal and Public Affairs

To support standardization of the product identification and package size identification components of the National Drug Code.

8515
CONTROLLED SUBSTANCES REGULATIONS
Source: Council on Legal and Public Affairs

To work with the Drug Enforcement Administration (DEA) to seek regulatory and policy changes to accommodate automatic data processing systems in individual hospitals within multihospital systems.

8516
SINGLE UNIT PACKAGES
Source: Council on Professional Affairs

To express concern about the following aspects of single unit packaging: (1) the small size of some single unit packages, which makes their labeling difficult to read; and (2) the variability in size and shape of outer cartons, which complicates inventory management; further,

To notify PMA of these concerns.

8517
STATEMENT ON INSTITUTIONAL PHARMACY RESEARCH
Source: Council on Professional Affairs

To approve the "ASHP Statement on Institutional Pharmacy Research."

8518
STATEMENT ON THE PHARMACIST'S ROLE IN INSTITUTIONAL PATIENT EDUCATION PROGRAMS
Source: Council on Professional Affairs

To approve the "ASHP Statement on the Pharmacist's Role in Institutional Patient Education Programs."

8519
HOSPITAL PHARMACY MANAGEMENT INFORMATION SYSTEM (HPMIS)
Source: House of Delegates Resolution

To reevaluate the current priority of, plans for, and need for the ASHP HPMIS; to promote more actively and prominently the HPMIS and the HPMIS national reporting program to all hospital pharmacies; and to discuss with AHA how HPMIS could be incorporated in the HAS/MONITREND reporting system used by over 2500 hospitals.

8520
BULK RESALE OF DRUG PRODUCTS
Source: House of Delegates New Business

To support legislation that would specifically prohibit bulk resale of drugs by pharmacies except for: (1) sales otherwise permitted by law to affiliated corporations in furtherance of a planned, integrated approach to delivery of health care within a health-care corporate structure; and (2) sales by bona fide group purchasing arrangements to members.

1984 Policies

8401
HEALTH-CARE FINANCING: STATE (MEDICARE) WAIVERS UNDER SOCIAL SECURITY ACT AMENDMENTS OF 1983
Source: Council on Administrative Affairs

To encourage ASHP's affiliated state chapters to involve themselves with state hospital associations, hospital financial management groups, other health professional organizations, and consumers to assure that state plans and hospital operations under state waiver plans authorized by the Social Security Act Amendments of 1983 reflect contemporary pharmaceutical services; further,

To encourage ASHP's affiliated state chapters to educate public coalitions interested in controlling health-care costs about the cost benefits of contemporary pharmacy practice.

8402
HEALTH-CARE FINANCING: DEPARTMENTAL STRATEGIES
Source: Council on Administrative Affairs

To form an interdisciplinary group to develop a modular study plan by June 1985. The purpose of this group would be:

- To evaluate the contribution of pharmaceutical services, especially clinical services, toward reduction of hospital inpatient costs in support of a prospective pricing health-care financing system.
- To evaluate contributions of pharmaceutical services to efficiencies in resource utilization in the health-care system as a whole.

Further, to include as components of the study plan, feasibility, design, budget, funding potential and sources, and implementation strategy.

8403
HOME HEALTH CARE
Source: Council on Administrative Affairs

To encourage hospital pharmacists to evaluate the need for and cost-effectiveness of participation in home health care through their institutions as a means to assure both a continuum and standard of patient care consistent with applicable standards of practice and to broaden the financial base of the institution.

8404
DRUG DIVERSION
Source: Council on Administrative Affairs

To encourage each institution to develop its own policy on how to identify, report, and deal with substance diversion by hospital employees; further,

To recommend that policies relating to substance diversion require reporting of relevant information to the director of pharmacy to permit evaluation by the pharmacy department and, if necessary, to make appropriate changes to the drug distribution and control system; further,

To request that the Council on Clinical Affairs, in due course, review and revise relevant Statements, Guidelines, and Technical Assistance Bulletins to account specially for the drug diversion problem.

8405
STATEMENT ON PHARMACY AND THERAPEUTICS COMMITTEE
Source: Council on Clinical Affairs

To approve the "ASHP Statement on the Pharmacy and Therapeutics Committee" as revised November 17, 1983; further,

To seek endorsement of the "ASHP Statement on the Pharmacy and Therapeutics Committee" by AHA, AMA, the American Osteopathic Association (AOA), and the American Pharmaceutical Association (APhA).

8406
PATIENT EDUCATION
Source: Council on Clinical Affairs

To reaffirm existing ASHP policy on patient education as summarized below.

The Society believes that efforts to provide patient information and educational services are maximized only when the multidisciplinary health-care team approach is used. A willingness to share pertinent patient information by all members of the team is the fundamental principle on which the success of these services is based. In discussions of patient drug education in institutions, it is important to have an appreciation of the institutional environment and an understanding of the philosophical framework in which education and information are provided in hospitals. While the *objectives* of health education are uniform among hospitals, the *method of executing* programs varies according to the requirements of each facility. Some hospitals may rely on multidisciplinary teams to deliver educational services; others may employ educational specialists. Programs use various media; some are developed inhouse and other media are provided commercially. No *one* method is best for integrating medication instruction into patient education programs.

Patient education is important from the perspectives of hospital accreditation, informed consent, consumer rights, and professional responsibility. An overview of pertinent legal and professional documents shows that patient education is a recognized component of high quality care, an integral part of professional services, a legitimate and growing demand of the consumer, and a mechanism to help prevent legal action that can result from medical procedures provided without a clear understanding of these procedures by the patient.

The needs of practitioners are reflected in the Society's official policies, statements, budgetary allotments, publications, and continuing education activities. With the expressed commitment to patient education on the part of its members in mind, ASHP plans to use all means available in its long-term efforts to alleviate deficiencies in the provision of drug information to patients and health-care professionals.

8407
ASHP PRACTICE STANDARDS AS AN INTEGRAL PART OF EDUCATIONAL PROCESS
Source: Council on Educational Affairs

To encourage faculties in schools of pharmacy and preceptors of ASHP-accredited residency training programs to use the ASHP standards of practice as an integral part of training programs and courses.

This policy was reviewed in 1996 by the Council on Educational Affairs and by the Board of Directors and was found to still be appropriate.

8408
DRUG PRICE COMPETITION ACT–POST-1962 ABBREVIATED NEW DRUG APPLICATION LEGISLATION

Source: Council on Legal and Public Affairs

To support legislation that would amend the Federal Food, Drug and Cosmetic Act to authorize an abbreviated new drug application for generic new drugs equivalent to approved new drugs (post-1962), as long as applicable standards of quality control, bioavailability, and patient care and safety are met.

8409
VETERANS ADMINISTRATION PERSONNEL LEGISLATION

Source: Council on Legal and Public Affairs

To oppose elimination of the director of pharmacy position in the Veterans Administration Central Office (as proposed in H.R. 2786).

8410
USE OF DRUGS IN CAPITAL PUNISHMENT

Source: Council on Legal and Public Affairs

To support the following concepts:

1. The decision by a pharmacist to participate in the use of drugs in capital punishment is one of individual conscience.
2. Pharmacists, regardless of who employs them, should not be put at risk of any disciplinary action, including loss of their jobs, because of refusal to participate in capital punishment.

8411
DISSOLUTION OF COUNCIL ON EDUCATIONAL AFFAIRS

Source: House of Delegates Resolution

To ask that the Board of Directors of ASHP reevaluate the objectives and purpose of the ASHP Council on Educational Affairs and that the Council on Educational Affairs be dissolved if appropriate responsibilities cannot be identified for it.

8412
AFFILIATED STATE CHAPTER MEMBERSHIP AND ASHP APPOINTMENTS

Source: House of Delegates Resolution

To urge that ASHP members who also hold membership in their state or regional affiliated chapters be given some priority when being considered for appointment to ASHP committees, councils, commissions, and SIGs.

1983 Policies

8301
FINANCIAL MANAGEMENT SKILLS

Source: Council on Administrative Affairs

To approve, as a major direction and effort, the development of programs and services aimed at improving financial management skills and awareness of ASHP members relative to cost containment, reimbursement, and management; further,

To consider development of the following specific services:

* Continuing education curricula for use by affiliated state chapters that would include detailed program outlines and regional listings of speakers or speaker bureaus.
* Correspondence courses or certificate programs or both (where possible, to be in conjunction with university systems).
* Focused attention on the financial management of hospital pharmacy departments through the residency accreditation process.

Further, to request that the SIG on Administrative Pharmacy Practice and affiliated state chapters give high programming priority to financial management topics.

8302
MEDICAID COST-CONTAINMENT OPTIONS

Source: Council on Administrative Affairs

To establish the following broad guidelines for formulation of the ASHP position(s) on specific Medicaid cost-containment options:

1. The option under consideration for implementation should not be unduly complex or involve costly administration.
2. As a result of an option's implementation, pharmacy should not be placed in an adversarial relationship with patients, physicians, or other professionals (e.g., the determination of patient financial eligibility should not be the responsibility of pharmacists).
3. The option should recognize the distinct differences between inpatient and outpatient settings. Elements of control that may be implemented must acknowledge these differences (e.g., co-payments or deductibles for inpatients should apply to the total cost of services rendered, not to discrete services or products).
4. The option should not impose any third-party restrictions on drug products or classes that compromise or preclude effective hospital formulary system management.

8303
MATERIALS MANAGEMENT

Source: Council on Administrative Affairs

To reiterate the following elements of ASHP's position on the topic of materials management (Board of Directors' minutes, November 15–16, 1979):

To alert hospital pharmacists of current trends in hospital materials management; further,

To advise AHA that a hospital's pharmacy department must be considered part of the institution's clinical services and should not be administered as a function of the materials handling department.

Further, to consider the following in an effort to

assist members in quantifying and dealing with this perceived problem:

- Development of a model survey questionnaire on the topic; this questionnaire would be used by ASHP's affiliated state chapters and would be designed to quantify and qualify the nature of this apparent trend.
- Expansion of communication and liaison with such groups as materials management associations and the American College of Hospital Administrators.
- Communication of the nature of this problem to the National Association of Boards of Pharmacy (specifically those instances in which pharmacy control of the drug-use process is seriously impaired).

8304
IMPAIRED PHARMACISTS
Source: Council on Administrative Affairs

To support APhA's program of activities to assist impaired (chemically dependent) pharmacists. These activities include:

- Survey state pharmaceutical associations and schools of pharmacy to determine the current level of interest and activity in developing programs for impaired pharmacists.
- Prepare a list of associations and schools of pharmacy that have programs, including short descriptions of these programs.
- Develop guidelines for associations and schools of pharmacy to use in planning and implementing their impaired pharmacists' programs.
- Distribute guidelines and other information in kit form to state associations and schools of pharmacy, with a recommendation that they develop programs for impaired pharmacists.
- Publish articles on the current level of program activity and other related areas in *American Pharmacy*.
- Ask Alcoholics Anonymous to hold sessions at the National Meeting of APhA's Academy of Pharmaceutical Sciences and at the APhA Annual Meeting.

Further, to disseminate information on impaired pharmacists' programs to members of ASHP through ASHP's meetings and publications.

8305
OUTPLACEMENT OF PHARMACY DIRECTORS
Source: Council on Administrative Affairs

To recognize the Society's responsibility for support of its members who seek employment information through such mechanisms as the ASHP Personnel Placement Service, informal networking, and dissemination of information regarding external assistance agencies.

8306
STATEMENT ON THE FORMULARY SYSTEM
Source: Council on Clinical Affairs

To approve the "ASHP Statement on the Formulary System" as revised November 18, 1982.

8308
"P.D." (PHARMACY DOCTOR) DESIGNATION FOR PHARMACISTS
Source: Council on Educational Affairs

To oppose the use of "P.D." or any other designation that implies an academically conferred degree where none exists; further,

To state the following reasons for this position:

1. ASHP believes that pharmacy is a clinical profession and that it meets a need in society that cannot be met by any other profession. ASHP believes that, to maintain pharmacy's position among the learned professions and the healing arts, pharmacists must strive to ensure that the academic preparation required for entry into the profession be maintained at the highest level possible.
2. The Doctor of Pharmacy (Pharm.D.) degree is well established and recognized as the profession's highest professional degree. The Society believes that it is in the best interest of the profession to move toward establishment of the Pharm.D. degree as the entry-level degree in pharmacy.
3. At a time when pharmacists are rapidly becoming recognized for their unique body of knowledge and their special contributions to patient care, ASHP believes that caution should be exercised to guard against erosion of our credibility in the eyes of the academic community, other health professions, and the public. ASHP believes that the adoption of such designations as P.D. does, indeed, put our credibility as a profession at risk.

Further, to continue to encourage colleges of pharmacy to make available reentry opportunities for midcareer practitioners who wish to pursue a Pharm.D. degree or other advanced program on a part-time basis.

This policy was reviewed in 1996 by the Council on Educational Affairs and by the Board of Directors and was found to still be appropriate.

8309
HEROIN LEGALIZATION FOR MEDICAL USE
Source: Council on Legal and Public Affairs

To approve support of any advancements in therapy and treatment that will allow improved control of pain, especially relief of chronic intractable pain; further,

To support educating pharmacists and other health professionals about contemporary techniques in pain management; further,

To oppose federal legislation legalizing heroin until it is clearly established that heroin legalization represents an advancement in the treatment of pain.

8310
SIZE, COLOR, AND SHAPE OF DRUG PRODUCTS
Source: Council on Legal and Public Affairs

To approve the authority of manufacturers to copy the size, shape, and color of generically equivalent drug products as a means of promoting better patient compliance (rational drug therapy), but only when the source and identity of the product are readily ascertainable from a uniform mark or symbol on the product.

8311
ASHP PLANNING PROCESS AND ASHP LONG-TERM GOALS
Source: House of Delegates Resolution

To encourage ASHP's long-range planning process and to inform the membership annually of the activities, conclusions, and outcomes of this process.

8312
DEA RECORDKEEPING REQUIREMENTS
Source: House of Delegates Resolution

To work in conjunction with DEA to establish regulations that provide alternative methods to the present recordkeeping requirements for less abused controlled substances.

1982 Policies

8201
PLAN OF ACTION FOR DEALING WITH PHARMACY REIMBURSEMENT MATTERS
Source: Council on Administrative Affairs

To pursue the following plan of action to deal with pharmacy reimbursement:

1. To educate members on the systems and mechanisms of reimbursement through such activities as:
   a. Sponsorship of a focused Institute on reimbursement.
   b. Development of a series of articles in *AJHP* focusing on existing major reimbursement models, using a case-study approach.
   c. Development of a glossary of key term definitions to ensure common understanding.
   d. Development of a manual of reimbursement for pharmaceutical services.
   e. Development of a checklist of information and documents that will assist pharmacist-administrators in understanding how pharmacy fits into the institutional fiscal structure of their own institutions.
   f. Focus of attention on reimbursement issues at all ASHP continuing education programs through a call for papers or other appropriate mechanisms.
2. To enhance understanding of pharmacy concerns relative to reimbursement among administrators, financial managers, fiscal intermediaries, and third parties through such activities as:
   a. Expansion of liaison activities with related organizations, including the Hospital Financial Management Association and Blue Cross/Blue Shield.
   b. Development of an article or series of articles in publications aimed at these audiences.
3. To initiate data gathering to establish an effective ASHP clearinghouse for reimbursement information through such activities as:
   a. Development of a geographical profile of current reimbursement mechanisms by region and state.
   b. Survey of institutions to determine those discrete pharmaceutical services currently being reimbursed separately for both inpatient and ambulatory care.
   c. Collection of qualitative and quantitative justification documentation successfully used in achieving reimbursement.
4. To continue to review and assess appropriate legislative and regulatory alternatives related to payment for pharmaceutical services.
5. To foster research in the area of cost justification of pharmaceutical services through solicited papers for continuing education programs, targeted research grants through the ASHP Research and Education Foundation, and other appropriate mechanisms.

8204
STATEMENT ON THE HOSPITAL PHARMACIST AND DRUG INFORMATION SERVICES
Source: Council on Clinical Affairs

To cease distribution of the "ASHP Statement on the Hospital Pharmacist and Drug Information Services."

(*Note*: The provision of drug information services as an integral part of institutional pharmacy practice is stated in Standard IV of the "ASHP Guidelines: Minimum Standard for Pharmacies in Institutions," thus eliminating need for the above statement.)

8205
STUDIES ON COSTS AND BENEFITS OF CLINICAL PHARMACY SERVICES
Source: Council on Clinical Affairs

To request that the ASHP Research and Education Foundation encourage studies to assess costs and patient benefits of various clinical pharmacy services in different types and sizes of institutions.

This policy was reviewed in 1996 by the Council on Educational Affairs and by the Board of Directors and was found to still be appropriate.

8207
MEDIATED CONTINUING EDUCATION PROGRAMMING
Source: Council on Administrative Affairs

To develop a pilot educational program for presentation to ASHP members sent through a video satellite network teleconferencing medium; further,

To consider the topic of reimbursement for pharmacy services for the first teleconferencing program; further,

To conduct the first program in 1982, if feasible; further,

To establish, within ASHP's organizational structure, a responsibility center to advise how electronic technologies can be used in continuing education and member communication activities and to recommend a timetable for implementing these applications.

8210

CONTINGENCY PLAN TO ASSIST STATE CHAPTERS' ADJUSTMENTS TO FEDERAL BUDGET REFORMS

Source: Council on Legal and Public Affairs

To develop, when appropriate, a contingency plan to commit existing ASHP resources to assist affiliated state chapters deal with new forms of Medicaid financing and the impact of budget constraints on hospitals if such constraints become too severe.

8211

PATENT TERM RESTORATION

Source: Council on Legal and Public Affairs

To support restoration of full patent term for pharmaceutical products to promote research and development, with consideration of the following:

1. That earnings attributable to such a restoration period are committed to research and development in new pharmaceutical products or prices that reflect the new monopoly period.
2. That regulatory barriers to market entry of pioneer and imitator drug products be eliminated to the extent they are not necessary to protect the public health.

(*Note*: Neither 1 nor 2 constitutes a specific legislative amendment but is to be accomplished through ongoing evaluations; item 2 might necessarily imply some regulatory action.)

8212

HOME HEALTH CARE

Source: Council on Legal and Public Affairs

To support, based on the following principles, the extension of home health services under Medicare and Medicaid as alternatives to institutionalization:

1. Pharmaceutical services should be covered specifically in any legislation.
2. Pharmaceutical services should be a required provision of all home health programs.
3. The responsibility for financial control and quality of services should be assumed through a centralized provider entity.

8213

PHARMACY CRIME

Source: Council on Legal and Public Affairs

To support making the theft or robbery of any controlled substance from any pharmacy, or from any area for which the pharmacist is responsible, a federal crime; further,

To encourage state societies to seek increased local vigilance by law enforcement to deter and punish such crimes when and as covered by state law.

8214

APPORTIONMENT/DELEGATE REPRESENTATION

Source: Council on Organizational Affairs

To reaffirm the following policy:

ASHP active members will be given the choice of which address (home or business) to be used to determine state delegate apportionment and delegate representation. If the member does not indicate a choice, representation will default to the state represented by the existing membership mailing address.

This policy was reviewed in 1996 by the Council on Organizational Affairs and by the Board of Directors and was found to still be appropriate.

8215

PROXY/ABSENTEE BALLOTS

Source: Council on Organizational Affairs

To oppose the resolution recommending the development of proxy/absentee balloting programs for the ASHP House of Delegates.

This policy was reviewed in 1996 by the Council on Organizational Affairs and by the Board of Directors and was found to still be appropriate.

8216

ANNUAL MEETING REGISTRATION FEES FOR DELEGATES

Source: Council on Organizational Affairs

To not waive or reduce registration fees for delegates attending the ASHP Annual Meeting.

This policy was reviewed in 1996 by the Council on Organizational Affairs and by the Board of Directors and was found to still be appropriate.

8219

AMERICAN HOSPITAL FORMULARY SERVICE

Source: House of Delegates Resolution

To proceed as rapidly as possible with developing improvements to the *American Hospital Formulary Service* and publishing spinoffs, based on sound market surveys and financial considerations, and to keep the membership frequently informed of the directions and plans of the Society with regard to improving and expanding the utility of the *American Hospital Formulary Service* database.

Index

A

Abbreviated new drug applications; generic drugs, 8408

Access to pharmacists, 9706

Accreditation; residencies, 8715

Administration devices; pharmacist's role, 8904

Administration process; pharmacist's role, 9112

Administration systems; manufacturer's role, 9202

Administrators, *see* Directors

Adulteration, *see* Counterfeit drugs

Advertising; direct-to-consumer, 9701

Adverse drug reaction; reporting, 9709

Affiliated chapters, *see* State chapters

AHA, *see* American Hospital Association

AHA and ASHP Statement on Clinical Pharmacy; discontinue, 8814

AHA/HIBCC Task Force on Implementation of Bar Code Standard; ASHP representation, 8503

AIDS, *see* Human Immunodeficiency Virus

Alcohol abuse, 8908

Alcoholics Anonymous; impaired pharmacists, 8304

Alternative delivery sites, *see* Nontraditional practice settings

Ambulatory care
see also Outpatient services
marketing, 8501

American Association of Colleges of Pharmacy (AACP); hospital practice sites, 8505

American College of Hospital Administrators; materials management, 8303

American Hospital Association (AHA)
discontinue ASHP and AHA Statement, 8814
Hospital Pharmacy Management Information System (HPMIS), 8519
materials management, 8303
pharmacy and therapeutics committees, 8405

American Hospital Formulary Service; development, 8219

American Medical Association (AMA); pharmacy and therapeutics committees, 8405

American Osteopathic Association (AOA); pharmacy and therapeutics committees, 8405

American Pharmaceutical Association (APhA)
education, undergraduate, 8506
impaired pharmacists, 8304
pharmacy and therapeutics committees, 8405

Analysis; body tissue/fluid, 8804

Annual Meeting; registration fees, 8216

Apothecary system; elimination, 8613

Appearance; generic drugs, 8310

Appointments; qualifications, 8412

Apportionment, 8214

ASHP name change, 9411

ASHP Personnel Placement Service; directors, 8305

ASHP practice standards
documenting pharmaceutical services, 8901
drug information services, 8204
education, 8407

ASHP Research and Education Foundation; cost-effectiveness, 8201, 8205

ASHP Statement on Continuing Education; approval, 9002

ASHP Statement on Goals for Institutional Pharmacy; discontinuance, 8710

ASHP Statement on Pharmaceutical Care, 9304

ASHP Statement on Pharmaceutical Research in Organized Health-Care Settings; approval, 9111

ASHP Statement on the Pharmacist's Clinical Role in Organized Health-Care Settings, 9611
approval, 8806, 8906

ASHP Statement on the Pharmacist's Responsibility for Distribution and Control of Drugs; approval, 9115, 9210, 9504

ASHP Statement on the Pharmacist's Role in Clinical Pharmacokinetic Services; approval, 8905

ASHP Statement on the Pharmacist's Role in Patient-Education Programs; approval, 9114

ASHP Statement on the Pharmacist's Role with Respect to Drug Delivery Systems and Administration Devices; approval, 8904, 9306

ASHP Statement on the Pharmacy and Therapeutics Committee, 9209

ASHP Statement on the Provision of Pharmaceutical Services in Ambulatory Care Settings; discontinuance, 9116

ASHP Statement on the Role of the Pharmacist in Patient-Focused Care; approval, 9505

ASHP Statement on Unit Dose Drug Distribution; approval, 8907

ASHP Statement on the Use of Medications for Unlabeled Uses, 9208

ASHP's organizational structure and governing process; review of, 8811

Automated systems, 9205

Automatic data processing; controlled substances, 8515

Aversive flavoring, 9207

B

Bar codes
see also Electronic data interchange
evaluation, 8503

Blue Cross/Blue Shield; reimbursement, 8201

Bulk resale; legislation, 8519

C

Capital punishment; ethics, 8410

Care MAPs; multidisciplinary action plans, 9403

Careers; counseling, 8507

Chemical dependence, *see* Impaired pharmacists

Clerkships; curriculum, 8506

Clinical pharmacy
cost-effectiveness, 8205
pharmacist's role in organized health-care settings, 8806, 8906

Clinical services; reimbursement, 8504

Clinical trials
geriatrics, 8711
models, 8712
pediatrics, 8711

Codes
dosage forms, 8709
National Drug Code, 8514

Colleges of pharmacy
career counseling, 8507
external degrees, 8508
hospital practice sites, 8505

Competency; education, continuing, 850, 9502

Compounding versus manufacturing, 9107

Computers
controlled substances, 8515
software vendors, 9119
standards, 8703

Consulting firms, external; communication with, 8902

Consumer education, 9705

Continuing education, *see* Education, continuing

Control, 8702, 9104, 9115
investigational drugs, 8616

Controlled substances
automatic data processing, 8515
crime, 8213
regulations, 8312

Cost containment, 8302
pharmacy services, 8402

Cost-effectiveness
clinical pharmacy, 8205
home health care, 8403
pharmacy services, 8402
research, 8201

Council on Educational Affairs; responsibilities, 8411

Council on Therapeutics; proposed creation of, 8809

Counterfeit drugs; legislation, 8609

Crime
  controlled substances, 8213
  laws, 8607

Curriculum; education, undergraduate, 8506

D

Data collection
  education, continuing, 8705
  manpower, 8704
  materials management, 8303
  reimbursement, 8201

Degrees
  external, 8508
  P.D. (Pharmacy Doctor), 8308
  Pharm.D., 8308, 9101

Delegate representation, 8214

Delegates; registration fees, 8216

Designer drugs, 8611

Directors
  employment, 8305
  staff development, 8706
  Veterans Administration Central Office, 8409

Discrimination, 9006

Dispensing; without prescription, 8511

Distribution, 8702, 8907, 9104, 9307

Dosage forms
  codes, 8709
  FDA review, 8512

Downsizing the pharmacy department, 8902

Drug abuse
  see also Impaired pharmacists
  alcohol, 8908
  education, 8713

Drug control, see Distribution

Drug costs, 9003

Drug delivery systems
  high technology, 9106
  pharmacist's role, 8904, 9112

Drug distribution, see Distribution

Drug diversion, 8404

Drug Enforcement Administration (DEA)
  automatic data processing, 8515
  records, 8312

Drug information services, 8204

Drug labeling, 9007

Drug naming, 9007, 9011

Drug packaging, 9007

Drug Price Competition Act; generic drugs, 8408

Drug pricing, 9003

Drugs; unapproved use, 9001

Drug samples, 9702

Drug testing, 8804, 9103, 9108

Drug therapy
  consensus documents, 8809
  pharmacokinetics, 8905

Dues rate, 9121, 9614

E

Economics, see Reimbursement, Cost containment, Cost-effectiveness

Education, 8407
  see also Consumer education; Patient education; Staff development
  compounding, 9107
  Council on Educational Affairs, 8411
  drug abuse, 8713
  human immunodeficiency virus, 8808
  pain control, 8309, 8805
  residency accreditation, 8715

Education, continuing
  ASHP Statement on Continuing Education, 9002
  ASHP support to affiliated state chapters, 8802
  competencies, 9502
  external degrees, 8508
  financial management, 8301
  needs, 8705
  non-traditional Pharm.D., 9502
  regulations, 9503
  reimbursement, 8201
  teleconferences, 8207
  use of tobacco at ASHP-sponsored events, 8807

Education, medical; funding, 8605

Education, postgraduate
  career counseling, 8507
  Pharm.D., 8308, 9101

Education, undergraduate
  curriculum, 8506
  hospitals, 8505

Elderly, see Geriatrics

Electronic communication, 9204

Electronic data interchange
  see also Bar codes
  standards, 8703

Electronic entry; medication orders, 9402, 9602

Employment
  external assistance agencies, 8305
  truth verification and integrity testing, 8804, 9108

Ethics
  capital punishment, 8410
  clinical trials, 8711
  code for Pharmacists, 9607
  nontraditional practice settings, 8501
  patient education, 8406

Expanded services, see Nontraditional practice settings

Expiration dating; pharmaceutical products, 9309

Externships
  curriculum, 8506
  hospital practice sites, 8505

F

FDA, see Food and Drug Administration

Financial management
  programs, 8301
  state chapters, 8210

Financing, see Reimbursement

Food and Drug Administration (FDA)
  counterfeit drugs, 8609
  new product review, 8512
  reform, 9606

Formulary system, 8306, 9501, 9601
  cost containment, 8302

G

Generic drugs
  evaluation, 9005
  legislation, 8408
  look-alike, 8310
  regulations, 8211
  selection, 9005

Geriatrics; clinical trials, 8711

Goals
  institutional pharmacy, 8710
  long-range planning, 8311

Governing process; ASHP, 8811

Government affairs; formation of political action committee, 8903

Group purchasing, see Purchasing; group

H

HAS/MONITREND; Hospital Pharmacy Management Information System (HPMIS), 8519

Health-care financing, see Reimbursement

Health-care reform, 9303

Health professionals; drug abuse education, 8713

Health risks; alcohol, 8908

Heroin; legislation, 8309

Home health care
  see also Nontraditional practice settings
  marketing, 8501
  need, 8403
  reimbursement, 8212, 9004

Home intravenous therapy; reimbursement, 9004

Hospital Financial Management Association; reimbursement, 8201

Hospital information systems; standardization, 9008

Hospital Pharmacy Management Information System (HPMIS); promotion, 8519

Hospitals; education, undergraduate, 8505

HPMIS, see Hospital Pharmacy Management Information System

Human Immunodeficiency Virus
    education of pharmacists, 8808
    testing, 9201

I

Identification
    dosage forms, 8709
    drug ingredients, 9011
    drug products by color, 9608
    generic drugs, 8310
    National Drug Code, 8514
Immunization; pharmacist's role, 9113
Impaired pharmacists, 8502
    programs, 8304, 9103
Indications, new, *see* New indications
Industry, *see* Manufacturers
Infection control, 8620
Information
    employment, 8305
    management, 8519, 9008
    reimbursement, 8201
Informed consent; clinical trials, 8711
Institutional pharmacy
    goals, 8710
    research, 8517
International System of Units (SI
    units); labeling, 8612
Internships; education, undergraduate,
    8506
Investigational drug studies, *see* Clinical
    trials
Investigational drugs
    control, 8616
    policies and procedures, 8712
Investigational review boards; liaisons,
    8616

J

Jails, *see* Correctional facilities
JCAH, *see* Joint Commission on
    Accreditation of Hospitals
Joint Commission on Accreditation of
    Hospitals (JCAH); purchasing, 8701

L

Labeling, 9007
    International System of Units, 8612
    single unit packaging, 8516
Laws
    enforcement, 8607
    patient education, 8406
Legislation
    bulk resale, 8520
    counterfeit drugs, 8609
    crime, 8213
    education, medical, 8605
    generic drugs, 8408, 9005
    heroin, 8309
    home health care, 8212
    reimbursement, 8201, 9004

Legislative affairs; function of political
    action committee, 8903
Long-range planning; goals, 8311

M

Management
    see also Financial management, Risk
        management, 9501
    Hospital Pharmacy Management
        Information System (HPMIS),
        8519
Manpower; data collection, 8704
Manufacturers
    clinical trial procedure, 8712
    codes, 8709
Manufacturing; generic drugs, 8310
Marketing; nontraditional practice
    settings, 8501
Materials management, 8303
MCM, 9506
Medicaid; cost containment, 8302
Medical education, *see* Education,
    medical
Medicare; state waivers, 8401
Medication distribution; unit dose,
    8907
Medications errors
    reporting, 9206, 9609, 9709
    risk management, 8614
Medication orders; electronic entry,
    9402
Membership; pharmacists in managed-
    care settings, 8801
Midyear Clinical Meeting, 9506
Misbranding, *see* Counterfeit drugs
Models; clinical trials, 8712
Multidisciplinary action plans; patient
    care MAPs, 9403

N

Name change; ASHP, 9411
National Association of Boards of
    Pharmacy
    materials management, 8303
    model regulations, 9503
National Drug Code, 8514
New drugs; regulations, 8211
New indications; FDA review, 8512
Nontraditional practice settings, 8619,
    8702
    see also Home health care
    marketing, 8501
Nutritional support pharmacy, *see*
    Pharmacy, nutritional support

O

Organ transplantation, *see* Transplanta-
    tion
Organizational resizing; pharmacy
    department, 8902

Organizational structure; ASHP, 8811
Outcome indicators, *see* Patient
    outcomes, 8901
Outpatient services
    see also Ambulatory care
    transplantation, 8510

P

Packaging, 9007
    single unit, 8516
Pain control; education, 8309, 8805
Patents; regulations, 8211
Patient assistance, 9703
Patient care
    multidisciplinary action plans (care
        MAPs), 9403
    nondiscriminatory, 9006
Patient education, 8406, 8518, 9114
    prescription drugs, 8513
Patient-focused care, 9401, 9505
Patient outcomes
    impact of pharmaceutical services,
        8901
    impact of productivity changes, 8902
Patients; right to choose, 9406
Pediatrics; clinical trials, 8711
Pediatric dosage forms, 9707
Pharmaceutical care
    definition of, 9304
    documentation of, 8901
    patient-focused care, 9401
Pharmaceutical Manufacturers
    Association (PMA); single unit
    packaging, 8516
Pharmaceutical services; documenta-
    tion of, 8901
Pharmaceutical testing; generic drugs,
    9010
Pharmaceutical waste, 9110
Pharmacist-industry relations, 9118
Pharmacist legend drugs, 8511
Pharmacists
    alcohol and professional responsibil-
        ity, 9120
    prescribing, 8202
Pharmacokinetic services; pharmacist's
    role, 8905
Pharmacy and therapeutics committee;
    endorsement, 8405
Pharmacy and therapeutics committees;
    investigational drugs, 8616
Pharmacy crime, *see* Crime
Pharmacy practice act; NABP model,
    9409
Pharmacy, managed-care settings;
    ASHP as a membership organization
    in, 8801
Pharmacy, nutritional support;
    recognition as a specialty, 8812
Pharmacy, organized health-care
    settings; promoting image of, 8810
PharmaTrend, 8902

Policies and procedures
  clinical trials, 8712
  drug diversion, 8404
  high-tech drugs, 9106

Political action committee, 8903

Polygraphs, 8804

Practice settings; nontraditional, 8619

Practice settings, managed-care; ASHP as a membership organization in, 8801

Practice settings, nontraditional; ASHP as a membership organization in, 8801

Practice settings, nutritional support; recognition as a specialty, 8812

Practice sites; hospitals, 8505

Preceptors, 8407

Prescribing
  pharmacists, 9404, 9410
  therapeutic purpose, 9708

Prescription drugs; advertising, 8513

Preventive care, 9407

Prices; drug product, 9003, 9105

Primary care, 9407

Productivity-monitoring system, 8902

Professional competency, *see* Competency

Professional image, *see* Public relations

Proxy/absentee ballots, 8215

Psychopharmacy; recognition as a specialty, 9122

Public relations
  organized health-care settings, 8810, 9710
  pharmacists' professional image, 8810, 9710

Publications
  American Hospital Formulary Service, 8219
  reimbursement, 8201

Purchasing, 8702, 9003, 9105
  group, 8701

 R

Records; Drug Enforcement Administration, 8312

Recruitment materials, 9710

Recycling, 9110

Registration fees; delegates, 8216

Regulations
  controlled substances, 8312, 8515
  drug approval process, 9010
  generic drugs, 8211
  new dosage forms, 8512
  new drugs, 8211

pharmacist legend drugs, 8511
  technicians, 8610

Reimbursement
  clinical services, 8504, 9004, 9308
  drugs, unapproved use, 9001
  education, continuing, 8207
  education, medical, 8605
  home health care, 8212, 9004
  home intravenous therapy, 9004
  Medicare, 8401
  programs, 8201
  prospective, 8402
  transplantation, 8510

Research, 8517, 9111
  cost-effectiveness, 8201, 8205

Residencies, 8407
  accreditation, 8715
  career counseling, 8507
  financial management, 8301
  funding, 8605

Resizing the pharmacy department, 8902

Right to choose; patients, 9406

Risk management; medication errors, 8614

Robbery, *see* Crime

Route of administration; FDA review, 8512

 S

Sales; bulk resale, 8519

Samples, *see* Drug samples

Self-review task force, 8811

SI units, *see* International System of Units

Single unit packaging; problems, 8516

Smoking; opposition to, 8807

Social Security Act Amendments of 1983; state Medicare waivers, 8401

Software vendors; standardized protocol, 9119

Specialties
  endorsement of nutritional support pharmacy, 8812
  endorsement of oncology pharmacy practice, 9310
  endorsement of psychopharmacy, 9122

Staff development; resources, 8706

Standards
  see also ASHP practice standards
  bar codes, 8503
  documenting pharmaceutical services, 8901
  drug information services, 8204
  electronic data interchange, 8703
  National Drug Code, 8514

State chapters
  ASHP appointments, 8412
  financial management, 8210
  state Medicare waivers, 8401
  statewide continuing education programs, 8802

Student membership dues, 9009

Substance abuse; alcohol, 8908

Supportive personnel, *see* Technicians

Surveys, *see* Data collection

 T

Tamper-evident packaging on topical products, 9211

Technicians
  see also Supportive personnel
  certificates, 9102, 9704
  education, 9603
  expanded role, 9613

Teleconferences
  education, continuing, 8207
  reimbursement, 8207

Testing; truth-verification, 8804

Theft, *see* Crime

Therapeutic interchange, 8708

Therapeutic substitution, *see* Therapeutic interchange

Therapeutics, Council on; proposed creation of, 8809

Third-party compensation, *see* Reimbursement

Tobacco; use and distribution in pharmacies, 8807

Training, *see* Education

Transplantation; outpatient services, 8510

Truth verification, *see* Polygraphs

 U

Undergraduate education, *see* Education, undergraduate

Unit dose drug distribution, 8907

 V

Vaccines; availability, 8707

Veterans Administration; directors, 8409

 W

Wholesalers; electronic data interchange, 8703